The History of Alternative Test Methods in Toxicology

The History of Alternative Test Methods in Toxicology

Edited by

Michael Balls

Robert Combes

Andrew Worth

 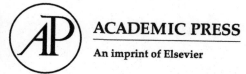

Academic Press is an imprint of Elsevier
125 London Wall, London EC2Y 5AS, United Kingdom
525 B Street, Suite 1650, San Diego, CA 92101, United States
50 Hampshire Street, 5th Floor, Cambridge, MA 02139, United States
The Boulevard, Langford Lane, Kidlington, Oxford OX5 1GB, United Kingdom

Library of Congress Cataloging-in-Publication Data
A catalog record for this book is available from the Library of Congress

British Library Cataloguing-in-Publication Data
A catalogue record for this book is available from the British Library

ISBN: 978-0-12-813697-3

For information on all Academic Press publications visit our website at
https://www.elsevier.com/books-and-journals

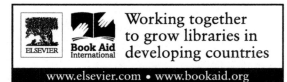

Working together
to grow libraries in
developing countries

www.elsevier.com • www.bookaid.org

Publisher: John Fedor
Acquisition Editor: Rafael E. Teixeira
Editorial Project Manager: Tracy Tufaga
Production Project Manager: Mohanapriyan Rajendran
Designer: Victoria Pearson Esser

Typeset by TNQ Technologies

Contents

Section 1
Setting the Scene

1.1 The Introduction and Influence of the Concept of Humane Experimental Technique

Michael Balls

1.2 Types of Toxicity and Applications of Toxicity Testing

Andrew P. Worth

1.3 The Key Technologies

Robert D. Combes

Section 2
Contributions From Countries, Regions and Organisations

2.1 Alternative Methods in Toxicity Testing in the UK

Michael Balls and Robert D. Combes

2.2 Contributions From the German-Speaking Countries

Horst Spielmann, Franz P. Gruber and Walter Pfaller

2.14 USA: Contributions From the Institute for *In Vitro* Sciences and the Animal Protection Community

*Rodger D. Curren, Erin H. Hill and
Martin L. Stephens*

2.15 Involvement of the Organisation for Economic Cooperation and Development

*Michael Balls, Andrew P. Worth and
Robert D. Combes*

Section 3
Important Issues Related to Types of Application

3.1 Animal-Free Cosmetics in Europe

Vera Rogiers

3.2 Safety Assessment of Pharmaceuticals

J Gerry Kenna and Rebecca Ram

3.7 Biologicals, Including Vaccines

Thea Sesardic and Philip Minor

3.8 The Use of Imaging, Biomonitoring and Microdosing in Human Volunteers to Improve Safety Assessments and Clinical Development

Tal Burt and Robert D. Combes

Section 4
Data Mining and Data Sharing

4.1 Scientific Journals as Beacons on the Journey Toward Global Three Rs Awareness

Susan Trigwell, Franz P. Gruber,
Sonja von Aulock and Koichi Imai

5.5 The Validation of Alternative Test Methods

*Michael Balls, Andrew P. Worth and
Robert D. Combes*

Section 6
Current Status of Alternatives and Future Prospects

6.1 Alternative Toxicity Test Methods: Lessons Learned and Yet to Be Learned

*Michael Balls, Robert D. Combes and
Andrew P. Worth*

6.2 The Current Situation and Prospects for Tomorrow: Toward the Achievement of Historical Ambitions

Andrew Rowan and Horst Spielmann

Contributors

Christopher P. Austin, National Center for Advancing Translational Sciences, Bethesda, MD, United States

Michael Balls, University of Nottingham, Nottingham, United Kingdom

Bas J. Blaauboer, Utrecht University, Utrecht, The Netherlands

Philip Botham, Product Safety, Syngenta, Jealott's Hill, United Kingdom

Tal Burt, Burt Consultancy, LLC, Durham, NC, United States

Warren Casey, National Institute of Environmental Health Sciences, Durham, NC, United States

Miroslav Červinka, Charles University Faculty of Medicine in Hradec Králové, Hradec Králove, Czech Republic

Shujun Cheng, Shanghai Jiao Tong University, Shanghai, China; Guangzhou Chn-Alt Biotechnology Co., Ltd., Guangzhou, China

Robert D. Combes, Independent Consultant, Norwich, United Kingdom

Raffaella Corvi, Joint Research Centre, European Commission, Ispra (VA), Italy

Mark T.D. Cronin, School of Pharmacy and Biomolecular Sciences, Liverpool John Moores University, Liverpool, United Kingdom

Rodger D. Curren, Institute for In Vitro Sciences, Gaithersburg, MD, United States

Isabella De Angelis, Istituto Superiore di Sanitá, Rome, Italy

Eva-Maria Dehne, TissUse GmbH, Berlin, Germany

John Doe, Parker Doe LLP, Stockport, United Kingdom

Chantra Eskes, 3RCC, Bern, Switzerland

Alexandre Feigenbaum, FCM, Rishon Lezyion, Israel

Zsolt Forgacs, Independent Researcher, Budapest, Hungary

Anna Forsby, Stockholm University, Stockholm, and SWETOX, Karolinska Institute, Stockholm, Sweden

Malcolm P. France, Consultant in Laboratory Animal Care and Management, Sydney, NSW, Australia

Simon A. Freeman Bain, Research Ethics Consultant, Canberra, ACT, Australia

Alan Goldberg, Johns Hopkins Bloomberg School of Public Health, Baltimore, MD, United States

Franz P. Gruber, Doerenkamp-Zbinden Foundation and ALTEX Edition, Kuesnacht ZH, Switzerland; ALTEX Editorial Office, ALTEX Edition, Kuesnacht, Switzerland

André Guillouzo, Rennes 1 University, Rennes, France

Thomas Hartung, Johns Hopkins Bloomberg School of Public Health, Baltimore, MD, United States; University of Konstanz, Konstanz, Germany

Tuula Heinonen, University of Tampere, Tampere, Finland

James Hickman, NanoScience Technology Center, University of Central Florida, Orlando, FL, USA

Erin H. Hill, Institute for In Vitro Sciences, Gaithersburg, MD, United States

Koichi Imai, Osaka Dental University, Osaka, Japan

Helena Kandarova, MatTek In Vitro Life Science Laboratories, Bratislava, Slovak Republic

Robert J. Kavlock, Washington, DC, United States

J Gerry Kenna, Safer Medicines Trust, Kingsbridge, United Kingdom

Lisbeth E. Knudsen, University of Copenhagen, Copenhagen, Denmark

Hajime Kojima, JaCVAM, NIHS, Tokyo, Japan

Roman Kolar, German Animal Welfare Federation - Animal Welfare Academy, Neubiberg, Germany

Marcel Leist, University of Konstanz, Konstanz, Germany

Brett A. Lidbury, NCEPH, ANU, Canberra, ACT, Australia

Anna Lowit, Environmental Protection Agency, Office of Pesticide Products, Arlington, VA, United States

Philip Minor, National Institute for Biological Standards and Control (NIBSC), Potters Bar, Hertfordshire, United Kingdom

Walter Pfaller, Medical University of Innsbruck, Innsbruck, Austria

Pilar Prieto, Joint Research Centre, European Commission, Ispra, Italy

Rebecca Ram, Safer Medicines Trust, Kingsbridge, United Kingdom

Guillermo Repetto, Universidad Pablo de Olavide, Sevilla, Spain

Vera Rogiers, Vrije Universiteit Brussel, Brussels, Belgium

Annett J. Roi, Joint Research Centre, European Commission, Ispra, Italy

Andrew Rowan, The Humane Society of the United States, Washington, DC, USA

Yasuyuki Sakai, University of Tokyo, Tokyo, Japan

Thea Sesardic, National Institute for Biological Standards and Control (NIBSC), Potters Bar, Hertfordshire, United Kingdom

Michael Shuler, Meinig School of Biomedical Engineering, Cornell University, Ithaca, NY, USA

Dariusz Śladowski, Medical University of Warsaw, Warsaw, Poland

Horst Spielmann, Freie Universität Berlin, Berlin, Germany

Martin L. Stephens, Johns Hopkins Bloomberg School of Public Health, Baltimore, MD, United States

Hanna Tähti, University of Tampere, Tampere, Finland

Noriho Tanaka, Hatano Research Institute, Hadano, Kanagawa, Japan

Emanuela Testai, Istituto Superiore di Sanitá, Rome, Italy

Raymond R. Tice, RTice Consulting, Hillsborough, NC, United States

Susan Trigwell, Fund for the Replacement of Animals in Medical Experiments (FRAME), Nottingham, United Kingdom

Catherine Verfaillie, Stem Cell Institute, Leuven, Belgium

Sonja von Aulock, ALTEX Editorial Office, ALTEX Edition, Kuesnacht, Switzerland

Andrew P. Worth, Joint Research Centre, European Commission, Ispra, Italy

Miyoung Yoon, ToxStrategies Inc., Cary NC, United States of America

Valérie Zuang, Joint Research Centre, European Commission, Ispra, Italy

Biographical Notes

CO-EDITORS

Michael Balls graduated in Zoology at Oxford University in 1960, and after post-graduate studies in Geneva, Switzerland, and post-doctoral research in Berkeley, California, and Portland, Oregon, USA, he returned to Britain in 1966, as a lecturer in the School of Biological Sciences at the University of East Anglia. In 1975, he moved to the University of Nottingham Medical School as a senior lecturer in the Department of Human Morphology, and subsequently became Professor of Medical Cell Biology. In 1995, he was made an emeritus professor of the University. Professor Balls became a Trustee of FRAME (Fund for the Replacement of Animals in Medical Experiments) in 1979, was Chairman of the Trustees from 1981 to 2013, and has been Editor-in-Chief of FRAME's journal, *ATLA (Alternatives to Laboratory Animals)*, since 1983. In 1993, Professor Balls became the first head of the European Centre for the Validation of Alternative Methods (ECVAM), established as part of the European Commission's Joint Research Centre, located at Ispra, near Lake Maggiore, in Italy. He retired from the Commission in June 2002.

Robert Combes graduated from the University of London (Queen Mary College; 1964–1970) with a BSc in Botany, and a PhD in Genetics, and has held posts in academia, industry and the charitable sector, including Reader in Toxicology at Portsmouth Polytechnic, Head of Mutagenicity and Cellular Toxicology at Inveresk Research International, Tranent, Edinburgh, Scotland, and Scientific Director, then Director, of FRAME (Fund for the Replacement of Animals in Medical Experiments), Nottingham (1994–2008). He has research interests in genetic toxicology, *in vitro* toxicology, xenobiotic biotransformation, *in silico* prediction systems, and the Three Rs (Reduction, Refinement and Replacement) approach to animal experimentation. Dr Combes has published numerous papers, book chapters and conference proceedings, given presentations at many conferences and workshops and served on many committees, including the ECVAM Scientific Advisory Committee (ESAC). He was elected a Fellow of the Institute of Biology (now the Royal Biological Society) in 1987, was Secretary of the United Kingdom Environmental Mutagen Society (UKEMS), was Secretary, then President, of the European Society of Toxicology *In Vitro* (ESTIV), later to be elected an Honorary Member (2010), and has served on the editorial boards of several journals, including *ATLA (Alternatives to Laboratory Animals, Toxicology in Vitro)* and *Mutation Research*. Dr Combes has acted as a co-editor for five scientific texts.

Andrew Worth is a Senior Scientific Officer at the European Commission's Joint Research Centre (JRC), where he leads the Predictive Toxicology Group within the Chemical Safety and Alternative Methods Unit. The unit incorporates the EU Reference Laboratory for Alternatives to Animal testing (EURL ECVAM) and is part of the JRC's Directorate for Health, Consumers and Reference Materials. The JRC provides independent scientific and technical support to the European Commission and other policy makers in the EU. Dr Worth has degrees in Physiological Sciences and in Linguistics from Oxford University, and a PhD in Computational Toxicology from Liverpool John Moores University. He has more than 180 publications in the area of predictive toxicology, and has a particular interest in the development and assessment of computational methods and their application in the regulatory assessment of chemical safety. During 2012, he held an ORISE fellowship while working at the US Food and Drug Administration's Center for Food Safety and Applied Nutrition (FDA CFSAN). Dr Worth is a member of the editorial boards of *ATLA (Alternatives to Laboratory Animals)* and *Computational Toxicology*.

CO-AUTHORS

Sonja von Aulock took up the position of Editor-in-Chief of *ALTEX — Alternatives to Animal Experimentation* in 2011, and started the journal *ALTEX Proceedings* in 2012. She studied biology in Germany at the University of Frankfurt and the University of Konstanz, and received her PhD in biochemical pharmacology at the University of Konstanz. She was an associate professor for pharmacology and cell biology at the University of Konstanz from 2007 to 2015. She is an author of more than 70 scientific papers.

Christopher Austin is Director of the National Center for Advancing Translational Sciences (NCATS) at the US National Institutes of Health. NCATS' mission is to catalyse the generation of innovative methods and technologies that will enhance the development, testing and implementation of diagnostics and therapeutics across a wide range of human diseases and conditions. Before becoming NCATS Director in September 2012, he was Director of the NCATS Division of Preclinical Innovation, which focuses on translating basic science discoveries into new treatments, particularly for rare and neglected diseases, and developing new technologies and paradigms to improve the efficiency of therapeutic and diagnostic development. In this role, he founded and directed numerous initiatives, including the NIH Chemical Genomics Center (NCGC), the Therapeutics for Rare and Neglected Diseases (TRND) programme and the Toxicology in the 21st Century (Tox21) programme. In 2016, he was elected Chair of the International Rare Disease Research Consortium (IRDiRC). Before joining the NIH in 2002, Dr Austin directed research programmes on genomics-based target discovery, pharmacogenomics, and neuropsychiatric drug development at Merck, with a particular focus on schizophrenia. He earned an A in biology from Princeton University and an MD from Harvard Medical School. He completed clinical training in internal medicine and neurology at Massachusetts General Hospital, and was a research fellow in genetics at Harvard.

Simon Bain is a Veterinarian and Consultant in Animal Ethics and Research Integrity, as well as a Member of the Australian and New Zealand College of Veterinary Scientists (Laboratory Animal Medicine and Management). He was employed at the Australian National University (ANU) for 33 years in several animal welfare roles, including 23 years as Executive Officer on the ANU Animal Experimentation Ethics Committee, and in the last eight years served as Director of the Office of Research Integrity. He was previously a member of the Code Writing and Code Reference Groups, Australian Code for the Care and Use of Animals for Scientific Purposes.

Bas Blaauboer received an MSc in biology and a PhD in toxicology at Utrecht University, where he led a group on *in vitro* toxicology (biochemical and cellular toxicology) at Utrecht University, and in 2008, was appointed to the Doerenkamp-Zbinden Chair on Alternatives to Animal Testing in Toxicological Risk Assessment. His research was focused on the use of *in vitro* toxicity data in combination with computer modelling as tools in risk assessments, and he is author or co-author of more than 180 scientific papers, editorials and book chapters. He was Director for Postgraduate Education in Toxicology from 2013 until his retirement from Utrecht University in 2014. Since his retirement, he has acted as a consultant, giving advice on the implementation of non-animal methods in risk and safety assessment strategies. He continues to be an Editor of *Toxicology in Vitro*, and is Vice-Chairman of the Central Authority for Scientific Procedures on Animals (CCD), which is the Dutch body which licences animal experimentation.

Phil Botham is currently Principal Science Advisor for Product Safety, Syngenta. Previously, he held senior leadership positions in Product Safety and toxicology for Syngenta and its legacy organisations based in the UK, initially at the company's Central Toxicology Laboratory (CTL) and then at its International Research Centre at Jealott's Hill. He has also led a number of research projects, both internally and in collaboration with academic and other industry partners, on the development and validation of alternative methods for acute toxicity, skin and eye irritation and skin sensitisation, and has more than 50 external publications in this area. He is a Fellow of the British Toxicology Society and the Royal College of Pathologists and has served as a Board Member of the UK National Centre for the 3 Rs (NC3Rs).

Tal Burt is a board-certified psychiatrist with more than 20-years experience in all phases of clinical development, with special expertise in the early-phase, proof-of-concept, and microdosing stages of clinical development. He has led clinical research and development programmes on drugs and devices in academia and in industry, leading him to appreciate the challenges of new treatment development, including the huge expenses, wastes, uncertainties and risks involved, and the considerable burden on public health and research ethics that ineffective translational and clinical research that result. He has worked with regulators, industries, academics, non-profit organisations and patient advocacy stakeholders to address these challenges to accelerate development of novel therapeutics. He has authored 45 manuscripts in clinical research and drug development, including original drug development methodologies such as Intra-Target Microdosing, randomised-withdrawal designs, assessment of the impact of false-negatives on the productivity of treatment development, the first publications of Vagus Nerve Stimulation in major depression, the first comprehensive review of Transcranial Magnetic Stimulation, and a textbook on outcomes measurement in clinical psychiatry. He has held Senior Medical Director positions at Pfizer Inc. and Eisai Inc., heading early-phase developmental programmes, and was the founding Medical Director of two state-of-the-art Point-of-Care research units, part of Duke's Global Research Network. He has established the microdosing programme and infrastructure at Duke University and the affiliated Investigational Medicine Unit in Singapore General Hospital, presented data, and chaired symposia and workshops on Phase-0/Microdosing in meetings of the relevant professional organisations.

Warren Casey is based at the NTP Interagency Center for the Evaluation of Alternative Toxicological Methods (NICEATM), and is Executive Director of the US Interagency Coordinating Committee on the Validation of Alternative Methods (ICCVAM). These groups work together to facilitate the development, validation, regulatory acceptance and industry adoption of non-animal test methods. Prior to assuming his current position, Dr Casey worked at GlaxoSmithKline for 15 years, in a variety of roles, including Manager of Pharmaceutical Microbiology, Head of *In Vitro* Biomarker Development, and Manager of Discovery and Investigative Toxicology. He received his undergraduate degree in biochemistry and his PhD in microbiology from North Carolina State University (NCSU), where he has been named a Distinguished Alumnus, and he also holds an adjunct professorship in the Department of Microbiology. He has been a Diplomate of the American Board of Toxicology (DABT) since 2007, received the 2016 Society of Toxicology Animal Welfare Award, and currently serves as the president-elect of the SOT *In Vitro* and Alternative Methods Specialty Section and co-chairs the OECD Validation Management Group — Non-Animal.

Miroslav Červinka studied animal physiology and medicine at Charles University in Hradec Králové and Prague and became a professor in the Faculty of Medicine in Hradec Králové in 2000 and dean in 2010. His research has been on the regulation of cell proliferation and cell death, the assessment of toxicity to cells cultured *in vitro* and mechanisms of chemoresistance in certain tumours. He has been active in a number of national and international scientific societies and a member of the editorial boards of *ALTEX* and *ATLA*.

Shujun Cheng is Director of the Toxicology Department of Guangdong Entry-Exit Inspection and Quarantine Bureau Technology Center. He has served as an adjunct professor at Sun Yat-sen University, Jinan University and Guangdong Pharmaceutical University. He has held positions in Chinese Laboratory Animal Society, Toxicology Testing and Alternatives Committee of the Chinese Society of Toxicology (CSOT). He is involved in research on the development, standardisation and expansion of alternative methods, and advocation of the regulatory acceptance of alternative methods in China. He created the Chinese Centre for Alternatives Research & Evaluation (CCARE), and founded the Conference of Alternative Methods in China, which has influenced hundreds of institutions and enterprises. He has issued or transferred more than 20 alternatives methods standards, which have been used widely. As Editor-in-Chief, he has published *Alternative Laboratory Animal Alternative Methods: Principles and Applications*, and *Guides on Alternative Methods Standards for Cosmetics*. He has more than 100 publications.

Raffaella Corvi is a Senior Scientific Officer at the European Commission's Joint Research Centre (JRC), where she is responsible for activities that evaluate innovative and integrated approaches to assess chemical safety, while also promoting the Three Rs across multiple regulatory sectors, within the Chemical Safety and Alternative Methods Unit. The unit incorporates the EU Reference Laboratory for Alternatives to Animal testing (EURL ECVAM) and is part of the JRC's Directorate for Health, Consumers and Reference Materials. The JRC provides independent scientific and technical support to the European Commission and other policy makers in the EU. She has a first degree in PhD in Biological Sciences from the University of Pavia (Italy) and the University of Heidelberg (Germany), respectively. During her PhD course, she worked at the German Cancer Research Centre in the Molecular Cytogenetics group. Then she moved to the International Agency for Research on Cancer (IARC) in Lyon, where her work focused on the molecular development of thyroid cancer. Since 2001, she has worked at the JRC, where she established the activities in the areas of genotoxicity and carcinogenicity testing.

Mark Cronin is Professor of Predictive Toxicology at the School of Pharmacy and Biomolecular Sciences, Liverpool John Moores University, UK. He has spent more than three decades in developing an understanding of how chemistry and physicochemical properties are related to the toxicity and fate of chemicals, most notably the development of (quantitative) structure—activity relationships ((Q)SARs) and other *in silico* approaches. His current research includes the application of chemical grouping and read-across to the assessment of human health and environmental endpoints, and in particular, the linking of the Adverse Outcome Pathways to category formation. This research effort has resulted in four books and more than 250 publications in all areas of the use of (Q)SARs, expert systems and read-across to predict toxicity.

Rodger Curren is CEO of the Institute for In Vitro Sciences, Inc., Gaithersburg, MD, USA. He received his BS (Biology) from Purdue University, an MS from Ohio University, and a PhD in Microbial Genetics from the Institute of Microbiology at Rutgers University. After more than 10 years of specialising in Genetic Toxicology at a contract research organisation, he created a separate division of *In Vitro* Toxicology, which was subsequently incorporated as the non-profit Institute for In Vitro Sciences (IIVS). Since 1997, the IIVS has provided educational and laboratory-based resources to industry, government and animal welfare organisations. Dr Curren has served on many national and international committees and science advisory boards, focused on the development, validation and practical use of *in vitro* methods. His efforts in optimising and promoting new alternative methods have earned him several honors, including the prestigious Russell and Burch Award, the Bjorn Ekwall Memorial Award, and the William and Eleanor Cave Award for outstanding achievements in the development, validation and advancement of humane alternatives for product testing.

Isabella De Angelis graduated in Biological Sciences at La Sapienza University of Rome and is a researcher at the Department of Environment and Health of the Italian National Institute of Health (Istituto Superiore di Sanità, ISS). Her research interests are focused on the application of cell culture in toxicology, covering both aspects of screening of toxic molecules and their mechanisms of action, with particular attention to the absorption processes of chemicals and nano-particles through epithelial barriers. She has been involved in national and European projects on *in vitro* toxicology and on the regulatory acceptance of *in vitro* methods. Since 2011, she has been Head of Delegation at the OECD Working Party of Manufactured Nanomaterials and a member of the ISS working group on Nanomaterials and Health. She also carries out a significant role in promoting the Three Rs principles and on the application of *in vitro* methods in many institutional courses organised by the ISS, universities, local authorities and scientific societies.

Eva-Maria Dehne is a biotechnologist who has worked in both academia and industry. She received her Diploma in Biotechnology from the Technische Universität Berlin, Germany, and an MSc degree in Biochemical Engineering from Dongseo University, Busan, Korea. She joined the Department of Medical Biotechnology, Technische Universität Berlin, in 2010, where her PhD was on the generation of a multi-organ-chip-based liver equivalent for toxicity testing. During this period, the spin-off company, TissUse GmbH, was founded. Her research interests include the design and development of microfluidic devices for multi-organ co-cultures, tissue engineering and bioartificial organs. She is currently leading research and development efforts at TissUse GmbH, developing the next generation of multi-organ microphysiological systems for systemic safety and efficacy testing.

John Doe joined ICI's Central Toxicology Laboratory (CTL) in the late 1970s, after having previously worked as a pharmacologist in the pharmaceutical industry in the areas of asthma, skin allergy and chronic obstructive pulmonary disease. He initially worked in inhalation toxicology, but then managed studies across the full spectrum of regulatory toxicology, including chronic, reproductive and developmental toxicology. He worked in industrial chemical and agro-chemical toxicology for many years, becoming Director of the CTL in 2003 and Head of Product Safety for Syngenta in 2006. He was Chairman of ECETOC Scientific Committee from 2006 until 2010. Dr Doe was a member of the UK Animal Procedures Committee from 2004 to 2012. He retired from Syngenta in 2010 and is now an independent consultant. He is a member of the UK Committee on Carcinogenicity.

Chantra Eskes has a bicultural Dutch and Brazilian origin, and has more than 20 years of experience in the development, optimisation, validation, peer-review and regulatory acceptance of alternative methods to animal toxicity testing conducted in Europe and in Brazil. Her activities contributed to the formal validation and international acceptance of several test methods and to the development of a number of international test guidelines. Chantra Eskes acts as a Nominated Expert for the OECD, is the Executive Secretary of the Animal Cell Technology Industrial Platform on the production of biopharmaceuticals (ACTIP), and is the past President of the European Society of *In Vitro* Toxicology (ESTIV). She has acted as Manager and Senior Consultant for SeCAM, a company offering independent consultation services on alternative methods. Since March 2018, she is Executive Director of the Swiss Competence Centre on 3Rs (3RCC). Finally, she is the editor, author and co-author of a number of books and scientific publications and acts as reviewer for several journals in the field of *in vitro* toxicology.

Alexandre Feigenbaum is an organic chemist, specialising in organic synthesis and physical chemistry. As a student, he has worked with Jean-Marie Lehn, Jean-Pierre Pete and Malcolm Green. As Director of Research at the Institut National de la Recherche Agronomique, Jouy-en-Josas and Reims, he set up the French research programme on Food and Packaging interactions and on food safety related to Food Contact Materials (FCM). He also coordinated several major EU research projects on migration control and modelling and on plastics recycling. His work provided major scientific support to the

EU legislation on FCM, which was then being developed. As Head of Unit at the European Food Safety Authority (EFSA; 2008–13), he managed the work of the CEF Panel on Food Contact Materials, Enzymes and Flavourings. When he chaired a European Scientific Cooperation Working Group, he was confronted with the need to propose approaches to solve the issue of thousands of substances which are used in the manufacture of FCM, but which had not been properly evaluated. This triggered his interest in alternative methods in toxicology, mainly in the Threshold of Toxicological Concern approach, to reduce the backlog. He currently elaborates global proposals for assessment of FCM.

Zsolt Forgács graduated at the Faculty of Pharmacy at Semmelweis Medical School, Budapest, Hungary, in 1988. His early scientific work was at the National Institute of Haematology and Blood Transfusion, Budapest, then at the National Institute of Occupational Health, which subsequently went through many reorganisations. His first *in vivo* experiments were to study endocrine disruptors and reproductive toxicants, but they were supplemented and later replaced by *in vitro* tests performed on cultures of steroidogenic primary gonadal cells and standardised cell lines. His PhD thesis was on the reproductive toxicology of nickel. He became the Head of the Division of *In Vitro* Toxicology in the National Public Health Centre, where several new OECD test methods were adopted, including 3-D tissue-based skin irritation/corrosion and eye irritation tests. After the closure of his GLP-certified laboratory during a reorganisation in 2017, he has continued his career in pharmacovigilance.

Anna Forsby gained a PhD in Animal Physiology at the University of Lund in 1994, and has been employed at the Department of Neurochemistry at Stockholm University since 1994. She has been Associate Professor of Neurochemistry with Molecular Neurobiology at the University of Stockholm since 2010, and has held a parallel position as Specialist for *in vitro* neurotoxicology at SWETOX (Karolinska Institutet) since 2014. Her research has a primary focus on the development and validation of *in vitro* methods for mechanistic studies and human health risk assessment, and she is interested in molecular and cellular toxicology with extrapolation to humans via physiologically-based toxicokinetic models. She developed the NociOcular *in vitro* assay for estimation of mild eye irritation and nociception and has experience of commissioned research for industry, participation in EU projects and teaching in toxicology and neurochemistry at all academic levels, as well as in information dissemination to the general public. She is a member of the Scandinavian Society for Cell Toxicology (SSCT) board, founded the Björn Ekwall Memorial Foundation in 2000, and received the Nordic Alternative Price in 2007, for promoting the development of alternatives to animal testing.

Malcolm France is a Consultant Veterinarian, specialising in the care and management of laboratory animals. Prior to his current role, he worked in private veterinary practice, then served on the academic staff of the Sydney Veterinary School, where he obtained a PhD in pathology before taking up an appointment as the Director of Laboratory Animal Services at the University of Sydney, a position which he held for 12 years. His current duties include serving as Chair of two Animal Ethics Committees.

Alan Goldberg obtained a bachelor's degree at the Brooklyn College of Pharmacy, continued his studies at the University of Wisconsin and holds a PhD (1966) from the University of Minnesota. He is currently a professor of Toxicology at the Johns Hopkins Bloomberg School of Public Health. He was the Founding Director (now Emeritus), and until 2014, Chairman of the Board, of the Center for Alternatives to Animal Testing (CAAT) and a Principal of the Global Food Ethics Project at Johns Hopkins University, Berman Institute of Bioethics. His current interest in Ethical Food issues developed when he accepted an appointment to the Pew Commission on the Impact of Industrial Farm Animal Production on Animal Welfare, Public Health, the Environment and Social Justice. He is actively pursuing a programme for the ethical certification of food.

Franz Paul Gruber, born in Aschau, Bavaria, studied Veterinary Medicine in Munich, and received his degree of DVM in 1968. After working as a practising veterinarian in Bavaria for a year, he joined School of Veterinary Medicine of the Free University Berlin and became a faculty member in 1977. In 1978, he joined the Faculty of Biology at the University of Konstanz, where he established the Animal Research Facility and was its first Director. In 1993, he moved to Zurich as Editor-in-Chief of the *ALTEX* journal, and in 2004, he was appointed President of the Doerenkamp-Zbinden Foundation (DZF) by its foundress, Hildegard Doerenkamp. He is currently President of the DZF and CEO of *ALTEX Edition*.

André Guillouzo is Emeritus Professor of Toxicology at the University of Rennes and a Senior Researcher at INSERM Unit U1241, Numecan, Site Pontchaillou-Villejean, Rennes. He graduated from the Universities of Rennes and Paris Unit 6 and was the Head of INSERM Units 49, 456 and 620 from 1986 to 2009. His research interests cover cellular and molecular toxicology, mainly related to human liver, using *in vitro* cell models (HepaRG cells and primary human hepatocytes). He has co-authored 320 publications. From 1997 to 2006, he was a member of the ECVAM Scientific Advisory Committee. He served as the Editor-in-Chief of *Cell Biology and Toxicology* (1997–2002) and as the President of the French Society of Pharmaco-Toxicology (1997–2001). He has also been a member of the editorial boards of *Toxicology in Vitro* and *ATLA (Alternatives to Laboratory Animals)*.

Thomas Hartung studied biochemistry at Tübingen and Konstanz, medicine at Tübingen and Freiburg, and mathematics/informatics at Hagen. He is the Doerenkamp-Zbinden Chair for Evidence-based Toxicology, with a joint appointment for Molecular Microbiology and Immunology, at Johns Hopkins Bloomberg School of Public Health, Baltimore, MD. He also holds a joint appointment as Professor for Pharmacology and Toxicology at the University of Konstanz and is Director of the Center for Alternatives to Animal Testing (CAAT) at both universities. CAAT hosts the secretariat of the Evidence-based Toxicology Collaboration, the Good Read-Across Practice Collaboration, the Good Cell Culture Practice Collaboration, the Green Toxicology Collaboration and the Industry Refinement Working Group. He headed the Human Toxome project funded as an NIH Transformative Research Grant. He is the former Head of the European Commission's Centre for the Validation of Alternative Methods (ECVAM), Ispra, Italy, and has authored more than 500 scientific publications.

Tuula Heinonen is a European Registered toxicologist with more than 25 years practical experience broadly in toxicology and alternative *in vitro* methods in the pharmaceutical industry and in academia. She established the Finnish Centre for Alternative Methods (FICAM), University of Tampere, Tampere, an expert centre that focuses on the development and validation of human cellular tissue and organ models for basic and applied research, as well as for regulatory testing, on the education of scientists and on the dissemination of information on the Three Rs. She holds Adjunct Professorships in the universities of Helsinki and Turku, and she is the Finnish EURL ECVAM's Network for Preliminary Assessment of Regulatory Relevance (PARERE) representative for the European Commission. In addition, she is President of the European Consensus Platform for Alternatives (ecopa) and the Scandinavian Society for Cell Toxicology (SSCT), and is a member of European Partnership for Alternative Approaches to Animal Testing (EPAA) Mirror Group.

James Hickman is the Founding Director of the NanoScience Technology Center and a Professor of Nanoscience Technology, Chemistry, Biomolecular Science, Material Science and Electrical Engineering at the University of Central Florida. Previously, he held the position of the Hunter Endowed Chair in the Bioengineering Department at Clemson University. He has a PhD from MIT in Chemistry. For the past 25 years, he has been studying the interaction of biological species with modified surfaces. While in industry, he established one of the first bioelectronics laboratories in the USA that focused on cell-based sensors and their integration with electronic and micro-electromechanical systems devices. He is interested in creating hybrid systems for biosensor and biological computation applications, and in the creation of functional *in vitro* systems for human body-on-a-chip applications. He has worked at the National Science Foundation and the Defense Advanced Research Projects Agency (DARPA) in the area of biological computation. He is also the Founder and Chief Scientist of Hesperos, with a focus on cell-based systems for drug discovery and toxicity.

Erin Hill is a Co-Founder, and currently President, of the Institute for In Vitro Sciences (IIVS), where she is responsible for planning, directing and coordinating activities to achieve the Institute's mission of increasing the use and acceptance of *in vitro* methods. For the last 20 years, she has actively engaged with industry, animal protection organisations and regulatory agencies, both domestic and international, to help coordinate efforts for the advancement of non-animal testing methods. After receiving her bachelor's degree in Cell Biology and Biochemistry from the University of California, San Diego, she joined a tissue engineering company and assisted in the business development, marketing and sales of 3-D human tissue constructs for toxicology testing. She expanded her interest in *in vitro* methods during work for a developer of hollow fibre bioreactors for the production of monoclonal antibodies. In 2010, she co-founded the American Society for Cellular and Computational Toxicology (ASCCT), where she now serves as board member and treasurer. She is also a board member of the *In Vitro* Testing Industrial Platform.

Koichi Imai was the Head of the Tissue Culture Facility at the Institute of Dental Research, Osaka Dental University, Osaka, Japan, from 1989 to 1997. During this time, he undertook collaborative research with the German Centre for Documentation and Evaluation of Alternatives to Animal Experiments (ZEBET) at the Federal Institute for Health Protection of Consumers and Veterinary Medicine (BgVV), Germany. From 2005, he was the Head of the Analytical Instrument Facility, Head of the Low Temperature Facility and Head of the Laser Facility at the Institute of Dental Research, Osaka Dental University. Since 2014, he has been a professor at Osaka Dental University in the Department of Biomaterials. His research interests include the biological evaluation of biomaterials in the dental field, and in particular, the development of *in vitro* methods for the evaluation of dental materials for embryotoxicity.

Helena Kandarova was awarded a Diploma in Food Engineering from the Slovak Technical University in Bratislava, Slovakia, and doctorate in Biology, Chemistry and Pharmacy from the Free University, Berlin, Germany. Her doctoral research, on *The Evaluation and Validation of Reconstructed Human Skin Models as Alternatives to Animal Tests in Regulatory Toxicology*, was at ZEBET under the supervision of Manfred Liebsch and Monika Schaefer-Korting. Since then, she has been involved in projects aimed at the pre-validation and validation of tests based on 3-D reconstructed human tissue models, including tests for skin corrosion and skin and eye irritation. In 2007, she joined MatTek Corporation as a Senior Scientist, and in 2009, she co-established the European subsidiary of MatTek in Slovakia, where she is now Executive Director. In 2010, she co-founded the In Vitro Toxicology Division of the Slovak Toxicology Society (SETOX), and since 2012, she has been Vice-President of SETOX. She co-authored more than 40 peer-reviewed papers, and serves on the editorial boards of several international journals. As chair of the communication committees of EUROTOX and the European Society of Toxicology In Vitro (ESTIV), she actively contributes to the dissemination of the information on the alternative methods to animal experiments and to their implementation in practical toxicology.

Robert Kavlock was the acting Assistant Administrator for the US Environmental Protection Agency (EPA) Office of Research Development (ORD), as well as the EPA Science Advisor, prior to his retirement in November 2017. The ORD is the scientific research arm of EPA, which helps provide the underpinning of science and technology for the Agency. He was responsible for overseeing the national research programmes for the Office, which has 1700 staff located in 13 facilities across the USA and an annual budget in excess of $500M. His previous positions included being Deputy Assistant Administrator for Science in the ORD, and he was founding Director of the National Center for Computational Toxicology (NCCT) within the EPA. The NCCT has pioneered the application of modern molecular biology and computational sciences through its ToxCast programme, to bring high-throughput methodologies to the study of chemical effects on biological systems. Prior to that, he spent 15 years as the Director of the Reproductive Toxicology Division in the ORD, where he focused on improving approaches to risk methods for non-cancer health outcomes.

Gerry Kenna is Pharmaceutical Director of the Safer Medicines Trust, an independent UK charity, and a drug safety consultant. He is a scientific adviser to Bioxydyn Ltd and Cosmetics Europe and Vice-President of the Evidence-Based Toxicology Collaboration. He has worked as a toxicologist in industry (at AstraZeneca, Syngenta and Zeneca). Prior to this, he led academic research teams that explored mechanisms underlying drug-induced liver injury and other serious human adverse drug reactions, at Imperial College and King's College London, UK, and also at the US National Institutes of Health. His focus is on developing and gaining regulatory acceptance of novel, human biology-based methods which can improve the human safety assessment of drugs and other chemicals.

Lisbeth Knudsen is Professor of Toxicology at the University of Copenhagen, where her main areas of research are in toxicology, genotoxicology, biomonitoring of environmental and occupational exposures, alternatives to animal experiments, and ethical aspects of genetic testing and biomonitoring. Her main current activities are in studies on the transplacental transport of chemicals by the human placental perfusion system and participation in the Human Biomonitoring for EU initiative. She was a member of the ECVAM Scientific Advisory Committee (ESAC) from 2000 to 2009, the EU implementation group on biomonitoring from 2003 to 2012, the Danish Consensus Platform for 3R Alternatives to Animal Experimentation (DACOPA) from 2003 to 2013, and the board the Danish 3R Centre from 2013. She received the Nordic Alternative Prize 2006 for promoting the development of alternatives to animal testing. She is also coordinator of the Danish *in vitro* toxicology network, past president of the European Consensus Platform for 3R Alternatives to Animal Experimentation (ecopa), and past president of the European Mutagenesis and Genomics Society (EEMGS).

Hajime Kojima worked in the safety department of the Research Institute of the Nippon Menard Cosmetic Company from 1983 to 2005. In 1984—86, he was a Fellow of the National Institute of Genetics and received a PhD from the University of Nagasaki in 1996. In 2005, he moved to the National Institute of Health Sciences as Secretary General of the Japanese Center for the Validation of Alternative Methods (JaCVAM), part of the Biological Safety Research Center (BSRC). He has received awards from the Japanese Society for Alternatives to Animal Experiments (JSAAE), and was President of the Society from 2013 to 2016. His current research topics are on assessment of the utility, limitations and suitability for use in regulatory studies of test methods for determining the safety of chemicals, pharmaceutical and other materials, and he is also involved in validation studies.

Roman Kolar is Director of the Animal Welfare Academy, the scientific affiliation to the German Animal Welfare Federation. He is also a board member of Eurogroup for Animals, the umbrella organisation of the major animal welfare associations in the EU. Since 1994, he has been involved in issues related to animal experimentation and alternatives.

His first activity was to further develop the database on alternatives to animal experiments of the Animal Welfare Academy. He is, or has been, a member of several national and international committees in that field and also has been member of various ethics committees. For more than two decades, he has strived to raise awareness of the need for animal protection in science and research, not least via numerous publications and conference presentations.

Marcel Leist studied biochemistry in Tübingen (Germany), and then obtained an MSc in toxicology at the University of Surrey, UK, in 1989, a PhD in pharmacology at the University of Konstanz in 1993, and a habilitation in toxicology/cell biology in 1998. Since 2006, he has been Head of the Department of *In Vitro* Toxicology and Biomedicine at the University of Konstanz (inaugurated by the Doerenkamp-Zbinden Foundation) and Co-Director of the Center for Alternatives to Animal Testing in Europe (CAAT-Europe), a joint venture with Johns Hopkins University, Baltimore, MD, USA. From 2000 to 2006, he worked as Head of the Department of Disease Biology on the discovery of neurology and psychiatry drugs in the Danish pharmaceutical company, Lundbeck A/S. The research of the department addresses stem cell differentiation to neuronal lineages, as well as the pharmacological and toxicological characterisation of test systems and *in vitro* disease models. The novel test methods are used both to reduce the use of animals in scientific research and to shift research applications towards the use of human cells. The laboratory is particularly well known for its test methods for developmental toxicity and neurotoxicity.

Brett Lidbury is Associate Professor in the National Centre for Epidemiology and Population Health at the Australian National University (ANU) College of Medicine, Biology and Environment, and serves as an advisor on the Three Rs and alternatives to the ANU Animal Ethics Committee. He is a member of the Editorial Board of *Applied In Vitro Toxicology*. His previous research was in fundamental biomedicine, specifically on questions of virus–host interaction and pathogenesis, which included animal models. In 2011, he was appointed to the position of Associate Professor in Animal Alternatives at the ANU, and focuses on statistical modelling and machine learning of human data as a strategy to provide replacement alternatives to mouse models in discovery and pre-clinical research environments. In recognition of these research contributions, he was admitted as a Fellow of the Faculty of Science, the Royal College of Pathologists of Australasia, in 2017.

Anna Lowit received her PhD in Environmental Toxicology from the University of Tennessee in 1998, where she was a Graduate Fellow in Sustainable Waste Management. She began her career with the US Environmental Protection Agency (EPA) in 1998, with the Office of Pesticide Programs, where she remains today. She is currently the Senior Science Advisor at the EPA's Office of Pesticide Programs, where she advises senior managers and leads multidisciplinary teams on a variety of cross-cutting topics. She is currently one of the Co-Chairs of the Interagency Coordinating Committee on the Validation of Alternative Methods (ICCVAM). She has extensive experience in developing cumulative risk assessments for groups of pesticides which share a common mechanism of toxicity (e.g. organophosphates, N-methyl carbamates). She is also interested in the integration of science along multiple lines of evidence (epidemiology, *in vivo* and *in vitro* experimental toxicology). She has a particular interest in improving the use of quantitative approaches in human health risk assessment, such as use of meta-analysis in deriving benchmark dose estimates and linking Physiologically-Based Pharmacokinetic (PBPK) models with probabilistic exposure models.

Philip Minor began to work at National Institute for Biological Standards and Control (NIBSC) in 1978, as a post-doctoral scientist in the Division of Virology, of which he became Head in 1985. NIBSC is deeply involved in measuring the potency and safety of vaccines, devising and evaluating tests, and developing reference materials to ensure comparability of results. The scope of his work included all virological issues related to biological medicines, including vaccines. Specific major programmes in which he was involved included live and killed polio vaccines, vaccines against influenza and live vaccines against mumps and measles, as well as more-recent vaccines based on recombinant proteins, such as those against Hepatitis B and Human Papilloma Virus. He retired from NIBSC in July 2017.

Walter Pfaller went to the Medical School of the Leopold-Franzens University in Innsbruck, Austria, from 1964 to 1971, ending with an MD. In 1971, he joined the Department of Physiology and Medical Physics at the Medical University of Innsbruck, where he became professor until he retired in 2013. He was head of a research group on experimental nephrology, and his main research topics were acute and chronic renal failure, nephrotoxicity and the development of *in vitro* testing strategies for nephrotoxicity. He was Founder of the Austrian National Platform for Alternatives to Animal Experiments, zet, and served as Chairman from 2000 to 2010. From 2006 to 2013, he was Austrian member of the ECVAM Scientific Advisory Committee (ESAC), and since 2010, he has been a Board Member of CAAT-Europe.

Pilar Prieto is a Senior Scientific Officer at the European Commission's Joint Research Centre (JRC), where she contributes to the Predictive Toxicology Group within the Chemical Safety and Alternative Methods Unit. She has a PhD in Pharmacy from the University of Salamanca, Spain, and held a post-doctoral position in the Department of Toxicology of Novartis Pharma AG, Basel, Switzerland. In 1996, she joined the JRC and became a member of the European Centre for the Validation of Alternative Methods (ECVAM, now called EURL ECVAM). She has more than 60 publications in the area of *in vitro* toxicology and has a particular interest in the development and evaluation of integrated approaches for systemic toxicity of regulatory concern. She is a member of the Spanish Network for the Development of Alternative Methods (REMA).

Rebecca Ram is a clinical data management and scientific research consultant with an MSc in Toxicology (with Bioinformatics) and a BSc in Applied Biology (specialising in Physiology & Pharmacology). After a decade working in phase I–IV clinical trials, within both the pharmaceutical and contract research organisation sectors, she became a scientific consultant to focus on the campaign to replace animal experiments with more-relevant, human-focused methods, as well as continuing to work in some clinical research projects, for example, the 100,000 Genomes Project. She has worked, or provided scientific support, for a number of organisations, including GlaxoSmithKline, University College London Hospital, Simugen, Genomics England, Cruelty Free International, People for the Ethical Treatment of Animals (PETA), Animal Defenders International, Vier Pfoten (Four Paws), Animal Aid, TRACKS Investigations, One Voice and most recently, the Lush Prize, the Safer Medicines Trust and the Alliance for Human Relevant Science.

Guillermo Repetto teaches at the University Pablo de Olavide of Seville, Spain. He leads the Area of Toxicology, which is responsible for training predoctoral and post-doctoral students in Toxicology and Risk Assessment, in parallel with research and toxicological evaluations. He has a Bachelor's degree in Medicine, a Masters in Toxicology and a PhD in Toxicology from the University of Seville. He has more than 80 publications in the area of *in vitro* toxicology, and has a particular interest in the development and assessment of non-animal methods and their application in the regulatory assessment of chemical safety, especially in relation to neurotoxicology, reproductive toxicology and ecotoxicology. He has been a member of the editorial board of *Alternatives to Laboratory Animals (ATLA)* and of various committees and workshops related to alternative methods. He is President of the Spanish Network for the Development of Alternative Methods (REMA).

Vera Rogiers is Professor of Toxicology at the Vrije Universiteit Brussel and organises international courses on Cosmetics and Risk Assessment in the EU. Her main research activity is on the development of *in vitro* models for pharmaco-toxicological purposes as an alternative to the use of experimental animals, with a particular focus on the differentiation of human skin-derived stem cells into functional hepatic cells and the application of this *in vitro* model to the detection of drug-induced liver injury. For several years, she was Co-Chair of the EU Scientific Committee on Consumer Safety (SCCS), then became an invited expert. She was a member of the ECVAM Scientific Advisory Committee (ESAC) and Co-Founder and Chair of ecopa, the European Consensus Platform on 3R-Alternatives, which aims to bring together academia, industry, animal welfare organisations and governmental institutes.

Annett Roi obtained her degree in Biology at the Martin Luther University in Halle-Wittenberg in 1986, followed by post-graduate training in chemical toxicology. She is a Senior Scientific Officer at the European Commission's Joint Research Centre (JRC), with long experience in chemical data sector evaluations and the coordination of scientific databases. She joined ECVAM in 1996 to establish its Scientific Information Service (SIS), and was responsible for leading activities on the dissemination of information on alternative and advanced non-animal methods via publicly accessible databases. To this was added the definition and publication of guidance on good practices for retrieving relevant information on alternatives on the Internet. She is also involved in teaching in post-graduate training courses, including courses for ethical committees on the availability and use of relevant information (systems).

Andrew Rowan, now Chief Scientific Officer of The Humane Society of the United States, founded and directed the Tufts University Center for Animals and Public Policy (1983–97), launched the first graduate degree in animal policy (1995) and chaired the Department of Environmental Studies at Tufts University School of Veterinary Medicine (1995–97). He was the founding editor of *Alternatives to Laboratory Animals (ATLA)* in 1977, the *International Journal for the Study of Animal Problems* (1979) and *Anthrozoos* (1987). He has received several awards in recognition of his work on alternatives to animals used in research and testing, and has contributed many publications on the use of laboratory animals and alternatives, on wildlife conservation, and on companion animal management and population control. He was born in Zimbabwe and raised in Cape Town, South Africa. He received a BSc (1968) from Cape Town University, and was the recipient of a Rhodes Scholarship (1969), and an MA and DPhil in Biochemistry from Oxford University (1975).

Yasuyuki Sakai received a PhD in chemical engineering from the University of Tokyo in 1993, then to work at the university's Institute of Industrial Science (IIS). In 1997—98, he was a visiting scientist at the University of Rochester, New York. From 2003—08, he worked as an associate professor in the Regenerative Medical Engineering Laboratory of the Graduate School of Medicine, University of Tokyo. He then returned to IIS as a professor and moved to be Professor of Chemical Bioengineering in 2015. He recently became a Fellow of the American Institute for Medical and Biological Engineering. His current research topics are the engineering of 3-D tissues/organs for clinical applications and cell-based assays, placing importance on realisation of good mass transfers and 3-D organisation of cells *in vitro*. He is President of the Japanese Society for Alternatives to Animal Experiments (JSAAE) for the period 2017 to 2018.

Thea Sesardic joined the National Institute for Biological Standards and Control (NIBSC) in 1990 as a senior scientist, after completing post-doctoral studies at the Department of Clinical Pharmacology, Imperial College London. She became Principal Scientist in 2004 and was head of a toxin, toxoid and antitoxin laboratory from 2009 until her retirement in June 2017. The remit of the group was the control and standardisation of biological products derived from bacterial toxins, including toxoid vaccines, therapeutic antitoxins and *Botulinum* toxin for injection. The research programme focused on development of assays that reduce, refine and replace the use of animals in biological testing. She has been an expert advisor to a number of national and international regulatory organisations and has contributed to more than 170 peer-reviewed publications and book chapters. She retired from the NIBSC in November 2017.

Michael Shuler is the Eckert Professor of Engineering in the Meing Department of Biomedical Engineering in the School of Chemical and Biomolecular Engineering at Cornell University, and director of Cornell's Nanobiotechnology Center. He has BS and PhD degrees in chemical engineering from Notre Dame and Minnesota, respectively, and has been a faculty member at Cornell University since 1974. His research includes the development of "body-on-a-chip" for testing pharmaceuticals for toxicity and efficacy, the creation of production systems for useful compounds, such as paclitaxel from plant cell cultures, and the construction of whole-cell models relating genome to physiology. He is CEO and President of Hesperos, a company founded to implement the "body-on-a-chip" system. With Fikret Kangi, he co-authored a popular textbook, *Bioprocess Engineering; Basic Concepts*, now in its third edition.

Dariusz Śladowski obtained an MD degree at the Medical University of Warsaw in 1987 and a PhD in 1990, and is now an Associate Professor in the Centre for Biostructure Research at the University. He was a visiting scientist in the FRAME Alternatives Laboratory at the University of Nottingham from 1991—92, and at ECVAM, at the European Commission's Joint Research Centre (JRC) Joint Research Centre at Ispra, from 1998 to 2003. He was a member of the ECVAM Scientific Advisory Committee (ESAC) from 2003 to 2009. He has been a board member of the European Society of Toxicology In Vitro (ESTIV), and was a member of the Polish National Committee for Ethics in Animal Experimentation from 2005 to 2013.

Horst Spielmann was born in Lublin, Poland, and studied at medical schools in Germany and Austria. He is currently Professor for Regulatory Toxicology at the Free University of Berlin and is head of the board of the TissUse GmbH, Berlin. He is also Secretary General of EUSAAT and Associate Editor of *ATLA (Alternatives to Laboratory Animals)* in Europe. He was Head of the German Centre for Alternative Methods (ZEBET) at the Federal Health Institute (BGA) and a member of the ECVAM Scientific Advisory Committee (ESAC). He chaired the management teams of several successful international validation studies, including those which became the first in vitro toxicity tests to gain regulatory acceptance, including the 3T3-NRU Phototoxicity Test, *in vitro* corrosivity tests, *in vitro* embryotoxicity tests, and skin irritation tests using human skin models.

Martin L. Stephens received a PhD in biology from the University of Chicago and is now a senior research associate at the Johns Hopkins Center for Alternatives to Animal Testing (CAAT), and a scientific consultant to the Alternatives Research & Development Foundation (ARDF). In both positions, he promotes animal-friendly methods in research, testing and education. At CAAT, he is deputy director of the Evidence-based Toxicology Collaboration, where he develops new approaches to assessing the performance of test methods. Prior to joining CAAT 2011, he was Vice-President for Animal Research Issues at The Humane Society of the United States. He served on the National Academy of Sciences committee that produced the landmark report on *Toxicity Testing in the 21st Century: A Vision and a Strategy*.

Hanna Tähti is emerita professor (biomedicine, environmental toxicology) at the University of Tampere (UTA), Finland, and her main area of interest is *in vitro* toxicology, especially neurotoxicology. In 1999, she established the Cell Research Centre in UTA with the goal to develop cell-based models for the needs of toxicological and biomedical research. After retiring officially in 2004, she has continued research at UTA and in the Finnish Centre for Alternative Methods (FICAM). She has been President of the Finnish Society of Toxicology and of the Finnish Consensus Platform for Alternatives, an executive committee member of EUROTOX and the Scandinavian Society for Cell Toxicology, and a member of the Scientific Advisory Board of ACUTETOX and of the Estonian National Institute of Chemical Physics and Biophysics (NICPB).

Noriho Tanaka was awarded a master's degree by Kagoshima University in 1972, and a PhD by the medical school of Kagoshima University in 1982. He worked at the Hatano Research Institute from 1976 to 2011, and was a visiting scientist at the US National Institute for Environmental Health Sciences from 1984 to 1986. His initial research field involved genetic toxicology using experimental animals and then he moved to the development of *in vitro* alternatives to animal experiment. From 2006 to 2011, he was leader for a national project for the development of alternative tests, under the auspices of the Ministry of Economy, Trade and Industry, Japan. He was President of the Japanese Society for Alternatives to Animal Experiments (JSAAE) from 2005 to 2007, and is now an Honorary Member of the Society.

Emanuela Testai studied biology at the University of Pisa, where her thesis was on xenobiotic metabolism by subcellular hepatic fractions. She then moved to the Istituto Superiore di Sanità in Rome, where she became part of the permanent staff in 1985. She has been involved in research and regulatory activities, as well as in teaching, in the area of toxicology, including the use of alternative methods, with a special interest in risk assessment for human health, involving toxicokinetics, xenobiotic metabolism, *in vitro* toxicology, molecular mechanisms of toxicity and metabolic biomarkers of individual susceptibility, associated with exposure to natural and synthetic chemicals. The author of more than 100 papers in peer-reviewed journals, she has been a member of a number of national and international scientific committees and working groups and a member of the editorial boards of *Drug Metabolism Reviews* and *Toxicology in Vitro*.

Raymond Tice has a PhD in Biology from Johns Hopkins University, Baltimore, MD. He was employed by the Medical Department at Brookhaven National Laboratory (Upton, NY) from 1976 to 1988, by Integrated Laboratory Sciences, Inc. (Durham, NC) from 1988 to 2005, and by the National Institute of Environmental Health Sciences (NIEHS) from 2005 to 2015. At the NIEHS, he served as the first Deputy Director of the National Toxicology Program (NTP) Interagency Center for the Evaluation of Alternative Toxicological Methods (NICEATM) and, in 2009, as the first Chief of the Biomolecular Screening Branch within the NTP, where he was the NTP lead on the US interagency Tox21 initiative. He retired from the NIEHS in January 2015. He served as President of the US Environmental Mutagen Society (EMS) and as Vice-President of the International Association of Environmental Mutagen Societies (IAEMS).

Susan Trigwell received a PhD in Biochemistry from the University of Nottingham in 1997 and worked in numerous academic research laboratories at the University of Nottingham, University of Leicester and University of Derby, applying cell culture, molecular biological and immunological techniques to a diverse range of studies on RNA polymerase, diabetes, breast cancer, plant tissue cryopreservation and DNA structure. She joined the Fund for the Replacement of Animals in Medical Experiments (FRAME) in 2006, to work on its journal, *Alternatives to Laboratory Animals (ATLA)*. She is currently Managing Editor of the journal.

Catherine Verfaillie received her Medical degree from the KU Leuven in 1982. She then trained as an internist/hematologist at the KU Leuven between 1982 and 1987. She went to the University of Minnesota in 1987 for a post-doctoral fellowship. After completing her post-doctoral fellowship, she was appointed consecutively as instructor, assistant professor, associate professor, and finally, full professor of Medicine in 1998. In 2001, she became the Director of the University of Minnesota's Stem Cell Institute. In 2006, she became the director of the Interdepartementeel Stamcel Instituut at the KU Leuven. She has a longstanding career in stem cell biology, initially focusing on normal hematopoietic stem cells and leukemic stem cells, and the role played by the microenvironment in regulating their self-renewal and differentiation ability. Since 1997, she has also focused extensively on more pluripotent stem cells. Her group described in 2002 a novel cell population culture from rodent and human bone-marrow samples with greater expansion and differentiation potency, named multipotent adult progenitor cells. The current research of the Verfaillie lab is focused on understanding what regulates self-renewal and (de)differentiation of adult, as well as, pluripotent, stem cells. She is testing the possible use of stem cell-based liver cell platforms for drug toxicity/metabolism, also including liver fibrosis in repeated-dose toxicity settings, and viral liver infections, as well as induced pluripotent stem cell-derived drug platforms for myelination, astrocyte-based and microglila-based defects, and neuronal defects in genetic and sporadic neurodegenerative and neuroinflammatory diseases. In 2014, she created the KUL-STEM platform to create induced pluripotent stem cells, isogenic lines and differentiated progeny, with the recent addition of an automated stem cell platform for stem cell differentiation, as well as high content screen and high content imaging purposes, for drug discovery using small molecule and CRISPR/Cas screens.

Miyoung Yoon, together with a multidisciplinary team at ToxStrategies, Cary, NC, USA, is dedicated to advancing chemical safety science by combining *in vitro* and computational tools, with a special emphasis on translating new streams of *in vitro* and *in silico* kinetics and toxicity data to estimate human safe exposure levels for risk-based assessment. Dr Yoon is an internationally-recognised expert in the field of quantitative *in vitro* to *in vivo* extrapolation (IVIVE), which is a crucial element of the National Academy of Science's vision for toxicity testing in the 21st century. Dr Yoon's list of more than 50 publications includes both peer-reviewed articles and book chapters in the fields of *in vitro* metabolism, physiologically-based pharmacokinetic (PBPK) modelling and IVIVE for drugs and chemicals. She is an active contributor to education and training for the toxicology and safety science communities. Her efforts include organising a series of workshops and continuing education courses on PBPK modelling and its applications, in particular, to IVIVE and children's risk assessment.

Valérie Zuang was awarded a Master's degree at the Free University of Brussels and a PhD by the University of Nottingham, UK. Formerly employed at the European Parliament's Scientific and Technological Options Assessment (STOA) programme, she provided scientific and technical advice to parliamentary committees to support their assessments of policy options. Since 1994, she has been employed at the European Commission's Joint Research Centre (JRC) in Ispra, Italy, where she has led the validation of alternative methods relevant to the cosmetics and chemicals legislation, especially in the key area on topical toxicity (skin irritation and corrosion, eye irritation and phototoxicity). From 2012, she has coordinated the validation workflow of EURL ECVAM. Since 2016, she has been responsible for the translation of validated alternative methods into the EU legislation and into international standards at the Chemical Safety and Alternative Methods Unit, and coordinates the EURL ECVAM network of regulators (PARERE) and the International Cooperation on Alternative Test Methods (ICATM).

Preface to the Series

In the realm of communicating any science, history, though critical to its progress, is typically a neglected backwater. This is unfortunate, as it can easily be the most fascinating, revealing and accessible aspect of a subject which might otherwise hold appeal for only a highly specialised technical audience. Toxicology, the science concerned with the potentially hazardous effects of chemical, biological and certain physical agents, has yet to be the subject of a full-scale historical treatment. Overlapping with many other sciences, it both draws from, and contributes to, them. Chemistry, biology and pharmacology all intersect with toxicology. While there have been chapters devoted to history in toxicology textbooks, and journal articles have filled in bits and pieces of the historical record, this new monographic series aims to further remedy the gap, by offering an extensive and systematic look at the subject from antiquity to the present.

Since ancient times, men and women have sought security of all kinds. This includes identifying and making use of beneficial substances, while avoiding the harmful ones, or mitigating harm already caused. Thus, food and other natural products, independently or in combination, which promoted well-being, or were found to have druglike properties and effected cures, were readily consumed, applied or otherwise self-administered, or made available to friends and family. On the other hand, agents found to cause injury or damage—what we might call *poisons* today—were personally avoided, although sometimes employed to wreak havoc on one's enemies.

While natural substances are still of toxicological concern, synthetic and industrial chemicals now predominate as the emphasis of research. Through the years, the instinctive human need to seek safety and avoid hazard, has served as an unchanging foundation for toxicology, and will be explored from many angles in this series. Although largely examining the scientific underpinnings of the field, chapters will also delve into the fascinating history of toxicology and poisons in mythology, arts, society and culture more broadly. It is a subject that has captured our collective consciousness.

The series is intentionally broad, thus the title *History of Toxicology and Environmental Health*. Clinical and research toxicology, environmental and occupational health, risk assessment and epidemiology, to name but a few examples, are all fair game subjects for inclusion. The opening volume of the series focuses on toxicology in antiquity, taken roughly to be the period up to the fall of the Roman empire and stopping short of the Middle Ages, with which period future volumes will continue. These opening volumes will explore toxicology from the perspective of some of the great civilisations of the past, including Egypt, Greece, Rome, Mesoamerica and China. Particular substances, such as harmful botanicals, lead, cosmetics, kohl and hallucinogens, serve as the focus of other chapters. The role of certain individuals as either victims or practitioners of toxicity (e.g. Cleopatra, Mithridates, Alexander the Great, Socrates, and Shen Nung) serves as another thrust of these volumes.

History proves that no science is static. As Nikola Tesla said, "The history of science shows that theories are perishable. With every new truth that is revealed we get a better understanding of Nature and our conceptions and views are modified."

Great research derives from great researchers who do not, and cannot, operate in a vacuum, but rely on the findings of their scientific forebears. To quote Sir Isaac Newton, "If I have seen further it is by standing on the shoulders of giants."

Welcome to this toxicological journey through time. You will surely see further and deeper and more insightfully by wafting through the waters of toxicology's history.

Phil Wexler

Preface for *The History of Alternative Test Methods in Toxicology*

In view of the time and space available to us, and given the wealth of literature and experience on the subject, we have not attempted to provide a fully comprehensive and all-embracing review of the history of alternative test methods in toxicology. For example, the application of alternative approaches in environmental toxicology and developments in nano-toxicology are out of the scope of this work. Instead we have gathered together a group of co-authors from a wide variety of geographical locations and with considerable scientific achievements in different areas, and invited them to give their impressions of how it all began, where we are now and what the future may hold.

We have tried assiduously not to impose our own experiences and prejudices on our co-authors, but this means that we are entitled to say that we do not necessarily agree with all that they have included in their chapters, or with the interpretations and views they have recorded.

To set the scene, we offer a quotation from Guinevere Glasfurd's novel, *The Words In My Hand*,[1] based on time spent in Amsterdam in the 1630s by the French philosopher, René Descartes. At a party held in his honour, Descartes is criticised for his belief that everything should be questioned and is asked what can be believed. He replies, *Truth — that which can be proven. Knowledge is insufficient. Knowledge is nothing without understanding.*

Our aim is to find better ways of searching for the truth, to increase understanding and thereby reduce uncertainty, to provide a relevant and reliable, valid and humane, basis for the policies and decisions which profoundly affect the well-being of humans and the world in which we live.

We believe that there is great value in historical perspectives, however subjective the individual accounts may be, as the collective lessons learned should guide us toward the truth.

Michael Balls
Robert Combes
Andrew Worth
Norwich, UK, and Ispra, Italy
March 2018

---

1. Glasfurd, G (2016). The Words in My Hand, 415pp. London, UK: Two Road Books.

Section 1

Setting the Scene

Chapter 1.1

The Introduction and Influence of the Concept of Humane Experimental Technique

Michael Balls

University of Nottingham, Nottingham, United Kingdom

SUMMARY

Since its publication in 1959, *The Principles of Humane Experimental Technique*, by Russell and Burch, which introduced the concept of the Three Rs (*Reduction*, *Refinement* and *Replacement*), has had a profound effect on attitudes, laws and practices related to the use of laboratory animals in education, research and testing. The search for more-relevant and more-reliable non-animal alternative procedures for predicting the potential hazards to humans represented by chemicals and cosmetics, pharmaceuticals and other products gained momentum in the 1970s, initially led by the Fund for the Replacement of Animals in Medical Experiments (FRAME) in the UK, later joined, in particular, by the Center for Alternatives to Animal Testing (CAAT) in the USA, the Center for Documentation and Evaluation of Alternative Methods to Animal Experiments (ZEBET) in Germany and the European Centre for the Validation of Alternative Methods (ECVAM) in Italy. The replacement of animal tests by alternative procedures and testing strategies is now the focus of scientific, political and administrative effort throughout the world.

1. INHUMANITY AND THE THREE RS CONCEPT

The use of animals as surrogates for humans in potentially painful experiments had been the subject of controversy and unresolved conflict for hundreds of years before William Russell and Rex Burch proposed a way forward in 1959, in their outstanding book, *The Principles of Humane Experimental Technique* (*The Principles*; (1)). Much of what they said is no less applicable today than it was almost 60 years ago, but, as has been discussed in a series of articles in *ATLA*, the wisdom of Russell and Burch has all too often remained unrecognised or been ignored (see Ref. (2)).

Their underlying philosophy concerned the concept, sources and incidence of *inhumanity* and its diminution or removal through implementation of the Three Rs, *Reduction*, *Refinement* and *Replacement*, as a way of promoting humanity 'without prejudice to scientific and medical aims'. They distinguished between *direct inhumanity*, 'the infliction of distress as an unavoidable consequence of the procedure employed', and *contingent inhumanity*, 'the infliction of distress as an incidental and inadvertent by-product of the use of the procedure, which is not necessary for its success'. Inescapably, toxicity testing in animals involves direct inhumanity, and the way to avoid it is replacement, i.e. 'any technique employing non-sentient material' to 'replace methods which use conscious living vertebrates'.

There are two main reasons for seeking to replace toxicity tests on animals: the insuperable inadequacy of animals as models for humans and the advantages afforded by the use of scientifically advanced, non-animal replacement tests and testing strategies.

As Russell and Burch pointed out, models must differ from what is being modelled, and the consequences of this difference depend on two major factors, *fidelity* (a high general similarity to what is being modelled) and *discrimination* (a high specificity to what is being modelled). They argued that a highly discriminative/poor fidelity model is more useful

The History of Alternative Test Methods in Toxicology. https://doi.org/10.1016/B978-0-12-813697-3.00001-9

than a high-fidelity/poorly discriminative model, and warned of the dangers of the *high-fidelity fallacy*. This can be described as follows: humans are placental mammals, so members of other mammalian species are more likely to be useful as models of man that would be fish, or still more markedly, bacteria, nematodes or insects. However, the stubborn assumption that laboratory mammals are the best models for use in fundamental biomedical research, drug development or toxicity testing, where humans are the focus of concern, fails to recognise that the phenomena under investigation are not sufficiently well understood in the models or in humans (i.e. that what may be happening in one black box is used to predict what might happen in another black box), that there are fundamental differences between animals and humans (species differences) and that there are major differences within animal species and in humans (intra-species variation).

The second reason for seeking replacement is that although the non-animal procedures have limitations, which must be taken into account, they can be used to provide information of more-direct relevance to human situations. They can offer advantages of scale (number of replicates), speed and manageability, more-tightly defined and more-mechanistic approaches, talking advantage of progress in cell and molecular biology and the use of human material, from 'normal' controls or individuals with particular characteristics, susceptibilities or disease histories.

Replacement can be categorised as *partial*, where an animal is exposed to chemicals, then killed and its cells and tissues are subjected to further tests (*ex vivo*), or *total*, where all the experimental procedures are applied to cells and tissues *in vitro*. However, more useful is the distinction between *direct* and *indirect* replacement. An example of direct replacement is the application of potential irritants to isolated rabbit eyes instead of to the eyes of intact rabbits where the *in vitro* approach still has the disadvantages of the *in vivo* one. Seeking genuine indirect replacement is much more intelligent — it involves defining the information it was hoped to get from the animal, then obtaining it from a different experimental approach, e.g. testing drugs on human hepatocytes, instead of administering them to rats or dogs, which have different complements of drug metabolising enzymes. Direct replacement offers the possibility of direct relevance.

Russell and Burch recognised toxicity testing as a particular problem, 'since this is one use [of animals] which is an urgent humanitarian problem, both numerically and in terms of severity, for it regularly involves a finite and large incidence of distress, which is often considerable and sometimes acute'. The problem that other mammals may only be superficially similar to humans 'is met in practice by erring on the side of caution, and by using more than one mammalian species; it cannot be fully met, for there may always be metabolic peculiarities specific to man'. They also referred to the fact that a very large number of substances are toxic at high doses, so 'the important concept is the therapeutic index of a drug, i.e. the ratio between its toxic doses and its therapeutically effective dosage: if this ratio is great, the use of the drug or preparation is prudent, since it allows for wide variations between human individual patients to sensitivity to the toxic effects'.

2. PROGRESS FOLLOWING THE PUBLICATION OF *THE PRINCIPLES*

An interesting chapter in *The Principles* deals with the factors governing progress. Russell and Burch divided them into *individual personality* factors, which they further subdivided into *authoritarian* and *revolutionary* factors, and *sociological* factors, which involved achieving a balance between efficiency or yield of information and humanity. They also warned against *rationalisation*, a mechanism of defence by which unacceptable actions are given acceptable reasons to justify them. Even today, despite all that happened since the publication of *The Principles*, there remains a struggle between authoritarian factors backed by rationalisation and revolutionary and sociological factors.

In the 1960s, very little attention was paid to the Three Rs concept, and Russell and Burch had gone off to further their own careers in different ways (3). However, in 1969, Dorothy Hegarty and her family and friends set up the Fund for the Replacement of Animals in Medical Experiments (FRAME), as a parallel development to the Three Rs concept, of which they seemed to be unaware (4). FRAME's aim was to benefit both man and animals by promoting 'the use of more reliable, accurate and relevant methods in biology and medicine which at the same time help to reduce the need for laboratory animals' and, in particular, by recognising that 'the exchange of information, and its ready availability, are or paramount importance, if new techniques are to be adopted rapidly'. To achieve this, in 1973, they introduced *ATLA Abstracts*, containing abstracts of relevant articles, selected and written by staff located at the British Library, Boston Spa, Wetherby, Yorkshire, and arranged in 17 subject sections. This way of informing scientists may look rather naïve today, but it should not be forgotten that, at that time, there were few abstracting services, no personal computers, no Internet or websites and limited access to electric typewriters and photocopiers. Scientists kept themselves informed by going to the library and looking through hard copies of the scientific journals.

In 1976, Andrew Rowan arrived at FRAME, and during his short time as Scientific Director, he revolutionised the work of the charity. He increased the non-abstract coverage of the journal through news, reviews and editorials, organised a meeting on the use of alternatives in drug research at the Royal Society in London and proposed the setting-up of a toxicity committee of experts, to consider the use of alternative methods in toxicology and toxicity testing. In an article on the early days of FRAME (4), he commented that he had come across a number of articles on problems with routine toxicity tests, such as the Draize irritancy tests and the LD50 test, which showed that toxicity testing in animals was a major problem, both in terms of animal suffering and the shaky science underlying it. For example, in 1971, Weil and Scala had published the results of a study involving intra- and inter-laboratory variability in the results of the rabbit eye and skin irritation tests (5). They had sent three test substances to 24 different universities and state laboratories and found that they reported significantly different results, from non-irritating to severely irritating, for the same substances.

In 1977—79, FRAME published two important publicity leaflets, entitled *What Price Vanity?* and *How safe is your medication?* (6). The first of the leaflets was timely, as the US cosmetic companies were coming under increasing pressure because of their use of animal tests, especially the rabbit eye irritation test. For example, on 15 April 1980, Henry Spira, founder of Animal Rights International, placed a full-page advertisement in the *New York Times*, with the header, *How many rabbits does Revlon blind for beauty's sake?* This prompted Revlon to donate $750,000 to a fund to investigate alternatives to animal testing, which was followed by substantial donations from other companies and led to the creation of the Center for Alternatives to Animal Testing (CAAT) at Johns Hopkins University in Baltimore. Meanwhile, back in the UK, FRAME developed a very fruitful collaboration with the Cosmetic, Toiletry and Perfumery Association (CTPA) and its member companies, which was to last for more than 30 years.

After achieving success in drawing attention to the Draize eye test, Spira turned his attention to the LD50 test, at about the time when Zbinden and Flury-Roversi published a highly critical review of the classical test (7). They said that, even with large numbers of animals, the LD50 value is influenced by many factors, such as animal species and strain, age and sex, diet, food deprivation prior to dosing, temperature, caging, season and experimental procedure. As a result, the LD50 value should not be regarded as a constant.

3. ALTERNATIVES

In 1978, *Alternatives to Animal Experiments* by David Smyth had been published by Scolar Press for the Research Defence Society (8). This was an important book, as it defined 'alternatives' to mean 'any change to established scientific procedures that will result in the replacement of animals, a reduction in the numbers used or a refinement of techniques that may minimize harms to the animals'. Since then, it has often been considered fashionable to criticise the use of the term in this way. However, as Smyth pointed out, the term had been used on 20 January 1971 by the Consultative Assembly of the Council of Europe when adopting 'recommendations about the use of animals in research', which included a clause 'to establish a Documentation and Information Centre … to collect data in … the alternatives to experiments on live animals'. In fact, the use of the term had been proposed much earlier than that, in a note dated 18 October 1954, when, commenting on the wording of a draft letter, Burch suggested to Russell that 'to suggest improvements' should be changed to 'to suggest some possible alternatives' (3). What was good enough for Burch should be acceptable to the rest of us.

4. PROGRESS IN THE 1980s

During the 1970s, the increasing activities of critics of animal experimentation on both ethical and scientific grounds had begun to encourage significant changes in attitudes, not least among politicians. For example, the British Government agreed to replace the *Cruelty to Animals Act 1876* and was willing to listen to proposals from animal welfare organisations. This was to result in the *Animals (Scientific Procedures) Act 1986*, which introduced a number of important stipulations, including the following:

Clause 5(5): *The Secretary of State shall not grant a project licence unless he is satisfied that the applicant has given adequate consideration to the feasibility of achieving the purpose of the programme to be specified in the licence by means not involving the use of protected animals.*

Clause 5(4): *In determining whether and on what terms to grant a project licence the Secretary of State shall weigh the likely adverse effects on the animals concerned against the benefit likely to accrue as a result of the programme to be specified in the licence.*

At about the same time, *Directive 86/609/EEC*, approved by the European Council and the European Parliament, spelled out its *Replacement* basis in *Article 7*, as follows: *An experiment shall not be performed, if another scientifically satisfactory method of obtaining the result sought, not entailing the use of an animal, is reasonably and practicably available.* Subsequently, this requirement resulted in the setting-up of the European Centre for the Validation of Alternative Methods (ECVAM).

FRAME had provided two members of a small group of experts who advised the British Government on the drafting and passage through Parliament of the 1986 Act. During this process, the responsible minister, David Mellor, having been reminded that the Government both required animal testing and sought to replace it, arranged for FRAME to be awarded the first government grant for alternatives research. This was used to support the establishment of INVITTOX, the *in vitro* toxicology databank, the development of the kenacid blue cytotoxicity test and the setting-up of the FRAME international test validation scheme.

A number of other significant events took place during the 1980s, including the establishment in 1989, of ZEBET, the Center for Documentation and Evaluation of Alternative Methods to Animal Experiments, the Japanese Society for Alternatives to Animal Experiments (JSAAE) and the European Research Group for Alternatives in Toxicity Testing (ERGATT).

5. INTO THE 1990s

By the end of the 1980s, the Three Rs concept was becoming more-widely accepted, and replacement alternatives were increasingly seen as ways of avoiding the ethical dilemmas and scientific inadequacies involved in routine regulatory testing in animals. The number of individuals, organisations and authorities involved was steadily increasing, and the Three Rs, and the desirability of replacement in particular, were enshrined in new international laws. ECVAM was about to be established in 1991, followed by the US Interagency Coordinating Committee on the Validation of Alternative Methods (ICCVAM) in 1997.

REFERENCES

1. Russell, W.M.S. & Burch, R.L. (1959). *The Principles of Humane Experimental Technique*, 238pp. London, UK: Methuen.
2. Balls, M. (2015). The Wisdom of Russell and Burch. 20. On replacing the concept of Replacement. *ATLA* **43**, P78—P79.
3. Balls, M. (2009). The origins and early days of the Three Rs concept. *ATLA* **37**, 255—265.
4. Rowan, A.N. (2009). FRAME: The early days. *ATLA* **37**(Suppl. 2), 7—12.
5. Weil, C.S. & Scala, R.A. (1971). Study of intra- and interlaboratory variation in the results of rabbit eye and skin irritation tests. *Toxicology and Applied Pharmacology* **19**, 276—360.
6. Balls, M. (2012). FRAME and the pharmaceutical industry. *ATLA* **40**, 295—300.
7. Zbinden, G. & Flury-Roversi, M. (1981). Significance of the LD50 test for the toxicological evaluation of chemical substances. *Archives of Toxicology* **47**, 77—99.
8. Smyth, D.H. (1978). *Alternatives to Animal Experiments*, 218pp. London, UK: Scolar Press.

Chapter 1.2

Types of Toxicity and Applications of Toxicity Testing

Andrew P. Worth

Joint Research Centre, European Commission, Ispra, Italy

SUMMARY

This chapter explains why toxicity testing is carried out for the purposes of protecting human health or the environment. The traditional reliance on animal testing and the challenges faced in the journey from developing to accepting non-animal methods are discussed, along with the roles of different players, including academia, industry, contract research organisations, governmental authorities and non-governmental organisations.

1. THE NEED FOR TESTING

Toxicity testing is carried out to characterise the potentially adverse effects of chemicals on human health, animal health or the environment, with a view to ensuring the safest possible use of chemicals and chemical-containing products. The majority of toxicity testing worldwide is conducted to comply with legal and regulatory requirements for the risk management of chemicals. In general, toxicity testing is carried out by industry or contract research organisations (on behalf of industry), and the resulting assessments are submitted to authorities (for notification/registration and, in some cases, marketing approval).

While the manner in which chemicals are assessed and managed varies according to geographical jurisdiction, the regulations applied typically address chemicals according to their manufacture, use, waste treatment and end-of-life disposal, or discharge to environmental media. Thus, toxicity testing is typically carried out on: (a) industrial chemicals (e.g. raw materials, processing aids, speciality chemicals, chemicals used in consumer products and articles); (b) chemicals with specific functions (e.g. detergents, pesticides); (c) chemicals used in certain kinds of product (e.g. cosmetics, medicines for human or veterinary use, toys, medical devices, tobacco-containing products); (d) chemicals that are intentionally added to, or inadvertently found in, food and feed, and (e) chemicals found in environmental media, with possible risks to human health and wildlife (e.g. surface, ground and marine waters, drinking water). In industrialised economies, legislation on chemicals originated in the 1960s (e.g. the *Dangerous Substances Directive* in the European Economic Community) or in the 1970s (e.g. the *Toxic Substances Control Act* in the USA).

Toxicity testing has traditionally been carried out on animals, with a wide variety of species being used. This tradition has its roots in the 'tools' that were available decades ago, and is based on the assumption that adverse effects seen at high doses in animal 'models' are relevant to human exposure scenarios (even at much lower exposures and often by different routes). For human health effects, not only have rodents been most-commonly used, but also larger animals, including rabbits, dogs and non-human primates. For environmental protection, with a view to capturing effects on a range of taxonomic levels, testing has typically been carried out, not only on algae, bacteria, plants, invertebrates and fish, but also on insects (e.g. bees), worms, amphibia and birds (1). Only some of these organisms (the vertebrate species) are protected by legislation on the use of animals for scientific purposes (e.g. (2)) and have been the focus of replacement efforts.

The History of Alternative Test Methods in Toxicology. https://doi.org/10.1016/B978-0-12-813697-3.00002-0

Increasingly, toxicity testing in animals is being supplemented with, or replaced by, non-animal (alternative) methods. This is not only to address animal welfare concerns, but also for reasons of scientific rigour (the need to maximise the relevance and credibility of safety assessments), practicality (including the need to manage the risks of tens of thousands of chemicals already in use) and competitiveness (the need to innovate new chemicals and products and satisfy ever-changing market demands). These research and development efforts are being carried out, not only by industry, but also by academic and governmental institutions. In addition, governmental organisations, such as the European Commission and the US Environmental Protection Agency, have developed large-scale research programmes to develop alternatives. Various non-governmental organisations (NGOs), with interests in protecting civil society, animal welfare or the environment, also play a forceful, sometimes constructive and sometimes provocative, role in the dialogue surrounding the regulatory use of alternative methods. Prominent NGOs with interests against animal testing include the European Coalition to End Animal Experiments (ECEAE), People for the Ethical Treatment of Animals (PETA) and the Physicians Committee for Responsible Medicine (PCRM), whereas organisations that advocate animal testing, or at least express concerns about the current readiness of alternative methods, include the European Animal Research Association (EARA) and PAN Europe.

There has been much discussion on the challenges faced in developing and gaining acceptance for non-animal approaches to toxicity testing (3–5). While the challenges of development and validation are largely scientific, technical and organisational, it is important to bear in mind that the challenge of acceptance is also related to the context of use and the associated practical and regulatory constraints, particularly the following:

1. The extent and nature of testing required depends on the application and jurisdiction. For example, medicines require more-extensive safety testing than food contact materials; active ingredients (of plant protection products and biocides) require more-extensive testing than their degradates and metabolites. In terms of the nature of testing, a largely prescriptive set of standard tests (e.g. Organisation of Economic Cooperation and Development [OECD] guideline tests) are applied to industrial chemicals and pesticides, whereas for cosmetic ingredients and products, the manufacturer has considerable flexibility in the choice of the methods used to meet the required safety standards.
2. The extent to which the burden of safety testing falls on manufacturers/importers/suppliers or authorities also varies according to region and sector, as does the scope of pre-marketing approval and post-marketing risk management procedures. For example, medicines, pesticides, biocides and chemicals intentionally added to food, typically require pre-market approval, whereas industrial chemicals and cosmetics typically do not (although there are exceptions, such as hair dyes, UV filters and preservatives in the EU).
3. There are regional and sectoral differences in the extent to which risk management is based on hazard, exposure or risk-based considerations (see below).

2. TYPES OF TOXICITY TEST

In the context of human health safety assessment, the main types of animal-based toxicity tests are conducted for: acute toxicity (skin and eye irritation/corrosion, acute systemic toxicity), allergenicity (skin and respiratory sensitisation), repeat–dose toxicity, genotoxicity and mutagenicity, carcinogenicity, reproductive and developmental toxicity, and biokinetics (also referred to as toxicokinetics or pharmacokinetics). The protection goal in these cases is the individual (i.e. the human). The historical development of alternatives for some of these endpoints is addressed in various chapters in this book.

3. APPLICATIONS OF TOXICITY TESTING

Toxicity testing is performed in the context of safety assessments for a diverse range of chemical and product types, and the historical development of alternatives for some of these applications is addressed in various chapters in this book.

Within the EU, a comprehensive suite of legislation has been built up since the 1960s, with the aim of protecting human health and the environment from the risks of chemical exposure. Today, the two main pillars of the chemicals 'acquis' are the Registration, Evaluation, Authorisation and Restriction of Chemicals (REACH) and Classification, Labelling and Packaging (CLP) Regulations, complemented by legislation that addresses chemicals with specific functions, such as biocides, plant protection products, fertilisers, detergents and medicines. In addition, product-related legislation, such as the *Toys Directive* or the *Medical Devices Directive*, aims to protect human health during the use of products, and various pieces of legislation on waste, recycling and emissions aim to protect both human health and the environment at the end of the product life cycle. Finally, occupational health and safety legislation has been adopted for worker protection.

The main types of animal-based toxicity tests conducted for environmental safety assessment are acute and chronic toxicity (including growth, survival and reproductive success) in fish, acute and chronic toxicity in crustaceans (typically daphnids), acute testing on birds, and bioaccumulation (typically in fish). The protection goal in these cases is the population, community or ecosystem.

4. RISK MANAGEMENT

The way in which information derived from toxicity testing is used varies according to geographical jurisdiction and regulatory application. However, in general terms, risk management is carried out on the basis of hazard, exposure or risk-based considerations.

Risk management is informed not only by scientific considerations but also by policy ones. This is distinguished from risk assessment, which is intended to be an entirely scientific process, consisting of four steps: hazard identification, hazard characterisation, exposure assessment and risk characterisation. The first two steps are collectively referred to as hazard assessment. Hazard identification is the identification of the type and nature of adverse effects that a chemical has an inherent capacity to cause, whereas hazard characterisation is the qualitative and, in some cases, quantitative description of the potential to cause adverse effects. Risk characterisation refers to the combined use of hazard characterisation and exposure assessment to reach conclusions on acceptable safety levels of exposure for human health or the environment.

The hazard assessment step has traditionally been based on animal testing. A dose—response curve is generated experimentally, to identify the lowest dose of the chemical of interest that produces a treatment-related adverse effect (in the whole organism) as well as the highest dose without an effect. The former is called the lowest observed adverse effect level (LOAEL), and the latter is called the no observed adverse effect level (NOAEL). The NOAEL is treated as a point of departure (POD) for the derivation of a safe exposure level (regulatory guidance value) for human or environmental protection.

In the case of threshold effects, safety (uncertainty) factors are applied to derive the guidance values in humans. These metrics are referred to in different ways, according to the sector. For example, in the food safety area, they include the acceptable daily intake (ADI) for food and feed additives and pesticides, the tolerable daily intake (TDI) for contaminants and chemicals in food contact materials, and for acute effects, the acute reference dose (ARfD). In the chemicals area, the terms Derived No Effect Level (DNEL) and Predicted No Effect Concentration (PNEC) are used for human health and environmental effects, respectively. In the case of genotoxic compounds (including genotoxic carcinogens), which are generally considered to occur without a threshold, a guidance value may be derived by linear extrapolation (to the dose causing no effect) or by the Margin of Exposure (MOE) approach, in which the POD is divided by the human exposure to indicate a level of concern.

In the interpretation of animal-based toxicity tests, a distinction is made between adaptive effects (effect levels) and those that are considered adverse (adverse effect levels), with the POD being based on the dose expected to cause no or minimal adverse effect (the NOAEL). In contrast, most alternative (non-animal) methods are designed for a mechanism-based assessment, and are not able (on their own) to distinguish between a treatment-related effect and an adverse effect. An advantage of non-animal tests, however, is that they are better able to distinguish between toxicokinetics (how the external dose translates into an internal one) and toxicodynamics (how the internal dose results in a toxic effect).

In the EU, some pieces of legislation (e.g. the CLP Regulation) manage chemical risks by a hazard-based approach. This is sometimes referred to as 'generic risk management', as generic exposure scenarios are taken into account. Other pieces of legislation (e.g. those for REACH, biocides and pesticides) supplement the hazard-based approach with risk-based considerations. In other words, a chemical-specific risk assessment is conducted for defined exposure scenarios. This is also referred to as a 'specific risk management' approach. Clearly, specific risk management requires more-precise information on chemical exposure, which is not always available.

It is worth noting that not all pieces of the EU legislation require new animal testing. Some rely instead on existing information and the data generated under other pieces of legislation. A notable example is the CLP Regulation, in which classification and labelling are carried out by using existing data, and in particular, data generated under the industrial chemicals, pesticides or biocides legislation. In the case of data gaps, non-testing methods and expert judgement can be applied. The CLP Regulation is the legal instrument used in the EU to apply the United Nations' Globally Harmonised System of Classification and Labelling of Chemicals (GHS), which aims to harmonise the rules for hazard classification and labelling worldwide.

5. THE REPLACEMENT OF ANIMAL TESTS

Looking to the future, it seems unlikely that the safety assessment framework will be organised around the same typology of animal-based toxicities. The replacement of animal studies to meet some regulatory requirements (in particular, local toxicity to the skin and eye, skin sensitisation, genotoxicity) has been achieved by demonstrating that non-animal methods provide equivalent information to that obtained in animal tests. However, the direct replacement of animal testing will not be possible, and would not be meaningful, for more-complex endpoints, including acute systemic toxicity, repeat—dose toxicity, carcinogenicity, and reproductive and developmental toxicity.

This is partly because a satisfactory understanding of the mechanisms involved in these forms of toxicity is lacking. However, the way forward is not the traditional approach, as the human relevance and reliability of the animal tests themselves are highly questionable because of differences within and between the species used, the tendency to use very high doses and an inability to take account of human variation resulting from various factors, including genetics, age, occupation and other health issues.

Moreover, the animal tests have been accepted and applied without formal validation studies of the kind now required for alternative tests, and their weaknesses stem primarily from poor reproducibility and lack of understanding of the fundamental nature and mechanistic basis of the effects that need to be predicted.

Thus, for the effective assessment and management of chemicals and products in the future, a huge investment should be made in both fundamental and applied research, to identify the key questions involved and how answers to them should be sought. It is here that non-animal studies will have a great deal to contribute by providing relevant, reliable and realistic solutions.

6. CONCLUSIONS

A diverse array of animal tests has been developed for the purposes of hazard assessment and risk management. The types of test, and the manner in which they are used, varies according to legislative sector and jurisdiction. Increasingly, the standard animal tests are being replaced by an ever-increasing selection of non-animal methods, but this poses technical, organisational, psychological and legal barriers, in terms of data integration and interpretation, as well as the credibility of the resulting safety assessments. Research on mechanistic toxicology and the development of non-animal methods will provide ways of overcoming these barriers.

REFERENCES

1. EC. (2013). *Seventh Report on the Statistics on the Number of Animals used for Experimental and Other Scientific Purposes in the Member States of the European Union. COM/2013/0859 final*, 14pp. Brussels, Belgium: European Commission..
2. EU. (2010). Directive 2010/63/EU of the European Parliament and of the Council of 22 September 2010 on the protection of animals used for scientific purposes. *Official Journal of the European Union* **L276**, 33−79.
3. Schiffelers, M.-J.W.A., Blaauboer, B.J., Bakker, W.E., *et al.* (2014). Regulatory acceptance and use of 3R models for pharmaceuticals and chemicals: Expert opinions on the state of affairs and the way forward. *Regulatory Toxicology and Pharmacology* **69**, 41−48.
4. Archibald, K., Drake, T. & Coleman, R. (2015). Barriers to the uptake of human-based test methods, and how to overcome them. *ATLA* **43**, 301−308.
5. Burden, N., Sewell, F. & Chapman, K. (2015). Testing chemical safety: What is needed to ensure the widespread application of non-animal approaches? *PLoS Biology* **13**, e1002156.

Chapter 1.3

The Key Technologies

Robert D. Combes

Independent Consultant, Norwich, United Kingdom

SUMMARY

A short introduction to the principal technologies that have had the most influence on the development and use of alternatives in toxicology and safety testing is provided. Advances in analytical and diagnostic methods, and a greater understanding of cell biology and molecular mechanisms of toxicity, have enhanced the range and detection of toxicity endpoints and, therefore, the relevance of test systems and data interpretation, as well as enabling an increased role for human studies.

1. INTRODUCTION

Replacement alternatives are being developed and used, to avoid the need to conduct tests for regulatory purposes or other scientific experiments on laboratory animals, for scientific and welfare reasons.

The areas where replacement alternative methods have had the greatest impact in toxicology include: (a) predictions based on the physical and chemical properties of molecules, including test material purity and the identification and quantification of impurities, and (quantitative) structure-activity relationship ((Q)SAR) modelling; (b) mathematical and computer simulation; (c) *in vitro* tissue culture methods; and (d) human studies.

This chapter provides a short overview of the key technologies, and their impact on the history of alternatives in toxicity testing, as a prelude to more-detailed discussions in later chapters.

This chapter is based on accounts in Refs. (1—3), which the reader should consult for further, more-detailed information.

2. TECHNOLOGY DRIVERS

2.1 Tissue Culture Systems

Several methods, systems and technologies are being applied in *in vitro* toxicology to overcome the problems of species differences and *in vitro* to *in vivo* extrapolation, and to cope with large amounts of data. Many of these new methods involve cultured human cells derived directly from tissues and organs as primary cells, by cellular immortalisation or genetic manipulation, or from embryonic and adult stem cells (a technology derived from the nuclear transplantation experiments with amphibian oocytes of Gurdon, which revealed the totipotency of differentiated cells), so that they exhibit the *in vivo* functional properties of the differentiated tissues from which they were derived.

Also, tissue cultures can be grown as simple monolayers of one cell type, or as more-complex 3-D organotypic systems, comprising different cell types, and involving interactions between them. They can also be grown, by tissue engineering, on scaffolds derived from extracellular matrix, to resemble, both architecturally and physiologically, whole tissues and organs (4).

2.2 Reporter Gene Assays and Biosensors

High-throughput screening is being achieved through the use of reporter gene assays, coupled with transcriptional activation. Mammalian cells are genetically engineered, by having DNA sequences coding for a specific receptor introduced into them on a vector molecule linked to the corresponding DNA response element sequence of a reporter gene, to which binding of the test material stimulates gene expression of a readily detectable product.

Biosensors are chemical detection devices in which a biologically derived recognition system (e.g. an enzyme, antibody or cell immobilised on a membrane) is coupled to a transducer, which generates a quantifiable electrical signal. Biosensors have been especially useful in ecotoxicity testing.

2.3 Miniaturised and Large-Scale Culture Systems

Microfabrication, micro-etching (soft lithography and hard micro-machining) and microfluidics have been adapted from the semi-conductor industry to generate organ-on-a-chip and organism-on-a-chip micro-scale culture systems, by using flexible, bio-compatible silicon and plastic wafer materials (5). Several chambers, each representing an organ, and containing mammalian cell cultures, interconnected by a fluid network, in microlitre, nanolitre and even picolitre volumes, can be constructed to permit intercellular communication and gaseous and nutrient exchange (6).

Miniaturisation facilitates the replication of experiments under identical conditions, requiring small amounts of test chemical and media.

At the other end of the size scale are large culture dynamic bioreactors comprising a 3-D network of interwoven hollow fibre membranes, which transport gases, nutrients, growth factors and by-products to and away from the cells, which can be in the form of mono-cultures or differentiated tissue constructs. Dynamic bioreactors show great promise for long-term toxicity testing (7).

2.4 Toxicogenomics and Proteomics

Other technologies broaden the range and improve the sensitivity and relevance of toxicity endpoints. Genomics and proteomics both arose from the Human Genome Project (8). In the former, differential transcription is measured by using microarrays of oligonucleotides to detect cDNA and cRNA copies of new transcripts via specific hybridisation. Toxicity affects gene expression differentially, which is measured at the transcriptional (genomic) level, or the translational (proteomic) level.

2.5 Other Enabling Technologies

Other technologies have improved the detection and interpretation of various toxicity endpoints, including cytogenetics using chromosome painting (via fluorescence *in situ* hybridisation [FISH], to detect and localise the presence or absence of specific DNA sequences), the use of quantum dot cell imaging (9) and the detection of biomarkers of endogenous exposure and effect. Biomarkers, together with highly sensitive analytical techniques, such as accelerated mass spectrometry (AMS), and the availability of non-invasive 'real-time' diagnostic imaging, have contributed to enabling earlier than usual first-in human studies of earlier first-in human studies (10).

Toxicokinetics can provide useful information for interpreting hazard data for risk assessment, by: (a) relating external and internal dose effects; and (b) facilitating interspecies extrapolation. In its more-elaborate form, physiologically based pharmacokinetic (PBPK) modelling involves representing organs or groups of organs as discrete compartments inter-connected with physiological volumes and blood flows into and out of which test chemicals and their metabolites partition, before being eliminated (11). *In vitro* biokinetics applies similar principles to tissue culture systems, to study test material availability to the target site, facilitating *in vitro* to *in vivo* extrapolation (12).

Finally, the vast amount of data generated by these collective approaches, and especially genomics, is being searched, analysed, compared and interpreted by using increasingly powerful bioinformatics procedures. These involve a range of computerised and statistical sorting, and cataloguing techniques.

3. DISCUSSION AND CONCLUSIONS

Advances in technology have provided many improvements in the sensitivity and resolving power of analytical and diagnostic methods, making them less invasive, and to an increased understanding of many of the major biological processes and mechanisms of toxicity of physical and chemical agents. This has resulted in improvements to both the detection of toxicity endpoints, and the range, and relevance to the target species of the available analytical systems, deployed as integrated testing strategies (13).

With the latter in mind, it is crucial that financial support for pure research continues to be provided, and that those interested in developing new alternatives continue to effectively exploit the results of their endeavours.

REFERENCES

1. Bhogal, N., Grindon, C., Combes, R., *et al.* (2005). Toxicity testing: creating a revolution based on new technologies. *Trends in Biotechnology* **23**, 299–307.
2. Balls, M., Combes, R. & Bhogal, N. (Eds.). (2011). *New Technologies for Toxicity Testing,* 258pp. Austin, TX, USA: Landes Bioscience & New York. NY, USA: Springer Science+Business Media.
3. Combes, R.D. (2013). Progress in the Development, Validation and Regulatory Acceptance of in Vitro Methods for Toxicity Testing. pp. 1–25. In J. Reedijk (Ed.), *Reference Module in Chemistry, Molecular Sciences and Chemical Engineering.* Waltham, MA, USA: Elsevier.
4. Heinonen, T. & Verfaillie, C. (2018). *The Development and Application of Key Technologies and Tools* (this volume).
5. Dehne, E.M., Hickman, J. & Shuler, M. (2018). *Biologically-inspired Microphysiological Systems* (this volume).
6. Benam, K.H., Novak, R., Nawroth, J., *et al.* (2016). Matched-comparative modelling of normal and diseased human airway responses using a micro-engineered breathing lung chip. *Cell Systems* **3**, 456–466.
7. Grindon, C., Combes, R., Cronin, M., *et al.* (2008). An integrated decision-tree testing strategy for repeat dose toxicity with respect to the requirements of the EU REACH Legislation. *ATLA* **36**, 93–101.
8. Kavlock, R., Austin, C. & Tice, R. (2018). *US Vision for Toxicity Testing in the 21st Century* (this volume).
9. Jaiswal, J.K. & Simon, S.M. (2015). Imaging live cells using quantum dots. *Cold Spring Harbor Protocols* **2015**, 619–625.
10. Burt, T. & Combes, R.D. (2018). *The use of non-invasive imaging and microdosing in volunteers to improve drug discovery and safety assessment* (this volume).
11. Cronin, M. & Yoon, M. (2018). *Computational methods to predict toxicity* (this volume).
12. Paini, A., Sala Benito, J.V., Bessems, J., *et al.* (2017). From *in vitro* to *in vivo*: Integration of the virtual cell based assay with physiologically-based kinetic modelling. *Toxicology in Vitro* **45**, 241–248.
13. Worth, A. & Blaauboer, B. (2018). *Integrated approaches to testing and assessment* (this volume).

Section 2

Contributions From Countries, Regions and Organisations

Chapter 2.1

Alternative Methods in Toxicity Testing in the UK

Michael Balls[1] and Robert D. Combes[2]

[1]University of Nottingham, Nottingham, United Kingdom; [2]Independent Consultant, Norwich, United Kingdom

SUMMARY

The challenge of the need for change was thrown down when Russell and Burch proposed the Three Rs in 1959, and, among others, Smyth responded by focusing on the concept of alternatives. The Fund for the Replacement of Animals in Medical Experiments (FRAME), formed in 1969 to seek the replacement of animal tests by better methods, played a major role, through its journal, *ATLA* (*Alternatives to Laboratory Animals*), its Toxicity Committee, its Research Programme, including the FRAME Alternatives Laboratory at the University of Nottingham, and its good relations with academia, government, industry and scientists in many parts of the world. FRAME played a pivotal role in the drafting and passage of the *Animals (Scientific Procedures) Act 1986*, which had a sound Three Rs basis, received the first government grant specifically for alternatives research, and also provided the first Head of the European Centre for the Validation of Alternative Methods (ECVAM). The National Centre for the Three Rs (NC3Rs), set up in 2004, rapidly established effective collaborations with science and industry, and its flagship initiative, CRACK IT, focuses on the development of new technologies to meet challenges put forward by its sponsors. Many other individuals and organisations have made major contributions to the promotion of the Three Rs, and, in particular, the Central Toxicology Laboratory, originally at Imperial Chemical Industries (ICI), and Unilever Research. Julia Fentem, now at Unilever, has had a notably unique career, including important periods at the University of Nottingham, FRAME and ECVAM.

1. EARLY DAYS

The 1970s seem to have been a time when attitudes to animal testing were changing in the UK, mainly because of growing awareness of the inadequacy of laboratory animals as models for humans, and the opportunities that could arise if *in vitro* systems were developed, rather than because of animal welfare concerns or the Three Rs concept put forward by Russell and Burch in 1959, in *The Principles of Humane Experimental Technique* (*The Principles*; 1). This is a strong underlying theme in David Smyth's 1978 book, *Alternatives to Animal Experiments* (2), which resulted from a survey he conducted on behalf of the Research Defence Society.

Smyth listed the 158 individuals he consulted, which included such influential figures as Mary Dawson, Anthony Dayan, Honor Fell, Roy Goulding, Dorothy Hegarty, John Paul, Andrew Rowan and Alistair Worden, but not William Russell or Rex Burch. He gave us the definition of 'alternatives', which still applies today (to include 'any procedures which do away with the use of animals altogether, lead to a reduction in the total number of animals used, or lead to less distress to the animals employed'), reviewed the alternative methods and enumerated leading questions about them, and summarised the activities of the interested parties, noting that the Fund for the Replacement of Animals in Medical Experiments (FRAME) deserved to be treated separately from other animal welfare organisations, because its 'main activities are quite different'. He included a whole chapter on toxicity testing, with comments on lethal toxicity and eye and skin irritation procedures, and on special kinds of toxicity, such as carcinogenicity and reproductive toxicity.

Anyone interested in the history of alternative methods in toxicity testing up to 1978, in the UK and beyond, should read this outstanding book, which ranks with that of Russell and Burch, in providing insight on what was to follow.

2. THE FUND FOR THE REPLACEMENT OF ANIMALS IN MEDICAL EXPERIMENTS

In the early 1960s, Dorothy Hegarty became increasingly dismayed by the total abolition demands of the antivivisection societies, which were easily countered by medical researchers, so she founded a positive campaigning group, Promoters of Animal Welfare (PAW). She sought the support of scientists, and was fortunate when Charles Foister, a recently retired agricultural biologist, together with her own scientist son and daughter-in-law, helped her to establish FRAME in 1969, to campaign for the use of alternatives instead of animals (3). PAW and then FRAME were run from the front room of her house, which became too small as FRAME got under way, so an office was set up in a former milliner's shop in the London suburb of Wimbledon. As David Smyth was to appreciate a few years later, FRAME had found a distinct niche, although totally independently of Russell and Burch's Three Rs concept, which had been put forward 10 years earlier.

FRAME's aim was 'to benefit both man and animals by promoting the use of more reliable, accurate and relevant methods in biology and medicine, which at the same time help to reduce the need for laboratory animals', and, in particular, by recognising that 'the exchange of information and its ready availability are of paramount importance, if new techniques are to be adopted rapidly'. This led to the launch of *Alternatives to Laboratory Animals (ATLA) Abstracts* in June 1973, published as an A4 single-column, camera-ready journal, with two issues per year. Initially, the abstracts were written by staff located at the British Library, Boston Spa in Yorkshire, and were arranged in 17 subject sections. Issue 1(1) had 149 pages (with two to three abstracts per page), plus an author index and a subject index.

This way of informing scientists may look rather naïve today, but it should not be forgotten that, in 1973, there were few abstracting services, no personal computers, no Internet or websites, and only limited access to electric typewriters and photocopiers. Scientists kept themselves informed by going to the library and looking through hard copies of the scientific journals.

Nevertheless, information services had begun to become available, and as the circulation of *ATLA Abstracts* remained very low, it was decided that it should be transformed into a more conventional scientific journal, *ATLA*, by including news, reviews and opinions. Andrew Rowan had joined FRAME as scientific director in 1976, and had spent 6 months patiently trying to persuade Mrs Hegarty that the change was necessary (4). One of the earliest reviews was by Mary Dawson, on the application of tissue culture to drug and toxicity testing (5).

Rowan also increased FRAME's scientific credibility, in various ways. He organised a symposium at the Royal Society of London in 1978, on *The Use of Alternatives in Drug Research* (6). The published proceedings remain very interesting today, but two chapters deserve special mention. Corwin Hansch's discussion of *computer-assisted enzyme studies in drug design* marked the beginning of recognition of the importance of quantitative structure—activity relationships, and Michael Balls and Ranjini Rao described their work on organ culture in pharmacology. Concerned by the weak scientific basis of much routine regulatory toxicity testing, Rowan also proposed that FRAME should establish an expert committee on animals and alternatives in toxicity testing, with Alastair Worden as its secretary. In addition, he raised questions with the Home Office about the use of monkeys in providing and testing polio vaccines, and about the LD50 test, and oversaw the publication of two important FRAME publicity leaflets, *What Price Vanity?* and *How safe is your medication?* (7).

Meanwhile, Michael Balls and his research group at the University of East Anglia had been using organ cultures since the early 1970s. Shortly after their move to the new University of Nottingham Medical School in 1975, they received a visit from David Smyth, who told them that they were working on 'alternatives', a term not previously known to them in that context. He suggested that they should approach animal welfare societies for financial support, which they did. A grant from the Humane Research Trust, and also a donation from Reckitt & Colman Ltd., supported Ranjini Rao's PhD project and the work they reported at the Royal Society Symposium.

By 1979, Rowan had departed for the Humane Society of the United States, and Balls had been invited to become a FRAME trustee. Mrs Hegarty asked him to represent FRAME on the toxicity committee that had been formed, and at their first meeting, its members asked him to be chairman, as he was the only member with no claim to be a toxicologist. When Mrs Hegarty decided to resign as chairman of the Trustees in 1981, Balls replaced her and immediately proposed that FRAME should move to Nottingham, to develop a practical research relationship with the University of Nottingham Medical School (8). FRAME had struggled to find a suitable scientific director to replace Rowan, and in early 1982, Balls became its honorary scientific director. He did this with the unwavering support of the vice-chancellor of the University of Nottingham, Sir Colin Campbell, and played that role until he left Nottingham in 1993, to become the first Head of the European Centre for the Validation of Alternative Methods (ECVAM; see also, Chapter 2.10). He was able to maintain his roles as chairman of the FRAME Trustees and editor of *ATLA* throughout his employment by the European Commission, to the benefit of both FRAME and ECVAM.

The 1980s was a decade of great achievements for FRAME (9). *ATLA* was relaunched as a typeset journal with an international editorial board. The FRAME Toxicity Committee produced its report in 1982, which was discussed with a distinguished audience at a conference held at the Royal Society. The Committee began to meet again in 1988, now under the chairmanship of James Bridges, and produced a second report in 1991, which was also discussed at a conference in London, this time at the Royal College of Physicians.

Meanwhile, FRAME had formed an alliance with the Committee for the Reform of Animal Experimentation (CRAE) and the British Veterinary Association (BVA). The recommendations for reform of the *Cruelty to Animals Act 1876* made by this Triple Alliance were used by the government in drafting its own proposals for a new law. The Alliance then provided the government's principal advisers during all stages of the preparation and passage through Parliament of what was to become the *Animals (Scientific Procedures) Act 1986*. An All-Party Parliamentary FRAME Group had been set up in Parliament in 1981, which also played an influential role during the passage of the new legislation.

Along the way, David Mellor, the home office minister responsible for the regulation of animal experimentation, had arranged for FRAME to receive the first government grant awarded to support research on alternatives. This was used for studies on cytotoxicity in human cell cultures, the establishment of an *in vitro* toxicology database, and the setting-up of the FRAME International Test Validation Scheme (10), which laid down many of the principles, which are now used in validation studies throughout the world (see also, Chapter 5.5).

In 1985, FRAME was a co-host of the first *Practical In Vitro Toxicology* (PIVT) conferences, held at the University of Reading, which led to the creation of a new journal, *Toxicology in Vitro*. Subsequently, FRAME hosted PIVT II and PIVT III at the University of Nottingham in 1989 and 1993, but the aims of the series were taken over by ECVAM. In 1986, with the assistance of Mary Dawson, FRAME organised the International Workshop on *In Vitro* Toxicology at Crieff, Scotland, the fourth in a series subsequently run by the European Society for Toxicology *In Vitro*. Much later, FRAME played a crucial role with ECVAM in organising the 3rd World Congress on Alternatives and Animal Use in the Life Sciences (Bologna, 1999), by participating in the financial management of the Congress and the editing and production of the proceedings. The proceedings of the 4th World Congress (New Orleans, 2002) were published as an *ATLA* supplement.

FRAME also played a leading role in the European Research Group for Alternatives in Toxicity Testing (ERGATT), which was recognised by Directorate General (DG) XI of the European Commission, and organised the 1990 workshop on the principles of validation (Amden I), in collaboration with the Center for Alternatives to Animal Testing (CAAT), and the 1990 Vouliagmeni workshop on the regulatory acceptance of validated alternative procedures. FRAME provided the secretariat for both workshops, and for a subsequent ECVAM workshop on practical aspects of validation (Amden II) in 1995.

Collaboration between FRAME and the German Center for Documentation and Evaluation of Alternative Methods to Animal Experiments (ZEBET) resulted from a long-standing friendship between Horst Spielmann and Michael Balls, partly developed through ERGATT, and led to many developments, including their collaboration as editors of *ATLA*, and in the background to the Amden I workshop on validation (11). Then, in 1991, a five-way partnership was established between FRAME, ZEBET, the University of Nottingham, the Free University of Berlin and Miroslav Cervinka at Charles University in Hradec Králové, Czech Republic, in a TEMPUS project, which played an important part in the introduction of the Three Rs concept in Eastern Europe. Later, relationships between ECVAM, FRAME and ZEBET were to be the basis of many positive developments in the EU and beyond.

FRAME's collaboration with the University of Nottingham was mutually very beneficial. The FRAME Research Programme and the FRAME Alternatives Laboratory (FAL) had collaborations with a number of laboratories and companies, including Avon Products, Bristol-Myers, Fisons-Boots, Hoechst, ICI, Johnson & Johnson, L'Oréal, May & Baker, Pfizer, Unilever and Huntingdon Research Centre. With a focus on cosmetics testing, a long-lasting relationship was established with the UK Cosmetic, Toiletry and Perfumery Association (CTPA) and the European Cosmetic and Perfumery Association (COLIPA). The FAL contributed to the development of a number of tests, including the kenacid blue cytotoxicity test and the fluorescein leakage test, although human cell culture took over from amphibian organ culture. Members of FRAME's scientific staff were successful as part-time PhD students.

After the success of the Amden I and Vouliagmeni workshops, DGXI and the UK Home Office contacted FRAME to manage an international, multicentre validation study on alternatives to the Draize eye irritation test (the EC/HO study). This was the first alternatives validation study outside the genotoxicity area, and its management was transferred to ECVAM in 1993.

When Michael Balls left for ECVAM, Richard Clothier succeeded him as Head of the FAL and maintained a very close relationship with ECVAM, including the supervision of ECVAM members of staff as part-time PhD students at the University of Nottingham. He managed the FAL's participation in a number of validation studies, including establishing the use of the neutral red phototoxicity test with human keratinocytes. Meanwhile, at FRAME, Robert Combes became scientific director in 1994, and the charity moved to its own new building, Russell & Burch House, which was officially opened by Bill Russell himself, in 1995. It should be noted that FRAME had many distinguished Trustees over the years, including Donald Straughan, a former Home Office Inspector, and two experts on Reduction and Replacement, Michael Festing and David Morton, respectively.

When this book is expected to be published, *ATLA* will be in its 46th year of publication. The history of the journal is itself remarkable. It has benefited from the services of many gifted editors, editorial staff, editorial board members and authors. It has covered key events in imaginative ways, some of which deserve special mention. Soon after ECVAM was formed, an agreement was reached, whereby *ATLA* would publish ECVAM workshop and task force reports, the outcomes of validation studies and official statements about alternative methods. *ATLA* has also published many challenging editorials and individual multiauthor comments on a number of key issues. In 1995, volume 23 was dedicated to Dorothy Hegarty, and many of its articles were truly memorable. They included reminiscences about FRAME itself, articles about the Three Rs, including separate contributions from Russell and Burch, the proceedings of the *Twelfth Congress on In Vitro Toxicology of the Scandinavian Society for Cell Toxicology*, and of *Poor Model Man*, the first PACE conference on experiments on chimpanzees, and eight ECVAM workshop reports, including that of Workshop 5 on *Practical Aspects of the Validation of Toxicity Test Procedures*. Of particular interest were the proceedings of ECVAM Workshop 11 on *The Three Rs: the Way Forward*, organised by FRAME for ECVAM at Sheringham in Norfolk, with Russell and Burch among the participants — the first meeting they had attended together since the publication of *The Principles of Humane Experimental Technique* in 1959.

Dorothy Hegarty had died in August 1995, and many of those who knew her offered their recollections of her and her achievements (12). Another issue deserving of special mention was volume 37, Supplement 2, 2009, the proceedings of a meeting held at the University of Nottingham to mark FRAME's 40th anniversary, organised with the support of Boots (UK) Ltd and the National Centre for the Three Rs (NC3Rs; 13). Its contributors included many individuals who have made great contributions to the Three Rs movement, including Rodger Curren, Michael Festing, Alan Goldberg, Thomas Hartung, Vicky Robinson, Andrew Rowan, Horst Spielmann and Martin Stephens. Mention should also be made of *ATLA*'s very high standard of production, not least in the accuracy of complex tables and mathematical formulae, largely due to the skills of Tony Marson of Four Sheets Design and Print, who has overseen the journal's production since 1982.

FRAME has also had another publication for many years, *FRAME News*, which was widely circulated and sometimes very influential, as during the passage through Parliament of the bill leading to the 1986 Act.

3. THE NATIONAL CENTRE FOR THE THREE Rs

The NC3Rs (the Centre) was established in 2004, in response to the suggestion of a House of Lords Select Committee on Scientific Procedures, in 2002 (14, 15), that: *"A centre for the Three Rs should be set up, consisting of a small, administrative hub which coordinates research units embedded in existing centres of scientific excellence, and the centre should coordinate the government spending on the Three Rs across all departments"*.

In its own words (www.nc3rs.org.uk), *"The Centre's mission is to replace, reduce and refine the use of animals in research and testing (the Three Rs). We use the Three Rs to accelerate scientific discovery, support innovation and technological developments and address societal concerns about animal research"*. The Centre also offers a Three Rs peer review and advice service to the UK's major funding bodies, including the Medical Research Council, the Biotechnology and Biological Sciences Research Council, the Wellcome Trust and the members of the Association of Medical Research Charities.

The Centre's activities are established and coordinated by a management board, comprising an externally appointed chairperson, the chief executive of the Centre, and several (currently 13) other scientists with expertise in animal and non-animal research, animal welfare and the Three Rs. Board members are appointed in a personal capacity for 3 years, with the possibility of an extension for a further 2 years. The board works closely with 20 or so other staff. When it first opened, the Centre received an annual budget of about £350,000, which has grown over the years to about £10 m.

The Centre's flagship initiative is called 'CRACK IT' (www.crack-it.org.uk). Its aim is to develop new technologies to benefit the Three Rs from challenges put forward by industry and academic sponsors. In essence, it is a mixing pot of industry, academic institutions and small- and medium-sized enterprises. CRACK IT combines funding with in-kind support from the sponsors, including equipment and data. Two examples of CRACK IT challenges in the *in vitro* testing area are the development of a cell-based/invertebrate approach to reproductive and toxicity screening to reduce and replace current mammalian methods, and the deployment of a system to supply and use human, rather than animal, dorsal root ganglia for testing potential analgesic drugs.

The Centre also undertakes office-based research investigations. All of these involve exploring opportunities for applying the Three Rs to specific areas of interest.

The Centre was involved in a research project on non-animal methods for cosmetics testing (16), in response to constraints to be imposed in 2013 by the EU-wide ban on the sale of any finished products or ingredients that are intended mainly for use in cosmetics.

Examples of other relevant office-based projects are as follows: (a) exposure-based waiving of testing; (b) cell transformation; (c) nanotoxicology; and (d) toxicokinetics.

It has been argued (17) that the best way to persuade scientists of the benefits of the Three Rs is to provide detailed evidence and clear examples of the scientific benefits to be gained, such as those from Reduction. It is suggested that this approach be seriously considered by the Centre.

In addition, the Centre needs to challenge the principal drivers for the increasing number of scientific procedures on genetically-modified animals and the extent to which they are successful in fighting human genetic diseases and other diseases.

In the 13 years since its inception, the NC3Rs has become a major player within the UK, promoting and facilitating the adoption of Refinement, Reduction and Replacement principles and methods. This is particularly the case with regard to networking, presentation and the coordinated provision of extensive research funding, all areas that will benefit the Centre in the years ahead (18).

Meanwhile, the Centre should conduct an annual detailed review of the UK statistics on animal procedures, to be able to assess more accurately the direct impact of the Centre on biomedical research and testing, and to allay possible criticism that it acts primarily as a buffer between those who want to preserve the *status quo* and others who wish to move forward, especially to achieve Replacement (19).

4. OTHER ORGANISATIONS

It would be wrong to give the impression that FRAME was the only UK organisation involved in the early days of the practical development of alternative methods. However, the main antivivisection societies, Animal Aid, the British Union for the Abolition of Vivisection (BUAV) and the National Antivivisection Society, were bitterly opposed to the concept of replacement alternatives, as they considered that it weakened their case for total abolition. The more progressive animal welfare societies, Dr Hadwen Trust and the Humane Research Trust, focused their activities on the replacement of laboratory animal use in fundamental biomedical research, whereas the RSPCA concentrated on refinement, leaving FRAME to deal with toxicity testing.

Subsequently, under the leadership of Chris Fisher and then Michelle Thew, the BUAV (now Cruelty Free International) became much more positive toward FRAME and the need for replacement, culminating much later in some outstanding works, led by Jarrod Bailey, on the inability of toxicity tests in animals to predict toxicity in any other species, including humans (20).

Despite the publication of *The Principles* and Smyth's book on alternatives, institutions such as the Medical Research Council Toxicology Unit and the British Industrial Biological Research Association (BIBRA), both located at Carshalton, showed little interest in alternatives, and the British Toxicology Society, strongly influenced by conventional toxicologists, did little, until much later when the *In Vitro* Toxicology Society (IVTS) was created. Meanwhile, the contract testing laboratories were content to continue to conduct *in vivo* tests, such as LD50, eye and skin irritation, skin sensitisation, repeated-dose tests, for their clients, and, apart from genotoxicity testing, preferred to wait for the day when alternative test methods would be accepted by the regulatory authorities. One notable exception to this was Huntingdon Research Centre (later Huntingdon Life Sciences), of which Worden was chairman, which had its own research programme and collaborated, for example, with FRAME and others in the development of the kenacid blue cytotoxicity test.

However, the laboratories of a number of British companies made, and are making, substantial contributions to the development and application of alternative test methods, including those at Unilever Research, Glaxo and the Central Toxicology Laboratory (CTL) at ICI (later Zeneca, then AstraZeneca, then Syngenta).

Under the direction of William Parish, the *ex vivo* isolated rabbit eye test for eye irritation, which was included in the EC/HO study in 1992, was developed at the Environmental Safety Laboratory (ESL) of Unilever Research at Colworth House, near Bedford. Many contributions were made under the leadership of David Clark, who was very supportive of FRAME and ECVAM, including participation in the ECVAM validation study on non-animal tests for phototoxicity, and many initiatives related to skin irritation and skin sensitisation.

In 1998, Julia Fentem joined Unilever Research, as the next step in a unique career, first as an academic (University of Nottingham), then with an animal welfare/medical research charity (FRAME), and then as an EU civil servant (at ECVAM). Having led the setting-up of ECVAM's validation study on non-animal tests for skin corrosivity, she led the management of the study from her new position at Colworth House. The ESL has been relaunched as the Safety and Environmental Assurance Centre (SEAC), of which she became the Head in 2007. For some time, SEAC had been considering the feasibility of assessing consumer safety without using animals at all (21), and this aim is now the driving force for Unilever's Scientific Research Programme (22).

The CTL has also been involved with alternatives in many ways, especially under the leadership of Iain Purchase, one of the originators of the PIVT conferences and of *Toxicology In Vitro*, and who provided toxicology profiles on substances used in the FRAME validation programme. Phil Botham and his colleagues were involved in many ECVAM activities, including the EC/HO validation study and studies on skin irritation and sensitisation. In the company's pharmaceutical laboratories nearby, Oliver Flint developed the micromass method for embryotoxicity and was an editor of *ATLA*, as well as a challenging discussant on issues related to test validation.

REFERENCES

1. Russell, W.M.S. & Burch, R.L. (1959). *The Principles of Humane Experimental Technique*, 238pp. London, UK: Methuen
2. Smyth, D.H. (1978). *Alternatives to Animal Experiments*, 218pp. London, UK: Scolar Press
3. Hegarty, T. (1995). Dorothy Hegarty and the founding of FRAME: A personal recollection. *ATLA* **23**, 15–17.
4. Rowan, A.N. (2009). FRAME: The early days. *ATLA* **37**(Suppl. 2), 7–12.
5. Dawson, M. (1976). The application of tissue culture to drug and toxicity testing. *ATLA Abstracts* **4**(2), 1–16.
6. Rowan, A.N. & Stratman, C.J. (1979). *The Use of Alternatives in Drug Research*, 190pp. London, UK: Macmillan
7. Balls, M. (2012). FRAME and the pharmaceutical industry. *ATLA* **40**, 295–300.
8. Balls, M. (2009). FRAME, animal experimentation and the Three Rs: Past, present and future. *ATLA* **37**(Suppl. 2), 1–6.
9. Annett, B. (1995). The Fund for the Replacement of Animals in Medical Experiments (FRAME): The first 25 years. *ATLA* **23**, 19–32.
10. Balls, M. & Clothier, R.H. (2009). FRAME and the validation process. *ATLA* **37**, 631–640.
11. Spielmann, H. (2009). Collaboration between ZEBET, FRAME and ECVAM: FRAME's contribution to establishing the Three Rs in Europe. *ATLA* **37**(Suppl. 2), 23–27.
12. Balls, M. (1995). On keeping your eyes on the prize: Dorothy Hegarty and acceptance of the concept of replacement of laboratory animal procedures in research, education and testing. *ATLA* **23**, 756–774.
13. Balls, M. (2009). Animal experimentation and the Three Rs: Past, present and future. *ATLA* **37**(Suppl. 2), 1–121.
14. House of Lords. (2002). *Select Committee on Animals in Scientific Procedures*, 82pp. Report volume I, HL paper 150-I. London, UK: The Stationery Office.
15. Home Office. (2004). *The Use of Animals in Scientific Procedures: Government Plans to Establish a National Centre for Research Into Reduction, Refinement and Replacement (the Three Rs) of Animal Use and Animal Welfare*. Press Release, 21 May 2004, 2pp. London, UK: Home Office
16. Adler, S., Basketter, D., Creton, S., *et al.* (2010). Alternative (non-animal) methods for cosmetics testing: Current status and future prospects-2010. *Archives of Toxicology* **85**, 367–485.
17. Combes, R.D. & Balls, M. (2014). The Three Rs — Opportunities for improving animal welfare and the quality of scientific research. *ATLA* **42**, 245–259.
18. Anon. (2015). *Our Vision 2015–2025*, 31pp. National Centre for the Three Rs. Available at https://www.nc3rs.org.uk.
19. Balls, M. & Combes, R.D. (2004). The UK National Centre for the Three Rs: Pathway to progress or mere fig leaf. *ATLA* **32**, 61–64.
20. Bailey, J., Thew, M. & Balls, M. (2015). Predicting human drug toxicity and safety via animal tests: Can *any* one species predict toxicity in any other, and do monkeys help? *ATLA* **43**, 393–403.
21. Fentem, J., Chamberlain, M. & Sangster, B. (2004). The feasibility of replacing animal testing for assessing consumer safety: A suggested future direction. *ATLA* **32**, 617–623.
22. Carmichael, P., Davies, M., Dent, M., *et al.* (2009). Non-animal approaches for consumer safety risk assessments: Unilever's scientific research programme. *ATLA* **37**, 595–610.

Chapter 2.2

Contributions From the German-Speaking Countries

Horst Spielmann[1], Franz P. Gruber[2,3] and Walter Pfaller[4]

[1]*Freie Universität Berlin, Berlin, Germany;* [2]*Doerenkamp-Zbinden Foundation and ALTEX Edition, Kuesnacht ZH, Switzerland;* [3]*ALTEX Editorial Office, ALTEX Edition, Kuesnacht, Switzerland;* [4]*Medical University of Innsbruck, Innsbruck, Austria*

SUMMARY

The Three Rs concept was welcomed in Austria, Germany and Switzerland, after the EEC had accepted *Directive 86/609/EEC on the protection of animals used for experimental and other scientific purposes*. However, it was implemented quite differently in each of the three countries. In 1985, Switzerland took the lead, because of generous funding by the Doerenkamp-Zbinden Foundation, by focusing on replacing the LD50 test, and in 2002, by establishing five chairs on alternatives in Germany, India, Switzerland, The Netherlands and the USA. In 1989, Germany established ZEBET at the Federal Health Institute (BGA) in Berlin, as the first national centre for alternatives, which significantly contributed to the international acceptance of the first *in vitro* OECD Test Guideline for local toxicity testing, for phototoxicity. Since 1992, the Austrian government has supported annual international Three Rs congresses in Linz, which are now organised by EUSAAT, the European Society for Alternatives to Animal Testing.

1. INTRODUCTION

The Three Rs concept, put forward in 1959 by William Russell and Rex Burch, was not greatly appreciated outside the UK for about 25 years. This changed in 1986, when the European Economic Communities adopted *Directive 86/609/EEC* (1) on the protection of animals used for experimental and other scientific purposes.

Previously, however, concern about toxicity tests in animals had been growing, and a highly critical review by Gerhard Zbinden and Marilena Flury-Roversi on the classical LD50 test, published in 1981 (2), had a great impact. They said that the LD50 value was affected by many factors and should no longer be accepted as a constant.

Zbinden was an internationally well-regarded toxicologist, and head of the Institute of Toxicology, located in Schwerzenbach near Zurich. In a 1982 radio interview, he stressed his opinion that tests on dogs should now be seen as obsolete. This encouraged a philanthropist, Hildegard Doerenkamp, and together they set up the Doerenkamp-Zbinden Foundation (DZF) in Chur, Switzerland, in 1985, to support the development of Three Rs approaches.

Later in the 1980s, the German Federal Government established the German Centre for Alternative Methods (ZEBET), at the Federal Health Institute (BGA) in Berlin. In the early 1990s, an Austrian platform for the development of animal-free *in vitro* methods for the toxicity testing of chemicals and pharmaceuticals emerged, the Zentrum für Ersatz- und Ergänzungsmethoden zu Tierversuchen (Zet).

In collaboration with the DZF, ZEBET and others, and with the support of the Austrian Federal Government, Zet organised a series of successful annual conferences in Linz, Austria. Meanwhile, the Swiss Fonds für versuchstierfreie Forschung (FFVFF, founded in 1976 and now known as AnimalFree Research) launched a journal, *Alternatives to Animal Experimentation* (*ALTEX*). Initially, the Linz meetings and ALTEX primarily used the German language, but there was a progressive change to English. In 2013, the European Society of Alternatives to Animal Testing (EUSAAT) took over organising the Linz conferences, and *ALTEX* is now closely associated with CAAT USA and CAAT Europe.

The History of Alternative Test Methods in Toxicology. https://doi.org/10.1016/B978-0-12-813697-3.00005-6

2. CONTRIBUTIONS FROM SWITZERLAND

In 1986, a second DZF was founded, to support research aimed at reducing the suffering of test animals. In 1993, after Gerhard Zbinden passed away, the two DZF foundations were combined, and the financial resources of the new foundation were significantly increased.

In 2002, the idea of a chair for alternative methods to animal testing was published (3), and in 2005, the first Doerenkamp-Zbinden Chair of In-vitro Toxicology and Biomedicine was established at the University of Konstanz, Germany, in cooperation with the Foundation for Science and Research of the Kanton of Thurgau, Switzerland. Up to 2009, four more chairs were established: the Doerenkamp-Zbinden Endowed Chair in Evidence-based Toxicology at Johns Hopkins University in Baltimore, MD (USA); the endowed Doerenkamp-Zbinden Chair, Alternatives to animal testing in toxicological risk assessment, at the University of Utrecht, The Netherlands; the Doerenkamp-Naef-Zbinden Chair for Alternative Methods at the University of Geneva, Switzerland, in cooperation with the Egon Naef Foundation; and at the Mahatma Gandhi-Doerenkamp Centre (MGDC) for Alternatives to Use of Animals in Life Science Education, at Bharathidasan University in Tiruchirapalli, Tamil Nadu, India.

Up to now, the DZF has supported projects to replace animal experimentation in the field of toxicology with around 30 million Swiss francs. Many of the projects supported have focused on replacing animals in neurotoxicology, beginning with Arie Bruinink's and Paul Honegger's work in the early 1990s, followed by Angelo Vedani and his tools for examining virtual test kits with computer-aided designs, and Barbara Rothen-Rutishauser in investigating the toxicity of nanoparticles *in vitro*. The highlights of the Foundation's work have been, of course, the DZ Chairs in Konstanz and Baltimore. Meanwhile, these two institutions have taken the lead in the field of *in vitro* toxicology, and have delivered outstanding, internationally-recognised results.

2.1 The Foundation Research 3R

On the initiative of the FFVFF, and with pressure from the public, the Swiss Government recognised the need for supporting research on alternatives to animal testing. As a result, the Foundation Research 3R was established in 1987, as a joint venture of the Parliamentary Group on Issues of Animal Experimentation, the Interpharma industry association and the FFVFF. The activities of the foundation were supervised by the Federal Home Office, and 146 projects, including about 20 toxicology projects, were funded from 1987 to 2015. During this period, more than 23 million Swiss francs of funding were provided on equal terms by the Swiss industry and the Swiss Government. A milestone in this process was a project in neurotoxicology, initiated by Gerhard Zbinden in 1988, which culminated in a project on nerve cell-mimicking liposomes as *in vitro* alternative to potency-testing of toxins with multistep pathways, such as *Botulinum* neurotoxins, by Oliver Weingart at the ETH Zurich. A list of INFO-Bulletins on all projects is provided on the website of the foundation (http://www.forschung3r.ch/de/publications/index.html).

In 2017, the Administrative Board of the Foundation Research 3R announced an end to its funding programme, and the two sponsors of the 3R Research Foundation, the Federal Food Safety and Veterinary Office and Interpharma, are now planning to establish a Swiss Three Rs Competence Centre.

2.2 The Swiss Institute for Alternatives to Animal Testing

Another player in the field of alternatives to animal experimentation in toxicology was the Swiss Institute for Alternatives to Animal Testing (SIAT), founded in 1990. It consisted of two groups. The first group, of Christoph Reinhardt, in Zürich, worked on *in vitro* teratology, *in vitro* neurotoxicology and cytotoxicity. The second group, chaired by Angelo Vedani, in Basel, worked on computer-assisted molecular modelling and receptor mapping, to predict the toxic potential of molecules even before they had synthesised, e.g. by applying the famous programmes, YAK and Yeti. The Zürich group ended its activity in 1995.

In 1997, Angelo Vedani's Basel group established a new foundation, the Biographics Laboratory 3R, to focus entirely on computational technologies to reduce and replace animal tests in the biomedical sciences. Its research is primarily concerned with the *in silico* prediction of the adverse/toxic effects of drugs and chemicals, which induce the most severe suffering of test animals. After Angelo Vedani's death in 2016, Peter Zbinden continued his work as president of the Biographics Laboratory 3R.

2.3 The Fondation Egon Naef Pour la Recherche *In Vitro*

Since 1998, the Fondation Egon Naef pour la recherché *in vitro* (FENRIV) has awarded a prize each year, to honour scientists in the French-speaking part of Switzerland and also from abroad. With funding from the Ligue Suisse contre la vivisection, FENRIV established a chair for alternative methods at the University of Geneva, in cooperation with the DZF.

2.4 Swiss Governmental Agency Support for the Three Rs Concept

It is important that, since the early 1980s, Swiss governmental agencies have supported activities to implement the Three Rs concept. Public institutions such as the Swiss Federal Institute of Aquatic Science and Technology (EAWAG) and the Swiss Federal Laboratories for Materials Science and Technology (EMPA) have not only shown a strong interest in alternatives to animal testing, but have also developed alternative methods in the fields of ecotoxicology and nano-toxicology. The scientists in these institutions have been networking with CAAT Europe at the University of Konstanz, which is financially supported by the Swiss DZF.

3. CONTRIBUTIONS FROM GERMANY

3.1 Zentralstelle zur Erfassung und Bewertung von Ersatz- und Ergaenzungsmethoden zum Tierversuch (ZEBET)

In 1989, Horst Spielmann, as the first head of ZEBET, defined the following mission for the German centre for alternatives:

- to establish a database and information service on alternatives at national and international levels;
- to develop alternatives according to the Three Rs principles of Russell and Burch;
- to fund research on alternatives;
- to coordinate validation studies;
- to cooperate with national and international funding agencies and validation centres; and
- to provide a forum for information on alternatives to animal testing.

Because the regulatory safety testing of cosmetics in animals, e.g. in the Draize eye and skin irritation tests, were heavily criticised by animal welfare organisations and consumers around the world, ZEBET collaborated with other organisations in focusing on reducing and replacing animal testing for local toxicity to the eyes and skin.

3.2 Reducing Animal Numbers in Regulatory Toxicity Testing

In the EU, the toxicity testing of chemicals, including cosmetic ingredients and finished products, had to comply with *Directive 67/548/EEC* (4) on the classification, packaging and labelling of dangerous substances, which involved animal tests, e.g. for skin and eye irritation and skin sensitisation.

The international harmonisation of toxicity tests by the OECD, in 1982 (5), was the first effective measure to reduce the unnecessary duplication of testing in animals for regulatory purposes, with result that tests conducted according to OECD test guidelines (TGs) are now accepted by the regulatory agencies of all major industrial countries.

To be acceptable as replacements for the accepted animal toxicity test, non-animal tests must provide at least the same level of safety as the established animal tests, and must be a basis for for classification and labelling. It has been agreed that alternative toxicity tests can be accepted for regulatory purposes only after they have been shown to be relevant and reliable in validation studies. At a meeting held in Berlin in 1989, some members of the European Research Group for Alternatives to Toxicity Testing (ERGATT), met with John Frazier of CAAT, and agreed to organise a workshop on validation. The CAAT/ERGATT workshop was held in Amden, Switzerland, in 1990, where an agreement was reached on a definition of experimental validation and on the essential steps in the process. An ECVAM workshop in 1995 recommended improvements to the process, and the importance of a prevalidation stage and of biostatistical prediction models came to be recognised. In 1996, the OECD accepted the progress that had been made, and agreed that validation should be regarded as necessary for new *in vitro* or *in vivo* tests (6).

In addition to its validation activities, ZEBET has critically analysed confidential data used for regulatory purposes, e.g. on the use of the dog as non-rodent test species in the safety testing of crop and plant protection products (7). As a result, the OECD has discouraged the use of dogs for the safety testing of plant protection products.

3.3 The Regulatory Acceptance of *In Vitro* Toxicity Tests Successfully Validated at ZEBET

The improved validation concept was immediately implemented in ongoing validation studies, such as the ECVAM/COLIPA validation study on *in vitro* phototoxicity tests. Because no standard guideline for the testing of photoirritation potential existed in 1991, ECVAM and COLIPA established a joint programme to develop and validate *in vitro* photo-irritation tests (PTs). In two formal validation studies, funded by ECVAM and coordinated by ZEBET, the *in vitro* 3T3 NRU PT, which involves the use of the mouse 3T3 fibroblast cell line and neutral red uptake (NRU) as the endpoint for cytotoxicity, was the only *in vitro* test in which all the test chemicals were correctly identified as positives or negatives (8). At the request of the Scientific Committee on Cosmetology, an ECVAM catch-up validation study managed by ZEBET was performed, which showed that the 3T3 NRU PT could reliably be used to identify phototoxic UN filter chemicals (9). Therefore, in 1998, the EU accepted the 3T3 NRU PT for regulatory purposes, and in 2004, the OECD accepted it as TG 432 at the world-wide level, as the first *in vitro* toxicity test in the OECD TG programme for the testing of chemicals (5). Meanwhile, the 3T3 NRU PT was accepted as the first *in vitro* toxicity test outside the OECD, in Brazil and China.

On the initiative of ECVAM and ZEBET in 2004, three additional *in vitro* toxicity tests were accepted by the OECD, namely, two experimentally-validated *in vitro* corrosivity tests, the rat skin TER test (TG 430) and the reconstructed human epidermis (RhE) test (TG 431), and one without experimental validation, an *in vitro* method for skin absorption (TG 428), with human or animal skin. Thus, by 2004, four *in vitro* toxicity tests have been accepted by the OECD (5). A major contributor to this success was Manfred Liebsch, from ZEBET, who provided his expertise during a sabbatical at the OECD in Paris in 2004.

From 2003 to 2007, ECVAM sponsored a formal validation study, coordinated by ZEBET, to replace the Draize skin irritation test with two RhE models, the EpiDerm and EPISKIN RhE models. Because of the success of this validation study, in 2010, the OECD accepted the In vitro Skin Irritation: RhE test method (TG 439), in which cytotoxicity is used as the endpoint (5).

From 2000 to 2004, ZEBET coordinated an ECVAM validation study of *in vitro* embryotoxicity tests, in which the mouse embryonic stem cell test (mEST), originally developed by ZEBET, was successfully validated (10), and was later improved by implementing reporter genes.

After Manfred Liebsch and Horst Spielmann, who had contributed to more than 20 OECD TGs and Guidance Documents, retired, ZEBET discontinued its validation activities and changed its name to German Centre for the Protection of Laboratory Animals (Bf3R).

3.4 The Funding of Research on *In Vitro* Toxicity Testing in Germany

Since 1981, the German Federal Ministry of Education and Research (BMBF) has continuously funded research on replacing the use of experimental animals, in a programme entitled Alternativen zum Tierversuch, with more than 160 million euros in support of about 500 projects. Most of the projects were joint projects with partners from industry, academia and regulatory agencies, including ZEBET. About 30% of them were devoted to reducing animal use in toxicity testing, including validation studies on the use of biostatistical methods for reducing animal numbers in toxicity testing and on implementing innovative molecular endpoints (11). Companies from the German drug, cosmetics and chemical industries have also actively participated in the BMBF research programme, and have contributed financially to it.

In 1986, the SET Foundation for the promotion of alternate and complementary methods to reduce animal experiments was initiated by the Federal Ministry of Food, Agriculture and Forestry (BMEL). The SET Foundation brought together the main stakeholders from animal welfare and industry, with the common goal of reducing or avoiding animal experiments, with initial funding of 1 million deutschmarks. The Foundation supports a wide range of scientific projects devoted to the Three Rs, with a focus on replacement and complementary methods, and on international cooperation, via, for example, the publication of *ALTEX* and the funding of national and international Three Rs workshops and congresses (12).

Since 1990, ZEBET, which is now part of the German Centre for the Protection of Laboratory Animals (Bf3R), has funded research in the area of the Three Rs for scientists in Germany, with an annual budget of 400.000€ and a focus on regulatory safety testing, including toxicology (13). An average of 10 projects have been funded each year, with a mean duration of three years. Many of these projects have achieved international recognition.

3.5 ZEBET's Wider Activities

ZEBET has made many substantial contributions outside Germany, the EU and Western Europe, notably, by promoting the Three Rs concept in Eastern Europe and in Asia, and, via the Alternatives Congress Trust, in the organisation of the World Congresses on Alternatives and Animal Use in the Life Sciences, the fifth of which was held in Berlin in 2005.

4. CONTRIBUTIONS FROM AUSTRIA

The importance of the Zet (Zentrum zum Ersatz von Tierversuchen = Austrian Centre for Replacing Animal Experiments) conferences at Linz, initially organised in collaboration with the DZF (Switzerland) and ZEBET (Germany), but now by EUSAAT, has already been mentioned.

Most of the activities of Zet, under the chairmanship of Walter Pfaller from 2000 to 2010, were directed toward the replacement of animal experiments by cell culture-based *in vitro* models. This research was conducted at the Division of Physiology of the Department of Physiology and Medical Physics of the Medical University of Innsbruck and by the Zet group in Linz. The research groups in Innsbruck were headed by Walter Pfaller, Gerhard Gstraunthaler and Paul Jennings, and the group in Linz was headed by Klaus Rudolf Schröder.

The Innsbruck groups actively participated in many key projects of the European Commission, dedicated to the development of alternatives to animal experiments (the BRIDGE programme, the SMT-programme, the Biotech II-programme, the Marie Curie Research Training Network — Pulmonet project, FP-6 Predictomics, FP-6 Carcinogenomics, FP-7 Predict-IV, FP-7 Detective, IMI-StemBANCC and horizon 2020-EUToxRisk). Walter Pfaller was also member of the ECVAM Scientific Advisory Committee, and is on the board of CAAT Europe in Konstanz, Germany.

Two important projects of the Austrian Three Rs platform have achieved international recognition: first, the establishment of Good Cell Culture Practice, a concept based on a series of presentations at the Linz congresses, which culminated in the establishment of a special Task Force on this topic at ECVAM, and second, the establishment of data repository on existing and purchasable serum-free cell culture media. This activity was initiated and completed by Zet, in collaboration with the groups in Innsbruck (14).

The contributions of Austria, and specifically of Innsbruck, to the development of alternatives, included the development of organotypic cultures for the epithelial cell systems of not only the kidney, but also the lung and liver, with the aim of identifying the mechanisms underlying chemically-induced and nanoparticle-induced cell injury. A number of strategies have been pursued and optimised, including the use of a defined medium with physiological glucose, the optimisation of medium volumes, the use of roller cultures and perfusion culture (15), the use of human platelet lysates as a serum replacement (16), and co-cultures with microvascular endothelial cells (17) and microporous supports.

The main cell culture models used in the Innsbruck laboratory are LLC-PK1 cells and MDCK cells. A number of other cell strains have been developed, including a gluconeogenic clone of LLC-PK1 cells and various wild type and mutant uromodulin-expressing LLC-PK1 cells (18). More-recently, the laboratory has focused on cells of human origin, and in particular, on RPTEC/TERT1 cells, which were immortalised from primary cells by overexpressing the catalytic unit of telomerase. The RPTEC/TERT1 cells are extremely stable and thus have been very useful for repeated-dose toxicity studies (19) and to demonstrate the importance of integrating kinetic data with transcriptomics, metabolomics and proteomics in acute and repeated-dose studies (20). The Innsbruck laboratories are now focusing on the use of human induced pluripotent stem cells for renal toxicological applications and as parts of integrated testing systems (21, 22).

5. CONCLUSIONS

The German-speaking countries have played a major role in implementing the Three Rs concept into regulatory toxicity testing both in Europe and internationally. Because of differences in the ethical, cultural and political perception of animal welfare issues, the contributions of the individual countries were quite different, but in the end they were all effective. The Swiss Doerenkamp-Zbinden Foundation established several chairs for alternatives at excellent international universities, the Federal German government established ZEBET as the first government, funded Three Rs and validation centre to reduce safety testing in animals, and the Austrian government has for more than 25 years provided an international platform for Three Rs research by funding the SET/EUSAAT congresses for alternatives to testing in animals in Linz.

REFERENCES

1. EEC. (1986). Directive 86/609/EEC on protection of animals used for experimental and other scientific purposes. *Official Journal of the European Communities* **L358**, 1−28.
2. Zbinden, G. & Flury-Roversi, M. (1981). Significance of the LD50 test for the toxicological evaluation of chemical substances. *Archives of Toxicology* **47**, 77−99.
3. Wendel, A. (2002). Do we need a "Chair of Alternatives Methods", and where? *ALTEX* **19**, 63−68.
4. EEC. (1983). Directive 83/467EEC adapting to technical progress for the fifth time Council Directive 67/548/EEC on the approximation of the laws, regulations and administrative provisions relating to the classification, packaging and labelling of dangerous substances. *Official Journal of the European Communities* **L275**, 1−33.
5. OECD. (2018). *OECD Guidelines for the Testing of Chemicals, Section 4, Health Effects.* Paris, France: OECD.
6. OECD. (2009). *Final report of the OECD workshop on "Harmonization of validation and acceptance criteria for alternative toxicological test methods" (Solna Report).* ENV/MC/CHEM/TG(96)9, 53pp. Paris, France: OECD.
7. Box, R.J. & Spielmann, H. (2005). Use of the dog as non-rodent test species in the safety testing schedule associated with the registration of crop and plant protection products (pesticides): present status. *Archives of Toxicology* **79**, 615−626.

8. Spielmann, H., Balls, M., Dupuis, J., *et al.* (1998). The international EU/COLIPA *In vitro* phototoxicity validation study: results of phase II (blind trial), part 1: the 3T3 NRU phototoxicity test. *Toxicology in Vitro* **12**, 305–327.

9. Spielmann, H., Balls, M., Dupuis, J., *et al.* (1998). A study on UV filter chemicals from Annex VII of European Union Directive 76/768/EEC, in the *in vitro* 3T3 NRU phototoxicity test. *ATLA* **26**, 679–708.

10. Seiler, A. & Spielmann, H. (2011). The validated embryonic stem cell test to predict embryotoxicity *in vitro*. *Nature Protocols* **6**, 961–978.

11. BMBF. (2018). *Alternativen zum Tierversuch*, 2pp. Berlin, Germany: Federal Ministry for Education and Research. Bundesministerium für Bildung und Forschung

12. SET. (2018). *Alternative Research Needs Support*, 1p. Frankfurt, Germany: SET. Available at http://www.stiftung-set.de/en/research-funding/overview

13. Anon. (2018). *Bf3R Funding in the Area of 3R − Replacement, Refinement and Reduction*, 1p. Berlin, Germany: Bundesinstitut für Risikobewertung (BfR)

14. Brunner, D., Frank, J., Appl, H., *et al.* (2010). Serum-free cell culture: the serum-free media interactive online database. *ALTEX* **27**, 3–62.

15. Felder, E., Jennings, P., Seppi, T., *et al.* (2002). LLC-PK(1) cells maintained in a new perfusion cell culture system exhibit an improved oxidative metabolism. *Cellular Physiology and Biochemistry* **12**, 153–162.

16. Rauch, C., Feifel, E., Amann, E.-M., *et al.* (2011). Alternatives to the use of fetal bovine serum: human platelet lysates as a serum substitute in cell culture media. *ALTEX* **28**, 305–316.

17. Aydin, S., Signorelli, S., Lechleitner, T., *et al.* (2008). Influence of microvascular endothelial cells on transcriptional regulation of proximal tubular epithelial cells. *American Journal of Physiology − Cell Physiology* **294**, 543–554.

18. Curthoys, N.P. & Gstraunthaler, G. (2014). pH-responsive, gluconeogenic renal epithelial LLC-PK1-FBPase+cells: a versatile in vitro model to study renal proximal tubule metabolism and function. *American Journal of Physiology − Renal Physiology* **307**, 1–11.

19. Aschauer, L., Gruber, L.N., Pfaller, W., *et al.* (2013). Delineation of the key aspects in the regulation of epithelial monolayer formation. *Molecular and Cellular Biology* **33**, 2535–2550.

20. Wilmes, A., Aschauer, L., Limonciel, A., *et al.* (2014). Evidence for a role of claudin 2 as a proximal tubular stress responsive paracellular water channel. *Toxicology and Applied Pharmacology* **279**, 163–172.

21. Rauch, C., Jennings, P. & Wilmes, A. (2014). Use of induced pluripotent stem cells in drug toxicity screening, pp.335–350. In A. Bal-Price, & P. Jennings (Eds.), *In Vitro Toxicology Systems*. New York, NY, USA: Springer.

22. Jennings, P. (2015). The future of *in vitro* toxicology. *Toxicology in Vitro* **29**, 1217–1221.

Chapter 2.3

Contributions to Alternatives From Italy and Spain

Isabella De Angelis[1], Emanuela Testai[1], Pilar Prieto[2] and Guillermo Repetto[3]
[1]Istituto Superiore di Sanitá, Rome, Italy; [2]Joint Research Centre, European Commission, Ispra, Italy; [3]Universidad Pablo de Olavide, Sevilla, Spain

SUMMARY

In Italy, a Coordination Group for *In Vitro* Toxicology was set up in 1984, to spread the Three Rs culture and improve *in vitro* models to be used in toxicity testing. In 1991, the group was formalised as the Italian Association for *In Vitro* Toxicology, named CELLTOX. It is still active in the organisation of meetings, and theoretical and practical courses, and in the publication of leaflets and books. The Italian Platform for Alternative Methods (IPAM) is another non-profit association dealing with alternatives in Italy, in which the four different parties involved in animal experimentation (academia, governmental institutions, industry and animal welfare organisations) are equally represented and cooperate to support the Three Rs philosophy. From 1980, Spanish research groups had shown increasing interest in the use of *in vitro* methods, and from 1992 to 2000, very intense activities were carried out to also include regulatory issues. In 1999, the Spanish Network for the Development of Alternative Methods (REMA) was created. It is a platform to connect the government administration, industry and the organisations interested in the reduction and the more-rational use of laboratory animals, by promoting the development, acceptance and application of alternative methods. REMA has become a recognised consultant for the Spanish Government in terms of the implementation of legal regulations on animal use and alternatives.

1. ACTIVITIES IN ITALY RELATED TO ALTERNATIVE METHODS

From the early 1980s, some academic and industrial researchers in Italy started to consider and discuss the application of the Three Rs principle and the use of animal-free methods in their studies (1, 2). In 1981, a review was published as a result of a screening of 51 scientific journals, covering the years 1976—79 (1): Only about 300 papers, involving the use of cell cultures as an experimental model, were found.

This picture did not improve very rapidly because, at that time, Italian attitudes toward the use of alternative methods were rather critical, although the use of animal models in such scientific disciplines as toxicology and pharmacology was the subject of a heated debate.

In 1984, the first coordination group for *in vitro* toxicology was created by researchers from universities and public research institutes, such as the Istituto Superiore di Sanità in Rome and the National Research Council (CNR). Annalaura Stammati and Flavia Zucco were the driving force of the group, whose aim was to spread the Three Rs culture among students and young researchers, and to develop and validate innovative *in vitro* models to be used in toxicity testing for evaluation of the safety of chemicals. The group organised several meetings in various Italian cities and established the basis for the first Italian network for alternative methods.

1.1 The Italian Association for *In Vitro* Toxicology

In 1991, the Group was formalised as the Italian association for *in vitro* toxicology, named CELLTOX, which is still active at the present time. Over the intervening 25 years, CELLTOX has carried out promotional and educational activities on the use of *in vitro* experimental models in toxicological research, in close collaboration with similar European societies. Indeed, CELLTOX was one of the first national societies to be affiliated to the European Society for Toxicology *In Vitro* (ESTIV). In particular, CELLTOX has been active in promoting alternative methodologies to investigate mechanisms of toxicity at the cellular and molecular levels, with special interest in cell culture models. Over the years, the association has favoured the dissemination of alternative methods by publishing leaflets and books (3) and organising scientific events and theoretical and practical training courses for young researchers on the use of *in vitro* methods in toxicology and pharmacology at national and international levels, such as the 1-week training course on *Cell Culture Models for In Vitro Toxicology*, organised in Brescia in 1997 by CELLTOX with the European Collection of Authenticated Cell Cultures (ECACC) and the Fondazione Iniziative Zooprofilattiche e Zootecniche. The contributions of the course teachers were then collected in a book (4) and were also published in a special issue in *Cell Biology and Toxicology* (5). One of the results of organising these events was to create a network beyond the Italian borders. Activity at the European level also resulted in the publication of a report prepared for the European Commission on the behalf of ESTIV (6).

The most recent courses were organised at the University of Milano Bicocca (2013) and at the University of Genoa (2016), during which the advantages of moving forward to animal-free testing, the emerging technologies and the future challenges in *in vitro* toxicology and in quantitative *in vitro in vivo* extrapolation (*QIVIVE*) were presented and discussed.

Another major CELLTOX activity has been the award of fellowships and reimbursement for the participation of young graduates in courses and conferences related to the association aims (7). Among the many scientific events organised by CELLTOX were three international Joint Meetings on *In Vitro Cytotoxicity Mechanisms* (1999, 2001, 2006), organised with the Italian Association for Cell Culture (AICC), the last of which was shared with the European Tissue Culture Society (ETCS), which were particularly relevant in terms of the scientific level of the speakers' contributions and the number of participants (7, 8). The CELLTOX-ESTIV satellite symposium, *From Tissue Engineering to Alternatives: Research, Discovery and Development*, which took place during the *7th World Congress on Alternatives and Animal use in the Life Sciences* (Rome, 2009), was particularly memorable. A congress, CELLTOX 1991-2011 Twenty Years of In Vitro Toxicology: Achievements and Future Challenges (9, 10), celebrated the 20 years of CELLTOX activities at the Istituto Superiore di Sanità in Rome, where there is an excellent tradition of research with alternative methods.

1.2 The Italian National Platform for Alternative Methods

Another player in Italy in the field of alternatives to animal experimentation is represented by the Italian National Platform for Alternative Methods (IPAM), a not-for-profit organisation founded in 2003 by 14 individuals, which, according to the founding principles of National Platforms, established during the *3rd World Congress on Alternatives and Animal Use in the Life Sciences* (Bologna, 1999), concerned four different parties, involved in various ways in animal experimentation, i.e. academia, government institutions, industries and animal welfare organisations. At present, IPAM manages participants and contributions from these four parties, based on *consensus*, i.e. the full agreement in opinions among all parties. IPAM's main goals are (1) to look, through a peaceful, responsible and informed dialogue, to overcome the conflicts and ideological barriers to get to a successful (and honest) discussion on animal testing; (2) to promote scientific information exchange and cooperation among the four parties; (3) to work toward a greater awareness by public opinion, government and investigators to promote acceptance and use of the available alternative methods within the scientific community; and (4) to disseminate as much as possible the Three Rs culture, particularly among young people, by promoting education and training initiatives on the scientific progress of alternative methods. One of the most important IPAM activities is the Farmindustria Award, which every other year is assigned to a young researcher making use of alternative methods in his or her studies.

In 2006, IPAM issued a training DVD, *Cell Cultures in Toxicology: Principles, Basic Technologies and Application*, aimed to introduce the topic of alternatives to animal testing to students from different disciplines, which was complemented by a text available in an interactive environment. The DVD was presented during specific events in various universities in Italy. Some special courses were also organised; the most recent of which, *Alternative Methods: Application to Dermatology*, was held in Rome in 2017, in collaboration with the Italian Dermatological Institute.

Recently, IPAM has arranged a didactic exhibition project, *Science and Awareness: A Journey inside the 3Rs*, and to which about 40 panels (more than 40 experts from different institutions have contributed to the project) ran through theoretical and practical aspects of the evolution of research methods based on Three Rs principles, in various biomedical research areas. The exhibition is intended to be a virtual journey to get to know the scientific value of the Three Rs. It came into being from the idea of tracing a path through time to show the gradual replacement of animals in testing, going on to predict a future in which a more-highly advanced science will no longer have any reason to use animals. It was designed and set up as an itinerant exhibition and has already been on display in a number of Italian universities and research institutes.

1.3 The Italian National Reference Centre

In 2011, as required by *European Directive 2010/63 on the Protection of Animals used for Scientific Purposes*, the Italian Ministry of Health established a National Reference Centre for Alternative Methods, Welfare and Care of Laboratory Animals. The Centre is located at the Istituto Zooprofilattico sperimentale della Lombardia e dell'Emilia Romagna, and it provides technical and scientific support for the Ministry of Health in the implementation of alternative methods and represents the Italian national contact point with the European Union.

Italian researchers involved in using alternative methods to animal testing have been often partners in EU-funded projects, e.g. AcuteTox, PredictIV on *in vitro* methods and many others related to *in silico* methodologies. They have a long tradition of collaboration with EURL ECVAM (via membership of the ESAC or ECVAM workshops or *ad hoc* working groups), and two Italian representatives are involved in the EURL ECVAM's PARERE (Preliminary Assessment of Regulatory Relevance) network, which provides advice on alternative methods according to regulatory needs. Over the years, Italian researchers have also contributed to the development of OECD guidelines related to the Three Rs and to their application, by organising specific information days for stakeholders and end-users at the Istituto Superiore di Sanità.

Other events are run by regional organisations or in some universities, but not in a systematic way. For example, the veterinary faculty of the University of Milan offered a practical course on *in vitro* toxicology, entitled *Toxicology an In Vitro Model*, to provide to the students with the basic knowledge of *in vitro* testing, coupled with information about innovative methodologies and applicability domains. At the same university, the attitude of veterinary science students toward the use of non-animal methods as tool for teaching has been investigated through the submission of a questionnaire. Although no complete agreement among the student responses was revealed, the majority of them supported the co-existence of traditional training methods with alternative approaches (11).

1.4 The Three Rs Declaration of Bologna

Not only was the 3rd World Congress in Bologna in 1999 one of the most enjoyable and most successful of the world congresses, on 31 August 1999, in the Aula Magna of the University of Bologna, Europe's oldest university, the participants accepted, unanimously and with acclamation, the Three Rs Declaration of Bologna, which says (12):

> *The participants in the 3rd World Congress on Alternatives and Animal Use in the Life Sciences strongly endorse and reaffirm the principles put forward by Russell and Burch in 1959. Humane science is a prerequisite to good science, and is best achieved in relation to laboratory animal procedures by the vigorous promotion and application of the Three Rs. The Three Rs should serve as a unifying concept, a challenge and an opportunity for reaping benefits of every kind — scientific, economic and humanitarian.*

The first participant to sign the Declaration was William Russell.

2. ACTIVITIES IN SPAIN RELATED TO *IN VITRO* PHARMACOTOXICOLOGY

During the 1980s, various research groups in Spain were showing increasing interest in the use of *in vitro* methods, particularly in pharmacology and toxicology. The main focus was on the development of cellular models to assess basal cytotoxicity, target-organ toxicity and drug metabolism in humans and in animals.

By the early 1990s, attention was being paid to regulatory aspects, and two meetings on the validation of alternative methods were organised in Valencia in 1992 and in 1994, by Maria Jose Gomez-Lechon and José Vicente Castell. A little later, Eduardo de la Peña and Guillermo Repetto encouraged the involvement of the pharmaceutical industry, by organising two workshops in Madrid in 1997, with Smithkline Beecham Pharmaceuticals and with Glaxo Wellcome.

2.1 The ICLAS/CSIC Working Group on Complementary Methods

In 1994, the International Council for Laboratory Animal Science (ICLAS), a non-governmental organisation for international cooperation in laboratory animal science, and the Spanish Research Council (CSIC) created a working group to promote complementary and alternative methods to reduce, refine and replace the use of laboratory animals.

An ICLAS/CSDIC Workshop on Complementary Methods was held in Toledo, Spain, in 1995 under the chairmanship of Eduardo de la Peña (13). The main focus was on the harmonisation of approaches to the development and validation of alternative methods. Several issues related to validation were discussed, including criteria, approaches and problems associated with previous studies. Several recommendations were also made, concerning the role ICLAS could take in fostering the development and implementation of alternatives.

2.2 The Spanish Working Group on Alternative Methods

A proposal was made in 1992 to the Board of the Spanish Society of Toxicology (AET), to create a Spanish working group on alternative methods (GTEMA). GTEMA was formally established in 1995, as a follow-up to the ICLAS/CSIC Workshop. Since then, the group's coordinator, Guillermo Repetto, has attended several meetings, among them the one organised by ECVAM in 1997, for representatives of European national centres for alternative methods. From 1995 to 2007, GTEMA issued three to four newsletters per year, which were distributed to all members of the AET.

2.3 The 3ERRES Mailing List on Alternatives

The mailing list was created in 1996, as a communication channel for researchers and as a forum to discuss and disseminate information in Spanish on the reduction, refinement or replacement of the use of animals for teaching and testing and for biomedical and environmental research. Today, experts from about 14 countries participate in the debates. Since 2000, there has been an electronic version of the list (RedIRIS).

2.4 Spanish Scientific Productivity Related to *In Vivo* and *In Vitro* Alternative Methods

To evaluate Spanish scientific productivity related to *in vivo* and *in vitro* experimental procedures, the numbers of relevant scientific publications were identified by searching the bibliographic database, Medline, from 1966 to 1998 (14, 15).

A relevant increase in Spanish scientific productivity was observed, reaching 2.13% of the worldwide publications. The increase on experimental studies was proportionally more important for the publications involving alternative methods (32%).

The species most used *in vivo* were rat, mouse and human. *In vitro* researchers preferred humans to rats and mice as the source of materials for their studies. The numbers of studies were parallel *in vivo* and *in vitro*, mainly involving the areas of physiology, genetics, pharmacology, biochemistry, toxicology, surgery and pathology.

2.5 The Inventory of the Spanish Institutions and Scientists Involved in Alternatives to the Use of Laboratory Animals

Thanks to a contract with ECVAM, the use of alternative methods to laboratory animals among Spanish researchers was reviewed in 1998, which included the number of scientific articles, the grants approved and the number of laboratory animals used (16).

Although Spanish scientific production in experimental approaches was only 2.13% of the overall international production, a substantial number of Spanish groups interested in alternatives were identified (98), of which 75% were very competitive, with a total of more than 340 scientists involved.

The total Spanish investment in R&D should be increased, and research tasks included in the National Programme of Health should be revised. In Spain, there is no fixed amount of investment for alternative methods. The total amount of private investment is low in comparison with other countries.

In relation to the type of institution, universities were the most active in the number of groups (46%), followed by governmental research facilities, including CSIC (15%), industry (13%) and hospitals and governmental service facilities (7%).

The main purpose of the work was basic research (29%), followed by non-regulated applied research (19%), development of methods (16%), regulatory testing (1%), alternatives in education and training (11%) and method validation (9%). In relation to the type of testing, the results were balanced, with screening tests (35%), complementary or adjunct tests (34%) and replacement tests (31%).

With regard to the main area of application, toxicology was clearly the most frequent (25%), followed by biochemistry (9%), molecular biology (9%), cell biology (9%), monitoring (7%), biology (6%), pharmacology (6%), pathology (6%) and nutrition (3%). Many types of test materials were evaluated, including pharmaceuticals (14%), pesticides (11%), environmental pollutants (11%), diverse chemical compounds (10%), wastes (9%), cosmetics (7%), toxins (4%), medical devices (4%), food additives (4%), hormones (4%), colourings (4%) and vaccines (2%).

The model systems most often employed were *in vitro* techniques (44%), followed by animals (28%), models in education and training (8%), embryos (6%) and plants and human volunteers (both 4%). With respect to the animals, 63% of the groups employed conventional animals, whereas 22% used invertebrates and 15% used transgenic animals. *In vitro* methods largely employed cell lines (34%), followed by primary cultures (25%), micro-organisms (19%) and cell-free systems (13%).

A wide variety of bioindicators were used with the *in vitro* models, including cell viability (19%), cell proliferation (14%), metabolic activity (14%), nucleic acids (9%), cytoskeleton enzyme release studies (8%), biotransformation systems (8%), morphology (7%), organ-specific endpoints (6%), defence systems (5%) and cell signalling (5%).

2.6 The Spanish Network for the Development of Alternative Methods

The Spanish Network for the Development of Alternative Methods (REMA) was created in 1999 as a way to bring together all the Spanish groups actively working on or interested in alternative methods (17, 18). The official foundation of REMA took place in the course of a scientific event at the Ministry of Health in Madrid. It came forward as a platform that helps to establish connections with the government, industries and groups, entities and societies interested in the reduction and more-rational use of laboratory animals and in promoting the development of alternative methods.

REMA was coordinated by Argelia Castaño from 1999 to 2011, and since then, by Guillermo Repetto. As an independent organisation, REMA has focused its activities on the Three Rs in research, testing and teaching in Spain. It provides information and encourages greater awareness of the use of alternative methods among the different interested parties. It organises courses, workshops and other activities related to the field of alternative methods and also seeks to maximise coordination, to avoid unnecessary repetition and undesirable overlapping of dates or topics.

REMA uses the well-established 3ERRES mailing list as the channel for communication. It also promotes alternatives through social networks in Facebook and Twitter.

REMA was among the first national platforms to become involved in ecopa, and two of its members have held the vice-presidency and the presidency of ecopa.

REMA has been involved in several relevant initiatives at both the national and international levels (e.g. the EU projects such as CONAM and ForInvitox). It has become a recognised consultancy for the Spanish Government in terms of the implementation of legal regulations on animal use (e.g. *Directive 2010/63/EU on the protection of animals used for scientific purposes*). In this regard, REMA collaborates with the Spanish Ministry of Agriculture, Fishery, Food and Environment (MAPAMA), which is the National Contact Point for the PARERE Network (Preliminary Assessment on Regulatory Relevance) in the context of *Directive 2010/63/EU*.

When asked by MAPAMA, REMA coordinates the replies of the PARERE consultations launched by EURL ECVAM on specific documents (e.g. draft EURL ECVAM Recommendations, selected test method submissions and draft EURL ECVAM strategy papers).

REMA has promoted publications on alternative methods (19) and continues to evolve, to be in touch with the progress and needs in the area of national and international alternative/new approaches to animal testing.

In conclusion, a number of Spanish researchers have successfully implemented the use of *in vitro* methods in basic and applied research. Many of their activities are related to alternatives, and those coordinated by members of REMA are particularly important. Nevertheless, there is a need to support the development and use of alternative approaches, via, for example, specifically targeted public funding. Furthermore, the creation of a centre dedicated to the Three Rs would also contribute significantly to the efficient and effective implementation of alternative approaches in Spain.

REFERENCES

1. Stammati, A.P., Silano, V. & Zucco, F. (1981). Toxicology investigations with cell culture systems. *Toxicology* **20**, 91–153.
2. Zucco, F., De Angelis, I., Testai, E. & Stammati, A. (2004). Toxicology investigations with cell culture systems: 20 years after. *Toxicology in Vitro* **17**, 153–163.
3. Zucco, F. & Bianchi, V. (Eds.). (1994). *Colture Cellulari in Tossicologia*, 276pp. Rome, Italy: Lombardo Editore.
4. Stacey, G.N., Doyle, A. & Ferro, M. (Eds.). (2001). *Cell Culture Methods for In Vitro Toxicology*, 153pp. Dordrecht, The Netherlands: Kluwer Academic Publishers.
5. Various authors. (2001). *Cell Biology and Toxicology* **17**, 4–5.
6. Zucco, F. & Vignoli, A.L. (1998). *In vitro* toxicology in Europe, 1986–1997. *Toxicology in Vitro* **12**, 745–928.
7. Testai, E., Stammati, A. & Blaauboer, B.J. (2002). Second International Celltox-AICC Joint Meeting 'In vitro Models and Toxicity mechanisms'. *Toxicology in Vitro* **16**, 329–330.
8. De Angelis, I., Arancia, G., Gómez-Lechón, M.J., Dal Negro, G. & Blaauboer, B.J. (Eds.). (2007). *In Vitro Cytotoxicity Mechanisms. Proceedings of the 46th ETCS International Meeting and the 3rd International Joint Meeting AICC and CELLTOX, Toxicology in Vitro* **21**, 175–334.
9. De Angelis, I., Gemma, S. & Caloni, F. (2010). CELLTOX: The Italian Association for *In Vitro* Toxicology. *ALTEX* **27**, 59–60. WC7 Proceedings.
10. Sambuy, Y., Caloni, F., Meloni, M., *et al.* (2012). CELLTOX 1991–2011: Twenty years of *in vitro* toxicology: achievements and future challenges. *ALTEX* **29**, 98–101.

11. Sachana, M., Theodoridis, A., Cortinovis, C., *et al.* (2014). Student perspectives on the use of alternative methods for teaching in veterinary faculties. *ATLA* **42**, 223–233.

12. Anon. (2000). The three Rs declaration of Bologna. *ATLA* **28**, 1–5.

13. de la Peña, E., Guadaño, A., Barrueco, C., Repetto, G., Gonzalez Menció, F. & Garcia Partida, P. (Eds.). (1995). *ICLAS/CSIC Working Group on Complementary Methods,* 101pp. *Comité Español del ICLAS/CICYT/CSIC, Dirección General de Investigación Científica y Técnica, Madrid.*

14. Repetto, G., del Peso, A. & Repetto, M. (1998). La Productividad científica española en relación con métodos experimentales alternativos in vivo e in vitro. *Revista de Toxicología* **15**, 101–104.

15. Repetto, G., Álvarez Herrera, C. & del Peso, A. (2014). Estrategias de identificación de planteamientos alternativos a la experimentación animal. *Revista de Toxicología* **31**, 108–114.

16. Repetto, G., del Peso, A., Salguero, M., *et al.* (1999). Inventory of the Spanish Institutions and Scientists involved in alternatives to the use of Laboratory Animals (Refinement, Reduction or Replacement). *Revista de Toxicología* **16**, 50–127.

17. de la Peña, E., Castell, J.V., Gargallo, D., *et al.* (1998). Documento de Trabajo sobre la Constitución de la Red Española para el Desarrollo de Métodos Alternativos (REMA). *Revista de Toxicología* **15**, 133–142.

18. de la Peña de Torres, E. (2014). *Actividades de promoción y difusión de alternativas en España Revista de Toxicología* **31**, 115–120.

19. Repetto, G. (2014). Monográfico sobre Planteamientos Alternativos a la Experimentación Animal. *Revista de Toxicología* **31**(2).

Chapter 2.4

Contributions to Alternatives From The Netherlands, Belgium and France

Bas J. Blaauboer[1], Vera Rogiers[2] and André Guillouzo[3]

[1]Utrecht University, Utrecht, The Netherlands; [2]Vrije Universiteit Brussel, Brussels, Belgium; [3]Rennes 1 University, Rennes, France

SUMMARY

In The Netherlands, important contributions to the development of alternative methods have been made by TNO, the RIVM and the universities of Leiden, Utrecht, Wageningen, Groningen, Maastricht and Amsterdam. The Dutch Platform for Alternatives was founded in 1987, and the National Centre for Alternatives was created in 1994. In 2014, national activities were taken over by the National Committee on Alternatives.

In Belgium, the Vrije Universiteit Brussel and the Université Catholique de Louvain were instrumental in establishing national activities aimed at the development and promotion of alternative methods across the Three Rs. Many of these activities were championed by HRH Prince Laurent. The Belgian Platform for Alternative Methods was established in 1999, and the Innovation Centre 3Rs in 2017.

In France, academic researchers have made significant contributions to the development of cell culture techniques, and skin and liver cell models in particular, while French cosmetic companies, especially L'Oréal, have played a major role in the development and validation of alternatives for the evaluation of cosmetic ingredients and finished products. The French Society of Cellular Pharmaco-Toxicology has played a central role in organising meetings, while the French platform, Francopa, was established in 2007.

In the mid-1980s, a number of European scientists, including individuals from The Netherlands, Belgium and France, created ERGATT (the European Research Group for Alternatives in Toxicity Testing), which made a number of important recommendations with regard to the validation and regulatory acceptance of alternative methods. In 1999, the national centres from Belgium, The Netherlands and Germany announced the creation of pan-European Consensus Platform (ecopa), which was subsequently joined by other European countries, leading to knowledge sharing activities and joint research projects.

1. DEVELOPMENT OF ALTERNATIVES TO TOXICITY TESTING IN THE NETHERLANDS

1.1 Early Years

The history of *in vitro* toxicology is naturally related to the developments in the field of cellular biology (1). Thus, when cell culture systems became available, toxicologists started to use these methods to study the toxic effects of chemicals. In The Netherlands, Jacob Hooisma and co-workers, working at the Netherlands Organisation for Applied Scientific Research (TNO), were among the first researchers to use cell lines in neurotoxicity studies, e.g. with compounds such as acrylamide in the mid-1970s (2). Together with Flavia Zucco and Edith Heilbronn, Hooisma was also very instrumental in organising a workshop on the application of tissue culture in toxicology, held in The Netherlands in 1980 (3–5). A series of workshops called INVITOX emerged from this initiative, and these have since evolved into the Congresses of the European Society of Toxicology *In Vitro* (ESTIV). Proceedings of these workshops and congresses are published, the most recent being in 2017 (6).

At the same time, in another branch of TNO, Herman Koëter and Menk Prinsen developed alternatives for the much criticised Draize eye irritation test on rabbits (7). Later, *in vitro* systems for skin absorption were developed by Han van de Sandt (8).

One of the earliest areas of toxicology in which *in vitro* methods were used was genotoxicity. In The Netherlands, this was mainly promoted by the work of Frits Sobels and co-workers at Leiden University. Interestingly, Sobels used the phrase "parallelogram approach", promoting the possibility of predicting the effects of compounds in man, by making use of *in vitro* systems from animals and man, and comparing the results with *in vivo* animal data (9).

In vitro skin toxicity systems were an initiative of Maja Ponec at Leiden University (10). This work was later extended by Susan Gibbs at the Vrije Universiteit Amsterdam (11). Other academic centres starting *in vitro* toxicology initiatives were at Utrecht, Wageningen and Groningen. At Utrecht University, the group chaired by Herman van Genderen mainly focused on improving understanding of the effects of environmental pollutants (e.g. pesticides). Joep van den Bercken and colleagues were leading the research on the mechanisms of neurotoxicity of compounds such as DDT and pyrethroids in a number of *in vitro* systems, e.g. isolated nerves (12). Bas Blaauboer and co-workers started to work on avian and mammalian red blood cells (13), later developing methods on hepatocyte cultures from rodents (14), domestic animals (15) and humans (16, 17). Another activity of this group was on keratinocytes, including studies on the effects of dioxins (18, 19).

At Wageningen University, the first *in vitro* systems were developed by Gerrit Alink and Ivonne Rietjens, who studied the effects of ozone in isolated lung cells (20). Geny Groothuis and colleagues at Groningen University worked on isolated liver cells and on precision-cut organ slices (21, 22).

Another interesting area was the work of Paul Peters and Aldert Piersma at the National Institute for Public Health and the Environment (RIVM), who developed a number of *in vitro* systems for studying developmental toxicity and embryotoxicity (23). At the same institute, Coenraad Hendriksen and colleagues were leaders in the development of alternatives in the field of vaccine development and efficacy and safety testing (24; see also Chapter 3.7).

1.2 Recent Technological Developments

More-recent developments in *in vitro* toxicology are manifold. One of these is the introduction of toxicogenomics (i.e. the application of 'omics' in toxicology) by the group of Jos Kleinjans at Maastricht University (25). Another is the application of culture systems derived from stem cells, e.g. in developmental toxicology (26), as well as the application of imaging techniques by Fred Nagelkerke and Bob van de Water at Leiden University (27).

1.3 Organisational Frameworks

1.3.1 National Initiatives

In the 1980s, the Dutch Society of Toxicology (NVT) created a speciality section on *in vitro* toxicology. This group organised annual meetings and cooperated with NVT in organising events in the wider framework of the discipline. The group discontinued specific activities after the mid-1990s, by which time one could perhaps state that *in vitro* methodologies had become mainstream toxicology, so there was no need for a speciality section.

Another initiative was the formation of the Platform for Alternatives (PAD). This organisation was founded in 1987 by the governmental ministry responsible for the law on animal experimentation and was the platform for discussion between government, academia, industry and animal welfare organisations. This was the first such platform in Europe; subsequently similar platforms were also founded in other countries, which now cooperate with *ecopa*.

In 1994, the National Centre for Alternatives (NCA), sponsored by PAD, was created, which served as the National Knowledge Centre for Alternatives. NCA was located at Utrecht University, and Jan van der Valk played an important role in this. Until 1998, PAD also had a (modest) budget to support research initiatives in the area of alternatives, and a number of the projects that were granted were in the area of toxicology. After 1998, the support of alternatives projects was taken over by the governmental organisation, ZonMW. By introducing the latest version of the EU directive on animal experimentation (*Directive 2010/63/EU*) that was implemented in Dutch law in December 2014, the knowledge centre activities were taken over by the National Committee on Alternatives (NCAD).

1.3.2 International Initiatives

As mentioned earlier, a groundbreaking first workshop on application of tissue culture in toxicology, held in Soesterberg in 1980, brought together a group of researchers who were very eager to cooperate in an international framework. One initiative resulting from this was the series of World Congresses on Alternatives, the first being held in Baltimore in 1993 and the second chaired by Bert van Zutphen in Utrecht in 1996. Another spin-off was the start, in the mid-1980s, of a group named European Research Group on Alternatives in Toxicity Testing (ERGATT), with one member from each of a number of European countries. The Dutch members were Herman Koëter and, at a later stage, Bas Blaauboer. One activity of this group was the creation of a data bank of alternative toxicity testing methods, INVITTOX (28; see also Chapter 4.2); another was the organisation of a series of workshops. The workshops with a major impact were the ones on the issue of validation of alternative methods (29, 30), the results of which eventually served as the starting point for the formation of ECVAM; see also Chapter 2.10).

Also noteworthy is an ERGATT workshop held in 1991 in Sweden, at which the first systematic research project on an integrated testing strategy was worked out (31, 32), which finally resulted in a research project sponsored by ECVAM. The integrated use of different types of information (33–36) is now the main trend in toxicity testing and assessment worldwide (see also Chapter 5.4). The main characteristics of these strategies are the combination of different pieces of information, typically including chemical-specific information on the compound(s) under study, their effects in selected *in vitro* systems and the use of biokinetic parameters to allow a quantitative *in vitro–in vivo* extrapolation (QIVIVE; 37).

Yet another Dutch initiative, together with Belgian colleagues, was the creation of the Dutch-Belgian Society for *In Vitro* Methods (INVITROM). Although not exclusively focusing on toxicology, many toxicology-related issues are being dealt with. INVITROM organises one or two meetings annually and is successful in attracting members from outside the two countries, so it is "International" rather than "Dutch-Belgian".

Also in the field of international research cooperation, a considerable number of activities took place with Dutch participation, especially in the EU Framework programmes. One example is the Predict-IV project, which focused on the use of *in vitro* methods to predict repeated-dose toxicity, one of the most challenging issues involved in aiming to replace regulatory animal testing (38, 39). In this project, considerable attention was given to the importance of biokinetic considerations not only in QIVIVE but also with regard to the biokinetic behaviour of compounds in *in vitro* systems (40).

1.4 Implementation of Alternatives

Already in 1984, Robert Kroes and Victor Feron, in a paper describing the by then state-of-the-art in regulatory toxicology and risk assessment procedures, stated that *Although at present a trend toward more extensive "protocol toxicology" can be noticed, this kind of toxicology will be replaced in the next decade by 'receptor toxicology'. A stepwise approach will become more and more accepted in toxicity testing. It can be anticipated that a decision tree approach based on systematic and sequential progression of investigation will become a recommended tool in the safety evaluation of chemicals. Deficiencies which may be associated with certain steps should be identified and investigated in order to resolve the problems which may arise* (41).

This optimistic — and to a certain extent Orwellian — prediction is still not completely fulfilled. However, the many significant initiatives taken, supported by vast technological developments, make it possible to take steps in this direction. Interesting first initiatives were taken under the auspices of ECVAM, e.g. by describing Integrated Testing Strategies (42), nowadays called Integrated Approaches to Testing and Assessment (IATA; see also Chapter 5.4). Other examples of strategies have been published by Bas Blaauboer in close cooperation with national and international colleagues (43–45). Further examples of such strategies, as first postulated in the ERGATT initiative described above (31), can be found in the work of Ivonne Rietjens at Wageningen University, e.g. the prediction of developmental toxicity of glycol ethers by Jochem Louisse (46).

These studies again make it clear that biokinetic considerations are of utmost importance (47). The more-recent work of Ans Punt in Wageningen (48, 49) strongly emphasises this. Groundbreaking was the work of Nynke Kramer and colleagues at Utrecht University on the biokinetic behaviour of chemicals in *in vitro* systems (40, 50, 51).

At the beginning of the 21st century, the Assuring Safety without Animal Testing (ASAT) initiative was started at Unilever Research in the UK by Unilever's Dutch Vice-President of Safety and Environmental Assurance, Bart Sangster, and his UK colleagues, Carl Westmoreland and Julia Fentem (52). The central principle in this initiative is that the safety assessment of chemicals should focus on identifying human health risks, to collect or generate knowledge on human biology related to health risks and to develop and use new *in silico* and *in vitro* methodologies to quantify these risks. Not only is this initiative now the leading principle at Unilever Research, but, after Sangster retired, he also succeeded in inspiring the Dutch government and the Dutch animal protection organisation, Proefdiervrij, to fund activities in this area (53, 54).

However, this vast development of *in vitro* toxicology does not automatically result in the acceptance of these strategies in regulatory procedures. Such implementation needs a good strategy of communication and perseverance, as shown by the work of Marie-Jeanne Schiffelers (55, 56).

1.5 Conclusions

In previous decades, many research and development activities in the area of *in vitro* toxicology were started in The Netherlands, and most of the work can be considered as pioneering and instrumental in the development of the area as a whole. Moreover, it could be stated that nearly all academic and other research activities in the field of toxicology research in The Netherlands are basically done *in vitro*. However, these endeavours should be seen within the international framework. Not all activities could succeed in isolation and need to be conducted in the European and wider international context.

2. DEVELOPMENT OF ALTERNATIVES TO TOXICITY TESTING IN BELGIUM

2.1 Early Years

One of the first initiatives in Belgium in the context of the development and promotion of alternative methods was the creation, under the auspices of HRH Prince Laurent of Belgium, of the *Group for the Reflection on the Quality of Life and the Environment*. This was realised in close collaboration with two professors at the Vrije Universiteit Brussel (VUB), Vera Rogiers, and the Université Catholique de Louvain (UCL), Marcel Roberfroid. The group organised an international symposium focusing on alternative methods in pharmaco-toxicological research, which was held in January 1991 (57).

As a further follow-up, the Minister of State, Philippe Busquin, who was responsible for Human Health and Social Affairs, started a working group chaired by honorary senator, Roland Gillet. The first success was a Royal Decree to ban the use of the acute systemic toxicity test in pharmaceutical dossiers submitted for national regulatory approval in Belgium. In addition, a platform was initiated with the aim of validating and promoting alternative methods, under the auspices of Prince Laurent. A prestigious symposium was organised in 1993 as a collaboration between the Department of Toxicology at VUB and DGXII of the European Commission. The focus was on the use of human cells for *in vitro* testing, and this resulted in a number of scientific publications (58–60).

Prince Laurent received the E.E. Noel Award for his efforts in contributing to the building up of a strong Europe. He was also invited to officially open the new building for ECVAM at the European Commission's Joint Research Centre, Varese, Italy, which was led by Michael Balls (see also Chapter 2.10).

In the mid-1980s, as mentioned earlier, a number of European individuals created ERGATT, and Prince Laurent was asked in 1997 to become its president. Meanwhile, the idea of creating a Belgian Platform for Alternative Methods (BPAM) was taking shape, and BPAM became a reality in February 1999, when the Prince accepted its presidency (61). This scientific Three Rs consensus platform involved four parties representing animal welfare and protection, legislation and regulation persons, industry and academia. The scientific activities of the platform were managed by Vera Rogiers and Sonja Beken. A newsletter was initiated, along with a comprehensive booklet entitled *Belgisch Platform voor Alternatieve Methoden. Ontwikkeling en strategie van alternatieve methoden voor Dierproeven in Belgie* (Belgian Platform for Alternative Methods. Development and strategy of alternative methods to animal experiments in Belgium). In addition, a brochure gave information on the actual status of alternatives in an EU context. Several research projects were supported. To commemorate this event, a book, *Alternative Methods to Animal Experiments - Actual status, development and approach in Belgium*, was compiled by Rogiers and Beken (62), to provide background information and to initiate discussions on the use of alternative methods. BPAM became an integral part of the Prince Laurent Foundation and was very active in organising meetings and raising more awareness of the importance of incorporating modern *in vitro* technology in research, regulatory testing and education.

During the *Third World Congress on Alternatives and Animal Use in the Life Sciences*, which took place in 1999 in Bologna, Italy, BPAM, SET (Stiftung zur Förderung der Erforschung von Ersatz- und Ergänzungsmethoden zur Einschränkung von TierversuchenStiftung) from Germany and NCA/ZON (Netherlands Centre Alternatives to Animal Use/Zorg Onderzoek Nederland) from The Netherlands officially announced the creation of the European not-for-profit organisation, namely, the pan-European Consensus Platform (*ecopa*).

The structure of *ecopa* consisted of a cooperating group of the EU national platforms that met the criterion of representation of all four main parties (academia, animal welfare, government and industry (63)). For 10 years, *ecopa* was chaired by Vera Rogiers, in close collaboration with José Castell (Co-chair) of the University of Valencia, Spain, and Bernward Garthoff (Secretary) of Bayer/Crop Protection, Germany. Two symposia per year were organized, and several European research projects were actively supported. All over Europe, national organisations based on the same four-party principle were created (e.g. Norcopa in Norway, Swecopa in Sweden, Hucopa in Hungary, and Polcopa in Poland) under the Belgian umbrella of *ecopa* (64–68). The *Ecopa* Science Initiative (e-SI) was initiated in November 2003 in Brussels. It was aimed at bringing together young scientists with senior researchers in a pleasant surrounding (e.g. Pueblo Acantilado in

Spain), to discuss new technology and its potential applicability for *in vitro* research and testing. The idea was to mix different scientific disciplines to let scientists think "about" and "for" alternatives. The e-SI workshops provided not only a state-of-the-art review but also discussions on future perspectives and the applications of innovative technologies that could be of importance for the field of *in vitro* research and alternative methods.

2.2 More-recent Three Rs Developments in Belgium

Over the years, many initiatives were taken by Belgian scientists in the field of alternative methods, often in a European or an international context. In particular, several Three Rs projects in the European Framework Programmes 5, 6 and 7 brought scientists together.

Besides the scientific activity in international scientific associations and societies involved in the Three Rs, researchers within VITO (Vlaams Instituut voor Technologisch Onderzoek) initiated an animal-free research programme, and in 2007, CARDAM (the Centre for Advanced R&D on Alternative Methods) was launched to meet the needs of industry and legislation in the field of alternative toxicology. It was a start-up company financed by VITO, in anticipation of the enormous testing needs under the new EU chemicals legislation, REACH.

In 2008, INVITROM (International Society for In Vitro methods) was started, which is a Dutch-Belgian Society organising annual symposia with a focus on the research of young scientists.

As in other European countries, *Directive 2010/63/EU* on the protection of experimental animals was implemented in the national legislation of Belgium, as a Royal Decree of 29 May 2013. With the Sixth State Reform, on 1 July 2014, a delegation of powers to the regional level took place, including animal welfare, so three regions are actually responsible for the implementation of the Three Rs. Initiatives have been taken by the three regions. In Flanders, a Minister, Ben Weyts, initiated a call for setting up a database on the available alternative methods and those under development in Flemish laboratories in research centres, universities and industries. This project, Re-Place, was just started under the auspices of WIV (Wetenschappelijk Instituut Volksgezondheid named now Sciensano) with Birgit Mertens, and VUB, with Vera Rogiers. In the Brussels-Capital Region, Bianca Debaets has followed this initiative and made finances available for a register of all alternatives available in Brussels. This work is also guided by VUB-WIV (Sciensano). As the same promoters are involved, the idea is to group all information from Flanders and Brussels and to add information from the third region, Wallonia, where a Minister, Carlo Di Antonio, organised Walcopa, a workshop on alternative methods, together with the Reflection Group of the University of Namen.

Parallel to these developments, the Innovation Centre 3Rs (IC-3Rs) was launched on 25 September 2017 at the Brussels Health Campus, VUB, located in Jette, chaired by Vera Rogiers (now professor emeritus). The plan to work at the regional level is important, as there are big gaps in communication and information on Three Rs alternatives, as highlighted in a recent EURL ECVAM study (69). IC-3Rs aims to bring Belgian scientists working with or interested in Three Rs methodology together, to work for a better visibility, communication and promotion of Three Rs alternatives and to use the platform as a means of showing relevant cutting-edge humane research and having an increased impact on education. For the academic year 2017—18, Maurice Whelan (current head of EURL ECVAM) and Vera Rogiers received the Francqui Chair in Belgium for the VUB and University of Antwerp, respectively. They both gave a series of lectures on the development and active use of alternative methods in toxicology and basic and applied research.

3. DEVELOPMENT OF ALTERNATIVES TO TOXICITY TESTING IN FRANCE

3.1 Early Years

The first French studies using cell cultures for toxicity studies were published in the 1960s and mainly used cell lines to study the toxicity of X-rays and antimitotic chemicals. These studies were limited in number and were mainly published in the French language up to the mid-1970s.

In the early years, several French groups became very active in the analysis of DNA damage induced by radiation, chemicals and metals, by using bacteria and yeast, and later, mammalian cells. Philippe Quillardet and Maurice Hofnung (Pasteur Institute, Paris) developed the SOS chromotest (70), while Raymond Devoret and his group (CNRS, Gif sur Yvette) showed that it was possible to detect potential carcinogens by prophage lambda induction (Inductest), and they described the role of the SOS signal in DNA repair (71), by using *Escherichia coli* (72). Ethel Moustacchi (Curie Institute, Paris) made major contributions on mutagenesis and DNA repair in yeast (73). Other groups were involved in the development and improvement of cell transformation tests for the detection of carcinogens, by using the sensitive Syrian hamster embryo cells, as well as other cell systems (74–76).

Before *Directive 86/609/EEC* on the protection of animals used for experimental and other scientific purposes was adopted, and even though no national centre for alternatives was established, an increasing number of French research groups started working on cell cultures from various tissues of animal and human origin and became increasingly interested in the use of *in vitro* cell models for cellular toxicity testing. They actively participated in the major progress made in the cultivation of various cell types, which included the development of new techniques for tissue disaggregation to isolate single viable cells and the definition of better conditions for the culture of cells retaining at least some of the specific functions of their tissues of origin.

Special efforts were aimed at the evaluation of cosmetics and hepatotoxic compounds. From an early stage, both academic groups and cosmetics companies were very active in developing original skin culture models and using them to test cosmetic ingredients. In particular, a new method for *in vitro* epidermalisation was established by Bernard Coulomb and Louis Dubertret in Paris. This consisted of inserting a punch biopsy as a source of epidermal cells into a dermal equivalent freshly made up by mixing fibroblasts in a collagen matrix (77). Several methods for the culture of keratinocytes on various dermal substrates at the air—liquid surface were also developed, e.g. the use of dead de-epidermised dermis by Michel Pruniéras and co-workers (78) and a human type IV collagen film covering a type I+III collagen layer developed by the Thivolet group in Lyon (79). This intensive research rapidly led to the development of commercially available reconstructed epidermis kits, and in particular, Episkin, a 3-D reconstructed epidermis with a functional stratum corneum, first distributed by Imedex and mass-produced as SkinEthic epithelial cell models, corresponding to reconstructed human tissues with specific properties, distributed by SkinEthic. The Episkin model and the SkinEthic company are now owned by L'Oréal. Many other French small companies are currently involved in the development, use and distribution of skin models for the evaluation of cosmetic ingredients and finished products.

Several multi-centre studies were conducted to compare and/or validate alternative methods to the Draize eye irritation test. An early study was financially supported by OPAL (Oeuvre pour l'Assistance aux Animaux de Laboratoire); it involved six laboratories and 40 test items. The data showed that even if interlaboratory agreement was relatively good, correlation with the Draize test markedly differed between the three alternative methods used (Griffith's test, the HET-CAM test and SIRC fibroblasts), supporting the need for improved cell models and assays (80).

The other major tissue of interest in the early development of alternative methods was the liver, as this plays a major role in xenobiotic metabolism and is a primary target for toxic compounds and their metabolites. Several groups started working with suspensions and primary cultures of rodent hepatocytes in the 1970s. The difficulty of maintaining *in vitro* the phenotype of adult hepatocytes under unsophisticated culture conditions (81), and the discrepancies between the results obtained in different laboratories, resulted in limitations in the definition of validated protocols. A multi-centre evaluation of acute *in vitro* drug cytotoxicity methods was financially supported by the French Ministry of Research, involving six French academic and pharmaceutical laboratories. This study, which used rat primary hepatocytes and hepatoma cells, highlighted a number of critical points that could lead to the poor prediction of *in vivo* effects or the misinterpretation of data (82). In the early 1980s, Christiane Guguen-Guillouzo (INSERM, Rennes) successfully developed an enzymatic method for the isolation of adult human hepatocytes (83) and invented the co-culture concept for hepatocytes that allowed the lifespan of hepatocytes to be increased from a few days to at least 2 months (84). Several French research groups have contributed to the improvement of culture conditions for human and animal hepatocytes and/or have used them for hepatotoxicity testing (85, 86). In 1998, Guguen-Guillouzo and her group also established the human HepaRG cell line, which exhibits functional properties close to those of mature hepatocytes (87). This cell line is now widely used for drug metabolism and hepatotoxicity studies (88), with more than 90 papers being published in 2017 (according to a Pubmed search).

Biopredic (Rennes), founded in 1987, was among the first companies to distribute fresh and cryopreserved human hepatocytes; it also distributes HepaRG cells.

In addition to skin and liver cell models, *in vitro* models from various other tissues were also developed in the 1980s (89–92), including human isolated glomeruli and mesangial cell cultures (93), polarised thyroid cells forming follicles in a collagen gel (94) and a blood—brain barrier model, developed by culturing brain capillary endothelial cells on one side of a filter and astrocytes on the other (95).

3.2 Recent Technological Developments

During recent years, considerable progress in the development and improvement of various *in vitro* cell models as well as their use in toxicity testing has been made by French laboratories. Many of their contributions are summarised in a recent book (96). Cell models from various tissues, including 3-D models with one or several cell types, cultures of differentiated cell types from stem cells, and cell cultures prepared by bioprinting, have been developed for diverse purposes, e.g. the pulmonary toxicity of nanoparticles, the evaluation of cosmetics with skin models, the evaluation of pollutants for reprotoxicity, and the screening of potential immunotoxic compounds. Modern 'omics' and cell imaging technologies are used by many of the laboratories involved in *in vitro* toxicity testing.

3.3 Organisational Frameworks

During the early years of the cell culture, Monique Adolphe played a crucial role in the dissemination of *in vitro* techniques and their use for toxicity testing in France. For many years (up to 1997), she organised annual courses with lectures and technical practice. Together with André Guillouzo and Benigne Chevalier, she created the French Society of Cellular Pharmaco-Toxicology (SPTC) that held its first meeting in 1987 in Paris. This 2-day meeting gathered more than 550 participants, indicating a strong interest in *in vitro* alternative methods in France. Since its first meeting, the SPTC has organised every year a 1-day or 2-day meeting dedicated to *in vitro* models and their use in toxicity testing; the 2016 meeting was organised jointly with ESTIV. Many proceedings of the early meetings were published in special issues of *Cell Biology and Toxicology*.

Other initiatives have led to the creation of the French Society of Genetic Toxicology (SFTG) in 1983 and the Association for Research in Toxicology, which is mostly focused on the toxicity of environmental contaminants, in 1989. Both these societies organise annual meetings, which include many presentations related to alternatives.

The Alfred Kastler prize was launched in 1984 for research development and applications of alternative methods to animal experimentation. Between 1985 and 2016, the prize has been awarded 11 times.

A platform named Francopa, headed in 2018 by Francelyne Marano, was founded in 2007 as a member of the *ecopa* network, with the aim of supporting the development, validation and dissemination of alternative methods. However, no budget has been allocated yet to projects on alternatives.

French scientists have also been involved in various European initiatives on alternatives, including membership of ERGATT and as the organisers of scientific meetings (e.g. INVITTOX in 1990, Seillac, and ETCS in 1993, Rennes).

3.4 Implementation of Alternatives

The Episkin model was validated for skin irritation by ECVAM in 2007 (97), and an OECD guideline (TG 439) was adopted. More recently, the commercially available reconstructed Human Corneal Epithelial model (SkinEthic HCE model) was evaluated for its ability to predict eye irritancy (98) and was subsequently validated by EURL ECVAM. In October 2017, the method was adopted as OECD TG 492, for the identification of chemicals (both substances and mixtures) not requiring classification and labelling for eye irritation or serious eye damage.

Even though no validated protocol has been adopted by the OECD for drug metabolism and hepatotoxicity investigations, some regulatory agencies (e.g. the FDA and the EMA) have published guidance or recommendations for the use of fresh and frozen human hepatocytes in preclinical drug metabolism studies. EURL ECVAM has recently coordinated a multi-study validation trial for cytochrome P450 (CYP) induction by using differentiated cryopreserved HepaRG cells and cryopreserved human hepatocytes. Notably, the AstraZeneca company has recently reported that it is routinely using HepaRG cells for evaluating the CYP3A4 induction potential of new drugs (99).

3.5 Conclusions

French academic laboratories and cosmetic companies, especially L'Oréal, have played a major role in the development and validation of alternatives for the evaluation of cosmetic ingredients and finished products. French academic researchers have also contributed to the development of human liver cell models (e.g. the first method for culturing primary human hepatocytes and the establishment of the HepaRG cell line) for investigating the metabolism and toxicity of drugs and other compounds. French teams are also leaders in the use of various other *in vitro* cell models for toxicity studies. All these alternative approaches for toxicity testing and other purposes have greatly contributed to reduction of animal use for experimentation.

REFERENCES

1. Blaauboer, B.J. (2015). The long and winding road of progress in the use of *in vitro* data for risk assessment purposes: from "carnation test" to integrated testing strategies. *Toxicology* **332**, 4—7.
2. Hooisma, J., de Groot, D.M.G., Magchielse, T., *et al.* (1980). Sensitivity of several cell systems to acrylamide. *Toxicology* **17**, 161—167.

3. Zucco, F. (1980). Introduction to the workshop on the application of tissue culture in toxicology. *Toxicology* **17**, 101–104.

4. Heilbronn, E. (1980). Summing up the international workshop on the application of tissue culture in toxicology. *Toxicology* **17**, 269–272.

5. Nardone, R.M. (1980). The interface of toxicology and tissue culture and reflections on the carnation test. *Toxicology* **17**, 105–111.

6. Jennings, P., Corvi, R. & Culot, M. (2017). A snapshot on the progress of *in vitro* toxicology for safety assessment. *Toxicology in Vitro* **45**, 269–271.

7. Prinsen, M.K. & Koëter, H.B.W.M. (1993). Justification of the enucleated eye test with eyes of slaughterhouse animals as an alternative to the Draize eye irritation test with rabbits. *Food and Chemical Toxicology* **31**, 69–76.

8. van de Sandt, J.J.M., Rutten, A.A.J.J.L. & Koëter, H.B.W.M. (1993). Cutaneous toxicity testing in organ culture: Neutral red uptake and reduction of tetrazolium salt (MTT). *Toxicology in Vitro* **7**, 81–86.

9. Sobels, F.H. (1989). Models and assumptions underlying genetic risk assessment. *Mutation Research: Fundamental and Molecular Mechanisms of Mutagenesis* **212**, 77–89.

10. Ponec, M. & Polano, M.K. (1979). Penetration of various corticosteroids through epidermis in vitro. *Archives of Dermatological Research* **265**, 101–104.

11. Gibbs, S., Backendorf, C. & Ponec, M. (1996). Regulation of keratinocyte proliferation and differentiation by all-trans-retinoic acid, 9-cis-retinoic acid and 1,25-dihydroxy vitamin D3. *Archives of Dermatological Research* **288**, 729–738.

12. Van Den Bercken, J. & Narahashi, T. (1974). Effects of aldrin-transdiol — A metabolite of the insecticide dieldrin — On nerve membrane. *European Journal of Pharmacology* **27**, 255–258.

13. Blaauboer, B.J., van Holsteijn, C.W.M. & Wit, J.G. (1979). Biochemical processes involved in ferrihemoglobin formation by monohydroxyaniline derivatives in erythrocytes of birds and mammals. *Comparative Biochemistry and Physiology – C* **62**, 199–203.

14. Wortelboer, H.M., de Kruif, C.A., de Boer, W.I., *et al.* (1987). Induction and activity of several isoenzymes of cytochrome P-450 in primary cultures of rat hepatocytes, in comparison with *in vivo* data. *Molecular Toxicology* **1**, 373–381.

15. Van't Klooster, G.A.E., Woutersen-Van Nijnanten, F.M.A., Klein, W.R., *et al.* (1992). Effects of various medium formulations and attachment substrata on the performance of cultured ruminant hepatocytes in biotransformation studies. *Xenobiotica* **22**, 523–534.

16. Blaauboer, B.J., van Holsteijn, I., van Graft, M., *et al.* (1985). The concentration of cytochrome P-450 in human hepatocyte culture. *Biochemical Pharmacology* **34**, 2405–2408.

17. Mennes, W.C., Wortelboer, H.M., Hassing, G.A.M., *et al.* (1994). Effects of clofibric and beclobric acid in rat and monkey hepatocyte primary culture: influence on peroxisomal and mitochondrial β-oxidation and the activity of catalase, glutathione S-transferase and glutathione peroxidase. *Archives of Toxicology* **68**, 506–511.

18. Van Pelt, F.N.A.M., Olde Meierink, Y.J.M., Blaauboer, B.J., *et al.* (1990). Immunohistochemical detection of cytochrome P450 isoenzymes in cultured human epidermal cells. *Journal of Histochemistry and Cytochemistry* **38**, 1847–1851.

19. Berkers, J.A.M., Hassing, G.A.M., Brouwer, A., *et al.* (1994). Effects of retinoic acid on the 2,3,7,8-tetrachlorodibenzo-p-dioxin-induced differentiation of *in vitro* cultured human keratinocytes. *Toxicology in Vitro* **8**, 605–608.

20. Rietjens, I.M.C.M., Alink, G.M. & Vos, R.M.E. (1985). The role of glutathione and changes in thiol homeostasis in cultured lung cells exposed to ozone. *Toxicology* **35**, 207–217.

21. Groothuis, G.M.M., Hulstaert, C.E., Kalicharan, D., *et al.* (1981). Plasma membrane specialization and intracellular polarity of freshly isolated rat hepatocytes. *European Journal of Cell Biology* **26**, 43–51.

22. Olinga, P., Meijer, D.K.F., Slooff, M.J.H., *et al.* (1997). Liver slices in *in vitro* pharmacotoxicology with special reference to the use of human liver tissue. *Toxicology in Vitro* **12**, 77–100.

23. Peters, P.W.J. & Piersma, A.H. (1990). *In vitro* embryotoxicity and teratogenicity studies. *Toxicology in Vitro* **4**, 570–576.

24. Hendriksen, C.F.M., van der Gun, J.W., Marsman, F.R., *et al.* (1991). The use of the *in vitro* toxin binding inhibition (ToBI) test for the estimation of the potency of tetanus toxoid. *Biologicals* **19**, 23–29.

25. Kienhuis, A.S., van de Poll, M.C.G., Dejong, C.H.C., *et al.* (2009). A toxicogenomics-based parallelogram approach to evaluate the relevance of coumarin-induced responses in primary human hepatocytes *in vitro* for humans *in vivo*. *Toxicology in Vitro* **23**, 1163–1169.

26. Theunissen, P.T. & Piersma, A.H. (2012). Innovative approaches in the embryonic stem cell test (EST). *Frontiers in Bioscience* **17**, 1965–1975.

27. Kruidering, M., van de Water, B. & Nagelkerke, J.F. (1996). Methods for studying renal toxicity. In J.P. Seiler, O. Kroftová & V. Eybl (Eds.), *Toxicology - From Cells to Man*. *Archives of Toxicology* (Suppl 18). Heidelberg, Germany: Springer.

28. Warren, M., Atkinson, K. & Steer, S. (1990). INVITTOX: The ERGATT/FRAME data bank of *in vitro* techniques in toxicology. *Toxicology in Vitro* **4**, 707–710.

29. Balls, M., Blaauboer, B., Brusick, D., *et al.* (1990). Report and recommendations of the CAAT/ERGATT workshop on the validation of toxicity test procedures. *ATLA* **18**, 303–337.

30. Balls, M., Blaauboer, B.J., Fentem, J.H., *et al.* (1995). Practical aspects of the validation of toxicity test procedures. The report and recommendations of ECVAM Workshop 5. *ATLA* **23**, 129–147.

31. Walum, E., Balls, M., Bianchi, V., *et al.* (1992). ECITTS: an integrated approach to the application of in vitro test systems to the hazard assessment of chemicals. *ATLA* **20**, 406–428.

32. Blaauboer, B.J., Balls, M., Bianchi, V., *et al.* (1994). The ECITTS integrated toxicity testing scheme: The application of *in vitro* test systems to the hazard assessment of chemicals. *Toxicology in Vitro* **8**, 845–846.

33. DeJongh, J., Nordin-Andersson, M., Ploeger, B.A., *et al.* (1999). Estimation of systemic toxicity of acrylamide by integration of *in vitro* toxicity data with kinetic simulations. *Toxicology and Applied Pharmacology* **158**, 261–268.

34. Blaauboer, B.J. (2003). The integration of data on physico-chemical properties, *in vitro*-derived toxicity data and physiologically based kinetic and dynamic as modelling a tool in hazard and risk assessment. A commentary. *Toxicology Letters* **138**, 161–171.

35. Blaauboer, B.J. & Andersen, M.E. (2007). The need for a new toxicity testing and risk analysis paradigm to implement REACH or any other large scale testing initiative. *Archives of Toxicology* **81**, 385–387.

36. Blaauboer, B.J. (2010). Biokinetic modeling and *in vitro-in vivo* extrapolations. *Journal of Toxicology and Environmental Health B: Critical Reviews* **13**, 242–252.

37. Yoon, M., Blaauboer, B.J. & Clewell, H.J. (2015). Quantitative *in vitro* to *in vivo* extrapolation (QIVIVE): An essential element for *in vitro*-based risk assessment. *Toxicology* **332**, 1–3.

38. Pfaller, W., Prieto, P., Dekant, W., *et al.* (2015). The Predict-IV project: Towards predictive toxicology using *in vitro* techniques. *Toxicology in Vitro* **30**, 1–3.

39. Wilmes, A., Limonciel, A., Aschauer, L., *et al.* (2013). Application of integrated transcriptomic, proteomic and metabolomic profiling for the delineation of mechanisms of drug induced cell stress. *Journal of Proteomics* **79**, 180–194.

40. Kramer, N.I., Di Consiglio, E., Blaauboer, B.J., *et al.* (2015). Biokinetics in repeated-dosing *in vitro* drug toxicity studies. *Toxicology in Vitro* **30**, 217–224.

41. Kroes, R. & Feron, V.J. (1984). General toxicity testing: Sense and non-sense, science and policy. *Toxicological Sciences* **4**, 298–308.

42. Blaauboer, B.J., Barratt, M.D. & Houston, J.B. (1999). The integrated use of alternative methods in toxicological risk evaluation: ECVAM Integrated Testing Strategies Task Force Report I. *ATLA* **27**, 229–237.

43. Gubbels-van Hal, W.M.L.G., Blaauboer, B.J., Barentsen, H.M., *et al.* (2005). An alternative approach for the safety evaluation of new and existing chemicals, an exercise in integrated testing. *Regulatory Toxicology and Pharmacology* **42**, 284–295.

44. Blaauboer, B.J., Boekelheide, K., Clewell, H.J., *et al.* (2012). The use of biomarkers of toxicity for integrating *in vitro* hazard estimates into risk assessment for humans. *ALTEX* **29**, 411–425.

45. Blaauboer, B.J., Boobis, A.R., Bradford, B., *et al.* (2016). Considering new methodologies in strategies for safety assessment of foods and food ingredients. *Food and Chemical Toxicology* **91**, 19–32.

46. Louisse, J., de Jong, E., van de Sandt, J.J.M., *et al.* (2010). The use of *in vitro* toxicity data and physiologically based kinetic modeling to predict dose-response curves for *in vivo* developmental toxicity of glycol ethers in rat and man. *Toxicological Sciences* **118**, 470–484.

47. Blaauboer, B.J., Bayliss, M.K., Castell, J.V., *et al.* (1996). The use of biokinetics and *in vitro* methods in toxicological risk evaluation: The Report and Recommendations of ECVAM Workshop 15. *ATLA* **24**, 473–497.

48. Punt, A., Schiffelers, M.J.W.A., Jean Horbach, G., *et al.* (2011). Evaluation of research activities and research needs to increase the impact and applicability of alternative testing strategies in risk assessment practice. *Regulatory Toxicology and Pharmacology* **61**, 105–114.

49. Punt, A., Freidig, A.P., Delatour, T., *et al.* (2008). A physiologically based biokinetic (PBBK) model for estragole bioactivation and detoxification in rat. *Toxicology and Applied Pharmacology* **231**, 248–259.

50. Kramer, N.I., Krismartina, M., Rico-Rico, Á., *et al.* (2012). Quantifying processes determining the free concentration of phenanthrene in basal cytotoxicity assays. *Chemical Research in Toxicology* **25**, 436–445.

51. Groothuis, F.A., Heringa, M.B., Nicol, B., *et al.* (2015). Dose metric considerations in *in vitro* assays to improve quantitative *in vitro-in vivo* dose extrapolations. *Toxicology* **332**, 30–40.

52. Fentem, J., Chamberlain, M. & Sangster, B. (2004). The feasibility of replacing animal testing for assessing consumer safety: a suggested future direction. *ATLA* **32**, 617–623.

53. Murk, A.J., Rijntjes, E., Blaauboer, B.J., *et al.* (2013). Mechanism-based testing strategy using *in vitro* approaches for identification of thyroid hormone disrupting chemicals. *Toxicology in Vitro* **27**, 1320–1346.

54. Weigand, K., Greupink, R., Bosgra, S., *et al.* (2015). Assuring Safety without Animal Testing concept (ASAT): Systems toxicology supported data infrastructure for human risk assessment. *The Toxicologist. Supplement to Toxicological Sciences* **144**, 127.

55. Schiffelers, M.-J.W.A., Blaauboer, B.J., Van Vlissingen, J.M.F., *et al.* (2007). Factors stimulating or obstructing the implementation of the 3Rs in the regulatory process. *ALTEX* **24**, 271–278.

56. Schiffelers, M.-J.W.A., Blaauboer, B.J., Hendriksen, C.F.M., *et al.* (2012). Regulatory acceptance and use of 3R models: A multilevel perspective. *ALTEX* **29**, 287–300.

57. Roberfroid, M. & Rogiers, V. (1991). Editorial. Brussels Symposium on Alternative Methods in Pharmaco-toxicological research. *ATLA* **19**, 367–368.

58. Rogiers, V. (1993). Cultures of human hepatocytes in in vitro pharmaco-toxicology. In V. Rogiers, W. Sonck, E. Shephard & A. Vercruysse (Eds.), *Human Cells in In Vitro Pharmaco-Toxicology*, pp. 77–115. Brussels, Belgium: VUB Press.

59. Rogiers, V. & Vercruysse, A. (1993). Rat hepatocyte cultures and co-cultures in biotransformation studies of xenobiotics. *Toxicology* **82**, 193–203.

60. Rogiers, V., Balls, M., Basketter, D., *et al.* (1999). Potential use of non-invasive methods in safety assessment of cosmetics. *ATLA* **27**, 515–537.

61. Rogiers, V. (1999). Launch of the Belgian platform for alternative methods. *ATLA* **27**, 485–487.

62. Rogiers, V. & Beken, S. (2000). *Alternative methods to animal experiments — actual status, development and approach in Belgium*, 124pp. Brussels, Belgium: VUB University Press.

63. Van der Valk, J., Garthoff, B., Schlitt, A., *et al.* (1999). Improving international co-operation between national organisations promoting the 3Rs. *ALTEX* **16**, 166–168.

64. Rogiers, V. (2002). Ecopa: A powerful concept in the way forward for alternative methods. *ATLA* **30**, 199–202.

65. Rogiers, V. (2003). Ecopa: actual status and plans. *Toxicology in Vitro* **17**, 779—784.

66. Rogiers, V. (2004). ECOPA: The European consensus platform on three Rs alternatives. *ATLA* **32**, 349—353.

67. Rogiers, V. (2005). Recent developments in the way forward for alternative methods: formation of national consensus platforms in Europe. *Toxicology and Applied Pharmacology* **207**, S408—S413.

68. Devolder, T., Rogiers, V., Garthoff, B., *et al.* (2007). *The Impact of REACH. Report of the CONAM/ecopa Chemical Policy Working Group.* March, 90pp. Brussels, Belgium: ecopa.

69. Holley, T., Bowe, G., Campia, I., *et al.* (2016). Accelerating progress in the replacement, reduction and refinement of animal testing through better knowledge sharing. *JRC Report EUR* **28234**, 64pp.

70. Quillardet, P., Huisman, O., D'Ari, R., *et al.* (1982). SOS chromotest, a direct assay of induction of an SOS function in *Escherichia coli* K12 to measure genotoxicity. *Proceedings of the National Academy of Sciences of the United States of America* **79**, 5971—5975.

71. Moreau, P., Bailone, A. & Devoret, R. (1976). Prophage lambda induction of *Escherichia coli* K12 envA uvrB: a highly sensitive test for potential carcinogens. *Proceedings of the National Academy of Sciences of the United States of America* **73**, 3700—3704.

72. Bailone, A., Sommer, S. & Devoret, R. (1985). Mini-F plasmid-induced SOS signal in *Escherichia coli* is RecBC dependent. *Proceedings of the National Academy of Sciences of the United States of America* **82**, 5973—5977.

73. Moustacchi, E. (2000). DNA damage and repair: consequences on dose-responses. *Mutation Research* **464**, 35—40.

74. Chouroulinkov, I. & Lasne, C. (1978). Two-stage (initiation-promotion) carcinogenesis in vivo and in vitro. *Bulletin du Cancer* **65**, 255—264.

75. Elias, Z., Poirot, O., Pezerat, H., *et al.* (1989). Cytotoxic and neoplastic transforming effects of industrial hexavalent chromium pigments in Syrian hamster embryo cells. *Carcinogenesis* **10**, 2043—2052.

76. Dhalluin, S., Elias, Z., Poirot, O., *et al.* (1999). Apoptosis inhibition and ornithine decarboxylase superinduction as early epigenetic events in morphological transformation of Syrian hamster embryo cells exposed to 2-methoxyacetaldehyde, a metabolite of 2-methoxyethanol. *Toxicology Letters* **105**, 163—167.

77. Coulomb, B., Saiag, P., Bell, E., *et al.* (1986). A new method for studying epidermalization in vitro. *British Journal of Dermatology* **114**, 91—101.

78. Pruniéras, M., Régnier, M. & Woodley, D. (1983). Methods for cultivation of keratinocytes with an air-liquid interface. *Journal of Investigative Dermatology* **81**, 28s—33s.

79. Tinois, E., Tiollier, J., Gaucherand, M., *et al.* (1991). In vitro and post-transplantation differentiation of human keratinocytes grown on the human type IV collagen film of a bilayered dermal substitute. *Experimental Cell Research* **193**, 310—319.

80. Blein, O., Adolphe, M., Lakhdar, B., *et al.* (1991). Correlation and validation of alternative methods to the Draize eye irritation test (OPAL project). *Toxicology in Vitro* **5**, 555—557.

81. Guguen-Guillouzo, C. & Guillouzo, A. (2010). General review on in vitro hepatocyte models and their applications. *Methods in Molecular Biology* **640**, 1—40.

82. Fautrel, A., Chesné, C., Guillouzo, A., *et al.* (1991). A multicentre study of acute in vitro cytotoxicity in rat liver cells. *Toxicology in Vitro* **5**, 543—547.

83. Guguen-Guillouzo, C., Campion, J.P., Brissot, P., *et al.* (1982). High yield preparation of isolated human adult hepatocytes by enzymatic perfusion of the liver. *Cell Biology International Reports* **6**, 625—628.

84. Guguen-Guillouzo, C., Clément, B., Baffet, G., *et al.* (1983). Maintenance and reversibility of active albumin secretion by adult rat hepatocytes co-cultured with another liver epithelial cell type. *Experimental Cell Research* **143**, 47—54.

85. Guillouzo, A. & Guguen-Guillouzo, C. (Eds.). (1986). *Isolated and Cultured Hepatocytes*, 408pp. Paris, France: Les Editions INSERM and John Libbey Eurotext.

86. Guillouzo, A. (Ed.). (1988). *Liver Cells and Drugs,* 497pp. Paris, France: Les Editions INSERM and John Libbey Eurotext.

87. Gripon, P., Rumin, S., Urban, S.L., *et al.* (2002). Infection of a human hepatoma cell line by hepatitis B virus. *Proceedings of the National Academy of Sciences of the United States of America* **99**, 15655—15660.

88. Guillouzo, A. & Guguen-Guillouzo, C. (2018). HepaRG cells as a model for hepatotoxicity studies. In T.P. Rasmussen (Ed.), *Stem Cells in Birth Defects Research and Developmental Toxicology*, pp. 309—339. Hoboken, NJ, USA: John Wiley & Sons, Inc.

89. Adolphe, M. & Barlowatz-Meimon, G. (Eds.). (1988). *Culture De Cellules Animals. Methodologies et Applications*, 898pp. Paris, France: Les Editions INSERM.

90. Adolphe, M. & Guillouzo, A. (Eds.). (1988). *Methodes In Vitro en Pharmaco-Toxicologie, Colloque INSERM* **170**, pp. 1—280.

91. Adolphe, M., Guillouzo, A. & Marano, F. (Eds.). (1995). *Toxicologie Cellulaire In vitro. Methodes et Applications*, 470pp. Paris, France: Les Editions INSERM.

92. Barlowatz-Meimon, G. & Adolphe, M. (Eds.). (2003). *Culture De Cellules Animals. Methodologies et Applications,* 2nd ed., 916pp. Paris, France: Les Editions INSERM.

93. Gonzalez, R., Redon, P., Lakhdar, B., *et al.* (1990). Cyclosporin nephrotoxicity assessed in isolated human glomeruli and cultured mesangial cells. *Toxicology in Vitro* **4**, 391—395.

94. Chambard, M., Gabrion, J. & Mauchamp, J. (1981). Influence of collagen gel on the orientation of epithelial cell polarity: follicle formation from isolated thyroid cells and from preformed monolayers. *Journal of Cell Biology* **91**, 157—166.

95. Dehouck, M.P., Méresse, S., Delorme, P., *et al.* (1990). An easier, reproducible, and mass-production method to study the blood-brain barrier in vitro. *Journal of Neurochemistry* **54**, 1798—1801.

96. Barlowatz-Meimon, G. & Ronot, X. (2014). *Culture De Cellules Animals,* 3rd ed., 916pp. Paris, France: Lavoisier Tec & Doc et Les Editions INSERM.

97. Spielmann, H., Hoffmann, S., Liebsch, M., *et al.* (2007). .The ECVAM international validation study on *in vitro* tests for acute skin irritation: report on the validity of the EPISKIN and EpiDerm assays and on the Skin Integrity Function Test. *ATLA* **35**, 559–601.

98. Cotovio, J., Grandidier, M.H., Lelièvre, D., *et al.* (2010). *In vitro* assessment of eye irritancy using the Reconstructed Human Corneal Epithelial SkinEthic HCE model: application to 435 substances from consumer products industry. *Toxicology in Vitro* **24**, 523–537.

99. Jones, B.C., Rollison, H., Johansson, S., *et al.* (2017). Managing the risk of CYP3A induction in drug development: a strategic approach. *Drug Metabolism & Disposition* **45**, 35–41.

Chapter 2.5

Contributions of the Scandinavian Countries to the Development of Non-Animal Alternatives in Toxicology

Anna Forsby[1], Lisbeth E. Knudsen[2] and Hanna Tähti[3]

[1]Stockholm University, Stockholm, and SWETOX, Karolinska Institute, Stockholm, Sweden; [2]University of Copenhagen, Copenhagen, Denmark; [3]University of Tampere, Tampere, Finland

SUMMARY

The development of cell methods for the toxicity evaluation of drugs and chemicals started in Scandinavia at the end of the 1970s. The pioneer *in vitro* toxicologist was Björn Ekwall (1940–2000), who published his basal cytotoxicity concept in 1983, and started the MEIC project in 1989, the first international project aiming to evaluate the competence of cell toxicity tests to predict human toxicity. The EU framework project, ACuteTox (2005–10), can be seen as a continuation of the MEIC study. Generally, the early use of *in vitro* methods in all Scandinavian countries initially began for cell toxicology and genotoxicology and then for neurotoxicology and other tissue-specific toxicities. The Scandinavian Society for Cell Toxicity, established in 1983, played an important role, not only in gathering the MEIC participants, but also by encouraging other *in vitro* toxicologists from Scandinavia to meet at its annual workshops. The EU framework programmes, Oculotox *in vitro*, ACuteTox, ReproTect, Sens-it-iv and NanoTest, secured the place of research on alternative methods to replace animal experiments in Scandinavia. After the implementation of *Directive 2010/63/EU*, governmental measures have promoted research and education on alternative methods in various countries, but without providing sufficient resources, especially for *Replacement*.

1. INTRODUCTION

The history of using cell models instead of traditional animal models for toxicity studies goes back to the 1970s in Scandinavia. In 1976, Erik Walum established an *in vitro* test laboratory at the Swedish Defence Research Agency (FOA), with the aim of establishing methods that were less expensive, faster and more accurate than the animal tests. In parallel with Erik Walum's activities at the FOA, Björn Ekwall studied the effects of pharmaceuticals on HeLa cells at Uppsala University (1, 2). These were probably the most important factors in the early development and implementation of cell-based assays for toxicity research and testing activities in Sweden.

Erik Walum and Björn Ekwall started the Scandinavian Society for Cell Toxicity (SSCT) in 1983 (3, 4). Its main objectives were: (a) to gather together scientists who were interested in cellular toxicity and the use of cell-based methodology for chemical risk assessment; and (b) to coordinate a validation project, which was going to become the Multicenter Evaluation of *In Vitro* Cytotoxicity (MEIC) project.

The SSCT organised annual workshops on cytotoxicity mechanisms, method development and test validation, in which scientists from Denmark (5, 6), Finland (7), Norway (8), Sweden and some other European countries participated. Most of the workshops were held in Sweden, but took place in another Scandinavian country every second year, including twice in Estonia and once in the Czech Republic, England, Germany and Poland. The workshop proceedings were usually published in *ATLA*. The SSCT still organises workshops, but the field of interest is now wider, including computational toxicology, along with *in vitro* test systems for medical and toxicological research and risk assessment. In 2001, the SSCT set up the Björn Ekwall Memorial Foundation (BEMF) to honour the memory of Björn Ekwall (9), who died in 2000. The BEMF gives the Björn Ekwall Memorial Award every year to a scientist who has significantly contributed to the field of cell toxicology, e.g. by developing new *in vitro* tests or carrying out mechanistic or validation studies (10).

The MEIC project can be seen as a pioneering international project aimed at developing and validating cell-based tests to replace animal experiments. During recent decades, international EU Framework projects, such as ACuteTox, Sens-it-iv and ReproTect, were involved in the development of robust testing strategies for the replacement of animal toxicity tests used for regulatory purposes. Several scientists from Scandinavian countries participated in these projects.

The Nordic countries also participated in the work of ECVAM, after its establishment in 1991 at the European Commission's Joint Research Centre in Italy, and in ECVAM's Scientific Advisory Committee (ESAC).

2. THE DEVELOPMENT AND USE OF ALTERNATIVE *IN VITRO* METHODS

2.1 Cell Toxicology

In Uppsala in 1981, the Swedish Board for Laboratory Animals (CFN) held a symposium on *Acute toxicity testing of new chemicals — necessary for safety evaluation or waste of animals?*, which was attended by Michael Balls, Björn Ekwall and Erik Walum, among others. Björn Ekwall gave a talk on *Correlation between cytotoxicity* in vitro *and LD$_{50}$ values*, and in his published paper, he wrote that 'the best way to evaluate tissue culture tests must be to compare *in vitro* toxicity with human toxicity' (4, 11). That principle was the basis of the MEIC project.

Björn Ekwall was convinced that health hazards to man should be estimated by using only human-relevant models (2). He introduced the basal cytotoxicity concept (12), and presented the hypothesis that the acute systemic toxicity induced by most compounds could be estimated by studying cytotoxicity and general endpoints in human cells. The basal cytotoxicity concept was confirmed in the MEIC study, which took place from 1989 to 1999. Fifty reference chemicals were tested in more than 60 non-animal assays by 100 laboratories worldwide (10). The reference chemicals were selected from the MEMO database of human blood concentrations of acutely toxic drugs and chemicals. Poisons centres in several countries were used as sources of these data. Eight papers featuring the results of the MEIC study were published in *ATLA*, where Michael Balls acted as their editor, with the help of Horst Spielmann as a referee (11). The MEIC project showed that human cell models could make a better prediction of human acute toxicity than could cell models from other species (13). However, the basal cytotoxicity concept did not correlate well for compounds that induced toxicity as a result of their interaction with specific molecular targets. Another obstacle was that the cytotoxic concentrations of a compound mimicked the toxic level at the target tissue and could not predict a toxic dose.

To overcome the two main obstacles of organ-specific toxicity and the issue of toxicokinetics, the Evaluation-guided Development of New In Vitro Test Batteries (EDIT) project was planned (14, 15). Unfortunately, the EDIT project was not completed, largely because of Björn Ekwall's death in 2000. However, the EDIT project was developed into an application for the EU Framework 5 research project call in 2004. In 2005, the ACuteTox project (2005–10) began, with scientific coordination by Björn Ekwall's former colleague, Cecilia Clemedson, and administrative coordination by Oulu University, Finland (16).

Basal cytotoxicity is now a fundamental reference point for all researchers and toxicologists who perform mechanistic studies, determine modes of action and estimate organ-specific toxicity risk assessments by using *in vitro* methodology.

2.2 Neurotoxicology

The early development of alternatives to animal experiments in Finland began at the end of the 1980s, when Hanna Tähti and her group at the University of Tampere Medical School started to develop *in vitro* methods for neurotoxicology. The aim was to elucidate the neurotoxic potency and neurotoxic mechanisms of organic solvents, pesticides and heavy metals. The first models for the evaluation of acute neurotoxicity were synaptosomes and neural cells isolated from embryonic rat brains. The targets of the organic solvents studied were cell membrane integral proteins and receptor functions (17), and the fluidity of the neural membrane (18). The specific neural membranes were excellent models to study, including receptor mechanisms. However, the source of the model was ethically not acceptable. The 1991 SSCT Workshop in Nagu (in the Turku Archipelago) was an important turning point for Hanna Tähti's research, especially because of the encouraging attitude of Björn Ekwall. The research group began to use cell culture techniques, including human cell lines. Both neural and glial effects of different toxicants were characterised, and neurotoxic markers, e.g. glutamate-uptake (20), glucose-uptake (20), mitochondrial metabolism and glial fibrillary acidic protein (21), were identified. An important outcome of these studies was that neural-specific markers showed their neurotoxic effects at a much lower dose than the basal cell toxicity dose (22). A novel technique involved analysing cultured living cells with a machine vision technique (Cell-IQ, developed by ChipMan Technologies and the Cell Research Centre (CRC) in Tampere). It permitted the quantitation of cell growth, changes in neurite length, cell migration and cell-cell contacts, which later were found to be important and sensitive markers of developmental neurotoxicity (23, 24). A 3-D blood—brain barrier (BBB) model for the neurotoxicity studies was developed by using co-culture techniques (25—28). The integration of a BBB toxicity and permeability model in the neurotoxicity assessment strategy was suggested in collaborative work with the group of Cecchelli at the University of Artois, France, and with ECVAM's participation (29). A 3-D culture technique was also developed, to detect metabolism-dependent neurotoxicity (30, 31).

Since the beginning of the 1980s, Tore Syversen's group at the Norwegian University of Science and Technology, Trondheim, studied the neurotoxic mechanism of methylmercury *in vivo* and *in vitro*. In several publications, the neural-specific targets of methylmercury have been elucidated, namely, protein synthesis (32), glutamate metabolism (33), mitochondrial activity and production of a reactive oxygen species (34—36).

Erik Walum and his group at the Department of Neurochemistry and Neurotoxicology, Stockholm University, studied mechanisms for the development of axonopathy by using differentiated neuroblastoma cell lines (37—39). Anna Forsby, a PhD student in Walum's group in the early 1990s, has carried on the neurotoxicity research on functional and structural endpoints, by using neuronal cell lines. The cell models were validated in the ERGATT/CFN *In Vitro* Toxicity Test Strategy (ECITTS) project and in the ACuteTox project, for their usefulness as indicators of neurotoxicity (40, 41). Some other hallmarks of Forsby's research are studies on axonopathy by using *in vitro* models (42, 43) and the estimation of acute neurotoxicity by using human neuroblastoma SH-SY5Y cells and the differentiated neural progenitor C17.2 cell model (44, 45). These cell lines have also been shown to be useful for the assessment of developmental neurotoxicity (DNT), e.g. for low dose gamma radiation (46) and for acrylamide (47).

Sandra Ceccatelli and her group at the Karolinska Institute, Stockholm, have used a wide array neuronal cell models in their research on DNT. They have provided substantial technical and mechanistic information about the primary cultures that are useful for the understanding of neurotoxicity modes of action (reviewed in Ref. 48).

Lennart Dencker and Michael Stigson at Uppsala University (SE) are other Swedish researchers who have used cell models for mechanistic studies of DNT. Early on, they elaborated the opportunity to use gene expression markers as indicators of adverse cell differentiation, as illustrated by valproic acid-exposed pluripotent P19 teratocarcinoma cells (49). Today, transcriptomic biomarker expression is one of the most used indicators in DNT.

At the beginning of 2014, the first International Stakeholder Network (ISTNET) was created for DNT testing, following an initiative by the Finnish Centre for Alternative Methods (FICAM) in the University of Tampere, to accelerate the development of alternative methods in neurotoxicity testing for regulatory purposes. The main focus is on bringing scientists, regulators and industry people together to define test requirements and to adapt test development and introduce standardisation for various toxicological endpoints.

2.3 Ocular Toxicology

At Tampere University, alternative methods for ocular toxicity were developed in the EU-Biomed project, Oculotox *in vitro* (BMH4-97-2324.1997-2001) in a collaboration between toxicologists and clinical experts from three other universities, namely, Tampere, Bremen (Germany), Pisa (Italy) and Ioannina (Greece), and two Finnish pharma companies. The project developed and standardised *in vitro* methods for the evaluation of topically dosed and systemic eye drugs with a panel of 18 test compounds. A corneal model involved the human corneal epithelial cell line, SV40 (50), and a retinal model used the retinal pigment epithelial (RPE) cell line, D407, and primary pig RPE cells (51). General cytotoxicity tests and tests based on sensitive biomarkers for eye-specific toxicity were proposed, to improve ocular safety research involving drugs (52). Today, RPE models from human pluripotent stem cells have been developed at Tampere University (53).

Anna Forsby's group at Stockholm University has implemented a mechanistic approach for the estimation of mild eye irritation. By using one initiator of neurogenic inflammation as a molecular initiating event, they studied the role of the Transient Receptor Potential vanilloid type 1 (TRPV1) ion channel in mild eye irritation and nociception (54, 55). Human neuroblastoma SH-SY5Y cells with stable expression of the TRPV1 channel can be used for the estimation of the eye stinging sensation in the so-called NociOcular assay (56). The research is now focused on the correlation between the activation of calcium ion influx in the TRPV1-expressing cell model and the categorisation of eye irritating chemicals.

In Denmark, the group of Eva Bonefeld-Jørgensen at Århus University has used the B4G12 cell line for testing for ocular toxicity (57).

2.4 Tissue Modelling

The field of tissue engineering and modelling is rapidly moving forward, and research groups in Scandinavia are making significant contributions. Since 2008, the research group of Tuula Heinonen at FICAM has been developing advanced tissue models relevant to human toxicology. These models combine several cell types of a tissue with supporting material, to mimic the normal functions of human tissues. The Adverse Outcome Pathway (AOP) is a leading principle in the strategy of model and assay development. The models are based on cells differentiated from human (adult) stem cells, iPS cells or human primary cells. The models developed so far are for vasculogenesis/angiogenesis (58, 59), a cardiovascular construct (60) and an adipose tissue model (61).

2.5 Reproductive Toxicology

At the end of the 1980s, the group of Kirsi Vähäkangas, now at the University of Eastern Finland, started to develop a research model for the placental barrier at Oulu University. The first experiments involved the use of rat placentas, but the use of human placentas was more successful (62). The model was characterised in several studies (63−66), and it was shown that the results achieved in animal experiments are not sufficient when considering the human situation (64). Important milestones in developing the placenta model have been studies showing xenobiotic metabolism (67, 68), the formation of DNA adducts and the determination of nanoparticle kinetics (69). The model was established in the ReProTect and NEWgeneris projects in the laboratory of Lisbeth Knudsen in Denmark, with the help of Kirsi Vähäkangas (70). The ReProTect project was aimed to substitute *in vivo* studies with *in vitro* assays (71). A preliminary interlaboratory comparison of the human placental model was published in 2010 (72). Studies on placental transport were extended to include the BeWo cell permeability assay (73). Under the leadership of Maria Dusinska at the Norwegian Institute for Air Research (NILU), Oslo, Norway, the BeWo cell assay was later included in the battery suggested for the safety testing of nanoparticles, as an outcome of the NanoTest project (74).

In vitro testing at the Danish National Food Institute is focused on endocrine disruptors, and a QSAR approach was developed in an international collaboration (75, 76).

The research group of Eva Bonefeld-Jørgensen, at Arhus University, Denmark, introduced the cell assay of dioxin-like activity in human biomonitoring (77), which was applied to the human biomonitoring of schoolchildren and their mothers (78).

2.6 Toxicokinetics and Biotransformation Modelling

From 1979 onwards, Olavi Pelkonen's group at Oulu University has studied human liver microsomes and other hepatic preparations, to elucidate the metabolism of drugs and other xenobiotics (79). They have evaluated human liver preparations as an *in vitro* model to predict the metabolism, interactions and clearance of drugs (80), pesticides (81) and various environmental chemicals (82). They have characterised the human, hepatoma HepaRG cell line, and have compared it to human hepatocytes (83).

At Uppsala University, Per Artursson has developed tools for studying drug absorption across the intestinal barrier. These *in silico* and *in vitro* cell models have been adopted by the pharma industry and have contributed to savings in costs, time and animals during drug development.

At Bergen University, Norway, Knut-Jan Andersen has developed *in vitro* kidney tubule models and LLC-PK1 proximal tubule cell spheroids for toxicity and fluid transport studies (8, 84). He organised the SSCT workshop at Ustaøset, Norway, in 1994.

2.7 Genotoxicity and Carcinogenicity Testing *In Vitro*

Many research groups used *in vitro* genotoxicity tests from the 1970s, and the development of high-throughput human and mammalian models for *in vitro* genotoxicity took place in Scandinavian countries.

The Institute of Public Health in Oslo established tests for DNA damage in the 1990s (85), and Andrew Collins established a laboratory for genotoxicity at the Department of Nutrition at Oslo University (86).

Maria Dusinska established a research team at NILU (87), which has played a leading role in *in vitro* testing for the cytotoxicity and genotoxicity of nanoparticles in a number of European projects for more than 10 years, including the NanoTest project (88, 89). She had worked on genotoxicology in Bratislava, then in Czechoslovakia, at the beginning of the 1990s, and collaborated with Ada Kolman at Stockholm University. She applied the Comet assay (single cell gel electrophoresis) for the analysis of DNA damage and for testing novel chemicals for genotoxicity.

In Denmark, Ulla Vogel and Håkan Wallin at the National Research Center for the Working Environment, Copenhagen, and Steffan Loft and Peter Møller at the University of Copenhagen, have also established *in vitro* methodologies for studying the genotoxicity of nanoparticles and air pollutants (90—92).

Ada Kolman and Dag Jenssen at Stockholm University have used cell assays for studies on inducers and protectors of DNA lesions and chromosomal aberrations, respectively. Kolman *et al.* (93) reviewed the genotoxic effects of ethylene oxide, propylene oxide and epichlorohydrin in humans, and included an evaluation of *in vitro* data obtained with mammalian cells. Starting at the end of 1970, the genotoxicity tests for monitoring cytogenetic changes in occupationally exposed humans were developed at the Institute of Occupational Health in Helsinki, Finland (94). Short-term *in vitro* bioassays, e.g. with Chinese hamster ovary cells, were also used as an *in vitro* test for monitoring occupational exposure to complex mixtures (95). The cytogenetic analyses from all the Nordic and some other European countries were validated against increased cancer risks, with results persisting even 20 years after testing (96).

In the 1970s, 1980s and 1990s, the group of Olavi Pelkonen studied benzo(a)pyrene metabolism in human preparations, to elucidate metabolic factors in polycyclic aromatic hydrocarbon carcinogenesis (97).

In the 1990s, the group of Kirsi Vähäkangas characterised human carcinoma cell lines as models for carcinogenicity testing, showing the importance of the expression of p53, because of its central role in the regulation of the cell cycle, apoptosis and DNA repair (98, 99). Later, because of the interest in fetal exposure, the research group used BeWo cells originating from human trophoblastic cancer cells (100).

Roland Grafström's research activities have taken place at the Karolinska Institute, Stockholm, and Åbo Academi University and Misvik Biology Oy, Turku, Finland. In the mid-1980s, he studied aldehyde-induced genotoxic effects in human cell cultures (101), and continued with studies on buccal epithelial cells and cell models of the respiratory tract as models for the evaluation of the genotoxic and carcinogenic potencies of chemicals (102,103), reviewed in 2004 (104). Later, his specific interests were also in *in silico* approaches in biomedical toxicogenomics and cancer research, and in the replacement of animal experiments through the bioinformatics-driven 'omics' data (105).

2.8 Ecotoxicology

In vitro ecotoxicology test models, especially for fish toxicity, have been developed by Boris Isomaa's research group at Åbo Academi University, Turku, Finland. Their studies were focused on fish (rainbow trout) gill epithelial cell cultures, as the gills are the primary target and uptake site for many water-borne toxicants (106). Primary hepatocytes from brown trout (*Salmo trutta lacustris*), fish cell lines (107) and zebrafish (108) were also used to study environmental endocrine disrupters.

Toxicologists from Estonia have long been in close contact with Scandinavian toxicologists. Anne Kahru organised the SSCT workshops in Tallinn in 1998 and in Toila in 2005. Her research group at the Estonian National Institute of Chemical Physics and Biochemistry (NICPB), Tallinn, is well known in the area of ecotoxicology of nanoparticles, and participated in the EU Nanovalid (2011—15) and Modern (2013—15) projects (109). The main goal of the group is to obtain new scientific knowledge on (eco)toxicity and the mechanisms of action of selected REACH-relevant chemicals and nanoparticles (e.g. titanium dioxide, zinc oxide and cupric oxide). Prokaryotic and simple eukaryotic organisms, and also human cell lines, are used as models. Special attention is focused on molecular mechanisms of toxicity and the bioavailability of xenobiotics as reviewed by Bondarenko *et al.* (110).

In the Nanovalid project, the applicability of conventional cytotoxicity assays for the toxicity evaluation of various nanoparticles was evaluated by Marika Mannerström *et al.* at FICAM (111).

Jette Rank established an ecogenotoxicology group at the Univeristy Centre in Roskilde, Denmark, working with fish cell lines (112). Åse Krøjke at Trondheim University, Norway, used cytogenicity testing for evaluating the genotoxic load in wildlife (113).

2.9 Skin Sensitisation

Erwin Roggen, Novozymes, Bagsvaerd, Denmark, coordinated the EU Sens-it-iv project, aimed at developing screening assays for sensitisation and contributed to the development of an AOP for sensitisation (114).

Malin Lindstedt's group at the University of Lund, Sweden, has developed a test strategy for the assessment of sensitising compounds, called the Genomic Allergen Rapid Detection (GARD) test (115). It is based on a transcriptomic fingerprint of approximately 300 genes in the human myeloma MUZT-3 cell line. The test is now undergoing validation via the OECD.

3. ALTERNATIVES IN INDUSTRY

The pharma industry uses *in vitro* cell models extensively, both for biological target hit screening and for early toxicity screening. Already in the 1970s, Vera Stejskal, an immunotoxicologist at Astra in Södertälje, Sweden, claimed, primarily for scientific reasons, that pre-clinical animal models were unsuitable for the prediction of immune effects in humans. She developed an *in vitro* assay for the diagnosis of drug-allergy in humans, by using primary human peripheral blood lymphocytes. This modified lymphocyte proliferation test, the Memory Lymphocyte Immunostimulation Assay (MELISA), precluded the use of fetal calf serum, as it induced false-positive lymphocyte proliferation, so human AB + serum was the serum of choice. Between 1980 and 1996, more than 1500 individuals were tested by using this assay. An immunotoxicologist, Karin Cederbrant, and a research engineer, Maritha Marcusson-Ståhl, continued this work at Astra/AstraZeneca from the mid-1990s. As a research strategy, human primary cells were the obvious alternative when developing new *in vitro* tests for the prediction of most possible types of immunotoxic effects by drugs in development. With the goal to cover both innate and acquired immune functions, a panel of human cell-based assays were developed and are today available and in use.

Per Kjellstrand and his group at GAMBRO AB in Lund, Sweden, were other pioneers in the implementation of *in vitro* methodology for safety assessments. Already in the 1980s, GAMBRO AB used basal cytotoxicity tests such as the neutral red uptake assay and the MTT test for screening dialysis biomaterial and fluids.

NOVO Nordic, Novozymes Lundbeck and other companies in Denmark have been introducing Three Rs initiatives, including *in vitro* and QSAR methodologies.

The pharmaceutical industry has participated in many international initiatives. For example, Orion Pharma, Espoo, Finland, took part in an Innovative Medicines Initiative (IMI) 5-year programme on developing mechanism-based methods and models, including cryopreserved primary human hepatocytes and stem cell-derived models, for the prediction of drug-induced liver injury (116–118).

4. FINANCING RESEARCH ON NON-ANIMAL ALTERNATIVES, 1980–2016

The Swedish Fund for Research without Animal Experiments, which is reliant on private donations, was established in 1964. The first research grants were given in 1971, since when the fund has awarded grants totalling more than 29 million Swedish kronor (SEK; approximately €3 million). Several scientists in Sweden, who played significant roles in the development and implementation of alternative methods for biomedical research and toxicity testing, were supported by the fund early in their careers. Since 1981, the Juliana von Wendt Fund has supported Finnish researchers in the development and application of humane methods.

In 1996, the Nordic Prize for Alternatives to Animal Experiments was established jointly by three organisations: the Swedish Fund, the Juliana von Wendt Fund and the Danish Alternativfondet.

The Swedish Government has supported Three Rs research projects since 1980, and since 2010, the Swedish Research Council has contributed approximately 15 million SEK annually. AstraZeneca and Pharmacia have invested about 1 million SEK annually, for alternative methods for use in drug development.

From 1986, the Finnish Ministry of Agriculture and Forestry supported research without experimental animals, by giving up to €34,000 annually. Since *Directive 2010/63/EU* came into force, the Ministry has provided €100,000–200,000 annually, to support the research and education programmes of FICAM, which also benefits from support by the Ministry of Education and Culture and the Finnish National Technology Agency.

The Danish Society for Protection of Laboratory Animals has existed since the 1970s and seeks the abolition of all painful experiments on animals, while supporting small research projects. In 2013, following negotiations between the Ministry of Food, the pharmaceutical industry and a number of animal welfare organisations, the Danish 3R-Center was established. Its aim is to be a leading contributor to the promotion of the Three Rs (119). Three Rs centres are also being set up in Norway and Sweden.

5. RESEARCH CENTRES ESTABLISHED FOR THE DEVELOPMENT AND VALIDATION OF NON-ANIMAL METHODS

The CRC was established in 1999 in the Medical School at the University of Tampere, at the instigation of Hanna Tähti and Timo Ylikomi. Its goal was to develop its activities toward being a national alternatives centre in Finland. In 2006, an expert group appointed by the Ministry of Agriculture and Forestry suggested that: 'A National Centre for Alternative Methods should be founded to promote, organise and coordinate research, communication and education on alternative methods. Long-term Government funding should be allocated to finance the establishment and operations of the Centre'. This was achieved in 2008, when the Finnish Centre for Alternative Methods (FICAM) was established under the leadership of Tuula Heinonen. FICAM is GLP-compliant and, since 2013, has acted as the Finnish reference laboratory for EURL ECVAM in the European Union Network of Laboratories for the Validation of Alternative Methods (EU-NETVAL), in compliance with *Directive 2010/63/EU*, according to which the use of experimental animals should be reduced and replaced with non-animal experimentation as soon as it is scientifically possible. Tuula Heinonen is the Finnish representative for the Preliminary Assessment of Regulatory Relevance (PARERE) network under Article 47(5) of the Directive, which evaluates the acceptance of alternative methods into regulatory guidelines.

The Cytotoxicity Laboratory in Uppsala (CTLU) was founded by Björn Ekwall in 1983 and was the main centre for the coordination of the MEIC project.

RISE Research Institute of Sweden (formerly the SP Sveriges Tekniska Forskningsinstitut) is a GLP-certified laboratory for *in vitro* toxicity testing and has been a member of the EU-NETVAL since 2013.

The Swedish Toxicology Sciences Research Center (SWETOX) was established in 2014 as a consortium, including 11 Swedish universities. The *in vitro* activities at SWETOX in Södertälje include research and a wide array of tests on immunotoxicity, neurotoxicity, eye irritation, hepatocyte toxicity, the sub-cellular bioaccumulation of compounds, nanoparticle toxicity, adverse toxicokinetic functions, impaired female fertility, and the epigenetic effects of endocrine disrupting chemicals. It also hosts an *in silico* group, which focuses on test optimisation, target prediction, QSARs, multivariate data analysis and physiologically based biokinetic (PBBK) modelling.

6. EDUCATION AND NON-ANIMAL METHODS

Erik Walum and Dag Jenssen, Stockholm University, and Leif Bjellin and Stina Oredsson, University of Lund, played fundamental roles in the establishment in Sweden of undergraduate education in the field of *in vitro* toxicology. Walum and Jenssen were two of the authors of one of the first tutorial books on *in vitro* toxicology, namely, *Understanding Cell Toxicology: Principles and Practice* (120). A course in toxicology at the University of Lund started in the late 1980s, and the Institute of Environmental Medicine at the Karolinska Institute provides a two-year masters programme on *in vitro* methodology and non-animal-based risk assessment.

Starting from 1980, special courses on alternatives to experimental animals took place in Finland but not on a regular basis. The CRC began such courses in 1999, which were taken over by FICAM and have continued since 2008. From 2007 to 2011, there was a national doctoral programme, the Finnish Graduate School in Toxicology, financed by the Ministry of Education and the Academy of Finland and led by Olavi Pelkonen. From 2012 to 2015, the programme continued as FinPharma Doctoral Program's Toxicology section, which resulted in 15 doctorates. From 2017, the Ministry of Agriculture and Forestry financed a new national education programme on alternative methods, organised by FICAM.

In Denmark, education on alternatives is part of animal welfare courses, but there are no independent courses.

7. CONCLUDING COMMENTS

During 1980s and 1990s, the personal impact of Björn Ekwall, the MEIC project and the SSCT meetings were particularly important in promoting the development of *in vitro* research and the development of alternative methods in all the Scandinavian countries. However, the principal focus of many research groups was on toxicity pathways (molecular mechanisms), not on the development of tests for regulatory purposes. Nevertheless, a change of emphasis toward test development could be detected during the 1990s, owing to several factors, including ECVAM's influence, the EU Framework programmes, new EU legislation, and the need for more-effective testing of chemicals and products of various kinds.

EU framework programmes promoted the networking of scientists and permitted the equipping of cell culture laboratories. Also, national technology programmes promoted the development of new technologies based on the use of cells, e.g. for the development of high-throughput technology for the pharmaceutical industry.

The incorporation of the requirements of *Directive 2010/63/EU* into national legislation has resulted in governmental measures for the promotion of Three Rs principles in several countries. This has led to the establishment of Three Rs and research centres and to the promotion and financial resourcing of research on alternative methods. Also, the importance of the education of scientists in new approaches to reduce the use of animals is now seen more clearly.

The focus on the Three Rs has affected the future development very positively, e.g. when scientists are made aware of the existence of *in vitro* and QSAR approaches. However, the cell culture background of scientists using animal experiments is often weak, and there is still much prejudice against the adoption of *in vitro* methods. More incentives to promote collaboration within the Three Rs is recommended, by, for example, the Danish 3-R Centre, in initiating a study on possibilities and barriers for replacement in animal science. Similarly, the national education programme of the Finnish Ministry of Agriculture and Forestry, has encouraged alternatives to animal experiments (with an emphasis on replacement), starting in 2017 as a FICAM project, is a sign of more-positive developments in the experimental biosciences.

The general opinion among the toxicologists concerning the possibility to replace the experimental animals with *in vitro* models and methods has changed during the past 20 years. In 1980s and at the beginning of the 1990s, *in vitro* testing was not of great interest at toxicology congresses among delegates working on animal tests. Today, *in vitro* toxicology is usually incorporated as part of the scientific programme of every toxicology congress, and knowledge of *in vitro* techniques has increased among toxicologists, which gives hope for more and more research without the use of experimental animals.

However, more education on alternative non-animal methods is needed, especially on advanced techniques, e.g. those based on functional human tissue models, which are more relevant for the evaluation of human effects than the traditional animal models. Substantial and permanent governmental resources are badly needed, both for education and research.

ACKNOWLEDGEMENTS

Scientists who provided information for this review, included: Erik Walum, Maria Dusinska (NILU), Tuula Heinonen (FICAM, Tampere University), Olavi Pelkonen (Oulu University), Kirsi Vähäkangas (University of East Finland) and Karin Cederbrant (Swetox).

REFERENCES

1. Ekwall, B. (1980). Screening of toxic compounds in tissue culture. *Toxicology* **17**, 127–142.
2. Ekwall, B. (1980). Preliminary studies on the validity of *in vitro* measurement of drug toxicity using Hela cells. II. Lethal action to man of 43 drugs related to the Hela cell toxicity of the lethal drug concentration. *Toxicology Letters* **5**, 319.
3. Bernson, V., Clausen, J., Ekwall, B., *et al.* (1986). Trends in Scandinavian cell toxicology. *ATLA* **13**, 162–179.
4. Walum, E. (2014). Scandinavian society for cell toxicology – thirty years of scientific pioneering. *Basic and Clinical Pharmacology and Toxicology* **115**, 88–92.
5. Hansen, K. & Stern, R.M. (1983). In vitro toxicity and transformation potency of nickel compounds. *Environmental Health Perspectives* **51**, 223–226.
6. Rasmussen, E.S. (1993). The role of *in vitro* experiments in animal welfare. *Human & Experimental Toxicology* **12**, 522–527.
7. Tähti, H. & Naskali, L. (1992). The effects of organic solvents on neural membrane integral proteins tested in neural cell cultures. *Neuroscience Research Communications* **10**, 71–77.
8. Andersen, K.J. & Vik, H. (1993). Use of renal epithelial cell lines for testing cellular toxicity. *Contributions to Nephrology* **101**, 227–234.
9. Kolman, A. & Walum, E. (2010). Bjorn Ekwall, an outstanding Swedish cell toxicologist. *Toxicology in Vitro* **24**, 2060–2062.
10. Walum, E., Tähti, H. & Kolman, A. (2011). The tenth anniversary of the Bjorn Ekwall memorial foundation. *ATLA* **39**, 389–402.
11. Balls, M. (2015). Scandinavia and the replacement of *in vivo* toxicity tests: Some personal reflections. The 2015 Bjorn Ekwall Memorial Award Lecture. *ATLA* **43**, 405–416.
12. Ekwall, B. (1983). Screening of toxic compounds in mammalian cell cultures. *Annals of the New York Academy of Sciences* **407**, 64–77.
13. Ekwall, B. (1999). Overview of the final MEIC results: II. The *in vitro–in vivo* evaluation, including the selection of a practical battery of cell tests for prediction of acute lethal blood concentrations in humans. *Toxicology in Vitro* **13**, 665–673.
14. Walum, E., Forsby, A., Clemedson, C., *et al.* (1996). Dynamic qualities of validation and the evolution of new *in vitro* toxicological tests. *ATLA* **24**, 333–338.
15. Ekwall, B., Clemedson, C., Ekwall, B., *et al.* (1999). EDIT: A new international multicentre programme to develop and evaluate batteries of *in vitro* tests for acute and chronic systemic toxicity. *ATLA* **27**, 339–349.
16. Clemedson, C., Kolman, A. & Forsby, A. (2007). The integrated acute systemic toxicity project (ACuteTox) for the optimisation and validation of alternative *in vitro* tests. *ATLA* **35**, 33–38.

17. Korpela, M. & Tähti, H. (1988). The effect of *in vitro* and *in vivo* toluene exposures on rat erythrocyte and synaptosome membrane integral enzymes. *Pharmacology & Toxicology* **63**, 30–32.

18. Naskali, L., Engelke, M. & Tähti, H. (1993). The neurotoxicity of organic solvents studied using synaptosomes and neural cell cultures. *ATLA* **22**, 175–179.

19. Raunio, S. & Tähti, H. (2001). Glutamate and calcium uptake in astrocytes after acute lead exposure. *Chemosphere* **44**, 355–359.

20. Mannerström, M. & Tähti, H. (2004). Modulation of glucose uptake in glial and neuronal cell lines by selected neurological drugs. *Toxicology Letters* **151**, 87–97.

21. Toimela, T.A. & Tähti, H. (1995). Effects of mercury, methylmercury and aluminium on glial fibrillary acidic protein expression in rat cerebellar astrocyte cultures. *Toxicology in Vitro* **9**, 317–325.

22. Toimela, T. & Tähti, H. (2004). Mitochondrial viability and apoptosis induced by aluminum, mercuric mercury and methylmercury in cell lines of neural origin. *Archives of Toxicology* **78**, 565–574.

23. Toimela, T., Tähti, H. & Ylikomi, T. (2008). Comparison of an automated pattern analysis machine vision time-lapse system with traditional endpoint measurements in the analysis of cell growth and cytotoxicity. *ATLA* **36**, 313–325.

24. Selinummi, J., Sarkanen, J.R., Niemisto, A., *et al.* (2006). Quantification of vesicles in differentiating human SH-SY5Y neuroblastoma cells by automated image analysis. *Neuroscience Letters* **396**, 102–107.

25. Toimela, T., Mäenpää, H., Mannerström, M., *et al.* (2004). Development of an *in vitro* blood-brain barrier model-cytotoxicity of mercury and aluminum. *Toxicology and Applied Pharmacology* **195**, 73–82.

26. Tähti, H., Nevala, H. & Toimela, T. (2003). Refining *in vitro* neurotoxicity testing — the development of blood-brain barrier models. *ATLA* **31**, 273–276.

27. Prieto, P., Blaauboer, B.J., de Boer, A.G., *et al.* (2004). Blood-brain barrier *in vitro* models and their application in toxicology. The report and recommendations of ECVAM Workshop 49. *ATLA* **32**, 37–50.

28. Nevala, H., Ylikomi, T. & Tähti, H. (2008). Evaluation of the selected barrier properties of retinal pigment epithelial cell line ARPE-19 for an *in vitro* blood-brain barrier model. *Human & Experimental Toxicology* **27**, 741–749.

29. Hallier-Vanuxeem, D., Prieto, P., Culot, M., *et al.* (2009). New strategy for alerting central nervous system toxicity: Integration of blood-brain barrier toxicity and permeability in neurotoxicity assessment. *Toxicology in Vitro* **23**, 447–453.

30. Mannerström, M., Toimela, T., Ylikomi, T., *et al.* (2006). The combined use of human neural and liver cell lines and mouse hepatocytes improves the predictability of the neurotoxicity of selected drugs. *Toxicology Letters* **165**, 195–202.

31. Mannerström, M., Mäenpää, H., Räty, S., *et al.* (2008). Metabolism-induced toxicity of selegeline and carbamazepine studied with an *in vitro* method. *The Open Toxicology Journal* **2**, 61–70.

32. Syversen, T.L. (1981). Effects of methyl mercury on protein synthesis *in vitro*. *Acta Pharmacologica et Toxicologica* **49**, 422–426.

33. Qu, H., Syversen, T., Aschner, M., *et al.* (2003). Effect of methylmercury on glutamate metabolism in cerebellar astrocytes in culture. *Neuro-Chemistry International* **43**, 411–416.

34. Kaur, P., Aschner, M. & Syversen, T. (2006). Glutathione modulation influences methyl mercury induced neurotoxicity in primary cell cultures of neurons and astrocytes. *Neurotoxicology* **27**, 492–500.

35. Kaur, P., Schultz, K., Heggland, I., *et al.* (2008). The use of fluorescence for detecting MeHg-induced ROS in cell cultures. *Toxicology in Vitro* **22**, 1392–1398.

36. Kaur, P., Evje, L., Aschner, M. & Syversen, T. (2009). The *in vitro* effects of selenomethionine on methylmercury-induced neurotoxicity. *Toxicology in Vitro* **23**, 378–385.

37. Walum, E. & Peterson, A. (1984). On the application of cultured neuroblastoma cells in chemical toxicity screening. *Journal of Toxicology and Environmental Health* **13**, 511–520.

38. Walum, E., Nordin, M., Beckman, M., *et al.* (1993). Cellular methods for identification of neurotoxic chemicals and estimation of neuro-toxicological risk. *Toxicology in Vitro* **7**, 321–326.

39. Odland, L., Romert, L., Clemedson, C., *et al.* (1994). Glutathione content, glutathione transferase activity and lipid peroxidation in acrylamide-treated neuroblastoma N1E 115 cells. *Toxicology in Vitro* **8**, 263–267.

40. DeJongh, J., Forsby, A., Houston, J.B., *et al.* (1999). An integrated approach to the prediction of systemic toxicity using computer-based biokinetic models and biological *in vitro* test methods: Overview of a Prevalidation Study Based on the ECITTS Project. *Toxicology in Vitro* **13**, 549–554.

41. Forsby, A., Bal-Price, A.K., Camins, A., *et al.* (2009). Neuronal *in vitro* models for the estimation of acute systemic toxicity. *Toxicology in Vitro* **23**, 1564–1569.

42. Nordin-Andersson, M., Walum, E., Kjellstrand, P., *et al.* (2003). Acrylamide-induced effects on general and neurospecific cellular functions during exposure and recovery. *Cell Biology and Toxicology* **19**, 43–51.

43. Axelsson, V., Holback, S., Sjogren, M., *et al.* (2006). Gliotoxin induces caspase-dependent neurite degeneration and calpain-mediated general cytotoxicity in differentiated human neuroblastoma SH-SY5Y cells. *Biochemical and Biophysical Research Communications* **345**, 1068–1074.

44. Lundqvist, J., El Andaloussi-Lilja, J., Svensson, C., *et al.* (2013). Optimisation of culture conditions for differentiation of C17.2 neural stem cells to be used for *in vitro* toxicity tests. *Toxicology in Vitro* **27**, 1565–1569.

45. Lundqvist, J., Svensson, C., Attoff, K., *et al.* (2017). Altered mRNA expression and cell membrane potential in the differentiated C17.2 cell model as indicators of acute neurotoxicity. *Applied In Vitro Toxicology* **3**, 154–162.

46. Bajinskis, A., Lindegren, H., Johansson, L., *et al.* (2011). Low-dose/dose-rate gamma radiation depresses neural differentiation and alters protein expression profiles in neuroblastoma SH-SY5Y cells and C17.2 neural stem cells. *Radiation Research* **175**, 185–192.

47. Attoff, K., Kertika, D., Lundqvist, J., *et al.* (2016). Acrylamide affects proliferation and differentiation of the neural progenitor cell line C17.2 and the neuroblastoma cell line SH-SY5Y. *Toxicology in Vitro* **35**, 100–111.

48. Tamm, C. & Ceccatelli, S. (2017). Mechanistic insight into neurotoxicity induced by developmental insults. *Biochemical and Biophysical Research Communications* **482**, 408–418.

49. Kultima, K., Nystrom, A.M., Scholz, B., *et al.* (2004). Valproic acid teratogenicity: a toxicogenomics approach. *Environmental Health Perspectives* **112**, 1225–1235.

50. Huhtala, A., Alajuuma, P., Burgalassi, S., *et al.* (2003). A collaborative evaluation of the cytotoxicity of two surfactants by using the human corneal epithelial cell line and the WST-1 test. *Journal of Ocular Pharmacology and Therapeutics* **19**, 11–21.

51. Mannerström, M., Zorn-Kruppa, M., Diehl, H., *et al.* (2002). Evaluation of the cytotoxicity of selected systemic and intravitreally dosed drugs in the cultures of human retinal pigment epithelial cell line and of pig primary retinal pigment epithelial cells. *Toxicology in Vitro* **16**, 193–200.

52. Tähti, H., Mäenpää, H., Salminen, L., *et al.* (1999). Retinal pigment epithelial cell cultures as a tool for evaluating retinal toxicity *in vitro*. *ATLA* **27**, 417–424.

53. Vaajasaari, H., Ilmarinen, T., Juuti-Uusitalo, K., *et al.* (2011). Toward the defined and xeno-free differentiation of functional human pluripotent stem cell-derived retinal pigment epithelial cells. *Molecular Vision* **17**, 558–575.

54. Lilja, J. & Forsby, A. (2004). Development of a sensory neuronal cell model for the estimation of mild eye irritation. *ATLA* **32**, 339–343.

55. Lilja, J., Lindegren, H. & Forsby, A. (2007). Surfactant-induced TRPV1 activity – a novel mechanism for eye irritation? *Toxicological Sciences* **99**, 174–180.

56. Forsby, A., Norman, K., EL Andaloussi-Lilja, J., *et al.* (2012). Prediction of human eye sting using the novel *in vitro* assay NociOcular. *Toxicological Sciences* **129**, 325–331.

57. Kruger, T., Cao, Y., Kjaergaard, S.K., *et al.* (2012). Effects of phthalates on the human corneal endothelial cell line B4G12. *International Journal of Toxicology* **31**, 364–371.

58. Sarkanen, J.R., Vuorenpää, H., Huttala, O., *et al.* (2012). Adipose stromal cell tubule network model provides a versatile tool for vascular research and tissue engineering. *Cells Tissues Organs* **196**, 385–397.

59. Huttala, O., Vuorenpää, H., Toimela, T., *et al.* (2015). Human vascular model with defined stimulation medium – a characterization study. *ALTEX* **32**, 125–136.

60. Vuorenpää, H., Ikonen, L., Kujala, K., *et al.* (2014). Novel *in vitro* cardiovascular constructs composed of a vascular-like network and cardiomyocytes. *In Vitro Cellular & Developmental Biology – Animal* **50**, 275–286.

61. Huttala, O., Mysore, R., Sarkanen, J.R., *et al.* (2016). Differentiation of human adipose stromal cells *in vitro* into insulin-sensitive adipocytes. *Cell and Tissue Research* **366**, 63–74.

62. Pienimaki, P., Hartikainen, A.L., Arvela, P., *et al.* (1995). Carbamazepine and its metabolites in human perfused placenta and in maternal and cord blood. *Epilepsia* **36**, 241–248.

63. Ala-Kokko, T.I., Pienimaki, P., Herva, R., *et al.* (1995). Transfer of lidocaine and bupivacaine across the isolated perfused human placenta. *Pharmacology & Toxicology* **77**, 142–148.

64. Lampela, E.S., Nuutinen, L.H., Ala-Kokko, T.I., *et al.* (1999). Placental transfer of sulindac, sulindac sulfide, and indomethacin in a human placental perfusion model. *American Journal of Obstetrics and Gynecology* **180**, 174–180.

65. Myllynen, P. & Vähäkangas, K. (2002). An examination of whether human placental perfusion allows accurate prediction of placental drug transport: studies with diazepam. *Journal of Pharmacological and Toxicological Methods* **48**, 131–138.

66. Annola, K., Karttunen, V., Keski-Rahkonen, P., *et al.* (2008). Transplacental transfer of acrylamide and glycidamide are comparable to that of antipyrine in perfused human placenta. *Toxicology Letters* **182**, 50–56.

67. Partanen, H.A., El-Nezami, H.S., Leppanen, J.M., *et al.* (2010). Aflatoxin B1 transfer and metabolism in human placenta. *Toxicological Sciences* **113**, 216–225.

68. Karttunen, V., Myllynen, P., Prochazka, G., *et al.* (2010). Placental transfer and DNA binding of benzo(a)pyrene in human placental perfusion. *Toxicology Letters* **197**, 75–81.

69. Myllynen, P.K., Loughran, M.J., Howard, C.V., *et al.* (2008). Kinetics of gold nanoparticles in the human placenta. *Reproductive Toxicology* **26**, 130–137.

70. Mose, T., Knudsen, L.E., Hedegaard, M., *et al.* (2007). Transplacental transfer of monomethyl phthalate and mono(2-ethylhexyl) phthalate in a human placenta perfusion system. *International Journal of Toxicology* **26**, 221–229.

71. Bremer, S., Brittebo, E., Dencker, L., *et al.* (2007). *In vitro* tests for detecting chemicals affecting the embryo implantation process. The report and recommendations of ECVAM Workshop 62: A strategic workshop of the EU ReProTect project. *ATLA* **35**, 421–439.

72. Myllynen, P., Mathiesen, L., Weimer, M., *et al.* (2010). Preliminary interlaboratory comparison of the ex vivo dual human placental perfusion system. *Reproductive Toxicology* **30**, 94–102.

73. Poulsen, M.S., Rytting, E., Mose, T., *et al.* (2009). Modeling placental transport: correlation of *in vitro* BeWo cell permeability and ex vivo human placental perfusion. *Toxicology in Vitro* **23**, 1380–1386.

74. Dusinska, M., Dusinska, M., Fjellsbo, L., *et al.* (2009). Testing strategies for the safety of nanoparticles used in medical applications. *Nanomedicine, London* **4**, 605–607.

75. Taxvig, C., Hadrup, N., Boberg, J., *et al.* (2013). *In vitro–in vivo* correlations for endocrine activity of a mixture of currently used pesticides. *Toxicology and Applied Pharmacology* **272**, 757–766.

76. van der Burg, B., Wedebye, E.B., Dietrich, D.R., et al. (2015). The ChemScreen project to design a pragmatic alternative approach to predict reproductive toxicity of chemicals. Reproductive Toxicology 55, 114–123.

77. Long, M. & Bonefeld-Jørgensen, E.C. (2012). Dioxin-like activity in environmental and human samples from Greenland and Denmark. Chemosphere 89, 919–928.

78. Mørck, T.A., Erdmann, S.E., Long, M., et al. (2014). PCB concentrations and dioxin-like activity in blood samples from Danish school children and their mothers living in urban and rural areas. Basic and Clinical Pharmacology and Toxicology 115, 134–144.

79. Puurunen, J., Sotaniemi, E. & Pelkonen, O. (1980). Effect of cimetidine on microsomal drug metabolism in man. European Journal of Clinical Pharmacology 18, 185–187.

80. Pelkonen, O., Turpeinen, M., Hakkola, J., et al. (2008). Inhibition and induction of human cytochrome P450 enzymes: current status. Archives of Toxicology 82, 667–715.

81. Abass, K., Lämsä, V., Reponen, P., et al. (2012). Characterization of human cytochrome P450 induction by pesticides. Toxicology 294, 17–26.

82. Pelkonen, O., Tolonen, A., Rousu, T., et al. (2009). Comparison of metabolic stability and metabolite identification of 55 ECVAM/ICCVAM validation compounds between human and rat liver homogenates and microsomes – a preliminary analysis. ALTEX 26, 214–222.

83. Turpeinen, M., Tolonen, A., Chesne, C., et al. (2009). Functional expression, inhibition and induction of CYP enzymes in HepaRG cells. Toxicology in Vitro 23, 748–753.

84. Andersen, K.J., Maunsbach, A.B. & Christensen, E.I. (1998). Biochemical and ultrastructural characterization of fluid transporting LLC-PK1 microspheres. Journal of the American Society of Nephrology 9, 1153–1168.

85. Bjørge, C., Brunborg, G., Wiger, R., et al. (1996). A comparative study of chemically induced DNA damage in isolated human and rat testicular cells. Reproductive Toxicology 10, 509–519.

86. Collins, A.R., Oscoz, A.A., Brunborg, G., et al. (2008). The comet assay: topical issues. Mutagenesis 23, 143–151.

87. Collins, A., El Yamani, N. & Dusinska, M. (2017). Sensitive detection of DNA oxidation damage induced by nanomaterials. Free Radical Biology & Medicine 107, 69–76.

88. Doak, S.H. & Dusinska, M. (2017). NanoGenotoxicology: present and the future. Mutagenesis 32, 1–4.

89. Dusinska, M., Boland, S., Saunders, M., et al. (2015). Towards an alternative testing strategy for nanomaterials used in nanomedicine: lessons from NanoTEST. Nanotoxicology 9 (Supplément, Le. 1), 118–132.

90. Wallin, H., Jacobsen, N.R., White, P.A., et al. (2011). Mutagenicity of carbon nanomaterials. Journal of Biomedical Nanotechnology 7, 29.

91. Mikkelsen, L., Jensen, K.A., Koponen, I.K., et al. (2013). Cytotoxicity, oxidative stress and expression of adhesion molecules in human umbilical vein endothelial cells exposed to dust from paints with or without nanoparticles. Nanotoxicology 7, 117–134.

92. Jantzen, K., Moller, P., Karottki, D.G., et al. (2016). Exposure to ultrafine particles, intracellular production of reactive oxygen species in leukocytes and altered levels of endothelial progenitor cells. Toxicology 359–360, 11–18.

93. Kolman, A., Chovanec, M. & Osterman-Golkar, S. (2002). Genotoxic effects of ethylene oxide, propylene oxide and epichlorohydrin in humans: update review (1990–2001). Mutation Research 512, 173–194.

94. Sorsa, M. (1980). Cytogenetic methods in the detection of chemical carcinogens. Journal of Toxicology and Environmental Health 6, 1077–1080.

95. Vainio, H. & Sorsa, M. (1985). Application of short-term tests in monitoring occupational exposure to complex mixtures. In M.D. Waters, S.S. Sandhu, J. Lewtas, L. Claxton, G. Strauss & S. Nesnow (Eds.), Short-term Bioassays in the Analysis of Complex Environmental Mixtures IV, pp. 291–302. New York, NY, USA: Springer.

96. Bonassi, S., Hagmar, L., Stromberg, U., et al. (2000). Chromosomal aberrations in lymphocytes predict human cancer independently of exposure to carcinogens. Cancer Research 60, 1619–1625.

97. Raunio, H., Husgafvel-Pursiainen, K., Anttila, S., et al. (1995). Diagnosis of polymorphisms in carcinogen-activating and inactivating enzymes and cancer susceptibility – a review. Gene 159, 113–121.

98. Rämet, M., Castren, K., Jarvinen, K., et al. (1995). p53 protein expression is correlated with benzo[a]pyrene-DNA adducts in carcinoma cell lines. Carcinogenesis 16, 2117–2124.

99. Zheng, A., Castren, K., Saily, M., et al. (1999). P53 status of newly established acute myeloid leukaemia cell lines. British Journal of Cancer 79, 407–415.

100. Kummu, M., Sieppi, E., Wallin, K., et al. (2012). Cadmium inhibits ABCG2 transporter function in BeWo choriocarcinoma cells and MCF-7 cells overexpressing ABCG2. Placenta 33, 859–865.

101. Grafstrom, R.C., Curren, R.D., Yang, L.L., et al. (1986). Aldehyde-induced inhibition of DNA repair and potentiation of N-nitrosocompound-induced mutagenesis in cultured human cells. Progress in Clinical & Biological Research 209A, 255–264.

102. Sundqvist, K., Kulkarni, P., Hybbinette, S.S., et al. (1991). Serum-free growth and karyotype analyses of cultured normal and tumorous (SqCC/Y1) human buccal epithelial cells. Cancer Communications 3, 331–340.

103. Hedberg, J.J., Hansson, A., Nilsson, J.A., et al. (2001). Uniform expression of alcohol dehydrogenase 3 in epithelia regenerated with cultured normal, immortalised and malignant human oral keratinocytes. ATLA 29, 325–333.

104. Staab, C.A., Vondracek, M., Custodio, H., et al. (2004). Modelling of normal and premalignant oral tissue by using the immortalised cell line, SVpgC2a: a review of the value of the model. ATLA 32, 401–405.

105. Grafstrom, R.C., Nymark, P., Hongisto, V., et al. (2015). Toward the replacement of animal experiments through the bioinformatics-driven analysis of 'omics' data from human cell cultures. ATLA 43, 325–332.

106. Sandbacka, M., Christianson, I. & Isomaa, B. (2000). Gill epithelial cells as in vitro models in aquatic toxicology. ATLA 28, 457–460.

107. Christianson-Heiska, I. & Isomaa, B. (2008). The use of primaryhepatocytes from brown trout (Salmo trutta lacustris and the fish cell lines RTH-149 and ZF-L for *in vitro* screening of (anti)estrogenic activity of wood extractives. *Toxicology in Vitro* **23**, 589−597.

108. Christianson-Heiska, I., Smeds, P., Granholm, N., *et al.* (2007). Endocrine modulating actions of a phytosterol mixture and its oxidation products in zebrafish (Danio rerio). *Comparative Biochemistry and Physiology. Toxicology & Pharmacology* **145**, 518−527.

109. Bondarenko, O.M., Heinlaan, M., Sihtmae, M., *et al.* (2016). Multilaboratory evaluation of 15 bioassays for (eco)toxicity screening and hazard ranking of engineered nanomaterials: FP7 project NANOVALID. *Nanotoxicology* **10**, 1229−1242.

110. Bondarenko, O., Juganson, K., Ivask, A., *et al.* (2013). Toxicity of Ag, CuO and ZnO nanoparticles to selected environmentally relevant test organisms and mammalian cells *in vitro*: a critical review. *Archives of Toxicology* **87**, 1181−1200.

111. Mannerström, M., Zou, J., Toimela, T., *et al.* (2016). The applicability of conventional cytotoxicity assays to predict safety/toxicity of mesoporous silica nanoparticles, silver and gold nanoparticles and multi-walled carbon nanotubes. *Toxicology in Vitro* **37**, 113−120.

112. Bokan, K., Syberg, K., Jensen, K., *et al.* (2013). Genotoxic potential of two herbicides and their active ingredients assessed with comet assay on a fish cell line, epithelioma papillosum cyprini (EPC). *Journal of Toxicology and Environmental Health* **A 76**, 1129−1137.

113. Fenstad, A.A., Bustnes, J.O., Bingham, C.G., *et al.* (2016). DNA double-strand breaks in incubating female common eiders (Somateria mollissima): Comparison between a low and a high polluted area. *Environmental Research* **151**, 297−303.

114. Rovida, C., Basketter, D., Casati, S., *et al.* (2007). Management of an integrated project (Sens-it-iv) to develop *in vitro* tests to assess sensitisation. *ATLA* **35**, 317−322.

115. Johansson, H., Albrekt, A.S., Borrebaeck, C.A., *et al.* (2013). The GARD assay for assessment of chemical skin sensitizers. *Toxicology in Vitro* **27**, 1163−1169.

116. Richert, L., Baze, A., Parmentier, C., *et al.* (2016). Cytotoxicity evaluation using cryopreserved primary human hepatocytes in various culture formats. *Toxicology Letters* **258**, 207−215.

117. Dragovic, S., Vermeulen, N.P., Gerets, H.H., *et al.* (2016). Evidence-based selection of training compounds for use in the mechanism-based integrated prediction of drug-induced liver injury in man. *Archives of Toxicology* **90**, 2979−3003.

118. Goldring, C., Antoine, D.J., Bonner, F., *et al.* (2017). Stem cell-derived models to improve mechanistic understanding and prediction of human drug-induced liver injury. *Hepatology* **65**, 710−721.

119. Danish 3R Center. (2017). *Vision, Mission and Tasks*, 1pp. Available at: http://en.3rcenter.dk/about-us/vision-mission-and-tasks.

120. Walum, E., Sternberg, K. & Jenssen, D. (1990). *Understanding Cell Toxicology: Principles and Practice*, 201pp. New York, NY, USA: Ellis Horwood.

Chapter 2.6

The Three Rs and Alternatives in the Visegrád (V4) Countries

Miroslav Červinka[1], Zsolt Forgacs[2], Helena Kandarova[3] and Dariusz Śladowski[4]

[1]*Charles University Faculty of Medicine in Hradec Králové, Hradec Králove, Czech Republic;* [2]*Independent Researcher, Budapest, Hungary;* [3]*MatTek In Vitro Life Science Laboratories, Bratislava, Slovak Republic;* [4]*Medical University of Warsaw, Warsaw, Poland*

SUMMARY

The Visegrád (V4) Group is a cultural and political alliance of four Central European nations, namely, the Czech Republic, Hungary, Poland and Slovakia. They have long had animal welfare interests and regulations, but their activities in relation to animal experimentation and alternative methods became more focused when they joined the EU in 2004 and adapted their national legislation for comply with *Directive 86/609/EEC* and later with *Directive 2010/63/EU*. Today, their scientists and institutions have many collaborations with others in the EU and beyond, but activities are also organised within the V4 Group itself.

1. CENTRAL EUROPEAN COUNTRIES JOIN WESTERN EUROPEAN COUNTRIES IN THE EU

The period covered by this book has seen profound political and social changes in Central Europe. When Russell and Burch's *The Principles of Humane Experimental Technique* (1) was published in 1959, the Soviet Union and seven of its satellite countries were united by a mutual defence treaty, the Warsaw Pact, in response to the perceived threat represented by the formation of NATO by the USA and the countries of Western Europe. However, by the late 1980s, the communist regimes had been overthrown in Bulgaria, Czechoslovakia, East Germany, Hungary, Poland and Romania. The Soviet Union itself was dissolved in 1991 and became 15 separate countries. On 1 January 1993, Czechoslovakia became two separate republics, the Czech Republic and Slovakia.

In 2004, eight former communist countries (the Czech Republic, Estonia, Hungary, Latvia, Lithuania, Poland, Slovenia and Slovakia) joined the EU, followed by Bulgaria and Romania in 2007 and Croatia in 2013.

The new EU Member States had to adapt their national laws to comply with *Directive 86/609/EEC* on the protection of animals used for experimental and other scientific purposes, and later, to comply with *Directive 2010/63/EU* (2), which replaced it. However, it should not be assumed that they had previously had no interest in animal welfare and that animal experimentation was not regulated.

As with adaptation to comply with other legislation, the European Commission gave advice and support to the new Member States. In the case of the Three Rs and alternative methods, this involved the European Centre for the Validation of Alternative Methods (ECVAM), in part via a series of events (3), including the following:

1. An international symposium on promotion of the Three Rs concept in Slovakia, Slovenia and the Czech Republic in June 2001 in Prague, Czech Republic, organised with the Charles University Faculty of Medicine in Hradec Králové, the National Institute of Public Health, Prague, and the Central Commission for Animal Welfare, Prague, and attended by 120 participants.

The History of Alternative Test Methods in Toxicology. https://doi.org/10.1016/B978-0-12-813697-3.00009-3

2. A workshop on the validation of alternative methods for regulatory toxicity testing, organised with ESTIV at ECVAM in November 2001.
3. A workshop on alternatives in higher education, in April 2002 in Piran, Slovenia.
4. A workshop on the promotion of the Three Rs concept in Estonia, Latvia, Lithuania and Poland, co-organised with the Department of Transplantology and Central Tissue Bank of the Medical University of Warsaw, in May 2002 in Warsaw, Poland.
5. A workshop on alternatives, in October 2002 in Balatonfüred, Hungary, in cooperation with the University of Veszprem, which involved participants from Bulgaria, Hungary, Romania and Slovenia.
6. A workshop on the use of computer models in chemical risk assessment, in October 2002 in Prague, Czech Republic, organised with the Czech National Institute of Public Health.
7. A training course on *in vitro* methods for pyrogenicity testing, in September 2003 in Budapest, Hungary.
8. Two training courses on the *in vitro* production of monoclonal antibodies, in March 2004 and 23–26 November 2004, organised in cooperation with Conraad Hendriksen and his team at The Netherlands Vaccine Institute, Bilthoven.
9. A JRC Enlargement Workshop for stakeholders, organised in cooperation with ecopa to promote the creation of national platforms on alternatives in accession countries, in June 2004 in Prague, Czech Republic.
10. A workshop on Three Rs approaches in the quality control of veterinary vaccines, from 29 November to 2 December, 2004 at Langen, Germany, organised by Klaus Cussler and his team at the Paul-Ehrlich-Institut.
11. A JRC Enlargement and Integration Workshop on promotion of the Three Rs, in September 2005 in Ljubljana, Slovenia, with 67 participants from Croatia, Macedonia, Serbia and Montenegro and Turkey.
12. A JRC Enlargement and Integration Workshop on alternative methods, in November 2007 at Ankara, Turkey, co-organised by ECVAM with Hacettepe University and the Turkish Pharmacological Society, and attended by 150 participants from Turkey.

Initially, new Member States were entitled to nominate a member of the ECVAM Scientific Advisory Committee, but the committee's organisation was subsequently reformed. ECVAM also received visiting scientists from Eastern Europe, including Dariusz Śladowski (Poland) and Lena Buzanska (Poland), national experts, including Sonja Jeram (Slovenia), and PhD students, including Agnieszka Kinsner (Poland, now a member of staff at ECVAM) and Iglika Lessigiarska (Bulgaria).

In this chapter, we focus on developments in what are now known as the four Visegrád countries, the Czech Republic, Hungary, Poland and Slovakia.

2. INITIAL THREE RS DEVELOPMENTS IN CZECHOSLOVAKIA

The international contacts made by Miroslav Červinka in the 1980s were crucial to the recognition of the Three Rs in Czechoslovakia. Since 1987, he had worked on *in vitro* methods of toxicity assessment at the Charles University Faculty of Medicine in Hradec Králové, primarily because of their scientific advantages, rather than in relation to animal protection. Between 1975 and 1989, he actively participated in several international scientific events in Hungary and Germany.

At that time in Czechoslovakia, there was only a small community of people working with cells cultured *in vitro*. The team in Hradec Králové collaborated closely with the group of Oldrich Nečas and Augustin Svoboda in the Department of Biology, Faculty of Medicine in Brno. Michael Balls had visited Prague and Brno in April 1988, as a result of which Miroslav Červinka was invited to participate in the *Second International Conference on Practical In Vitro Toxicology*, which took place in Nottingham in July 1989, where he met Horst Spielmann, Richard Clothier and Björn Ekwall, among others.

Soon after the revolution in 1989, and in an attempt to change the attitudes of teachers and students, a Committee for the Proper Use of Laboratory Animals was established at the Faculty of Medicine in Hradec Králové. Special rules for using laboratory animals in education and research at the university were adopted, which are still valid today, although very few animals are now used.

3. THREE RS ACTIVITIES IN THE CZECH REPUBLIC

3.1 The TEMPUS Joint European Project

During a visit to Michael Balls and Richard Clothier in the Department of Human Morphology at the University of Nottingham Medical School in January 1991, Miroslav Červinka prepared a proposal for a TEMPUS Joint European Project, which was accepted as Project No. 1485 on *Alternatives to Experiments with Animals in Medical Education*.

The project ran from 1993 to 1995, and was based on collaboration between the Charles University Faculty of Medicine in Hradec Králové (Department of Biology), Nottingham University Medical School, FRAME, the Free University of Berlin, and ZEBET.

The primary goal of this project was to introduce the Three Rs concept and practical approaches to alternatives to animal experiments into the whole educational system at the universities of the Czech Republic. The results were significant improvements in the curricula at medical faculties; the establishment of committees for the proper use of animals at medical faculties; the preparation of new rules and regulations for controlling the use of animals in education and research at medical faculties; training in the practical use of alternative methods; and the production and exchange of the new teaching materials concerning alternatives.

The TEMPUS project promoted cooperation with several West European institutions and very substantially affected the situation at the Faculty of Medicine in Hradec Králové. The main long-lasting achievement of the project was to change the attitudes of staff and students and make them aware of the scientific and ethical value of alternative approaches.

The results of the project were discussed at a meeting held in Hradec Králové in May 1994, the proceedings of which were published in Czech and English (4).

3.2 World Congresses on Alternatives

Crucial to developments in the Czech Republic was participation in *The First World Congress on Alternatives and Animal Use in the Life Sciences*, held in Baltimore, Maryland, in 1993. The Czech participants gained an overall view of what was happening in the world of alternatives. Several important personal contacts were made, including contact with Nick Jukes, who subsequently made valuable educational materials available from InterNICHE. A meeting with William Russell was particularly memorable.

Czech scientists also participated in subsequent world congresses, including those in Utrecht (1996), Bologna (1999) and New Orleans (2002).

As a result of the increasing involvement of Czech scientists in the development and application of alternative methods, the *9th World Congress on Alternatives and Animal Use in the Life Sciences* took place in Prague on 24–28 August 2014. The Congress Co-chairs were Dagmar Jirová and Horst Spielmann, and the theme of the Congress was *Humane Science in the 21st Century*. At the Gala Dinner, Michael Balls gave a memorable speech, in which he said that *The time has come to plan for a future where the Three Rs will have served their purpose, animal experimentation will have been consigned to history, and humane biomedical science in research, testing and education will have become the norm, for the benefit of humans and animals alike* (5).

3.3 Visit of Professor William Russell in 1997

After the meeting in Baltimore in 1993, William Russell was invited to visit the Czech Republic in October 1997, where he gave lectures at meetings of the J.E. Purkyne Society in the Faculty of Medicine in Hradec Králové and in the Carolinum Hall at Charles University, Prague. Reminiscences of this much-appreciated visit were published in *ATLA* (6).

3.4 Alternatives Conference in Prague, 2001

An international symposium on promotion of the Three Rs concept in Slovakia, Slovenia and the Czech Republic took place in Prague in 2001. The meeting was organised by the Charles University Faculty of Medicine in Hradec Králové, the National Institute of Public Health, Prague, and the Central Commission for Animal Welfare, Prague, as a result of an initiative by ECVAM to promote the Three Rs concept in what were then known as the PECO countries (Countries of Central and Eastern Europe).

This was the first meeting of its kind in that part of the world, with the aim of bringing together representatives of academia, industry, animal welfare and government. It was not easy to achieve this aim, as there had been few previous contacts between the various stakeholders in some of the countries. Nevertheless, the meeting was successful. It was attended by 120 participants from 10 countries and was covered by the main news programme on Czech television, and Miroslav Červinka and Michael Balls were invited to take part in a live television discussion programme.

3.5 SSCT Meeting, 2009

A request by the Scandinavian Society of Cell Toxicology (SSCT) that its 27th annual meeting should be held in the Czech Republic received a positive response, and Zuzana Červinková was the principal organiser of the workshop, which took place on 16–19 September 2009 at Lázně Sedmihorky, in the beautiful Bohemian Paradise region close to Hradec Králové. During the workshop, which was attended by 120 participants from 15 countries, the Björn Ekwall Memorial Award was presented to Dr Annalaura Stammati from Italy.

3.6 Major Collaborations

Czech scientists have long had good relations with ECVAM, and Dagmar Jirová is currently a member of the ECVAM Scientific Advisory Committee. Miroslav Červinka participated in a number of ECVAM workshops, of which that on Good Laboratory Practice in *in vitro* studies (7) was particularly important.

Cooperation between Horst Spielmann and Manfred Liebsch, at ZEBET, and Zuzanna Červinková and Miroslav Červinka, at Hradec Králové, began with the TEMPUS project, and later, they together organised the first German-Czech Animal Welfare Symposium, held in Prague in March 1999. This collaboration also resulted in the annual international Three Rs meetings held each year since 1992 in Linz, Austria, which are now organised by the European Society for Alternatives to Animal Testing (EUSAAT).

Collaboration with FRAME and the University of Nottingham was particularly important, initially via the TEMPUS project, but then when Michael Balls became Head of ECVAM in 1993. Miroslav Červinka has been a member of the Editorial Board of FRAME's journal, *ATLA*, for many years.

Another interaction of the Czech Republic has been with ecopa. In 2003, 10 scientists established a Czech branch, called CZECOPA, the main aims of which are to circulate information on alternative methods and stimulate contacts between the various stakeholders — in academia, government, industry and animal welfare.

3.7 Government Organisations

The head of the Centre for Toxicology and Health Safety at the National Institute for Public Health is Dagmar Jirová. The activities of the Centre are focused on topics covered by *Act No. 258/2000 Coll. Law*, on public health protection and related requirements on health and safety for consumer products and their ingredients. The research units of the Centre develop new test methods, conduct validation studies on these methods, and cooperate on a national and international basis with other scientific institutes (including the Joint Research Centre of the EU). The laboratories of the Centre conduct some physical, chemical, microbiological and toxicological tests at the request of the regulatory authorities. Experts from the Centre represent the Czech Republic in the expert committees and regulatory bodies of the EU and the Council of Europe.

The Centre's Unit for Alternative Toxicological methods performs *in vitro* laboratory tests and participates in the development, validation and implementation of alternative toxicological test methods.

3.8 The State Veterinary Administration

The State Veterinary Administration is a public administration body related to the Ministry of Agriculture of the Czech Republic, which was established according to *Veterinary Act No. 166/1999*.

Its purpose is primarily the protection of consumers from products of animal origin which are likely to be harmful to human health, the monitoring of animal health and veterinary protection, via supervision of the protection of farm animals, companion animals and wild animals and of the breeding and use of experimental animals.

A committee for protection of animals used for scientific purposes was established by Ministry of Agriculture under *Act No 246/1992 Sb*, and provides advisory information related to experimental animals and to the fulfilment of the requirements of *Directive 2010/63/EU on the protection of animals used for scientific purposes* (2).

4. ACTIVITIES IN SLOVAKIA

4.1 Early Developments in Slovakia

A number of universities and several institutes of the Slovak Academy of Sciences had already started to use *in vitro* cell culture techniques during the Czechoslovak era. One of the pioneers, who brought these techniques to Slovakia and significantly contributed to their practical implementation, was Ivan Stanek. His early work was an inspiration to many of his pupils and followers (8). *In vitro* cell cultures were also used by the Slovak pharmaceutical industry. For example, by the late 1950s, the IMUNA company, founded in 1953 in Šariské Michaľany, recognised the benefits of *in vitro* techniques in the production of vaccines and biologicals.

The use of cell cultures in research was mainly due to their scientific and practical benefits, rather than to ethical considerations. The Three Rs concept was recognised in Slovakia much later, mainly in connection with the legislative changes made during the process of joining the EU. These changes included the ban on testing cosmetic products in animals, the acceptance of validated alternative methods into the EU legislation and regulatory toxicology, and the requirements of *Directive 86/609/EEC* on the protection of animals used for experimental and other scientific purposes. When Slovakia joined the EU in 2004, the number of animals used for experimental purposes started to decline.

The international symposium on promotion of the Three Rs concept in Slovakia, Slovenia and the Czech Republic that took place in Prague in 2001, greatly increased understanding of the importance of alternative tests and the need for their independent validation. The discussion also focused on the implementation of the Three Rs in basic research and education. Slovakia was represented on the scientific programme, with four lectures from the Slovak University of Technology, the Slovak Academy of Sciences and the private pharmaceutical sector (the VULM company).

4.2 The National Scientific Network on Alternative Methods

The Slovak Ministry of Agriculture and Rural Development was appointed as the single contact point under Article 47 (5) of *Directive 2010/63/EU* on the protection of animals used for scientific purposes.

The Ministry established a national scientific network on alternative methods (the NOVS Committee), to actively support Slovak's representation in EURL ECVAM's Network for Preliminary Assessment of Regulatory Relevance (PARERE). The membership of the national network includes representatives of the Ministry of Agriculture and Rural Development, the State Veterinary and Food Administration, the Ministry of the Environment, the Public Health Authority, the Slovak Academy of Sciences, the Slovak Technical University and the private sector, including MatTek In Vitro Life Science Laboratories (MatTek IVLSL) and Hameln rds. Members of the NOVS are regularly updated about EURL ECVAM activities and provide their scientific expertise and comments to the documentation circulated to the PARERE network. Some of the NOVS Committee experts also work on OECD Test Guidelines expert panels.

4.3 The Slovak Toxicology Society

The most active organisation in Slovakia in relation to toxicology is the Slovak Toxicology Society (SETOX), which was established in 2006 by splitting from the Slovak Medical Society. SETOX is a member of the Federation of European Toxicologists and the European Societies of Toxicology (EUROTOX).

SETOX has four divisions, namely, experimental toxicology, clinical toxicology, industrial toxicology and *in vitro* toxicology. The *in vitro* division was established by Helena Kandarova in 2011 and became a platform to promote alternative methods within the Slovak scientific community. The mission of the *in vitro* division is

- to promote *in vitro* toxicology and its development;
- to support the practical implementation of *in vitro* methods;
- to stimulate, support and promote the use of *in vitro* tests in the field of education;
- to serve as an information channel between national and international groups interested in toxicology *in vitro*; and
- to organise scientific seminars on *in vitro* methods.

Every 2 years, SETOX organises the TOXCON conferences in Slovakia. This conference series has gained an international reputation and has become one of the renowned, most highly appreciated conferences in central and eastern European countries, with the complimentary attribute of "having a family atmosphere". In addition to its regular participants, many outstanding specialists from Austria, Estonia, Germany, Hungary, India, Iran, Israel, Italy, Poland, Spain, Sweden, Turkey and the USA have participated in TOXCON. It is rather encouraging that the number of participants has been steadily growing (9). The programme of the conference traditionally includes a session that discusses the alternative methods and the Three Rs concept.

SETOX, in collaboration with its corporate member, MatTek IVLSL, organises courses on methods that can be used to replace animal procedures. The courses include hands-on training, as well as theoretical discussions, allowing trainees to experience the technology in practice, under the supervision of experts.

The members of SETOX are also actively involved in various national and international committees related to toxicology and pharmacology. There is a very close and long-lasting collaboration with Czech societies active in the toxicology and with EUROTOX. One of the major achievements of SETOX was the organisation of the EUROTOX 2017 congress in Bratislava, Slovakia, which was attended by more than 1200 participants from 53 countries and included many sessions that were focused on *in vitro* toxicology.

In February 2018, members of NOVS and external invited experts on alternative methods endorsed the establishment of the Slovak National Platform for Three Rs (SNP 3Rs). The platform was officially launched at the the annual SETOX meeting at High Tatras on 21 June 2018, on the occasion of the TOXICON 2018 conference. The SNP 3Rs will operate with the support of SETOX, and will stimulate the development and implementation of alternative methods which can replace, reduce and refine animal experimentation in Slovakia.

4.4 Interdisciplinary Toxicology

Since 2008, SETOX, in close cooperation with the Institute of Experimental Pharmacology and Toxicology of the Slovak Academy of Sciences, has published an international journal, *Interdisciplinary Toxicology*, which is indexed in several world scientific databases. *Interdisciplinary Toxicology* publishes original papers, review articles and clinical reports on research related to the toxicity of chemicals and their mixtures at the molecular, cellular, tissue, target organ and whole body levels *in vivo* (by all routes of exposure) and *in vitro/ex vivo*. The focus is on all aspects of modern toxicology, including pharmacotoxicological and metabolic mechanisms, toxicogenomics and proteomics, pharmacokinetics, developmental toxicity, carcinogenesis and mutagenesis, environmental toxicity and environmental health concerning humans (including epidemiological studies), forensic toxicity, immunotoxicity, pesticides, predictive toxicology, risk assessment, and the use of alternative methods in toxicity testing.

4.5 The State Veterinary and Food Administration of the Slovak Republic

The State Veterinary and Food Administration of the Slovak Republic (SVFA SR) is the Slovakian administrative authority concerned with the laws on veterinary care and protection, *Act of the Slovak National Council No 39/2007 Coll.*, and on food products, *Act of the Slovak National Council No 152/1995 Coll.* The SVFA SR is the national contact point for the implementation of *Directive 2010/63/EU.* As the sole competent authority, it evaluates, regulates and approves proposals for animal experiments. It also approves and regulates animal breeding houses, conducts inspections and ensures the compliance of breeders and suppliers, as well as the users of the animals, with the national and EU legislation. By means of its web-page, the SVFA SR informs about new EU legislation related to animal protection. The SVFA SR is the expert guarantor of educational seminars and training courses in the areas of animal use and animal protection.

4.6 The Private Sector

There are two private organisations with significant input in relation to the concept of Three Rs in Slovakia.

Hameln rds, located in Modra, Slovakia, is a well-known pharmaceutical service provider for the health-care industry. It focuses on various stages in the development and production of pharmaceutical products, including quality control and good manufacturing practice, and preclinical and toxicological testing *in vivo* and *in vitro*. Hameln has been a member of EURL ECVAM's Network of Laboratories for the Validation of Alternative Methods (NETVASL) since 2015, and is also a member of the NOVS Committee.

Toxicology services in Modra had already started in the 1970s, when the Drug Research Institute was established there. In 1996, the state institute was transformed into VULM, a joint-stock company, with Slovakofarma as its main shareholder. In 2006, Hameln rds acquired all the VULM shares.

The second private organisation, MatTek IVLSL, was established in 2009 in Bratislava, as a wholly-owned subsidiary of the MatTek Corporation, Ashland, MA, USA, a world-leading pioneer in the development and application of reconstituted human tissue models, such as Epiderm and EpiOcular. MatTek is actively involved in *in vitro* toxicology throughout the world (10). The facility in Bratislava is very active in European validation studies and research projects leading to the development of new alternative methods. In addition to production and research activities, it also provides training for scientists in the application of selected OECD test methods and, in general, tissue and cell culture practice. MatTek IVLSL is a corporate member and supporter, not only of SETOX, but also of the European Society for Toxicology in Vitro (ESTIV), the European Society for Alternatives to Animal Testing (EUSAAT) and the Italian Association of In Vitro Toxicology (CellTox).

4.7 International Collaboration

There have long been very good relationships between Czech and Slovak scientists, involving collaborations which were not significantly affected by the division of Czechoslovakia in 1993. There is extensive cooperation between SETOX and the Toxicological Section of the Czech Society for Experimental and Clinical Pharmacology and Toxicology of the Czech Medical Association of J.E. Purkyně, aimed mainly at the joint organisation of conferences and specialised educational courses.

With the now-open borders, it is easier for many students and young scientists to establish contacts and acquire knowledge at renowned institutions and universities. For example, Helena Kandarova had a unique opportunity in 2003, to visit ZEBET and participate in the development and validation of *in vitro* skin irritation test projects sponsored by ECVAM and the German Federal Institute for Risk Assessment, and led by Manfred Liebsch and Horst Spielmann. The visit, initially planned for 1 year, was prolonged to 3 years and resulted in a PhD thesis on the use of reconstructed tissue models in the regulatory toxicology (11). The knowledge gained at ZEBET on the conduct of multi-centre validation studies on alternative methods, significantly helped in other projects on other reconstructed tissue. Unfortunately, so far, no Slovak scientists have had the opportunity to work directly at EURL ECVAM.

5. ACTIVITIES IN HUNGARY

5.1 Organisations

The Toxicological Section of the Hungarian Society for Experimental and Clinical Pharmacology was established in 1984, and in 1992, a new and separate organisation, the Hungarian Toxicology Society, was created. In 1995, the union of these two organisations formed the Hungarian Society of Toxicologists (MTE), which was transformed into the Society of Hungarian Toxicologists (MTT) in 2003. MTT is a member of the Federation of European Toxicologists and European Societies of Toxicology (EUROTOX) and of the International Union of Toxicology (IUTOX). The Society's activities cover chemical carcinogenesis, clinical toxicology, environmental toxicology, immunotoxicology, neurotoxicology, occupational toxicology, pesticide toxicology, pharmacotoxicology, teratology, toxicokinetics and toxicological biochemistry. Two separate sections are for drug safety and environmental toxicology specialists, but there is no section for *in vitro* toxicology. The Society organises an annual scientific conference, where members active in *in vitro* toxicology have an opportunity to present their latest achievements.

5.2 Governmental Institutions

In Hungary, there is currently no state reference laboratory or any other significant testing facility which specialises in the development or performance of *in vitro* toxicology tests. In the National Public Health Center (NPHC), part of the National Public Health and Medical Officer Service (NPHMOS), there was a small, GLP-certified research laboratory (Division of In Vitro Toxicology), which had started in the early 1990s in the National Institute of Occupational Health. It focused on the culture of various steroidogenic primary gonadal cell cultures for studies on endocrine disruptors and reproductive toxicants. Later, several OECD validated cell line and 3-D tissue-based test methods were adopted, including local skin irritation/corrosion and eye irritation tests. For the promotion of the 3-D tissue-based test methods in Hungary, they reviewed the latest research of this field in a Hungarian scientific journal (12). In 2017, during a reorganisation, this laboratory was closed, but some basic *in vitro* tests (for cytotoxicity and genotoxicity) are available in the National Public Health Institute (the reorganized NPHC).

In the Department of Hygiene at the Plant Protection Institute of Pannonian University (Keszthely), the eye irritation effects of chemicals (mainly agrochemicals) have been studied *in vitro* since the 1990s, with the HET-CAM test (13, 14). Several diploma theses and science degrees were based on this research, and the results have been consistently incorporated into the teaching materials of a graduate and doctoral training and doctoral programme (e.g. on alternative methods in toxicology).

5.3 The Private Sector

Three main contract research organisations (CROs) are involved in the provision of alternatives toxicity tests in Hungary.

Toxi-Coop Ltd. is a European, non-clinical CRO with two research sites in Hungary, at Dunakeszi and Balatonfüred. It was founded in 1982 as a joint venture of eight, formerly state-owned Hungarian pharmaceutical companies. Today, Toxi-Coop is a fully privately-owned CRO, which serves the chemical, agrochemical and pharmaceutical industries. It is certified and complies with GLP and ISO 9001. Its studies are conducted in accordance with the regulatory requirements of the OECD, ICH, FDA, EMEA and OPPTS. In addition to *in vivo* studies, a wide range of OECD-accepted *in vitro* genotoxicology and topical irritation/corrosion tests are offered to clients.

CitoxLAB is an international CRO (with laboratories in Canada, Denmark and France, as well as in Hungary), which was created through the merger of CIT and LAB-Research. In GLP-compliant and AAALAC (Association for Assessment and Accreditation of Laboratory Animal Care International)-certified facilities, the company conducts non-clinical *in vivo* and *in vitro* safety studies for the agrochemical, biotechnology, chemical, cosmetics, food, medical device and agrochemical industries. It has extensive experience in test development, managing international validation studies, writing OECD test guidelines, and performing *in vitro* toxicology studies to meet international requirements for regulatory labelling purposes (including CLP/GHS). The Hungarian affiliate is located in Veszprém-Szabadságpuszta. Among their in vitro studies, there are several OECD-accepted genotoxicology and topical irritation/corrosion tests.

ATRC Aurigon Ltd., established in 2000, is an independent, privately-owned CRO, dedicated to providing preclinical services for food, chemicals and human and veterinary pharmaceuticals. The company provides a full range of advisory and experimental services in pharmacology, bio-analytics and toxicology. With its international headquarters in Munich, Germany, Aurigon operates GLP-compliant and/or GMP-compliant facilities in Dunakeszi. The company also conducts some *in vitro* toxicology tests (for genotoxicity and cytotoxicity).

5.4 International Collaborations

As mentioned above, an ECVAM workshop on alternative test methods took place in October 2002, in Balatonfüred, Hungary, in cooperation with the University of Veszprem, which involved participants from Bulgaria, Romania and Slovenia, as well as from Hungary. Also, a training course on *in vitro* methods for pyrogenicity testing took place, in September 2003, in Budapest, Hungary.

The Division of In Vitro Toxicology in the NPHC had two successful collaborations with Slovakian partners. For more than two decades, they worked together with Department of Animal Physiology in the Slovak University of Agriculture, Nitra, on *in vitro* reproductive toxicology. Several Slovakian PhD students began their research by working with cell cultures in Budapest. The results of the collaborative experiments were published in various international scientific journals (e.g. 15–17) and were also presented at the annual international scientific conferences on *Risk Factors of Food Chain*. The 18th conference took place in Żmiąca, Poland, in September 2017, under the auspices of the Slovak University of Agriculture, the Pedagogical University of Kraków, Poland, the University of Rzeszów, Poland, and the Szent István University Gödöllő, Hungary.

Another major collaboration has been with MatTek IVLSL in Bratislava, where Hungarian scientists were trained to perform the 3-D tissue-based *in vitro* skin irritation test according to OECD TG 439.

5.5 Journal

Egészségtudomány is the journal for science and continuing education of the Hungarian Hygiene Society, which publishes four issues per year in the Hungarian language, with English abstracts. The Journal publishes original papers and review articles related to toxicology, including *in vitro* methods.

Acta Veterinaria Hungarica is a quarterly publication of the Hungarian Academy of Sciences. It publishes original research papers and a limited number of reviews and clinical case reports, on veterinary physiology, clinical veterinary science, microbiology, parasitology, pathology and reproduction. In addition, the journal sometimes publishes articles on toxicology, including *in vitro* toxicology.

6. THREE RS DEVELOPMENTS IN POLAND

6.1 Animal Experimentation in Poland

The first regulations on the protection of animals used for food and in research in Poland were introduced between 1918 and 1939. After the end of the First World War, when Poland regained its independence after almost 123 years, the State Temporary Committee for Nature Conservation at the Ministry of Religious Denominations and Public Education was established. The Regulation of the President of the Republic of 22 March 1928 on the protection of animals prohibited cruelty to animals. It forbade 'any kind of suffering to be inflicted on animals without a valid and just need'. Experiments on animals for scientific purposes were only allowed, if they were necessary for the conduct of fundamental and applied science.

The progress being made stalled during the Second World War and during the communist period (1945−89), since human beings had limited freedom and animal welfare was viewed to be of relatively little importance. There was little recognition of human rights, let alone animal rights. The adoption in 1977 by UNESCO of the World Declaration of Animal Rights was undoubtedly an important event.

In 1997, the Polish Parliament stated that 'An animal, being a living creature capable of suffering, is not a thing. Man owes him respect and protection'. In September that year, as a contribution to the harmonisation of Polish legislation with that of other European countries, the Polish Parliament adopted the *Animal Protection Act*, which was compliant with the principles of *Council of Europe Convention ETS 123 1986* and *Directive 86/609/EEC. Chapter 9, Article 28*, of the Act, clearly stated that experiments on animals can be justified for scientific purposes, for teaching in universities and for the protection of human and/or animal health, but only when no appropriate alternative methods are available. No animal experimentation is allowed without the positive approval of the appropriate ethical committee, and such experiments can only be performed at accredited institutions. In September 1999, the head of the State Committee for Scientific Research appointed 17 Local Ethics Committees and the National Animal Ethics Committee, consisting of 15 members, 12 members representing the biological sciences, medical sciences, veterinary sciences and the humanities and three members from non-governmental animal welfare organisations. The system was substantially improved in 2005, when a new law was enacted, which was fully implementing *Directive 86/609/EEC* on the protection of animals used for experimental and other scientific purposes, which was before Poland joined the EU. This system included a requirement for attendance at a Three Rs course for those who wanted to perform animal experiments and an in-depth analysis of the availability of alternative methods.

From the moment when Poland joined the EU, the number of animal procedures in Poland decreased steadily until 2014, and has then remained at an almost constant level of about 170,000 animals per year. This can be attributed to the rapid development and modernisation of Polish industries and represents a tendency similar that in Europe as a whole.

In 2015, a new Animal Protection Act (implementing *Directive 2010/63/EU*) was adopted by the Polish Parliament, putting more emphasis on the implementation of the Three Rs. The Act requires a limit to the number of animals used in a given procedure, that animals be kept under conditions appropriate for their species, and that pain, suffering and prolonged stress are eliminated or kept to an unavoidable minimum. The introduction of new regulations and the availability of European funds has resulted in a thorough modernisation of existing animal facilities. Laboratory animals in Poland are now maintained under conditions that meet the highest European standards. Some of the challenges experienced in the transposition of the EU Directive into Polish law, along with perspectives of Polish scientists on the state-of-play of the Three Rs in Poland, were described by Zwolińska (18).

6.2 The Promotion of Alternatives

As with initial developments in Czechoslovakia, the early stages of recognition of the significance of the Three Rs in Poland began as a result of personal contacts among scientists. Through their respective roles as Vice-President and Secretary-General of the European Cell Biology Organisation, a friendship developed between Kazimierz Ostrowski, of the Department of Histology, Warsaw Medical University, and Michael Balls, of the University of Nottingham Medical School. As a result, two young medical scientists, first Witek Lasek and then Dariusz Śladowski, both spent a year in Nottingham, where they also interacted with FRAME (19, 20).

Then, between 1998 and 2003, Śladowski made three extended work experience visits to ECVAM, where, with Marlies Halder and ECVAM's support, he organised *Alternatives 2002* in Warsaw, an international workshop on the promotion of the Three Rs concept in Estonia, Latvia, Lithuania and Poland. Shortly afterwards, he was chairman of the organising committee for *INVITOX 2004*, the 13th international workshop of the European Society for Toxicology *In Vitro*, held in cooperation with the Scandinavian Society for Cell Toxicology in Zergrze, near Warsaw. The workshop was attended by about 200 participants and resulted in numerous future international project involving Polish laboratories.

In 2003, Śladowski also organised the Conference on Alternatives to the Use of Animals in Higher Education (18—20 October 2003 in Warsaw), which resulted in numerous collaborations among scientists in Poland. Shortly afterwards, Konrad Rydzyński and Maciej Stępniac, from the Nofer Institute, Łódz, established the National Centre for Alternative Methods in Toxicity Assessment (NCAM). They created a website devoted to the Three Rs, *Vitryna*, which became the primary source of knowledge about alternatives for Polish-speaking scientists and animal rights activists. The Nofer Institute is still involved in the development of alternative methods, as a member of the EU Network of Laboratories for the Validation of Alternative Methods (EU-NETVAL). A second Polish member of the Network is a private commercial company, Selvita S.A., which was founded in 2007. It is now one of the largest drug discovery companies in Europe. It currently employs more than 400 scientists, of whom 30% have PhDs. The company's headquarters are in Krakow, with a second research site in Poznan, and foreign offices located in Cambridge, MA, and the San Francisco Bay Area, California, USA as well as in Cambridge, UK.

In 2005, The Polcopa Founding Committee was established. The platform has involved representatives of the governmental institutions such as the National Ethics Committee on Animal Experimentation (Dariusz Śladowski), NCAM (Maiej Stępniac), the Polish Academy of Sciences (Barbara Pastuszewska), as well as cosmetic companies such as the Dr Irena Eris Cosmetic Laboratories (Renata Dębrowska), Procter & Gamble (Mikolai Józefowicz) and animal welfare groups, namely, the Polish Society for Protection of Animals (Wojciech Muża) and the GAJA Association for Animal Protection (Pawel Grzybowski).

The involvement of industry and academia in various activities has resulted in several meetings to promote the Three Rs concept widely in Poland. This was of crucial significance during the phasing out of the acceptance animal testing for cosmetics purposes in the EU.

6.3 International Scientific Collaboration

It should be recognised that the cooperation with FRAME in the early 1990s, and later with ECVAM, resulted in the establishment in Poland of the first on-line access system for INVITTOX protocols and ECVAM reports via Warsaw Medical University. The service was provided for several years, until the establishment of DB-ALM, when its contents were transferred to ECVAM. Several students were involved with Dariusz Śladowski in the project, including Kamil Lipski, Sebastian Majewski and Agnieszka Kinsner. These young scientists were also involved in laboratory work on alternative methods.

Warsaw Medical University was an important partner in the EU AcuteTox project, for which a database was set up at the Department of Medical Informatics by Robert Rudowski (21, 22). The In Vitro Methods Laboratory at the Department of Transplantology and Central Tissue Bank, Warsaw Medical University, was one of the partners in the first successful validation of an alternative method, the 3T3 NRU Phototoxicity Test (23). Scientists from Poland were involved in the project from its very beginning. In 1993, Śladowski became a member of the European Research Group for Alternatives in Toxicity Testing (ERGATT), long before Poland joined the EU in 2004. This informal group of scientists, devoted to the practical application of the Three Rs in the biosciences, initiated many activities which shaped the course of the development and application of alternative test methods. Thus, through Śladowski, Poland was involved in the process of defining the principles of validation of alternative safety test procedures (24) and also in several ECVAM workshops, including those on phototoxicity testing (25), on the use of human cells and tissue for research (26), and on long-term toxicity testing *in vitro* (27).

Joining the EU in 2004 meant that Poland could nominate a member of the ECVAM Scientific Advisory Committee (ESAC), and Śladowski was nominated to represent his country. He was actively involved in the ESAC until July 2009, when the ESAC was reorganized. Since this time, there has been no Polish representative in the ESAC, as the committee is no longer composed of representations of the EU Member States. However, several Polish scientists have been working at ECVAM.

Lena Buzanska, a visiting scientist at ECVAM, was involved in the development of a humanised organoid system (cord blood-derived differentiated human stem cells) for *in vitro* neurotoxicity studies (28–30).

Agnieszka Kinsner-Ovaskainen joined the European Commission's Joint Research Centre (JRC) in 2002 and is now a permanent staff member. Between 2002 and 2010, she was working at ECVAM in the field of *in vitro* neurotoxicity and acute toxicity (22, 31). During that period, she also spent six months at the OECD, working for the Test Guideline Programme and, in particular, on issues related to alternative methods. Since 2010, she has been responsible for the optimisation and standardisation of *in vitro* methods for the assessment of nanomaterials (32). She has participated in the activities of the OECD Working Party for Manufactured Nanomaterials, and has coordinated and/or contributed to several research projects related to *in vitro* methods for assessing nanomaterials.

Anna Price joined the JRC in 2002 and is now a member of the JRC's permanent staff. Working at ECVAM, she has been responsible for developing and evaluating *in vitro* methods for neurotoxicity testing, including developmental neurotoxicity (33), involving human cell-based models derived from pluripotent stem cells (34). She is a co-editor of two books (35, 36).

6.4 Concluding Comment

It must be emphasised that the application of the Three Rs in Poland has been greatly influenced by the country's accession to the EU in 2004. Animal experimentation is strictly regulated and monitored, and the housing conditions of laboratory animals have dramatically improved. What is particularly important is that the concept of the Three Rs is widely accepted and implemented by the scientific community in Poland. This was achieved in a relatively short time, because of the EU support and international collaboration. FRAME and ECVAM played a particularly important role, by supporting the transfer of knowledge and ideas during the crucial years of Polish transformation at the beginning of the 21st century.

REFERENCES

1. Russell, W.M.S. & Burch, R.L. (1959). *The Principles of Humane Experimental Technique*, 238pp. London, UK: Methuen.
2. EU. (2010). Directive 2010/63/EU of the European Parliament and of the Council of 22 September 2010 on the protection of animals used for scientific purposes. *Official Journal of the European Union* **L276**, 33–79.
3. Sladowski, D. & Halder, M. (2002). ECVAM's activities in the EU candidate countries, pp. 203–205. *ATLA* **30**(Suppl. 2)
4. Cervinka, M. & Balls, M. (1995). *Alternatives to Animal Experimentation*, 99pp. Hradec Králové, Czech Republic: NUCLEUS HK for TEMPUS JEP 1485. Charles University Medical Faculty.
5. Balls, M. (2014). Animal experimentation and alternatives: Time to say goodbye to the Three Rs and hello to Humanity? *ATLA* **42**, 327–333.
6. Červinková, Z. & Červinka, M. (2006). Professor W.M.S. Russell: Some personal reminiscences from the Czech Republic. *ATLA* **34**, 481–482.
7. Cooper-Hannan, R., Harbell, J.W., Coecke, S., *et al.* (1999). The principles of good laboratory practice: Application to in vitro toxicology studies. *ATLA* **27**, 539–577.
8. Stanek, S. (1947). Benefits and drawbacks of in vitro tissue cultures (Výhody a nedostatky kultivácie tkanív in vitro). *Bratislavské Lekárske Listy,* Roč **XXVII**(č. 10), 4. fol.
9. Ujházy, E., Navarová, J., Zemánek, M., *et al.* (2016). Twenty-year history of the organization of the international interdisciplinary toxicological conferences TOXCON. *Neuroendocrinology Letters* **37**(Supplément, Le 1), 3–8.
10. Sheasgreen, J., Klausner, M., Kandárová, H., *et al.* (2009). The MatTek story   how the Three Rs principles led to 3-D tissue success! *ATLA* **37**, 611–622.
11. Kandarova, H. (2006). *Evaluation and Validation of Reconstructed Human Skin Models as Alternatives to Animal Tests in Regulatory Toxicology* (PhD Dissertation). Berlin, Germany: Free University of Berlin.
12. Csizmarik, A., Szivósné Rácz, M. & Forgács, Z. (2016). A háromdimenziós, mesterségesen felépített, szervspecifikus szövetkultúrák alkalmazása a toxikológiában [Application of reconstructed three-dimensional organospecific tissue cultures in toxicology] *Egészségtudomány* **60**, 59–87.
13. Budai, P. & Várnagy, L. (2000). In vitro ocular irritation toxicity study of some pesticides. *Acta Veterinaria Hungarica* **48**, 221–228.
14. Budai, P., Lehel, J., Tavaszi, J., *et al.* (2010). HET-CAM test for determining the possible eye irritancy of pesticides. *Acta Veterinaria Hungarica* **58**, 369–377.
15. Knazicka, Z., Forgacs, Z., Lukacova, J., *et al.* (2015). Endocrine disruptive effects of cadmium on steroidogenesis: Human adrenocortical carcinoma cell line NCI-H295R as a cellular model for reproductive toxicity testing. *Journal of Environmental Science and Health, Part A* **50**, 348–356.
16. Bistakova, J., Forgacs, Z., Bartos, Z., *et al.* (2017). Effects of 4-nonylphenol on the steroidogenesis of human adrenocarcinoma cell line (NCI-H295R). *Journal of Environmental Science and Health, Part A* **52**, 221–227.
17. Jambor, T., Tvrda, E., Tusimova, E., *et al.* (2017). In vitro effect of 4-nonylphenol on human chorionic gonadotropin (hCG) stimulated hormone secretion, cell viability and reactive oxygen species generation in mice Leydig cells. *Environmental Pollution* **222**, 219–225.
18. Zwolińska, J. (2018). The use of animals in contemporary medical research   If not animals, then who or what? *ATLA* **46**, 43–51.
19. Steer, S., Lasek, W., Clothier, R.H., *et al.* (1990). An in vitro test for immunomodulators? *Toxicology in Vitro* **4**, 360–362.
20. Sladowski, D., Steer, S.J., Clothier, R.H., *et al.* (1993). An improved MTT assay. *Journal of Immunological Methods* **157**, 203–207.
21. Rudowski, R., Śladowski, D., Radomski, R., *et al.* (1997). The development of a multimedia database, INVITTOX (in vitro methods for toxicology, and an associated World-Wide Web information service provider. In L.F.M. Van Zutphen, & M. Balls (Eds.), *Proceedings of the 2nd World Congress on Alternatives and Animal Use in the Life Sciences*, pp. 499–503. Amsterdam, The Netherlands: Elsevier.
22. Kinsner-Ovaskainen, A., Rzepka, R., Rudowski, R., *et al.* (2009). Acutoxbase, an innovative database for in vitro acute toxicity studies. *Toxicology in Vitro* **23**, 476–485.
23. Spielmann, H., Balls, M., Dupuis, J., *et al.* (1998). The international EU/COLIPA In vitro phototoxicity validation study: results of phase II (blind trial), part 1: the 3T3 NRU phototoxicity test. *Toxicology in Vitro* **12**, 305–327.
24. Balls, M., Blaauboer, B.J., Fentem, J.H., *et al.* (1995). Practical aspects of the validation of toxicity test producers. The report and recommendations of ECVAM Workshop 5. *ATLA* **23**, 129–147.
25. Spielmann, H., Lovell, W.W., Holzle, B.E., *et al.* (1994). *In vitro* phototoxicity testing. The report and recommendations of ECVAM Workshop 2. *ATLA* **22**, 314–348.
26. Anderson, R., O'Hare, M., Balls, M., *et al.* (1998). The availability of human tissue for biomedical research: The report and recommendations of ECVAM Workshop 32. *ATLA* **26**, 763–777.
27. Pfaller, W., Balls, M., Clothier, R., *et al.* (2001). Novel advanced in vitro methods for long-term toxicity testing. The report and recommendations of ECVAM Workshop 45. *ATLA* **29**, 393–426.
28. Hogberg, H.T., Buzanska, L., Lenas, P., *et al.* (2009). In vitro developmental neurotoxicity (DNT) testing: relevant models and endpoints. *Neurotoxicology* **31**, 545–554.
29. Crofton, K.M., Mundy, W.R., Lein, P.J., *et al.* (2011). Developmental neurotoxicity testing: recommendations for developing alternative methods for the screening and prioritization of chemicals. *ALTEX* **28**, 9–15.

30. Buzanska, L., Sypecka, J., Nerini-Molteni, S., *et al.* (2009). A human stem cell-based model for identifying adverse effects of organic and inorganic chemicals on the developing nervous system. *Stem Cells* **27**, 2591–2601.

31. Prieto, P., Cole, T., Curren, R., *et al.* (2013). Assessment of the predictive capacity of the 3T3 Neutral Red Uptake cytotoxicity test method to identify substances not classified for acute oral toxicity (LD50>2000 mg/kg): results of an ECVAM validation study. *Regulatory Toxicology and Pharmacology* **65**, 344–365.

32. Kinsner-Ovaskainen, A., Colpo, P., Ponti, J., *et al.* (2014). Nanotoxicology. In A. Bal-Price, & P. Jennings (Eds.), *In Vitro Toxicology Systems*, pp. 481–500. New York, USA: Humana Press.

33. Bal-Price, A., Crofton, K.M., Leist, M., *et al.* (2015). International STakeholder NETwork (ISTNET): creating a developmental neurotoxicity (DNT) testing road map for regulatory purposes. *Archives of Toxicology* **89**, 269–287.

34. Pistollato, F., Canovas-Jorda, D., Zagoura, D., *et al.* (2017). Nrf2 pathway activation upon rotenone treatment in human iPSC-derived neural stem cells undergoing differentiation towards neurons and astrocytes. *Neurochemistry International* **108**, 457–471.

35. Bal-Price, A. & Jennings, P. (2014). *In Vitro Toxicology Systems*, 583pp. New York, NY, USA: Humana Press.

36. Aschner, M., Sunol, C. & Bal-Price, A. (2011). *Cell Culture Techniques*, 497pp. New York, NY, USA: Humana Press.

Chapter 2.7

Australia and New Zealand

Malcolm P. France[1], Simon A. Freeman Bain[2] and Brett A. Lidbury[3]

[1]Consultant in Laboratory Animal Care and Management, Sydney, NSW, Australia; [2]Research Ethics Consultant, Canberra, ACT, Australia; [3]NCEPH, ANU, Canberra, ACT, Australia

SUMMARY

Animal-based toxicology is only conducted on a small scale in Australia and New Zealand. Initiatives to develop alternatives to animal tests have arisen most often in the economically important agriculture sector, and in environmental monitoring. Stringent controls restricting the use of the Draize and LD_{50} tests emerged as far back as 1985. While the animal testing of cosmetics is banned in New Zealand, and a similar ban is expected soon in Australia, these moves are considered to be largely symbolic because there is virtually no history of such testing in either country. A 1989 Australian Senate report recommended the establishment of a government fund for research into alternatives, but no such entity yet exists in Australia or New Zealand. Progress in New Zealand may be facilitated in some areas because regulatory control lies within a single layer of government, whereas in Australia, state boundaries can be an impediment.

1. INTRODUCTION

Animal-based toxicology is only conducted on a small scale in Australia and New Zealand. Australia was placed only 14th, and New Zealand, 54th, in a ranking of research output in pharmacology, toxicology and pharmaceutics (1), and neither Australia nor New Zealand is an active participant in the REACH programme (2). Another ranking, which looks at relative expenditure on pharmaceutical research and development, places Australia behind more than 20 other countries (3); New Zealand is not included in this listing.

In both Australia and New Zealand, the regulation of animal-based toxicology is governed by broader animal research legislation, which dates back to the 1980s. Common to both countries is a requirement that all animal-based scientific procedures must be approved in advance by an Animal Ethics Committee. The membership of Animal Ethics Committees in Australia and New Zealand is unique in that it must include external representatives with credentials relating to animal welfare; this is in addition to a membership category that must be filled specifically by a veterinarian.

Both regulatory systems have long included a requirement that animals may only be used when no suitable alternatives are available. The Australian regulatory framework is united by a national, legally-binding code, the current version of which states that *'Methods that replace or partially replace the use of animals must be investigated, considered and, where applicable, implemented'* (4). Similarly, the section of New Zealand's Animal Welfare Act dealing with animal research is underpinned by a commitment to the Three Rs (5).

An index prepared by World Animal Protection classifies countries according to their commitment to animal protection. Both Australia and New Zealand rank within the highest classification with respect to 'Protecting animals used in scientific research'. New Zealand is also placed within the highest welfare classification for most other aspects of animal use and regulation, but Australia is only ranked in the second or third classifications for areas other than the use of animals in research (6).

The History of Alternative Test Methods in Toxicology. https://doi.org/10.1016/B978-0-12-813697-3.00010-X

2. THE 1989 AUSTRALIAN SENATE REPORT

While the militancy of the animal protection movement over the last few decades has perhaps been greater at times in New Zealand, community concerns regarding animal industries in Australia in the 1980s had become sufficient to prompt the establishment of a federal Senate Select Committee into Animal Welfare.

First appointed in 1983, the committee considered various animal industries and issued a report focusing on animal experimentation in 1989 (7). This had drawn on information from a questionnaire sent to universities, hospitals and research institutions as well as the outcomes of hearings and inspections of animal facilities. One of the report's 16 chapters was devoted to animals in toxicological testing and provides essential historical reading on the situation at the time and a context for the situation today.

Submissions to the Committee by the federal health department provide an account of a governmental position on animal toxicology at the time. Statements in these submissions included the following: (a) *Animal studies are not required unless they will contribute worthwhile information on the new medicine; … The LD$_{50}$ test as such is not required … The use of* in vitro *screening tests is recognised and accepted;* (b) *Non-human primates were required in some studies, but this requirement as such has now been deleted;* (c) *The Australian guidelines are very similar and consistent with many overseas requirements so that any additional animal testing for some medicines is kept to a minimum;* (d) *The Australian Department of Health accepts data generated overseas without any requirement for animal studies to be repeated in Australia.*

The report goes on to say that, (a) *Toxicological tests using live animals are not done on a large scale in Australia and that most tests are conducted overseas where the products are developed.… Some chemical evaluation studies are performed in Australia using animals. The purpose of additional testing is to generate data on the performance of the chemical under Australian conditions, e.g. insects or internal or external parasites.* (b) *Probably because of the small amount of toxicity testing actually undertaken in Australia little work has been done to develop non-animal toxicological tests by Australian scientists.*

The report made a number of recommendations specific to animal toxicology: (a) *That the Draize test be banned in Australia;* (b) *That there be a ban on the classical LD$_{50}$ test in Australia, but that acute toxicity tests be allowed with ministerial approval.*

While most Australian states later implemented controls over these procedures, the state of New South Wales, which remains the only Australian state to have specific legislation to govern animal research, had already restricted the Draize test to the assessment of substances intended for application to the human eye and only permitted LD$_{50}$ testing if approved by the Minister.

The report also recommended *That the Commonwealth Government establish a separate fund for research into the use of alternatives to animal experimentation….*

More than 25 years on, there is still no government funding in either Australia or New Zealand, specifically for research into the development of non-animal alternatives in toxicology, or other branches of biomedical research.

3. LOCAL FACTORS

While toxicological testing has only ever been conducted on a limited scale in Australia and New Zealand, local economic and environmental features have prompted some interesting developments to address specific needs. The relative geographic isolation of both countries has also probably helped to foster local solutions for local problems.

3.1 The Australian Anti-Venom Industry

Australia is home to several species of highly venomous terrestrial snakes, spiders and marine species. Not surprisingly, the development and testing of anti-venoms have a long local history, and much of this has relied heavily on animal use. For example, Charles Kellaway, while serving as director of one of Australia's premier medical research institutes, conducted a number of animal studies into the pathogenesis of envenomation (8), and, in a single paper published in 1938, makes reference to the use of cats, dogs, monkeys, rabbits and guinea-pigs (9).

The first specific therapy for envenomation developed in Australia was a tiger snake anti-venom released in 1930. In the half century that followed, anti-venoms were developed to treat envenomation from a wide range of species (10). Animal-based batch testing for potency was always central to the manufacturing process, and this continues to be the case today, not just in Australia but worldwide (11). While it appears that the current scope for animal replacement in this area is limited, there has been some research into the use of recombinant technologies for anti-venom production (12). It remains to be seen whether this will deliver opportunities for reducing the current reliance on animal testing during batch testing.

3.2 Facial Eczema in Sheep

An illustrative example highlighting how toxicological testing can progress from animal-based to non-animal-based methods emerges in the comprehensive account by DiMenna *et al.* (13) of the history of research into facial eczema, a locally important disease of sheep in New Zealand.

Facial eczema (pithomycotoxicosis) is a form of photosensitivity resulting from chronic liver damage, which had a substantial, but unpredictable, impact on the New Zealand sheep industry for several decades of the 20th century. It was eventually shown that the underlying liver damage was caused by a fungal toxin produced on decaying pasture.

Prior to this discovery, pasture toxicity was assessed by bioassay. This initially involved the use of 'indicator' lambs obtained from districts known to be free of facial eczema, which would be grazed on suspect pasture, then killed to be examined for the presence of characteristic liver lesions. In the 1950s, this method was replaced by a guinea-pig bioassay, which, in addition to pasture assessment, contributed significantly to the characterisation of the toxic principle.

A serendipitous finding with the guinea-pig bioassay was that glassware used during solvent extraction of the still-unidentified toxin developed a white film. This observation was exploited to develop a crude *in vitro* assay, which became known as the beaker test. An important breakthrough occurred when samples of a black dust, collected while mowing a field adjacent to a facial eczema trial plot, were found to produce a strongly positive reaction in the beaker test. Further samples of the dust were identified as spores of the saprophytic fungus, *Pithomyces chartarum,* which was shown subsequently shown to be the source of the toxin.

Although further research following the identification of the toxin permitted the development of a range of *in vitro* assays, animal-based studies continued to be deployed in a complementary manner for a considerable number of years. Ironically, it was found that the beaker test itself did not detect the toxin, but detected a non-toxic component of the spores that co-purified with the toxin, instead.

The history of facial eczema research in New Zealand stands as an important example of how local needs can drive scientific progress. But perhaps more broadly, it is a reminder that the development of alternatives is often part of a process in which the integration with animal-based research is complex and, at times, mutually dependent.

4. PARALYTIC SHELLFISH TOXIN

Paralytic shellfish poisoning is a syndrome caused by the consumption of filter-feeding bivalve molluscs contaminated with algal-derived toxins. These toxins include more than 30 analogues based on a parent compound, saxitoxin, which is among the most toxic compounds known (14). The risk of exposure to paralytic shellfish toxins, therefore, presents a public health concern, and a threat to shellfish aquaculture in many parts of the world, including New Zealand, where seafood has a high profile, both domestically, and as a part of the country's reputation for quality food exports.

Until recently, the reference method for safety and quality assurance, to prevent paralytic shellfish poisoning, was a mouse bioassay. However, increasing ethical concerns, and ongoing technical limitations have prompted the development of *in vitro* assays. One of these, known as the Lawrence method, involves the pre-chromatographic oxidation of samples, followed by liquid chromatography with fluorescence.

New Zealand's Cawthron Institute operates a testing service for the detection of paralytic shellfish toxins, and has updated the Lawrence method to provide more rapid analysis. Responding to the ethical and technical concerns associated with the mouse bioassay, the Institute had implemented the Lawrence method at a non-regulatory level in 2002, and used it to fully replace the mouse bioassay following an evaluation conducted in 2010 (15, 16).

In 2011, a major algal bloom occurred, which resulted in the closure of some of New Zealand's commercial shellfish harvesting areas for up to 3 months. Deployment of the modified Lawrence test in managing that incident proved successful, with no reports of human illness or recalls of exported product (16).

In another New Zealand innovation, the corporatised government research body, AgResearch, developed a prototype assay for shellfish toxins that measures the effects of toxins and other compounds in about an hour, compared with the several days required for the mouse bioassay.

These lines of research were recognised in 2004 and 2008, through the Three Rs award co-ordinated by New Zealand's National Animal Ethics Advisory Committee.

5. ENVIRONMENTAL MONITORING

In addition to developments prompted by economic or environmental factors that are, to varying degrees, unique to Australia or New Zealand, local research has supported the development of alternatives in areas of toxicology with broader applications.

Occupational exposure to agricultural chemicals is a matter of concern in many countries where there is a substantial economic reliance on agriculture. Chlorpyrifos is an organophosphate, which is widely used to control insect pests in food crops. A team at Griffith University, in the Australian state of Queensland, has developed an approach for setting safety guidelines for exposure to chlorpyrifos, which has the potential to replace animal use (17). The acute Reference Dose for chlorpyrifos, recommended by the United States Environmental Protection Agency (500 m g/kg/d), is based on the dose that causes cholinesterase inhibition in rat plasma. However, this has been criticised as too conservative and not reliably-linked to clinical evidence of exposure. Therefore, the objective was to develop methods to set guideline values via the direct utilisation of human data, and to avoid surrogate test animals. Human data were used to assist the development of dose–response relationships, as well as drawing on data from the scientific literature on human populations and their adverse responses. Subsequent to the change to direct human data assessment, it was concluded that the guidelines should set the values at 0.5 and 3 μg/kg/d for chronic and acute exposures, respectively.

Work to replace animals in the toxicological assessment of airborne pollutants has been conducted by the UNSW Sydney's Chemical Safety and Applied Toxicology Laboratories (18). Conventional tests of the toxicity of gases and vapours, in which laboratory animals are exposed to lethal or sub-lethal doses of chemicals, have been criticised as expensive, unethical, inhumane, and time-consuming. Hayes *et al.* (19–21) used Snapwell permeable polyester membrane technology to grow a range of human cells. The cell types represented human organ systems pertinent to airborne toxin exposure and/or detoxification, namely, lung cells, liver cells and skin fibroblasts. This application of Snapwell technology was more-predictive than traditional *in vitro* testing. The range of toxins tested included ammonia, cyanide, formaldehyde, hydrogen sulphide, nitrogen dioxide, toluene and xylene, with IC_{50} *in vitro* values corresponding well to published acute inhalation data for animals. This line of *in vitro* toxicology research also extended successfully into the investigation of 11 airborne pollutants commonly generated by fires (22).

Further examples of advances in environmental toxicology from both Australia and New Zealand could probably be found to represent most of the technologies applicable to the replacement of animal-based methods. However, in the absence of a major centralised programme to promote non-animal alternatives, it is likely that such developments will continue to be driven primarily by economic and practical factors, rather than by a primary demand to reduce animal testing.

6. COSMETICS TESTING

There appears to be no evidence that animal-based testing of cosmetics has ever taken place in New Zealand (23), and in Australia, such testing has probably only ever been conducted on a very small scale. The report from the Australian Senate in 1989 included a submission from the Cosmetic Toiletry and Fragrance Association of Australia, which stated that '*In this country, the cosmetic industry consists largely of subsidiaries of overseas companies, and as a consequence most research resulting in toxicological validation is carried out abroad ...*' (7). More-recently, Australian government consultation established that no applications were received by Animal Ethics Committees to test cosmetics, and/or their ingredients from 2013 to 2015, and that there is agreement between industry and animal protection groups that this sort of testing no longer takes place in Australia (24).

Despite animal testing of cosmetics being non-existent in both countries, proposals to implement formal bans have attracted political interest in recent years. In 2015, amendments to New Zealand legislation effectively banned the animal-testing of finished cosmetic products or ingredients that are intended exclusively for this purpose. Subsequently, the deliberations and stakeholder submissions underpinning that move formed the basis of recommendations for similar legislative provisions in Australia.

In practice, Australia's current regulatory framework does not actually require any cosmetic product to be tested on animals. Animal test data are only required if a company is introducing a new chemical ingredient into Australia, and if no validated non-animal alternative tests are available (25).

Bills aimed at formalising a ban on the animal testing of cosmetics have been tabled in the Australian Parliament by all the major political parties over recent years (26). The latest of these bills is expected to pass into law in 2018. While this bill has been promoted as a strategy to support animal welfare through a ban on cosmetics testing, its primary purpose is much broader. Currently, titled the *Industrial Chemicals Bill*, it actually stems from a bipartisan reform commenced in 2011, which aims to streamline Australia's complex framework of chemical regulations, which are currently spread across some 140 pieces of legislation, and multiple agencies (27).

7. ORGANISATIONS

The small scale of animal-based toxicology in Australia and New Zealand means that organisations and resourcing for the development of non-animal alternatives are correspondingly limited.

At present, the only body with a charter directed specifically to the development of alternatives in either country is the Medical Advances Without Animals (MAWA) Trust. The MAWA Trust is an Australian-based not-for-profit organisation, established in 2000 by Ms Elizabeth Ahlston and Associate Professor Garry Scroop, with Professor Stephen Leeder, then University of Sydney Dean of Medicine, and later Editor-in-Chief of the *Medical Journal of Australia*, as its first Chair.

The Trust has issued more than 100 grants to Australian universities and research institutions, in support of initiatives, such as research Fellowships, equipment grants, travel bursaries and human tissue banks. Another initiative has been to establish a partnership with The Australian National University, as a strategic move toward establishing an Australian Centre for Alternatives to Animal Research.

While the focus of the MAWA Trust is on basic research, it has lent its support to a number of programmes that could have future applications in toxicology. Examples include the refinement of cell culture methods for *in vitro* drug screening.

In 2006, a consortium for health risk assessment held a symposium, which saw the founding of the Australasian College of Toxicology and Risk Assessment. This body was established to support the professional development of toxicologists in Australia and New Zealand. The *Journal of Toxicology and Environmental Health* subsequently published a special issue containing 14 papers from the symposium, focusing on local perspectives. While some of these described, or advocated the development of *in vitro* alternatives to animal-based toxicology, this was generally prompted by technical goals rather than to support a specific animal welfare agenda (28).

Neither Australia nor New Zealand has established the sort of partnerships between government, industry and the broader community to pursue the development of alternatives that have emerged in the UK, the USA, Canada, the EU and several other individual European countries. Nevertheless, a Three Rs programme in New Zealand is supporting links between Massey University, government and non-government organisations, to facilitate collaboration and awareness, and the release of details of a government initiative to promote the Three Rs is expected shortly in Australia.

8. CURRENT REGULATORY INTEREST

Given the importance of primary industry to the economies of Australia and New Zealand, much of the toxicology in both countries is driven by the needs of that sector. For example, Johnston *et al.* (29) mention that testing is mandatory for biological products produced in Australia, the majority of which are livestock vaccines for local use and export. The same authors mention that, in New Zealand, the use of 20% of animals involved in research was for commercial purposes (Johnson, P., Einstein, R., Chave, L. *et al.* [2005], unpublished).

Australia's regulatory body for such products, the Australian Pesticides and Veterinary Authority (APVMA), states in its application guidelines (29): *Applicants are encouraged to submit data obtained from OECD Guidelines for the Testing of Chemicals (or other recognised test guidelines)* in vitro *assay systems or alternative methods, which use fewer animals according to the "3Rs" principle (reduce, refine, replace).* Similarly, in New Zealand, the 1997 *Agricultural Compound and Veterinary Medicine Act* has established the Agricultural Compound and Veterinary Medicines (ACVM) Group, which aligns with international regulatory guidelines, and organisations that set standards aimed at harmonising technical requirements for the registration of veterinary products to minimise the use of testing in animals (30, 31). However, searches of the APVMA and ACVM websites failed to produce examples of significant alternatives to the use of animals in toxicological research.

Australian regulatory approval of products for use in humans is controlled by the Therapeutic Goods Administration (TGA; see Ref. 32). The technical data requirements for the registration of medicines evaluated by the Drug Safety Evaluation Branch of the TGA have been aligned with those required for applications for marketing authorisation by the EU. A search for an alternative to animal methods failed to produce any TGA examples. Medsafe is the New Zealand medicine and medical devices authority, and again, a search failed to produce evidence that alternative methods were being used. For the TGA and Medsafe, this is most likely because of the reliance on the EU directives and innovations, rather than on local innovations.

9. DISCUSSION AND CONCLUSIONS

Animal-based toxicology is only conducted on a very small scale in Australia and New Zealand, and is mainly driven by the local needs of primary industry and environmental health. Most testing of pharmaceuticals is conducted overseas, where the products are developed, with animal testing in Australia or New Zealand only being performed occasionally, to ascertain activities of the product under local conditions. There is no evidence that animal testing of cosmetics has ever been undertaken in New Zealand, whereas in Australia, the evidence suggests that only very limited testing has ever occurred, and that this has not happened for many years. Although regulatory moves to ban animal-based cosmetics testing have taken place recently in both countries, the lack of such testing essentially renders these moves to be symbolic in nature.

The New Zealand public have a history of strong animal welfare consciousness, and the single-tiered government has been responsive to public sensitivities in this area. In contrast, the Australian public have not displayed the same degree of sustained concern over animal welfare issues. The constitutional devolving of Australian animal welfare legislation to the states can also create an impediment to collective progress nationally. While Australia's 1989 Senate Committee Report recommended that the government establish a separate fund for research into the development of alternatives, this has yet to happen.

Notwithstanding all of this, some commitment to innovative animal replacement technologies relevant to toxicology exists in both countries, and there is local expertise across the range of methods applicable to animal-free technologies. Even in the absence of coordinated national approaches, these resources have supported, and can be expected to continue to support, progress in the replacement of animal-based toxicology in specific areas of importance to local economic and environmental conditions.

REFERENCES

1. Anon. (2017). *Scimago Journal & Country Rank (Pharmacology, Toxicology and Pharmaceutics, 1996–2016)*. Available at http://www.scimagojr.com.
2. EC. (2006). Regulation (EC) No 1907/2006 of the European Parliament and of the Council of 18 December 2006 concerning the Registration, Evaluation, Authorisation and Restriction of Chemicals (REACH), establishing a European Chemicals Agency, amending Directive 1999/45/EC and repealing Council Regulation (EEC) No 793/93 and Commission Regulation (EC) No 1488/94 as well as Council Directive 76/769/EEC and Commission Directives 91/155/EEC, 93/67/EEC, 93/105/EC and 2000/21/EC. *Official Journal of the European Union* **L396**, 1–849.
3. OECD. (2015). *Health at a Glance 2015*, 220pp. Paris, France: OECD.
4. Health and Medical Research Council. (2013). *Australian Code for the Care and Use of Animals for Scientific Purposes*, 8th ed., 46pp. Canberra, ACT, Australia: National Health and Medical Research Council.
5. Wells, N. & Nicholson, J. (2004). Five plus three: legislating for the five freedoms and the Three Rs — Animal Welfare Act 1999 (New Zealand). *ATLA* **32**(Suppl. 1B), 417–421.
6. World Animal Protection. (2017). *Animal Protection Index*. London, UK: World Animal Protection.
7. Parliament of the Commonwealth of Australia. (1989). *Animal Experimentation. Report by the Senate Select Committee on Animal Welfare*, 16pp. Canberra, ACT. Australia: Australian Government Publishing Service.
8. Burnet, F.M. (1983). Kellaway, Charles Halliley (1889–1952). *Australian Dictionary of Biography* **9**, 1.
9. Feldberg, W., Holden, H. & Kellaway, C.H. (1938). The formation of lysocithin and of a muscle-stimulating substance by snake venoms. *Journal of Physiology* **94**, 232–248.
10. Winkel, K.D., Mirtschin, P. & Pearn, J. (2006). Twentieth century toxinology and antivenom development in Australia. *Toxicon* **48**, 738–754.
11. WHO. (2010). *WHO Guidelines for the Production, Control and Regulation of Snake Antivenom Immunoglobulins*, 141pp. Geneva, Switzerland: WHO.
12. Laustsen, A.H., Johansen, K.H., Engmark, M., *et al.* (2017). Recombinant snakebite antivenoms: A cost-competitive solution to a neglected tropical disease? *PLoS Neglected Tropical Diseases* **11**(2), e0005361.
13. Di Menna, M.E., Smith, B.L. & Miles, C.O. (2009). A history of facial eczema (pithomycotoxicosis) research. *New Zealand Journal of Agricultural Research* **52**, 345–376.
14. Mackenzie, A.L. (2014). The risk to New Zealand shellfish aquaculture from paralytic shellfish poisoning (PSP) toxins. *New Zealand Journal of Marine and Freshwater Research* **48**, 430–465.
15. Holland, P.T., McNabb, P., Van Ginkel, R., *et al.* (2010). *Saxitoxins in Seafood: Assessment of Test Methods to Replace the PSP Mouse Bioassay*. Cawthron Institute Report No. 1717, 29pp. Nelson, New Zealand: Cawthron Institute.
16. Harwood, D.T., Boundy, M., Selwood, A.I., *et al.* (2013). Refinement and implementation of the Lawrence method (AOAC 2005.06) in a commercial laboratory: Assay performance during an Alexandrium catenella bloom event. *Harmful Algae* **24**, 20–31.
17. Phung, D.T., Connell, D. & Chu, C. (2015). A new method for setting guidelines to protect human health from agricultural exposure by using chlorpyrifos as an example. *Annals of Agricultural and Environmental Medicine* **22**, 275–280.
18. Potera, C. (2007). More human, more humane: a new approach for testing airborne pollutants. *Environmental Health Perspectives* **115**, A148.
19. Bakand, S., Winder, C. & Hayes, A. (2007). Comparative *in vitro* cytotoxicity assessment of selected gaseous compounds in human alveolar epithelial cells. *Toxicology in Vitro* **21**, 1341–1347.
20. Bakand, S., Winder, C., Khalil, C., *et al.* (2006). An experimental *in vitro* model for dynamic direct exposure of human cells to airborne contaminants. *Toxicology Letters* **165**, 1–10.
21. Bakand, S. & Hayes, A. (2010). Troubleshooting methods for toxicity testing of airborne chemicals in vitro. *Journal of Pharmacological and Toxicological Methods* **61**, 76–85.
22. Lestari, F., Hayes, A.J., Green, A.R., *et al.* (2005). *In vitro* cytotoxicity of selected chemicals commonly produced during fire combustion using human cell lines. *Toxicology in Vitro* **19**, 653–663.

23. Guy, N. (2015). *Law Change to Ban Cosmetic Testing on Animals*. News Release 1 April 2015, 1p. Wellington, New Zealand: Beehive.govt.nz.

24. Anon. (2017). *Ban on the Testing of Cosmetics on Animals*. Consultation Paper, March 2017, 16pp. Canberra, ACT, Australia: Australian Government Department of Health.

25. Anon. (2017). *Ban on the Testing of Cosmetics on Animals*. Background Paper, 8pp. Canberra, ACT, Australia: Australian Government Department of Health.

26. Petrie, C. (2017). *The Commonwealth's Role in Animal Welfare*, 1p. Canberra, Australia: Parliament of Australia.

27. Anon. (2012). *Discussion Paper. Review of the National Industrial Chemicals Notification and Assessment Scheme (NICNAS)*, 56pp. Canberra, ACT, Australia: Australian Government Department of Health and Ageing and Department of Finance and Deregulation.

28. Priestly, B.G., Di Marco, P., Sim, M., *et al.* (2007). Environmental toxicology in Australasia (2007) *Journal of Toxicology and Environmental Health, Part A* **70**, 1577–1711.

29. Anon. (2017). *APVMA Application Guidelines, Toxicology (Part 3)*. Symonston, ACT, Australia: Australian Pesticides and Veterinary Medicines Authority.

30. Anon. (2017). *Agricultural Compounds and Veterinary Medicines Act 1997*. Reprint of 1 March 2017, 119pp. Wellington, New Zealand: New Zealand Government.

31. Anon. (2015). *Use of Animals in the Registration of Veterinary Products in New Zealand*. Occasional Paper No. 11, 12pp. Wellington, New Zealand: National Ethics Advisory Committee.

32. Anon. (2017). *Therapeutic Goods Administration*. Canberra, ACT, Australia: Australian Government Department of Health.

Chapter 2.8

Japanese Contributions to the Development of Alternative Test Methods

Hajime Kojima[1], Yasuyuki Sakai[2] and Noriho Tanaka[3]

[1]JaCVAM, NIHS, Tokyo, Japan; [2]University of Tokyo, Tokyo, Japan; [3]Hatano Research Institute, Hadano, Kanagawa, Japan

SUMMARY

There are two organisations in Japan that have been instrumental in promoting the development of alternatives to test methods that use animals: the Japanese Society for Alternatives to Animal Experiments (JSAAE) and the Japanese Center for the Validation of Alternative Methods (JaCVAM). The JSAAE is a scientific organisation that promotes international acceptance of the replacement, reduction and refinement of animal use (the Three Rs) as a guiding principle in scientific testing. The Society's members are science professionals, who are active in the research, development and surveillance of alternative methods, and who make an effort to educate other professionals, as well as to enhance public awareness of alternatives to animal testing. For more than a quarter of a century, the JSAAE has built a reputation, both in Japan and around the world, for sponsoring significant professional activities, including the 2007 *6th World Congress on Alternatives and Animal Use in the Life Sciences* in Tokyo, and the 2016 *Asian Congress on Alternatives and Animal Use in the Life Sciences* in Karatsu and Saga. In contrast to the JSAAE, JaCVAM is a public agency that was established in 2005 as part of the Biological Safety Research Center (BSRC) at the National Institute of Health Sciences (NIHS). JaCVAM's stated mission is to promote the use of alternative methods to animal testing in regulatory studies, while meeting the responsibility of the BSRC to ensure the protection of the public by assessing the safety of chemicals and other materials, as stipulated in NIHS regulations. JaCVAM plays an active role in the approval process for permission to manufacture and sell pharmaceutical and other products, as well as in revising standards for cosmetic products. JaCVAM also participates in International Cooperation on Alternative Test Methods (ICATM), under which it has organised a number of international validation studies that have led to the issuance of nine test guidelines and one guidance document from the Organisation for Economic Cooperation and Development (OECD).

1. THE JAPANESE SOCIETY FOR ALTERNATIVES TO ANIMAL EXPERIMENTS

The Japanese Society for Alternatives to Animal Experiments (JSAAE) is a scientific organisation that promotes the international acceptance of the Three Rs as a guiding principle for the proper use of animals in scientific testing, through activities such as research, development, education and surveillance (1). The Society's members are science professionals, who are active in the research, development and surveillance of alternative methods, and who make an effort to educate other professionals, as well as to enhance public awareness of alternatives to animal testing.

The Three Rs were first described by Russell and Burch in 1959 (2) and were officially endorsed by the *3rd World Congress on Alternatives and Animal Use in the Life Sciences* in 1999, by affirmation of the Declaration of Bologna (3). The Three Rs have now been incorporated into the laws and official policies in countries all over the world, as well as into international standards for the welfare of animals used in experiments.

The JSAAE's roots lie in a research group established by Professor Tsutomu Sugawara in 1982, and the Society itself was established as a scientific association in 1988 and accepted as a member of the Science Council of Japan in 2002. For more than 25 years, the JSAAE has earned a reputation in Japan and around the world, for sponsoring significant professional activities. We are particularly proud of the fact that JSAAE's annual meetings consistently attract 500 professionals, with programmes that feature the latest findings from state-of-the-art research. Although Japanese researchers are highly regarded for their diligent teamwork, there remains a general lack of awareness in Japan about the benefits available from alternatives to animal testing. Thus, a great many of the JSAAE's activities focus on scientific research into the replacement of animal testing with alternative methods, and cooperation with other international organisations promoting research and development in this area, particularly with regard to the use of *in silico* techniques, is an important part of our regular activities. Also, while *Reduction* and *Refinement* have not always received the emphasis that they deserve, we are now renewing our efforts to advance understanding and awareness of achievements in these areas. The JSAAE is proud of its collaboration with other professionals performing research into or providing support for the welfare of laboratory animals, as part of its efforts to promote the Three Rs.

1.1 JSAAE Activities

JSAAE members undertake the following activities:

1. An annual meeting of the society.
2. Ad hoc symposia and workshops.
3. Publications, namely: (a) its journal, *Alternatives to Animal Testing and Experimentation* (AATEX), which reports on Japanese Three Rs research, including that related to validation studies in Japan; past issues are available in PDF format to both members and non-members, except for the most recent issue, which is available to members only; (b) *Newsletters*, published two or three times per year; and (c) a website and e-mail news (30 times per year).
4. Funding for relevant research.
5. Evaluation and validation of newly developed alternative methods.
6. Acquisition of relevant information.
7. Communication with other international organisations.
8. Support of international meetings; collaboration with other scientific associations, such as the Tissue Culture Association and the Mutagenicity Association, and others; communication with animal protection groups.

1.2 International Cooperation

The *6th World Congress on Alternatives and Animal Use in the Life Sciences* (WC6) was held in Tokyo from 21 to 25 August 2007 at Hotel East 21, with support from the JSAAE, the Science Council of Japan, and the Alternatives Congress Trust (ACT), which had in the past hosted the World Congresses.

The objectives of WC6 were:

1. to review progress made in promoting reduction, refinement and replacement in education, research and testing;
2. to develop a realistic understanding of the status of alternative methods;
3. to create the understanding that research and animal studies, together with clinical studies and *in vitro* methods, are all necessary;
4. to advance the science, to contribute to our basic understanding of biology and diseases; and
5. to encourage constructive discussions between animal protection groups and the scientific community.

WC6 was attended by some 1030 professionals, including 440 non-Japanese from 34 countries and regions, and as the first of the World Congress series to be held in East Asia, was as an excellent opportunity to review animal welfare issues and to encourage research on alternative methods in this region. Chinese and Korean scientists organised satellite symposia in Beijing and Seoul that were held just prior to WC6 in Tokyo, and other satellite symposia were held in Kyoto and Nagoya shortly thereafter. A follow-up symposium was also held in Tokyo some six months later. WC6 in Tokyo was a tremendous success, thanks to support from its many affiliated organisations and related companies.

The Asian Congress 2016 on Alternatives and Animal Use in the Life Sciences was held jointly with the 29th Annual Meeting of the JSAAE at the Karatsu Civic Hall in Karatsu, Saga, and at Kyushu University in Fukuoka, Fukuoka, from 15 to 18 November 2016. As the first conference of its kind for researchers from Asia, the Asian Congress 2016 was an excellent opportunity to promote the Three Rs and the use of alternative test methods to researchers in this region. Attended by some 530 professionals, including 80 non-Japanese participants from 17 countries and regions throughout Asia, the tremendous success of this Congress was due in large part to support received from the ACT. Looking ahead, China will host the upcoming Asian Congress in 2018, and Korea will host the next Congress after that. The JSAAE welcomes this collaboration from other countries throughout Asia in maintaining Asia's standing in the Three Rs.

The JSAAE is now working to form ties with like-minded organisations, to increase opportunities for Japanese researchers to promote their findings and to gain greater worldwide recognition of Japan's efforts in this field. The JSAAE now has cooperative agreements in place with the Korean Society for Alternatives to Animal Experiments (KSAAE), the European Society for Alternatives to Animal Experiments (EUSAAT), and the American Society for Cellular and Computational Toxicology (ASCCT).

1.3 What Is Next for the JSAAE?

The JSAAE considers interdisciplinary collaboration to be the key to increasing its membership, and hopes to cooperate with other academic societies in promoting annual meetings and other events where new members can be recruited from both the private and academic sectors. The focus of research into alternatives to animal testing is now shifting away from the study of localised effects toward gaining an understanding of long-term, systemic effects. This will require, not only enhancement of *in vitro* test methods, but also proper integration with a variety of analytical and numerical methodologies. The JSAAE has a major role to play in promoting future ideal systems for the non-animal evaluation of toxicological effects in humans through objective-oriented integration of diverse disciplines and technologies. But to achieve this, the JSAAE must also develop its ability to organise multidisciplinary collaboration with other professionals in closely related fields. Specifically, the JSAAE is now planning a series of experimental seminars that will focus on alternative test methods proposed by JSSAE members or recently issued as either guidance or test guidelines by the Organisation for Economic Cooperation and Development (OECD; (4)). Events such as these are eagerly awaited by Japanese manufacturers.

Unfortunately, the actual use of alternative methods by Japanese manufacturers is still not as widespread as it could be. Therefore, the JSAAE is also strengthening its efforts to promote the use of strategies for *Refinement* and *Reduction* in Japan. These efforts must include collaboration with animal rights and animal welfare groups, as well as the proactive promotion of the use of alternative methods in research. In addition, greater awareness of these issues by the general public overall, and by younger Japanese, in particular, should be promoted.

In terms of contributing internationally to the promotion of the Three Rs, the JSSAE proactively supports the activities of the Japanese Center for the Validation of Alternative Methods (JaCVAM), and is working toward establishing a counterpart in the Chinese scientific community, in addition to further developing existing relationships with KSAAE, EUSAAT and ASCCT.

Another important development is to open new possibilities for the JSAAE's official journal, *AATEX*, through registration with the web-based database, PubMed Central. The JSAAE's contributions to promoting the Three Rs have been very much appreciated by the international community. In particular, the 6th World Congress Tokyo in 2007, and the 1st Asian Congress in Karatsu in 2016 were well attended and well received by the international community.

The nurturing of a new generation of junior researchers is a fundamental problem for any scientific organisation dedicated to the promotion of research activities, and the JSAAE is no exception. The recruitment of junior researchers from both the private and academic sectors is an essential part of ensuring that the JSAAE continues to grow as a scientific organisation, and measures are needed to streamline its own management, so that younger professionals can participate actively in the JSAAE, without sacrificing precious time devoted to research.

2. THE BACKGROUND TO JACVAM

A complete ban on the marketing in the EU of cosmetic products and cosmetic ingredients tested on animals has been in effect since March 2013 (5). In view of this, some Japanese manufacturers have also abandoned the use of animal testing in the in-house development of cosmetic products and ingredients. Just as in the EU, Japanese regulatory agencies generally have not required permits for the production and distribution of new cosmetic products or ingredients, other than positive and negative listed ones.

In contrast, the manufacture and sales of cosmetic products or quasi-drugs containing new ingredients (those included in the positive list) does require the submission of results from safety testing on animals. In such cases, the test methods must ordinarily conform to notifications regarding drug safety, OECD Test Guidelines (TGs) and other publicly recognised standards. They must also appear in the *keshohin-iyakubu gaihin seizou hanbai gaidobukku 2011–2012* (the 2011–2012 *Guidebook on the Manufacture and Sales of Cosmetics and Quasi-Drugs*; (6)) Also, all animal testing must conform to *koseirodousho non shokan suru jisshikikan ni okeru doubutsu jiken tou no jisshi ni kan suru kihonhoushin* (basic policies regarding implementation of animal and other testing at organisations under the jurisdiction of the Ministry of Health, Labour and Welfare (MHLW)) as well as all other laws and regulations relevant to animal and other testing (7).

In addition, an administrative notice (8) issued in July 2006 by the MHLW Evaluation and Licensing Division indicated that the inclusion of results from alternative test methods as documentary evidence in an application was acceptable, provided that the alternative test methods conformed to accepted OECD alternative test methods or had been similarly validated in a suitable manner. The administrative notice further stipulated that, even in cases where animal testing was to be performed, if information about the physicochemical properties of the test chemical itself or similar chemical substance as well as the results of *in vitro* testing led to the reasonable expectation that the test chemicals could induce distress or suffering in test animals, efforts were to be made to dilute such test chemicals and thereby mitigate the distress or suffering of the test animals.

On 4 February 2011, the MHLW issued a notification that data obtained with alternative testing methods approved by JaCVAM could be used for the submission of quasi-drug applications or for petitions to include ingredients in the Standards for Cosmetics (9). Information is available on the JaCVAM website (10), to help ensure proper preparation of the documentary evidence to be included with applications for approval of manufacturing and sales of quasi-drugs, as well as in requests for revisions to positive lists for cosmetics. This information has been conveyed to the appropriate businesses and other concerned parties.

In addition, administrative notices issued in April 2012 and May 2013 by the MHLW Evaluation and Licensing Division publicised the availability of alternative test methods for phototoxicity testing and skin sensitisation testing for use in safety evaluations of cosmetics and quasi-drugs (9). Additional information on other alternatives to animal testing will be issued as it becomes available.

Even though alternative test methods developed for OECD TGs are useful for the potential hazard evaluation of chemicals, they are not always suitable for providing the wide range of information needed for risk assessment and other safety evaluations. Thus, many Japanese manufacturers will find it difficult to gain approval for cosmetic products or quasi-drugs containing new ingredients, without animal testing.

2.1 What Is JaCVAM's Role?

JaCVAM was established to promote the use of alternative methods to animal testing in regulatory studies, thereby replacing, reducing or refining the use of animals wherever possible, while meeting the responsibility of the National Center for Biological Safety and Research (BSRC) to ensure the protection of the public by assessing the safety of chemicals and other materials, as stipulated in the regulations of the National Institute of Health Sciences (NIHS) in November 2005. JaCVAM activities are also beneficial to the application and approval for the manufacture and sale of pharmaceutical, chemical, pesticide and other products, as well as to revisions to standards for cosmetic products (9).

To this end, JaCVAM assesses the utility, limitations and suitability for use in regulatory studies of test methods for the safety assessment of chemicals and other materials, and performs validation studies, when necessary. In addition, under the framework of the International Cooperation on Alternative Test Methods (ICATM; (11)), JaCVAM co-operates and collaborates with similar organisations worldwide, to ensure that new or revised tests are validated through comparison with domestically-developed or internationally-certified standard tests, undergo peer review and are officially accepted by the regulatory agencies. JaCVAM is affiliated with a number of agencies overseas, including the European Union Reference Laboratory for Alternatives to Animal Testing (EURL ECVAM), the United States NTP Interagency Center for the Evaluation of Alternative Toxicological Methods/Interagency Coordinating Committee on the Validation of Alternative Methods (NICEATM/ICCVAM), Health Canada and the Korean Center for the Validation of Alternative Methods (KoCVAM).

Japanese scientists, laboratories and companies have been involved in the development or validation of a number of non-animal toxicity test procedures, many of which are now the subject of OECD TGs, and some of which have been subjected to independent peer review under the ICATM framework.

To ensure the proper management of JaCVAM activities, an Advisory Council, Steering Committee and Regulatory Acceptance Board are being established. The Steering Committee requests the organisation of Peer Review Panels and Validation Management Teams, when necessary. Members of each of these bodies are appointed by the NIHS director general for renewable 2-year terms. A secretariat to provide administrative support for these organisations is to be provided by the Section for the Evaluation of the Novel Methods, Division of Pharmacology, the BSRC and the NIHS. A quorum of two-thirds of the membership of a body is required to transact the business at a meeting, and in principle, decisions are made by consensus among those in attendance. In cases where a consensus cannot be reached, decisions can be made by a two-thirds majority vote of those in attendance. Meeting reports include information on issues for which a consensus was not achieved. These procedures were recommended by the JaCVAM Steering Committee after the decision by the JaC-VAM Regulatory Acceptance Board, which was based on material summarised by the JaCVAM Editorial Committee, as outlined in the Regulations on the Foundation of JaCVAM.

2.2 Regulatory Acceptance and Ongoing Studies

In the 11 years that JaCVAM has been active, it has assisted in the development and acceptance in Japan of a number of non-animal test methods, as shown in Table 1. With the 2011 MHLW notification, JaCVAM decided to take advantage of the opportunity to strongly impact testing throughout Japan by accelerating the development of new *in vitro* test methods. JaCVAM also supports and collaborates with other international organisations on ongoing method validation studies.

TABLE 1 Test Methods Proposed to MWLH (Ministry of Health, Labour and Welfare) by JaCVAM

No.	Test Method
1	*In vitro* skin corrosion: reconstructed human epidermis (RHE) test methods: epiCS, EpiDerm, Episkin, SkinEthic and Vitrolife-Skin
2	*In vitro* skin irritation: RHE test methods: Episkin, Epiderm, LabCyte EPI-Model and SkinEthic
3	Bovine corneal opacity and permeability (BCOP) test method for identifying: (a) chemicals inducing serious eye damage; and (b) chemicals not requiring classification for eye irritation or serious eye damage
4	Isolated chicken eye (ICE) test method for identifying: (a) chemicals inducing serious eye damage; and (b) chemicals not requiring classification for eye irritation or serious eye damage
5	Fluorescein leakage (FL) assay for identifying ocular corrosives and severe irritants
6	Short time exposure (STE) *in vitro* test method for identifying: (a) chemicals inducing serious eye damage; and (b) chemicals not requiring classification for eye irritation or serious eye damage
7	Reconstructed human cornea-like epithelium (RhCE) test method for identifying chemicals not requiring classification and labelling for eye irritation or serious eye damage
8	Acute eye irritation/corrosion (updated TG 405, 2012): use of anaesthetics, analgesics and humane endpoints for routine use in TG 405
9	Skin sensitisation: local lymph node assay (LLNA)
10	Skin sensitisation: local lymph node assay, non-radioactive method: (LLNA-DA)
11	Skin sensitisation: local lymph node assay, non-radioactive ELISA method: BrdU-ELISA
12	*In chemico* skin sensitisation: direct peptide reactivity assay (DPRA)
13	*In vitro* skin sensitisation: ARE-Nrf2 luciferase test method
14	*In vitro* skin sensitisation assays addressing the key event on activation of dendritic cells on the adverse outcome pathway for skin sensitisation: h-CLAT (human Cell Line Activation Test)
15	Skin absorption *in vitro* method
16	Reactive oxygen species (ROS) assay: *in chemico* method for identifying the phototoxic potential of chemicals
17	Use of *in vitro* cytotoxicity tests for estimating starting doses for acute oral systemic toxicity tests
18	Performance-Based Test Guideline for stably transfected transactivation *in vitro* assays to detect oestrogen receptor agonists and antagonists: The Stably Transfected Transcriptional Activation (STTA) assay using the (h)ERα-HeLa-9903 cell line
19	Performance-Based Test Guideline for stably transfected transactivation *in vitro* assays to detect oestrogen receptor agonists and antagonists: The VM7Luc ER TA assay using the VM7Luc4E2 cell line1, which predominately expresses hERα with some contribution from hER

JaCVAM is currently coordinating or participating in the validation or peer review of several tests in accordance with the ICATM framework (Table 2). As a result, JaCVAM has proposed a number of test guidelines to the OECD or the International Conference on Harmonisation of Technical Requirements for Registration of Pharmaceuticals for Human Use (ICH). There are 10 test methods developed and validated in Japan that have been approved and issued as test guidelines or guidance documents by the OECD. In addition, new test methods are being developed for endpoints such as skin sensitisation and endocrine disruption. The proposed test methods currently submitted to the OECD include the reactive oxygen species (ROS) assay for screening substances for phototoxicity, the Vitrigel-EIT (eye irritation test) for identifying eye irritants, the LabCyte Cornea Model-EIT for identifying eye irritants, and the Hand-1 Luc assay for identifying reproductive toxicants.

Since its establishment, JaCVAM has contributed to a number of OECD TGs for alternatives to animal testing. Furthermore, a number of test methods, either developed by Japanese researchers or having undergone a JaCVAM-coordinated validation study, have been considered for regulatory acceptance as ICH guidelines or as OECD TGs. JaCVAM is committed to promoting the regulatory acceptance of these and other assays that have been validated and have undergone peer-review studies according to the ICATM framework.

TABLE 2 The International Acceptance Status of Test Methods Developed in Japan

Test Method	Organisations Conducting Validation Study	Organisations Conducting Peer Review	Accepted TG	Date
Skin sensitisation: Local lymph node assay: DA	JaCVAM	ICCVAM	OECD TG442A	2010
Skin sensitisation: Local lymph node assay: BrdU-ELISA	JaCVAM	ICCVAM	OECD TG442B	2010
In vitro skin irritation: reconstructed human epidermis test method, LabCyte EPI-Model	JaCVAM	OECD experts for skin irritation	OECD TG439	2013
Reactive oxygen species assay	JaCVAM, NICEATM	JaCVAM	ICH harmonised tripartite guideline: Photosafety Evaluation of Pharmaceuticals S10	2013
In vivo comet assay	JaCVAM, ECVAM, ICCVAM	OECD experts for genotoxicity	OECD TG489	2014
Short-time exposure *in vitro* test method	JaCVAM	ICCVAM	OECD TG 491	2015
Stably-transfected TA assay using the (h)ERα-HeLa-9903 cell line	JaCVAM	OECD EDTA VMG-NA	OECD TG 455	2015
Stably transfected transactivation *in vitro* assays to detect oestrogen receptor (AR-Ecoscreen)	JaCVAM	OECD EDTA VMG-NA	OECD TG458	2016
In vitro skin sensitisation, Human cell line activation test (h-CLAT)	ECVAM	ECVAM	OECD TG442E	2016
In vitro Bhas 42 cell transformation assay (Bhas 42 CTA)	JaCVAM, ECVAM, ICCVAM	ECVAM	OECD GD231	2016
In vitro skin sensitisation, IL-8 Luc assay	JaCVAM, ECVAM, ICCVAM, KoCVAM	JaCVAM	OECD TG442E	2017
Vitrigel-EIT (eye irritation test)	JaCVAM, ECVAM, ICCVAM, KoCVAM	JaCVAM	OECD work plan	
Reconstructed human cornea-like epithelium (RhCE) test method: LabCyte EIT Cornea Model-EIT	JaCVAM	JaCVAM	OECD work plan	
Hand-1 Luc assay for identifying reproductive toxicants	JaCVAM, ECVAM, ICCVAM, KoCVAM	JaCVAM	OECD work plan	

REFERENCES

1. JSAAE. (2017). *The Japanese Society for Alternatives to Animal Experiments*. Available at: http://www.asas.or.jp/jsaae/eng/index.html.
2. Russell, W.M.S. & Burch, R.L. (1959). *The Principles of Humane Experimental Technique*, 238pp. London. UK: Methuen.
3. Anon. (2000). The Three Rs declaration of Bologna. *ATLA* **28**, 1–5.
4. OECD. (2017). *OECD Guidelines for the Testing of Chemicals. Section 4: Health Effects*. Paris, France: OECD.
5. EC. (2004). *Time Tables for the Phasing-out of Animal Testing in the Framework of the 7th Amendment to the Cosmetics Directive (Council Directive 76/768/EEC)*. Commission Staff Working Documents, (SEC82004)1210. Brussels, Belgium: European Commission.
6. Anon. (2011). *Guidebook on the Manufacture and Sales of Cosmetics and Quasi-Drugs,* pp. 159–182. [In Japanese]. Tokyo, Japan: Yakuji Nippo Ltd.
7. Anon. (2005). *Guide for the Care and Use of Laboratory Animals* [In Japanese]. Tokyo, Japan: Ministry of Health, Labour and Welfare.
8. Anon. (2006). *Cosmetics Standard Amendment Request and Manufacturing and Marketing Approval of Quasi-Drugs* [In Japanese]. Tokyo, Japan: Ministry of Health, Labour and Welfare.
9. PMDA. (2017). *Homepage* [In Japanese]. Tokyo, Japan: Pharmaceuticals and Medical Devices Agency. Available at: https://www.pmda.go.jp/review-services/drug-reviews/about-reviews/q-drugs/0002.html.
10. JaCVAM. (2017). *Homepage*. Tokyo, Japan: Japanese Center for the Validation of Alternative Methods. Available at: http://www.jacvam.jp/en/index.html.
11. Barroso, J., Ahn, I.Y., Caldeira, C., *et al.* (2016). Validation of alternative methods for toxicity testing. *Advances in Experimental Medicine & Biology* **856**, 343–386.

Chapter 2.9

Contributions to the Development of Alternatives in Toxicology in China and Brazil

Rodger D. Curren[1], Chantra Eskes[2], Shujun Cheng[3,4] and Erin H. Hill[1]

[1]Institute for In Vitro Sciences, Gaithersburg, MD, United States; [2]3RCC, Bern, Switzerland; [3]Shanghai Jiao Tong University, Shanghai, China; [4]Guangzhou Chn-Alt Biotechnology Co., Ltd., Guangzhou, China

SUMMARY

China and Brazil are two of the largest international economies now attempting to incorporate non-animal, *in vitro*, testing methods into their regulatory systems. While Brazil has a government mandate to replace certain animal tests with alternative methods in a stated time-frame, China has no such requirement, but is none-the-less pursuing a similar goal. China lacks the internal infrastructure to provide *in vitro* testing and easy access to validated human tissue constructs, and Brazil lacks financial support to develop new alternative methods and has difficulty in commercialising human-based materials, e.g. cells and reconstructed tissues. However, both countries are embracing offers for training and other technical assistance, when needed. It is expected that formal regulatory acceptance of non-animal test results will continue and expand in both China and Brazil.

1. INTRODUCTION: ALTERNATIVES IN CHINA AND BRAZIL

In this chapter, we explore the developing acceptance of alternatives in toxicology testing for two rapidly growing economies — China and Brazil, especially with respect to cosmetics and specialty ingredients. Although they are using slightly different approaches, both countries are actively forging their way toward the adoption of alternatives, starting with cosmetics regulations.

As this chapter is being written, there remains the mandatory animal testing of cosmetics in China to register many domestically produced cosmetics, imported cosmetics and new ingredients. Additionally, the national and provincial governments reserve the right to conduct the random surveillance, which can include animal toxicity testing, of marketed products. Pressure for China to adopt alternatives for cosmetics regulations comes primarily from the US and EU cosmetics manufacturers and governments, which wish to allow cosmetic companies to assess safety without the use of animals, thus retaining their "cruelty-free" status. Also, the substantially increasing market for the production and consumption of cosmetics makes the transition to rapid non-animal testing appealing, if not a necessity. The regulatory adoption and availability of alternatives in China would not only benefit foreign companies wishing to sell in China, but would also allow Chinese cosmetics companies access to the lucrative European market by meeting the requirements of the EU ban on animal testing. China is currently building capacity and infrastructure related to alternatives, by spending resources to retrain its provincial government laboratories in the conduct of these new methods and in the review of data for regulatory safety decisions. The China Food and Drug Administration (CFDA) has stated that regulations with regard to the acceptance of alternatives will not change until this infrastructure is in place, but, although progress has been made, the timelines for this process have not been revealed.

By contrast, Brazil has current and pending legislative requirements for alternatives for cosmetics, and is now working to build capacity and infrastructure within the country. The process of adoption and associated timelines is transparent, but also somewhat overwhelming, due to a lack of certain key methodologies (e.g. reconstructed human tissue equivalents). However, as outlined in this chapter, Brazil has organised a network of laboratories, and is working with the international community to assist in the training and development of methods within the country. The process of adoption and implementation of alternatives in Brazil will stand as the prime example for other countries in the region — adding pressure to ensure success.

While the impetus to adopt alternatives for cosmetics differs somewhat between these two countries, certain important similarities remain. Both regions are in a capacity-building mode and are turning to the international community to help them with training needs. Although not currently members, representatives of China and Brazil attend OECD meetings and International Co-operation on Alternative Methods (ICATM) meetings as observers, to learn from the successes of other countries. Furthermore, Brazil also adheres to the Mutual Acceptance of Data (MAD) procedure of the OECD Test Guidelines (TGs) programme. As the regulations change, new market opportunities are arising for test method developers, equipment manufacturers, contract research laboratories and consultants. Most importantly, both countries have embarked on the path to fully adopt alternatives for the regulatory safety assessment of cosmetics and have turned to the international community to assist them along the way.

2. ALTERNATIVES IN CHINA

2.1 History of Animal Use Regulations in China

In ancient traditional Chinese medicine (TCM) books, there are references to the experimental use of animals. After industrialisation, Ji Chang Qing, of Peking University, reported the earliest record of China's use of animal testing as having been in 1918. He used mice in his research on the prevention of infectious diseases. After the Regulation for Administration of Laboratory Animals was issued in 1988, the utilisation of laboratory animals came to be supervised by the Ministry of Science and Technology (MOST), and Local Science and Technology Departments are responsible for supervision within their jurisdictions. In the 1990s, the Three Rs principles and animal welfare started to emerge, but it took about 20 years for this to be widely recognised by Chinese scientists. Recognition of the importance of the Three Rs was stimulated by the 2014 publication in China of an abridged version (written by Michael Balls and called *The Three Rs and the Humanity Criterion* (1)) of the famous Russell and Burch book, *The Principles of Humane Experimental Technique*" (2). This activity was truly an international collaborative effort, with Chinese contributors providing the translation from English into Mandarin, the US-based Institute for In Vitro Sciences (IIVS) organising the project, and the European Partnership for Alternative Approaches to Animal Testing providing the funding. A copy of the book was supplied free-of-charge to libraries and universities in China. In 2006, the Three Rs principles were incorporated into MOST guidance documents, and in 2016, the laboratory animal institute accreditation system was established. Academic progress was also made, as indicated by the establishment during the last decade of animal welfare ethics committees founded via the Chinese Association for Laboratory Animal Science (CALAS; 3), and the Sino-British International Seminar on Laboratory Animal Welfare & Ethics, held annually since 2014.

2.2 The Regulatory Framework in China

At present, China's animal use involves scientific research, including medicine and vaccine development, health and bioscience research and toxicity testing. The CFDA, reorganised in 2013, is responsible for the supervision of drugs, medical devices, cosmetics and food. Local (provincial) FDAs are the supervisors and administrators within their jurisdictions, under the direction of the CFDA. The National Institute for Food and Drug Control (NIFDC) and local IFDCs, as technology supporting departments, are responsible for the toxicity testing of products administrated by the CFDA. The pre-General Administration of Quality Supervision, Inspection and Quarantine (pre-AQSIQ) was in charge of the toxicity testing of a selected amount of the imported and exported chemicals and other products, including cosmetics. The Ministry of Environmental Protection (MEP) is mainly responsible for examining and approving the application and registration of new chemicals. There is some overlap of authority between the various organisations, which sometimes makes the final responsibility unclear. The area of cosmetics is a good example. The CFDA is responsible for the pre-market approval of cosmetics, post-marketing surveillance and new ingredient registration, whereas the pre-AQSIQ was responsible for assuring the safety of imported and exported cosmetics and some post-marketing surveillance. Currently, China relies on the assessment of the finished product for regulatory safety decisions on cosmetics.

In 2014, the CFDA announced that animal testing could be waived for the safety evaluation of domestically produced, non-special-use cosmetics, if other safety data could be provided. However, this did not mean that data from non-animal or *in vitro* tests would be accepted. Subsequently, the CFDA guidance, *Cosmetic Safety Technical Specifications*, did formally adopt the 3T3 NRU Phototoxicity Assay (OECD TG 432) and the Transcutaneous Electrical Resistance (TER) Assay (OECD TG 430). However, the adoption of these methods for the regulatory assessment of other commodities, such as food, medicines and medical devices, has not been announced.

2.3 Movement Toward the Use and Validation of Alternative Methods in China

In China, the concepts of the Three Rs and laboratory animal welfare are relatively new. The cosmetic industry is motivated by the scientific and business advantages that alternative tests provide (e.g. the formulation of milder products and rapid test results) and the increased accessibility to markets where animal testing is prohibited. The Chinese cosmetics industry can play an important role in informing the Chinese Government of the advantages non-animal methods provide. In the most-recent decade, several companies have focused on developing and providing alternative methods and a platform of *in vitro* test systems for the Chinese market (4). The ChnAlt Biotechnology Company, Guangdong Biocell Biotechnology Ltd. and Shanghai EPISKIN Biotech (a subsidiary of EPISKIN France) are three key tissue-engineering manufacture companies in China that produce and commercialise 3-D human reconstructed-skin models to Chinese users for alternative testing. The only Chinese alternative platform validated in a multicentre study of *in vitro* skin irritation test method is the China EpiSkin model. The study was organised by pre-AQSIQ, and was conducted by five participating laboratories from 2011 to 2013. Based on the successful result of this study, an SN standard (SN/T 4577-2016) was approved and published, which encourages the use of the *in vitro* skin irritation testing method in China (5, 6).

Since 2010, several prominent universities and institutes have taken steps to develop new methods in harmony with OECD guidelines and the Toxicity Testing in the 21st Century (TT21C) and adverse outcome pathway (AOP) concepts. For example, the Academy of Military Medical Sciences, Guangzhou ChnAlt, Shanghai Jiaotong University and Beijing Technology and Business University (BTBU), have established alternative educational programmes, which include training. Some academic progress has been made in the *in vitro* fields of mitochondrial toxicity (7) and embryonic stem cell differentiation toxicology (8). Notably, the Toxicological Alternatives and Translational Toxicology (TATT) subsection of the China Society of Toxicology (CSOT) was founded in 2014, along with the Society of Toxicity Testing and Alternatives (STTA), a subgroup of the Chinese Environmental Mutagen Society. With more than 500 members in 2017, the TATT has already held three international conferences (independent of the annual CSOT meetings). The most historic and influential Chinese alternative conference is sponsored by the Guangdong CIQ and Guangzhou Chn-Alt. Initiated in 2013, the annual conference has grown in terms of numbers in attendance and in the participation of international experts.

2.4 Support for, and Regulatory Implementation of, Alternatives Within China

Following their duty to promote international trade and risk control, pre-AQSIQ and its branches usually accept global regulations and cooperate internationally on research and technology, including that on alternatives (9). AQSIQ has accepted several international alternative methods since 2005, and makes efforts to incorporate alternative test methods into their safety evaluations. They have issued more than 17 SN standards of chemicals and cosmetics toxicology testing methods and principles within their inspection and quarantine standard system (Table 1). The MEP directly adopted the OECD TGs, and transferred them to the chemicals national testing standards (GB standard) as their testing methods. In recent years, the MEP has also made more-positive efforts to adopt and accept alternative methods, such as QSAR and read-across methods.

The CFDA has stated that, before the regulations can change, the authorities must have confidence that the methods they approve are available within the provincial government system. To achieve this goal, the NIFDC entered into a Memorandum of Understanding (MoU) with the IIVS, a US-based non-profit laboratory, to collaborate in promoting the use of non-animal tests in the regulation of cosmetic products and ingredients in China. A key component of this work is an annual hands-on training course in China, provided by IIVS scientists. To date, the IIVS has provided five intensive hands-on trainings for scientists from the provincial IFDCs, as well as hosting visits by Chinese regulatory scientists at IIVS in the USA. The success of this approach can be observed in the Zhejiang IFDC, which is not only proficient in many methods, but also serves as a training hub for other regulatory scientists and provides services to Chinese and international cosmetic companies.

TABLE 1 Standards Issued by China's Regulatory Authorities

ID of Standard (1)	Name
GB/T 21827-2008	Skin Allergy Test — Local Lymph Node Assay[a]
GB/T 21769-2008	*In Vitro* 3T3 NRU Phototoxicity Test
GB/T 21757-2008	Acute Oral Toxicity — Acute Toxic Class Method[a]
GB/T 21804-2008	Acute Oral Toxicity — Fixed Dose Procedure[a]
GB/T 21826-2008	Acute Oral Toxicity: Up-And-Down Procedure[a]
GB/T 27829-2011	*In Vitro* Membrane Barrier Test Method for Skin Corrosion
GB/T 27818-2011	Skin Absorption: *In Vitro* Method
GB/T 27828-2011	Rat Skin Transcutaneous Electrical Resistance Test
GB/T 27830-2011	*In Vitro* Human Skin Model for Skin Corrosion
SN/T 2245-2009	Chemicals: *In Vitro* Skin Corrosion; Transcutaneous Electrical Resistance Test
SN/T 2285-2009	Cosmetics: GLP for *In Vitro* Alternative Tests
SN/T 2328-2009	Cosmetics: Cytotoxicity tests to estimate starting doses for acute Oral Acute Toxicity Tests
SN/T 2329-2009	Cosmetics: Ocular Corrosive and Irritant HET-CAM Test
SN/T 2330-2009	Cosmetics: Embryotoxicity and Developmental Toxicity Test: EST (Embryonic Stem Cell) Test
SN/T 3084.1-2012	Cosmetics: Neutral Red Uptake Assays for eye irritation
SN/T 3084.2-2014	Cosmetics: Red Blood Cell Test for eye irritation
SN/T 3527-2013	Chemicals: Embryotoxicity Test Post Implantation Embryo Culture Method
SN/T 3715-2013	Cosmetics: Developmental Toxicity Test: WEC (Whole Embryo Culture) Test
SN/T 3824-2014	Cosmetics: Phototoxicity: Combined RBC (Red Blood Cell) Test
SN/T 3882-2014	Chemicals: Skin Sensitization of Chemicals: LLNA (Local Lymph Node Assay) for Brdu-ELISA[a]
SN/T 3898-2014	Cosmetics: Validation Procedures for *In Vitro* Alternative Tests
SN/T 3899-2014	Cosmetics: GLP for *In Vitro* Alternative Tests: Cell Culture and Sample Preparation
SN/T 3948-2014	Chemicals: *In Vitro* Skin Irritation Reconstructed Human Epidermis Test Method
SN/T 4150-2015	Chemicals: Method for Isolated Chicken Eye Test
SN/T 4153-2015	Chemicals: Bovine Corneal Opacity and Permeability Tes
SN/T 4154-2015	Chemicals: Skin sensitization Local Lymph Node Assay:DA[a]
SN/T 4577-2016	Cosmetics: *In Vitro* Skin Irritation Reconstructed Human Epidermis Test Method

GB, Guo Biao — National Standards for Chemicals; *SN/T*, Professional Standards for Inspection and Quarantine system.
[a]*Not non-animal methods, but tests which give Three Rs benefits of refinement and reduction compared with standard animal tests.*

Contract research organisations and consulting firms are also emerging in response to the growing demand for alternatives. As an example, the Chn-Alt was established as a third-party company specialising in non-animal testing, technical training and the development of new *in vitro* methods for the testing of cosmetics and chemicals. There are five R&D centres in the Chn-Alt, which individually focus on organ-on-a-chip systems, skin sensitisation, the safety of TCM and plant-based medicine, integrated testing and Big Data analytics. In addition to toxicology services, this organisation also offers efficacy testing and innovative methods based on industry's needs (10–12).

2.5 Special Difficulties or Hurdles to Accepting and/or Using Alternative Methods

The CFDA has stated its concern about the applicability of OECD TG methods to cosmetic products, because those guidelines were validated for ingredients and China regulates cosmetics based on the final formulation. In addition, the CFDA wishes to explore the utility of these methods for TCMs, which are also used widely as cosmetic ingredients. Access to certain reagents and equipment can also be difficult.

Until the regulations are changed, many potential technology providers are in a wait-and-see mode, unwilling to expend resources until they have confidence in the acceptance of the new methods by the regulatory authorities.

2.6 Future Outlook for Alternatives in China

The development and application of alternative methods in China has made great progress, and there is the exciting prospect that there will be a breakthrough in the near future in the innovation of alternative methods and their recognition in laws and regulations (13, 14). In 2017, Chinese stakeholders have launched multiple projects. For example, an *in vitro* method laboratory accreditation guidelines project was launched in August 2017, which will be set up within three years, ultimately to achieve the mutual recognition of data. Translational toxicology courses were first set up in Shanghai Jiaotong University in September 2017. Finally, a cosmetic *in vitro* database project, led by Guangzhou Chn-Alt Co., has been established. It is encouraging to note that the Chinese Government will make the inspection and testing, certification and accreditation and metrology and standards a part of the national quality infrastructure, which will benefit future alternative testing.

3. ALTERNATIVES IN BRAZIL

3.1 History of Animal Use Regulations in Brazil

Brazil's legislation for animal protection began in 1934, with a law against animal cruelty which was general in nature. It included all animals and recognised them as protected by the state (15, 16). Subsequently, a law dealing with environmental crimes established, for the first time, a duty of care to anyone involved in the use of animals, including their use in experimentation and in teaching (16).

However, it was only in 2008 that Brazil adopted *Law 11,794*, which specifically regulates the use of laboratory animals in experimentation and in education (17). This law represented an invaluable advance in the country (18) and implemented two important actions, namely: (a) the creation of the National Council of the Control of Animal Experimentation (Conselho Nacional de Controle da Experimentação Animal (CONCEA)); and (b) the obligation for all institutions using animals for experimentation or education to have an Ethics Committee on Animal Use (Comissão de Ética no Uso de Animais (CEUA)).

CONCEA is a multi-institutional council, with representatives from different government ministries, associations, scientific societies and non-governmental organisations (NGOs), and possesses among its competences the duty to control and monitor the implementation of alternative methods (17).

3.2 The Regulatory Framework in Brazil

In Brazil, a central regulatory agency, the National Health Surveillance Agency (Agência Nacional de Vigilância Sanitária (ANVISA)), along with its other duties, is responsible for the registration and authorisation of various kinds of products. Established in 1999, ANVISA is a governmental agency, characterised by its administrative independence and financial autonomy and the stability of its directors (ANVISA is ruled by a Collegiate Board of Directors composed of five members). ANVISA's primary goal is to protect and promote public health by exercising health surveillance over products and services, including processes, ingredients and technologies that may pose health risks. The agency is also responsible for health control in ports and airports and at borders, as well as for establishing relations with the Ministry of International Affairs and with foreign organisations and institutions, to deal with international affairs regarding health surveillance. The various areas regulated by ANVISA comprise cosmetics, food, medical devices, pharmaceuticals, plant protection products, sanitising products, blood-tissues-organs, tobacco and customs regulations.

3.3 Movement Toward the Use and Validation of Alternative Methods in Brazil

Since 2003, ANVISA has recognised the use of *in vitro* test methods as pre-clinical tests for the safety assessment of cosmetics products (19). This guideline was subsequently revised in 2012, and currently accepts a number of Three Rs methods, including *in silico* evaluation, *in vitro* test methods, the use of existing data and bridging principles (20). In particular, the use of pre-clinical *in vitro* testing is suggested for the assessment of eye hazards, skin irritation and corrosion, phototoxicity and skin absorption.

Furthermore, in 2012, ANVISA established a co-operative agreement with the Oswaldo Cruz Foundation (FIOCRUZ), a research institution under the auspices of the Ministry of Heath, to establish the Brazilian Center for the Validation of Alternative Methods (BraCVAM). BraCVAM, subsequently created in 2013, is currently managed under the auspices of the National Institute of Quality Control in Health (Instituto Nacional de Controle de Qualidade em Saúde (INCQS)).

BraCVAM represents the first Latin American centre dedicated to the development and validation of alternative methods. Its objectives are to promote national and international harmonisation on the acceptance of alternative methods and to be responsive to regional needs, such as the need to develop alternatives for the quality controls of biological produced for specific Brazilian threats (e.g. antivenoms against the effects of venomous snakes, spiders, scorpions and frogs). In particular, the validation process in Brazil follows OECD Guidance Document No. 34 (21). Furthermore, BraCVAM aims at collaborating with Brazilian and international partners, including ICATM (22). In 2015, the first Brazilian validation study was initiated on the Hen's Egg Test — Chorion-Allantoic Membrane test (HET-CAM) for eye hazard identification, sponsored by the Brazilian Ministry of Science, Technology and Innovation (Ministério da Ciência, Tecnologia e Inovação (MCTI)). Finally, BraCVAM makes recommendations on the scientific validity of alternative test methods to CONCEA, which is then responsible for the official adoption of alternative methods in the legislation and regulations.

3.4 Support for, and Regulatory Implementation of, Alternatives Within Brazil

In 2012, the National Network on Alternative Methods (Rede Nacional de Métodos Alternativos (ReNaMA)) was established, completing the three pillars responsible for the validation (BraCVAM), regulatory acceptance (CONCEA) and implementation (ReNaMA) of alternative methods in Brazil (15). ReNaMA was created by the MCTI and is composed of three central laboratories and associated laboratories that work with alternative methods, including official and private laboratories in academia and in industry. The three central laboratories are the INCQS; the National Institute of Metrology, Quality and Technology (Instituto Nacional de Metrologia, Qualidade e Tecnologia (INMETREO)) and the Brazilian Biosciences National Laboratory (LNBio). The network aims to: (a) provide training and stimulate the implementation of alternative methods to animal testing; (b) monitor the proficiency of laboratories conducting alternative test methods in Brazil; (c) provide high quality reference materials to promote the quality of alternative test methods; (d) promote the implementation of Good Laboratory Practices; and (e) promote the development, validation and adoption of novel alternative methods to animal testing.

From a regulatory point of view, CONCEA officially adopted in 2014 a total of 17 alternative methods to animal use having international regulatory acceptance, and established a 5-year term for the replacement of the traditional methods by the adopted alternative test methods (23, 24). These methods were subsequently approved by ANVISA in 2015. Furthermore, in 2016, an additional seven alternative test methods were officially adopted by CONCEA, also with a 5-year term for the replacement of the traditional method (24). Table 2 lists the 24 alternative test methods officially recognised by CONCEA in Brazil.

3.5 Special Difficulties or Hurdles to Accepting and/or Using Alternative Methods

From a research and developmental point of view, only a few projects have benefited from public funding to develop alternative test methods in Brazil. These include the development of a reconstructed human epidermis, the development of *in silico* methods to predict the toxicity and pharmacokinetics of small candidate molecules for pharmaceuticals and cosmetics, and the development of a human-on-a-chip model. Further investment on the research and development of alternative methods would certainly favour the further implementation of such methodologies. Another major bottleneck, preventing a broader use of *in vitro* test methods in Brazil, remains the commercialisation of the consumables and cells needed for conducting *in vitro* assays. Legislation in Brazil entails a very strict control on human-derived products, and that may hamper the accessibility and commercialisation of cell-based and tissue-based products of human origin, as well as some critical reagents. In addition, import requirements can lead to delays at the borders, and products can be retained without appropriate storage conditions. Finally, the existing high import tax costs may discourage Brazilian researchers from acquiring materials from abroad and could prompt them to make use of foreign contract research facilities instead.

TABLE 2 Alternative Test Methods Officially Endorsed by CONCEA

Endpoint	OECD	Name	Year of Endorsement
Skin irritation and corrosion	TG 430	*In Vitro* Skin Corrosion: Transcutaneous Electrical Resistance Test	2014
	TG 431	*In Vitro* Skin Corrosion: Reconstructed Human Epidermis Test Method	2014
	TG 435	*In Vitro* Membrane Barrier Test Method for Skin Corrosion	2014
	TG 439	*In Vitro* Skin Irritation	2014
Eye irritation and corrosion	TG 437	Bovine Corneal Opacity and Permeability Test Method	2014
	TG 438	Isolated Chicken Eye Test Method	2014
	TG 460	Fluorescein Leakage Test Method	2014
	TG 491	Short-Term Exposure *In Vitro* test for ocular hazard	2016
	TG 492	Reconstructed Human Cornea-like Epithelium	2016
Phototoxicity	TG 432	*In Vitro* 3T3 NRU Phototoxicity Test	2014
Skin absorption	TG 428	Skin Absorption: *In Vitro* Method	2014
Skin sensitisation	TG 429	Skin Sensitisation: reduced Local Lymph Node Assay	2014
	TG 442A & 442B	Non-radioactive versions of the Local Lymph Node Assay	2014
	TG 442C	*In Chemico* Skin Sensitisation	2016
	TG 442D	*In Vitro* Skin Sensitisation	2016
Acute toxicity	TG 420	Acute Oral Toxicity − Fixed Dose Procedure	2014
	TG 423	Acute Oral Toxicity − Acute Toxic Class	2014
	TG 425	Acute Oral Toxicity − Up and Down Procedure	2014
	GD 129	Estimation of starting dose for Acute Oral Systemic Toxicity Testing	2014
Genotoxicity	TG 487	*In Vitro* Mammalian Cell Micronucleus Test	2014
Reproductive toxicology	TG 421	Reproduction/Developmental Toxicity Screening Test	2016
	TG 422	Combined Repeated Dose Toxicity Study with the Reproduction/Developmental Toxicity Screening Test	2016
Pyrogenicity	Not applicable	Bacterial Endotoxin Test from Brazilian Pharmacopoeia	2016

3.6 Future Outlook for Alternatives in Brazil

The further use of alternative methods in toxicology in Brazil (and in South America, in general) has been encouraged by cooperation in training within South America. Mercosur is a South American common market and trade union, comprising Argentina, Brazil, Paraguay and Uruguay as Member Countries, as well as Bolivia, Chile, Peru, Colombia, Ecuador and Suriname as Associate Member Countries. The creation of Mercosur's Regional Platform on Alternative Methods (Plataforma Regional de Métodos Alternativos ao Uso de Animais do Mercosul (PReMASul)) was endorsed in 2015. PReMASul aims to establish a trained infrastructure of laboratories and a workforce specialised in, and able to implement, alternative methods to animal testing within the respective countries. The first step of the project is to train and qualify personnel and laboratories, for which Brazil has offered a series of training courses within the central laboratories of ReNaMA, in, for example, the areas of genotoxicity and ocular and skin irritation and corrosion, as well as on the regulatory acceptance of alternative methods.

REFERENCES

1. Balls, M. (2014). *The Three Rs and the Humanity Criterion* (in Mandarin), 106pp. Beijing, China: PRC Science Press.
2. Russell, W.M.S. & Burch, R.L. (1959). *The Principles of Humane Experimental Technique*, 238pp. London, UK: Methuen.
3. Zhengming, H. & Guanmin, L. (2003). *Introduction to Alternative Methods of Animal Experiment*, 302pp. Beijing, China: Academy Press.
4. Cheng, S., Hong, J. & Yao, Q. (2008). The preliminary study of *in vitro* constructing new skin model inspectskin I for cosmetics inspection. *Journal of Toxicology* **22**, 428−431.
5. Nan, L., Yanfeng, L., Jie, Q., *et al.* (2017). *In vitro* skin irritation assessment becomes a reality in China using a reconsturcted human epidermis test method. *Toxicology in Vitro* **41**, 159−167.
6. Qiu, J., Zhong, L., Zhou, M., *et al.* (2016). Establishment and characterization of a reconstructed Chinese human epidermis model. *International Journal of Cosmetic Science* **38**, 60−67.
7. Guo, J., Peng, H., Wang, Y., *et al.* (2012). Significance of mitochondrial toxicity testing in the safety evaluation of innovative drugs. *Chinese Journal of New Drugs* **16**, 1867−1871.
8. Cheng, S., Yao, Q., Huan, Y., *et al.* (2016). Progress for alternatives methods predict the embryotoxicity by embryonic stem cell test. *Chinese Journal of Comparative Medicine* **26**, 81−85.
9. Cheng, S. & Jiao, H. (2010). *Alternative Laboratory Animal Methods, Principles and Application*, 655pp. Beijing, China: PRC Science Press.
10. Qiu, T., Cheng, S., Jiancong, H., *et al.* (2014). Integrated CAMVA and BCOP methods to predict eye irritation caused by cosmetics. *Chinese Journal of Comparative Medicine* **24**, 78−82.
11. Yu, C., Huan, Y., Cheng, S., *et al.* (2016). Research on bovine corneal opacity and permeability test integrating with histopathological evaluation. *Detergents & Cosmetics* **46**, 106−110.
12. Yihui, K., Yu, C. & Cheng, S. (2016). Preliminary study for integrating DPRA with h-CLAT to predict skin sensitizers. *Acta Laboratorium Animalis Scientia Sinica* **24**, 613−619.
13. Cheng, S. (2017). *Guides of Alternative Methods Standards for Cosmetics Assessment*, 362pp. Beijing, China: Standard Press.
14. Cheng, S., Qu, X. & Qin, Y. (2017). Harmonisation of animal testing alternatives in China. *ATLA* **45**, 333−338.
15. Presgrave, O., Moura, W., Caldeira, C., *et al.* (2016). Brazilian Center for the Validation of Alternative Methods (BraCVAM) and the process of validation in Brazil. *ATLA* **44**, 85−90.
16. Cardoso, C. & Presgrave, O. (2010). Princípios éticos na experimentação animal. In A. Andrade, M. Andrade, A. Marinho, & J. Filho (Eds.), *Biologia, Manejo e Medicina de Primatas Nao Humanos na Pesquisa Biomedica*, pp. 435−449. Rio de Janeiro, Brasil: Fiocruz.
17. Presidência da República. (2008). *Lei n. 11.794, de 08 de outubro de 2008. Diário Oficial, Seção 1, 09.10.2008*. Brasilia, Brasil: Republica Federativa do Brasil.
18. Marques, R.G., Morales, M.M. & Petroianu, A. (2009). Brazilian law for scientific use of animals. *Acta Cir rgica Brasileira* **24**, 69−74.
19. ANVISA. (2003). *Guideline for the Safety Evaluation of Cosmetic Products*, 43pp. Basillia, Brazil: Brazilian Health Surveillance Agency.
20. ANVISA. (2012). *Guia para Avaliação de Segurança de Produtos Cosméticos*, 2nd ed., 71pp. Brasilia, Brazil: Brazilian Health Surveillance Agency.
21. OECD. (2005). Guidance document on the validation and international acceptance of new or updated test methods for hazard assessment. In *OECD Series on Testing and Assessment No. 34*, 96pp. Paris, France: OECD.
22. Barroso, J., Ahn, I.Y., Caldeira, C., *et al.* (2016). International harmonization and cooperation in the validation of alternative methods. *Advances in Experimental Medicine & Biology* **856**, 343−386.
23. Ministério da Ciência, Tecnologia e Inovação. (2014). *Resolução Normativa n. 18 de 24 de setembro de 2014* (Diário Oficial da União 185, 9). Brasilia, Brasil: Republica Federativa do Brasil.
24. Ministerio da Ciência, Tecnologia e Inovação. (2016). *Resolução Normativa n. 31 de 18 de Agosto de 2016* (Diário Oficial da União). Brasilia, Brasil: Republica Federativa do Brasil.

Chapter 2.10

The Role of ECVAM

Valérie Zuang[1], Andrew P. Worth[1] and Michael Balls[2]

[1]Joint Research Centre, European Commission, Ispra, Italy; [2]University of Nottingham, Nottingham, United Kingdom

SUMMARY

Established in 1991 by a Commission Communication and in the context of *Directive 86/609/EEC*, ECVAM was given the mandate to coordinate the EU-level validation of non-animal methods and to promote dialogue between legislators, industries, biomedical scientists, consumer organisations and animal welfare groups, with a view to the development, validation and international recognition of alternative test methods. In 2011, these duties were reaffirmed under *Directive 2010/63/EU*, which also formalised ECVAM as an EU Reference Laboratory. In the 1990s, ECVAM's scientific activities were focused mainly on the needs of EU cosmetics legislation, with the new EU chemicals legislation, REACH, becoming important in the early 2000s. In the 2010s, additional cross-sector policy areas, such as chemical mixtures and endocrine disruptors, have become important drivers of ECVAM's activities. From its establishment, ECVAM has also played an important role in promoting the uptake of the Three Rs in the biologicals area. ECVAM's training, dissemination and stakeholder engagement activities have also served to promote better regulatory science through alternatives to animal testing.

1. THE EARLY YEARS OF ECVAM, 1991–2002

The background to the establishment of the European Centre for the Validation of Alternative Methods (ECVAM), and its contributions and achievements during its first 10 years, are outlined in the proceedings of two symposia, which took place in 1994 and in 2002 (1, 2).

ECVAM was established in 1991 (Table 1), as a unit of the Environment Institute of the European Commission's (EC's) Joint Research Centre (JRC), at Ispra, Italy, by a Communication from the Commission to the Council and the Parliament (3), pointing to *Article 23* of *Directive 86/609/EEC* (4), which required that 'The Commission and the Member States should encourage research into the development and validation of alternative techniques which could provide the same level of information as that obtained in experiments using animals, but which involved fewer animals or less painful procedures'. Also of particular importance was *Article 7.2* of the Directive, which stated that 'An experiment shall not be performed, if another scientifically satisfactory method of obtaining the result sought, not entailing the use of an animal, is reasonably and practically available'.

ECVAM was given specific duties, namely: (a) to coordinate the validation of alternative test methods at the European Union level; (b) to act as a focal point for the exchange of information on the development of alternative test methods; (c) to set up, maintain and manage a database on alternative procedures; (d) to promote dialogue among all the stakeholders; and (e) to help expand the JRC's role in prenormative research.

A number of significant earlier developments had occurred, including the establishment of the Fund for the Replacement of Animals in Medical Experiments (FRAME) in the UK in 1969, the Center for Alternatives to Animal Testing in the USA in 1981, and the Center for Documentation and Evaluation of Alternative Methods to Animal Experiments (ZEBET) in Germany in 1989. Also of great importance were the activities of the European Research Group for

The History of Alternative Test Methods in Toxicology. https://doi.org/10.1016/B978-0-12-813697-3.00013-5

TABLE 1 Summary Timeline for European Centre for the Validation of Alternative Methods

Date	Event
1986	Adoption of *Directive 86/609/EEC* (4)
1991	European Commission Communication establishes ECVAM (3)
1993	Michael Balls becomes first Head of ECVAM
1994	ECVAM Opening Symposium 'The Validation of Replacement Alternative Methods' (1) Establishment of the first ECVAM Scientific Advisory Committee (ESAC)
1999	Third World Congress on Alternatives and Animal Use in Life Sciences organised by ECVAM with signing of the Three Rs Declaration of Bologna
2002	ECVAM Status Seminar (2) Michael Balls retires from the JRC Thomas Hartung takes over as Head of ECVAM
2005	European Partnership for Alternative Approaches to Animal Testing (EPAA) established with EC membership
2008	Joachim Kreysa takes over as Head of ECVAM
2009	Establishment of the International Cooperation on Alternative Test Methods (ICATM)
2010	Adoption of *Directive 2010/63/EU* (13) ECVAM becomes EURL ECVAM, the EU Reference Laboratory for Alternatives to Animal Testing
2011	Establishment of the Preliminary Assessment of Regulatory Relevance (PARERE) network and the ECVAM Stakeholder Forum (ESTAF)
2012	Maurice Whelan takes over as Head of EURL ECVAM
2014	Establishment of the European Union Network of Laboratories for the Validation of Alternative Methods (EU-NETVAL)
2015	European Commission Communication on the European Citizens' Initiative 'Stop Vivisection'

Alternatives in Toxicity Testing (ERGATT), an *ad hoc* group of experienced and committed European individuals, recognised by the EC for their contributions to the development, validation and acceptance of alternative methods.

The Communication stipulated that an ECVAM Scientific Advisory Committee (ESAC) be formed, comprising representatives of the Member States, European industry associations, animal welfare organisations and ECVAM's partner services within the EC. ECVAM's interactions with Directorate General (DG) XI (later renamed DG Environment), was particularly important, as DGXI was responsible for the administration of *Directive 86/609/EEC*. Initially, ECVAM was given a protected budget, competent staff were appointed, and a purpose-designed building was constructed at Ispra.

In 1998, ECVAM was moved from the JRC's Environment Institute to the newly formed Institute for Health and Consumer Protection.

1.1 Validation

ECVAM's main activity during its first 10 years involved the definition of the principles of validation (the process whereby the relevance and reliability of a method are established for a particular purpose) and their practical application in the ECVAM validation process (5), which involved the following five main stages: (a) test development; (b) prevalidation; (c) formal validation; (d) independent assessment (peer review); and (e) progression toward regulatory acceptance. Stages 1–2 involve the definition of a prediction model, an unambiguous algorithm for converting the result from the test into a prediction of a pharmacotoxicological endpoint in humans or animals. On the completion of an ECVAM study, a report on its outcome was considered by the ESAC, which considered whether ECVAM's criteria for test development and validation had been satisfied. If so, the ESAC endorsed the scientific validity of the method, and this was communicated to the EC and others by ECVAM and DGXI.

By 2002, ESAC statements had been made for 10 tests: the 3T3 NRU phototoxicity test; the application of the 3T3 NRU phototoxicity test for UV filter chemicals; the EPISKIN, Epiderm, rat TER skin corrosivity and CORROSITEX tests for skin corrosivity testing; the local lymph node assay for skin sensitisation; and the embryonic stem cell, whole embryo culture and micromass tests for embryotoxicity.

Three further important principles emerged along the way. First, that defining the structural and performance criteria for a test would facilitate the validation and acceptance of any method that satisfied those criteria (6). This would also avoid the situation where the patenting of method could prevent the development and acceptance of a similar and competing method for the same purpose. Second, that each study should have an independent statistician, who would give advice on the design of the study, with particular emphasis on the way in which the results were calculated and expressed, and on the prediction models for the application of the outcome. Third, that catch-up validation, by a rapid and simplified process, is possible for a method similar to a validated method or the use of the same method for a different purpose, such as application to a different class of chemicals, as in the case of the use of the phototoxicity test for UV filter chemicals.

ECVAM was not directly involved in the regulatory acceptance of validated test methods, as this was handled by DGXI for the EC, within the EU in relation to Annex V of *Directive 67/548/EEC* on classification and labelling of hazardous chemicals, and at the OECD in relation to the OECD Test Guidelines (TGs) Programme. By 2002, the EU had accepted the *in vitro* phototoxicity test, the first formally validated *in vitro* toxicity test to be accepted into Annex V, and two *in vitro* corrosivity tests, and draft OECD TGs had been published for these three tests for consideration for worldwide acceptance and use (7).

1.2 Workshops and Task Forces

ECVAM began its workshop programme in 1994, and 51 workshops had been held by 2002. They usually involved about 15 participants and were held at the Hotel Lido, Angera, on the shore of Lake Maggiore. There, the quiet solitude and calming views of the lake, together with good food, wine and grappa, encouraged thought and discussion, so that what often began with suspicion and even hostility, ended with mutual understanding and agreement. The principal aim of the workshops was to consider the current status of replacement alternative tests and to suggest ways forward to maximise their development and realise their potential.

ECVAM also set up eight task forces, where smaller groups of experts focused on specific issues, including prevalidation, biostatistics, nephrotoxicity, skin irritation, metabolism, integrated testing strategies, quality control of hormones and alternative databases.

By 2002, as reviewed by Combes (8), 46 workshop reports and 7 task force reports had been published in *ATLA*, in line with an agreement that the journal would publish ECVAM reports and news, and ESAC statements. The workshops had involved 490 participants from 22 countries, who had produced more than 800 agreed conclusions and recommendations. Of particular importance were Workshop 2, on phototoxicity, which led to the successful validation of the 3T3 NRU phototoxicity test; Workshop 5 (Amden II), on practical aspects of validation; Workshop 11, on the way forward for the Three Rs (held in Sheringham, UK, with Russell and Burch among its participants); and Workshop 37, on the application of the principles of GLP in *in vitro* toxicological studies. Task force reports on prevalidation and on good cell culture practice were also of particular value.

As Combes (8) concluded, these reports 'have had a substantial effect on the development and implementation of alternative methods, and have been a major factor in contributing to the success of the first 9 years of ECVAM's existence'.

1.3 Biologicals

ECVAM's activities have not been confined to chemicals and chemical products, as it was agreed at the first meeting of the ESAC that they should also involve biologicals. As a result, nine workshops on biologicals had taken place by 2002, and eight reports had been published in *ATLA* (9); six ESAC statements were made and publicised, on: the *in vitro* production of monoclonal antibodies; an ELISA test and the ToBI test for batch potency testing of tetanus vaccines for human use; an ELISA test for batch potency testing of inactivated swine erysipelas vaccines; the relevance of the target animal safety test for batch safety testing of vaccines for veterinary use; and the deletion of a test in polycythaemic mice for the potency testing of erythropoietin concentrated solution. This involved successful collaborations with the relevant authorities in Germany, The Netherlands and the UK; and the European Directorate for the Quality Control of Medicines.

1.4 In-house Research

In 2002, as described in the ECVAM Status Seminar report (2), ECVAM's internal research activities were focused on the following subjects: barriers, nephrotoxicology and chronic toxicity testing *in vitro*; a testing strategy for embryotoxicity; haematotoxicology; metabolism and neurotoxicity; topical toxicity and human studies; biologicals; genomics and *in vitro* toxicology; and computer modelling and integrated testing.

1.5 Collaboration in Education and Training

ECVAM successfully developed effective collaborations with a number of academic institutions in Austria, Belgium, France, Germany, Italy, Poland, Spain, The Netherlands and the UK (10). By 2002, 13 students had been awarded higher degrees for research conducted at ECVAM, and the research of another 13 students was in progress.

The collaborations with the Free University of Berlin and the University of Nottingham were particularly significant, as they also involved ZEBET and FRAME, including participation in validation studies, as well as in the TEMPUS Project with Charles University, Hradec Králové, Czech Republic.

In 2000, ECVAM was awarded a special grant, as part of the JRC Enlargement Project, for collaborative projects on alternative/advanced testing methods with 11 Candidate Countries for membership of the EU (11). This resulted in short-term training visits on validation, GLP in *in vitro* toxicology, the embryonic stem cell test, and extended visits by students from Poland and Bulgaria. Three ECVAM-sponsored international workshops on alternatives were held in 2002 in Prague, Czech Republic; Warsaw, Poland and Veszprem, Hungary. Three other workshops, held in 2001 and 2002, focused on regulatory testing, chemical risk assessment and alternatives to the use of animals in higher education.

1.6 The ECVAM Scientific Information Service

The Scientific Information Service (SIS) was set up in 1996 (see also, Chapter 4.2), to fulfil one of the duties laid down for ECVAM by the Commission, with its own Advisory Board comprising members from the University of Utrecht, FRAME, ZEBET and the University of Graz. It was decided early on that the service would provide evaluated and factual (i.e., ready-for-use) information. It was a matter of concern that the information required was not readily available and that it existed in many different forms, often with serious deficiencies. Two complementary projects were therefore undertaken to establish the SIS databases and an ECVAM Thesaurus on Advanced Alternative Methods (TAAM).

The SIS databases were designed to provide full method descriptions, including the INVITTOX protocol collection, originally set up by ERGATT and FRAME with support from the UK Government, but now taken over by ECVAM. Where possible, test results and validation status were to be included, and the initial priority topics were *in vitro* hepatotoxicity, metabolism-mediated toxicity, percutaneous absorption and neurotoxicity.

By 2002, the SIS databases contained 39 method summary descriptions, 130 INVITTOX protocols, 13 evaluation/validation studies, 1585 test results for 1104 test compounds, and 2474 bibliographic references.

The first version of TAAM was produced in 2001, in collaboration with the Thesaurus Section of the US National Library of Medicine.

1.7 Collaborations

ECVAM built up an extensive network of partners in industry, academic and government. The progress made would not have been possible without effective collaboration with, for example, ERGATT, FRAME, ZEBET, the European Cosmetics Toiletry and Perfumery Association (COLIPA), and companies such as L'Oréal, Procter & Gamble, Syngenta and Unilever.

A different kind of collaboration was represented by ECVAM's contributions to the first two World Congresses on Alternatives and Animal Use in the Life Sciences in 1993 and 1996, and in particular, to the third Congress, held in 1999, which was organised by ECVAM with the support of other EC services and FRAME.

1.8 Summary

The first part of ECVAM's history was dominated by the cosmetics testing issue, but a new EU chemicals policy, on the Registration, Evaluation, Authorisation and Restriction of Chemicals (REACH), had emerged by 2001 (12), and ECVAM was ready to make its contribution (13). The REACH regulation was adopted in 2006 (14) and entered into force in 2007.

2. THE EVOLUTION OF ECVAM AND ITS NETWORKS

On 22 September 2010, the EU adopted *Directive 2010/63/EU* (15), which updated and replaced *Directive 86/609/EEC* on the protection of animals used for scientific purposes. The aim of the new directive is to strengthen legislation and improve the welfare of those animals that still need to be used, as well as to firmly anchor the principle of the Three Rs, to Replace, Reduce and Refine the use of animals, in EU legislation. The new Directive became fully effective on 1 January 2013.

Directive 2010/63/EU formally established ECVAM as the European Union Reference Laboratory for Alternatives to Animal Testing (EURL ECVAM; Table 1) and defined its duties in Article 48 and Annex VII. These duties are in line with the original EC Communication of 1991 (3), while explicitly mandating EURL ECVAM to address areas of basic and applied research, in addition to regulatory testing.

Other provisions of *Directive 2010/63/EU* have had an impact on ECVAM's work. For instance, as a response to Article 47(2), which requires that Member States assist the EC in identifying and nominating suitable specialised and qualified laboratories to carry out validation studies, ECVAM set up a European Union Network of Laboratories for the Validation of Alternative Methods (EU-NETVAL) in 2014. In June 2017, this network was comprised of 37 members (from 15 EU Member States and EFTA countries). EU-NETVAL increases the European Union's validation capacity for *in vitro* methods by providing a laboratory network experienced in the routine implementation of good *in vitro* practices for regulatory use in human safety assessment. The EU-NETVAL members support validation studies through the execution of one or more specific tasks, and also contribute to the development of guidance documents and training materials in support of good *in vitro* method development and application.

In addition, Article 47(5) requires that Member States nominate a single point of contact to provide advice on the regulatory relevance and suitability of alternative approaches proposed for validation. Accordingly, ECVAM established the *Preliminary Assessment of Regulatory Relevance* (PARERE) network in 2011. It is composed of regulators nominated by the EU Member States, and representatives from EU regulatory agencies, such as the European Medicines Agency (EMA), the European Chemicals Agency (ECHA) and the European Food Safety Authority (EFSA), and from relevant EC services. To expedite the process of regulatory acceptance of alternative methods, it was considered that regulators should be involved as early as possible in providing a preliminary view on the potential regulatory relevance of methods submitted to ECVAM for validation.

Finally, Article 47(6) tasks the EC with taking appropriate actions to obtain international acceptance of alternative approaches validated in the EU. Besides involving regulators early on in the evaluation process of new tests and approaches, ECVAM continued to support the OECD TGs Programme by participating in the annual meetings of the Working Group of National Coordinators of the OECD TGs Programme and by leading the drafting of several new OECD TGs or Guidance Documents (GDs). The Mutual Acceptance of Data (MAD) Agreement is the main legal instrument used by the OECD to ensure a globally harmonised approach to the testing and assessment of chemicals. This is estimated to reduce costs and save thousands of animals every year. The OECD is also the default route for taking new test methods into the EU Test Method Regulation No 440/2008 (16). Only when there is 'undue delay' in the OECD process is the EU likely to decide to use a unilateral streamlined procedure for adoption of test methods. In addition to the OECD TGs Programme, ECVAM has also contributed extensively to the OECD Working Party on Hazard Assessment and to the OECD Extended Advisory Group on Molecular Screening and Toxicogenomics.

International cooperation has also been promoted through the International Cooperation on Alternative Test Methods (ICATM), which was established in 2009. ICATM includes governmental organisations from the EU (EURL ECVAM), the USA (ICCVAM), Japan (JaCVAM), Canada (Health Canada), South Korea (KoCVAM), Brazil (BraCVAM) and China (CFDA and Institute of Toxicology, Guangdong Provincial Center for Disease Control and Prevention), which are working together to promote enhanced international cooperation and coordination on the scientific development, validation and regulatory use of alternative approaches.

In relation to medicinal products, including biologicals, ECVAM has been represented in meetings of the EMA JEG 3Rs (the Joint Committee for Medicinal Products for Veterinary Use [CVMP]/Committee for Medicinal Products for Human Use [CHMP] *ad hoc* Expert Group on the Application of the 3Rs in Regulatory Testing of Medicinal Products), now called the J3RsWG (CVMP/CHMP Working Group on the Application of the 3Rs in Regulatory Testing of Medicinal Products). ECVAM has continued to collaborate with the International Council for the Harmonisation of Technical Requirements for Pharmaceuticals for Veterinary Use (VICH), in particular on the development of guidelines for the harmonisation of criteria to waive the target animal batch safety testing for inactivated and live vaccines for veterinary use, and on an *ad hoc* basis with the International Council for Harmonisation of Technical Requirements for Pharmaceuticals for Human Use (ICH) in the area of pharmaceuticals. In addition, ECVAM has initiated or supported a range of activities aimed at introducing alternative methods in the quality control of vaccines for human use (17), including workshops on the consistency approach (18, 19) and the validation of two serological methods for potency testing of whole cell pertussis vaccines (20). ECVAM's partnership with the EPAA has also been an important means of promoting the Three Rs in the biologicals area (21).

Ad hoc collaborations have also taken place with the World Health Organisation (WHO) through its International Programme on Chemical Safety (IPCS) and through the International Pharmacopoeia (Ph. Int.), which aims to achieve a global harmonisation of quality specifications for selected pharmaceutical products, excipients and dosage forms, thereby contributing to the safety and efficacy of medicines.

In line with Annex VII (e) of *Directive 2010/63/EC*, ECVAM also established in 2011 the ECVAM Stakeholder Forum (ESTAF), to maintain dialogue with the Stakeholder community and involve industrial associations, research organisations and civil society.

In 2010, the ECVAM Scientific Advisory Committee (ESAC) was re-formed and restructured in line with new Comitology procedures in the EC, aimed at ensuring a clear and consistent separation of the provision of independent scientific advice from any vested interests. The ESAC's main role is to conduct independent peer reviews of validation studies of alternative test methods, assessing their scientific validity for a given purpose, although they can be requested to provide advice on any matter under ECVAM's remit.

Notably, over the years, the number of validation studies carried out externally, i.e. not coordinated or carried out by ECVAM and submitted to ECVAM for evaluation and ESAC peer review, has considerably increased. The ESAC's advice to ECVAM is formally provided as ESAC working group reports and ESAC opinions at the end of the peer review process. ESAC's advice serves as the basis for the development of EURL ECVAM Recommendations that summarise ECVAM's view on the validity of a test method and advise on its possible regulatory applicability, limitations and proper scientific use. EURL ECVAM Recommendations also identify knowledge gaps and define follow-up actions. Developed in close dialogue with regulators (PARERE), stakeholders (ESTAF) and international partners (ICATM), EURL ECVAM Recommendations prepare and support the international recognition and regulatory use of alternative methods, as well as their application by end users.

Even though there is no specific mandate under the Directive, a number of Member States have set up, or are in the process of setting up, dedicated Three Rs centres, to advance alternatives through co-ordinated action. ECVAM has convened two meetings of the Three Rs centres, to identify areas for which further collaboration and strategic planning of activities between the different Three Rs centres could speed up the development and uptake of alternatives, including reduction and refinement alternatives.

With regard to the coordination and promotion of the development and use of alternatives in the areas of basic and applied research, ECVAM has continued to disseminate knowledge in the field of research through its publicly accessible DataBase service on ALternative Methods (DB-ALM; see also, Chapter 4.2). In addition to providing evaluated information on alternatives, ECVAM published a Search Guide to help scientists and committees during project preparations and evaluations to identify relevant sources of biomedical information.

ECVAM is also one of the EC services that are members of the European Partnership for Alternative Approaches to Animal Testing (EPAA), which was established in 2005. The EPAA is a public-private collaboration between the EC, European trade associations and companies from seven business sectors. The overall aim is to promote the Three Rs in regulatory testing. The *ad hoc* expert group described in the next section was a forerunner to the establishment of the EPAA.

3. ECVAM ACTIVITIES IN THE CONTEXT OF EU POLICY DRIVERS FOR ALTERNATIVES

3.1 EU Legislation on Cosmetic Products

As mentioned earlier, the Cosmetics Directive (and its subsequent amendments, and in particular, the seventh Amendment) was the main driver for ECVAM's initial activities because it involved an animal testing ban for cosmetic ingredients and products, as well as an EU marketing ban for cosmetic products, which included ingredients tested on animals or where the final product had been tested on animals.

The seventh Amendment to the Cosmetics Directive, adopted in 2003 (22), made several other provisions related to the development, validation and acceptance of alternative methods. One of those was that the EC should establish timetables for the implementation of the bans, including deadlines for the phasing out of the various animal tests. The EC therefore set up an *ad hoc* group including the relevant EC services, the EC Scientific Committee on Cosmetic Products and Non-Food Products (SCCNFP), stakeholder representatives from industry, animal welfare and consumer associations and the OECD. The members of the *ad hoc* group nominated experts on the 11 human health effects of concern related to cosmetics. ECVAM coordinated and contributed to the scientific work. The participating experts were requested, in a first step, to provide an inventory of the most valuable and/or advanced alternative methods currently known to be available in the respective toxicological areas. Based on this inventory, they were requested, in a second step, to: (a) estimate the time necessary to achieve ESAC endorsement of the identified methods assuming that optimal conditions were met (e.g. sufficient human and financial resources); (b) identify the gaps left by the *in vitro* methods compared with the animal test; (c) make recommendations for achieving full animal replacement; and (d) estimate the time necessary, including that for regulatory acceptance, to achieve full replacement of the animal test, assuming that all the necessary conditions were optimally met. The outcome of this exercise was reviewed in 2005 (23).

A similar exercise took place again in 2010, because the seventh Amendment also foresaw that the 2013 deadline for prohibiting the marketing of cosmetics tested on animals could be further extended for more-complex endpoints, if alternative and validated methods were not available in time. The EC invited stakeholder bodies (industry, non-governmental organisations, EU Member States and the EC's Scientific Committee on Consumer Safety) to identify scientific experts in five toxicological areas, namely, toxicokinetics, repeated-dose toxicity, carcinogenicity, skin sensitisation and reproductive toxicity. These experts were asked to analyse the status and prospects of alternative methods and to provide a scientifically-sound estimate of the time necessary to achieve full replacement of animal testing. ECVAM chaired the different endpoint working groups and, as in 2005, coordinated the whole process (24).

Since 2005, ECVAM has also provided annual technical reports on the progress made in the development, validation and regulatory acceptance of alternative methods, as an input to the EC's yearly report on progress and compliance with the deadlines of the Directive.

Since 2009, *Regulation (EC) N° 1223/2009* on cosmetic products (25) has replaced *Directive 76/768/EC* and its revisions. The marketing bans complementing the animal testing bans of the Cosmetics Regulation came into force, in March 2013.

3.2 The EU Chemicals Policy – REACH

In 2001, the EC adopted a White Paper on a *Strategy for a Future Chemicals Policy* (12), the main objective of which was to ensure a high level of protection for human health and the environment, while ensuring the efficient functioning of the internal market and protecting the competitiveness of the EU's chemical industry. The White Paper proposed to harmonise the testing requirements for new and existing substances by introducing a new regulatory system, REACH.

The new chemicals policy took legal effect through the REACH regulation, which was adopted on 18 December 2006 and entered into force on 1 June 2007 (13). REACH requires that animal tests are only used as a very last resort when no other validated and approved non-animal tests are available. Recent updates of the REACH annexes for more-advanced endpoints (26, 27) make the use of validated and accepted non-animal tests the default information requirement for assessing whether chemicals have the potential to cause these hazards, irrespective of the tonnage level of production.

Following the publication of the White Paper, the JRC played an advisory role in the formulation of the EU Chemicals Policy, by contributing to inter-service discussions within the EC that were aimed at elaborating the details of the new policy. This support was carried out by both ECVAM and the European Chemicals Bureau (ECB; (28)). To support the process, ECVAM established a Working Group on Chemicals in July 2001, with the remit to propose, by the end of 2001, a strategy on alternative (non-animal) methods in relation to the emerging Chemicals Policy.

The ECVAM Working Group produced a detailed review of the status of alternative methods for chemicals testing, which also included proposals for the strategic use of alternative tests and a three-stage action plan, containing proposals reflecting the short-, medium- and long-term prospects for the development and validation of alternative tests. To help with the production of the review document, nine ECVAM Focus Groups were established that concentrated their efforts on the most relevant toxicological endpoints. The outcome of this work was published in 2002 (13).

During the same period, the ECB managed a series of REACH Implementation Projects (RIPs) to develop, with Member State authorities and industry, what would subsequently become the tools and guidance for REACH. Both ECVAM and the ECB also made scientific contributions to these projects. In particular, RIP 3.3 developed guidance for industry on how to fulfil the REACH information requirements, while respecting the Three Rs provisions of the REACH legal text on alternative methods. This work formed the basis of the ECHA guidance on information requirements and chemical safety assessment (29).

In 2012, ECHA commissioned ECVAM to prepare an updated review on the status of alternatives for REACH (30).

3.3 Other EU Chemicals Policies Relevant to Alternatives

While REACH and the Cosmetics Regulation had the largest impact on the Three Rs by increasing the pace and the number of methods which were developed, validated and accepted, it is important to note that other pieces of chemicals and products legislation refer to alternative approaches and allow them to be used in hazard and risk assessments. Examples include: (a) *Regulation (EC) No 1272/2008* on Classification, Labelling and Packaging of substances and mixtures (CLP); (b) *Regulation (EC) No 1107/2009* concerning the placing of plant protection products on the market;

(c) *Regulation 283/2013* on data requirements for active substances; (d) *Regulation 284/2013* on data requirements for plant protection products; (e) *Regulation 528/2012* concerning the making available on the market and use of biocidal products; (f) *Directive 2001/83/EC* (and its amendments) on the Community code relating to medicinal products for human use; and (g) *Directive 2001/82/EC* (and its amendments) on the Community code relating to medicinal products for veterinary use.

Two other policies have also been important drivers of ECVAM's work, namely, the Community Strategy on combined exposures ('mixtures') (31, 32) and the Community Strategy on Endocrine Disrupters (33, 34). These policies inevitably cut across the product sectors and present significant opportunities for the use of non-animal methods.

3.4 The European Citizens' Initiative 'Stop Vivisection'

A European Citizens' Initiative (ECI), called 'Stop Vivisection', signed by 1.17 million citizens, was submitted to the EC on 3 March 2015. It was the third ECI that collected sufficient signatures to be considered by the EC. The ECI asked for the abrogation of *Directive 2010/63/EU* and for the adoption of a new legislative framework that fully phased out animal experiments by 2020. The organisers emphasised that *There are clear ethical objections of EU citizens to animal experiments* and claimed that *The animal model is not suitable to predict human responses and that animal testing hinders the development of new and more efficient methods in research.*

In response to the ECI, the EC published a communication on 3 June 2015 (35), which welcomed the mobilisation of citizens in support of animal welfare. The ECI had provided an opportunity to critically examine how the EU can reinforce its efforts in moving from animal-based to non-animal-based research and testing. It underlined that, while working toward the ultimate goal of full replacement of animals, *Directive 2010/63/EU* was an indispensable tool at the EU level for protecting those animals that are still required. The EC also identified four actions which could accelerate the development and uptake of non-animal approaches in research and testing. In addition to the continuous support in the development, validation and implementation of alternative approaches for regulatory and research use (Action 2), the EC proposed an action to assess the current situation regarding the sharing of knowledge, which is relevant to the Three Rs (Action 1). In this context, ECVAM conducted a public survey to identify: (a) the availability of knowledge sources relevant to the Three Rs; (b) how such knowledge is currently used, disseminated or shared; and (c) opportunities to fill knowledge gaps and enhance knowledge sharing (36).

4. ECVAM'S CONTRIBUTIONS TO INTERNATIONAL HARMONISATION ACTIVITIES WITHIN THE OECD

Through ECVAM, the European Commission has been leading or contributing to many projects within the OECD Chemical Safety and Biosafety Programme. These projects fall, in particular, within the OECD Test Guidelines (TGs) Programme, the OECD Working Party on Hazard Assessment (WPHA) and the OECD Extended Advisory Group for Molecular Screening and Toxicogenomics (EAGMST). ECVAM's more-recent contributions to these OECD projects are described in the EURL ECVAM status reports (37–41).

4.1 OECD Projects of the TGs Programme Currently (Co-)led by ECVAM

In the area of aquatic toxicity and bioaccumulation, ECVAM is currently working on the development of two OECD TGs (in collaboration with the USA), which involved the use of trout S9 and hepatocytes to determine *in vitro* hepatic clearance. Extrapolated to whole body metabolism, this information can be used to improve prediction models for fish bioaccumulation and to avoid unnecessary bioaccumulation tests requiring large numbers of fish. Another project, which ECVAM is co-leading with the International Council on Animal Protection in OECD Programmes (ICAPO), relates to the update of GD 23 on the aquatic toxicity testing of difficult substances and mixtures, with a view to minimising the need for solvent control experiments.

ECVAM has also made significant contributions to projects led by other OECD Member Countries, such as the revision of TG 203 on acute fish toxicity testing, which is one of the few guidelines still involving death (of fish) as an endpoint. This project, co-led by Switzerland and UK, aims at including the use of non-lethal endpoints (i.e. a moribund state) to reduce the suffering of the fish. Another contribution was the revision of GD 126 on the threshold approach for acute fish toxicity to include the fish embryo acute toxicity (FET) test (TG 236) in a step-wise approach for determining acute fish toxicity. ECVAM coordinated the validation of the FET in collaboration with the OECD, and issued an EURL ECVAM recommendation in 2014 (42) that the method should be considered as an alternative to the acute fish toxicity test. Its use will result in an overall reduction of the numbers of juvenile and adult fish required for aquatic toxicity testing.

In the area of skin allergy testing, ECVAM has led or co-led the production of three recently-adopted skin sensitisation TGs, including the Direct Peptide Reactivity Assay (DPRA; TG 442); the ARE-Nrf2 Luciferase Test Method (KeratinoSens; TG 442D); and the human Cell Line Activation Test (h-CLAT; TG 442E). Other methods, such as the U-SENS, the SENS-IS and the GARD assays, which were submitted to ECVAM for evaluation and were peer reviewed by the ESAC, have also been included in the work plan of the OECD TGs Programme. The U-SENS and the IL-8 LUC (a method proposed by Japan) test methods have recently been included in TG 442E, which was renamed as 'Key Even Based Test Guideline 442E'. A new project proposal based on the LuSens test method, which was evaluated by ECVAM and peer reviewed by the ESAC in 2016, has subsequently been included in the OECD work plan, with Germany as the lead country.

The currently adopted *in chemico* and *in vitro* methods address specific key events in the skin sensitisation Adverse Outcome Pathway (AOP), published by the OECD in 2014, and in isolation cannot provide the same type of information as that generated by the animal models. Combinations of non-animal data are therefore needed, in so-called Defined Approaches (DAs), to provide comparable or better information than that provided by the animal tests. Various approaches for integrating data within DAs, and in particular, data generated with the officially adopted *in vitro* methods, have been proposed as valid components of Integrated Approaches to Testing and Assessment (IATA) and documented in GD 256 (43), using harmonised templates for their reporting (provided in GD 255 (44)). The drafting of these two documents was led by ECVAM within the OECD WPHA (see the following section).

In the EU, this progress was the driver for the 2016 revision of the REACH information requirements for the skin sensitisation endpoint, with *in chemico* and *in vitro* methods becoming the default route instead of the animal-based test (26), and of the December 2016 update of the REACH Guidance on Information Requirements and Chemical Safety Assessment, in relation to the skin and respiratory sensitisation endpoints (29).

As discussed later, ECVAM submitted, together with two of its ICATM partners (Canada and the USA), a new project proposal in 2016 on a Performance-Based TG (PBTG) for DAs and test methods for skin sensitisation, which should put these new types of approaches at least on an equal footing with the current animal-based test (TG 429).

The need for alternative methods to assess eye irritation has been a major driver of ECVAM activities since its establishment (45, 46). Under some EU regulations (e.g. the Cosmetics Regulation, REACH), this information is now required to be generated without the use of animal tests. Therefore, ECVAM co-led (with the USA) the development of a GD on an IATA for serious eye damage/eye irritation, which was approved by the Working Group of National Co-ordinators (WNT) of the OECD TGs Programme in April 2017. ECVAM also led the drafting of a TG based on a reconstructed human cornea-like test method, the EpiOcular EIT test method, for the identification of chemicals not requiring classification for serious eye damage/eye irritation, which was approved by the WNT in 2014 (TG 492). A second, similar method, the SkinEthic Human Corneal Epithelium Eye Irritation Test, that had been submitted to ECVAM for evaluation and had been peer reviewed by ESAC, was included in TG 492 in 2017.

The integration of new technologies, such as *in vitro* methods and computer models, permits the prediction of absorption, distribution, metabolism and excretion (ADME), the four underlying processes driving toxicokinetic (TK) behaviour. However, the lack of standardisation of these methods is still hampering their regulatory acceptance and use. The need for better ADME and TK prediction methods has been a driver of ECVAM activities since its establishment (47–49). The ECVAM-validated human cytochrome P450 (CYP) induction *in vitro* test method was the first formally validated *in vitro* method for generating ADME information in human cells. Current efforts are focused on the characterisation and description of human *in vitro* ADME methods (e.g. for human hepatic metabolic clearance) and on the establishment of good modelling practices.

In line with the EC's Community Strategy on Endocrine Disrupters (EDs; (50)), ECVAM has been supporting OECD activities on the testing and assessment of endocrine disrupters, in particular via the Endocrine Disruptors Testing and Assessment Advisory Group (EDTA), the Validation Management Group on Non-Animal Methods (VMG NA) and the Validation Management Group on Ecotoxicity (VMG Eco). For the detection of the endocrine disrupting potential of chemicals, several androgen receptor transactivation assays have been developed and are currently undergoing validation. To develop an OECD PBTG for Androgen Receptor Transactivation Assays (ARTAs), ECVAM is carrying out a validation study on the AR-CALUX *in vitro* method with three EU-NETVAL test facilities. Besides the AR-CALUX method, the PBTG on ARTAs and related Performance Standards will also be based on other ARTAs, either already validated or in the process of a validation: the AR STTA, involving the AR-EcoScreen cell line (led by Japan, recently accepted and issued as TG 458) and an ARTA involving the 22Rv1/MMTV cell line (led by Korea). In 2017, ECVAM initiated a large-scale validation study of 17 *in vitro* assays for the detection of chemicals that disrupt thyroid function. The experimental work is being carried out in collaboration with EU-NETVAL members. In addition, ECVAM is currently contributing to the update of the OECD GD 150, which is a key document for the identification and assessment of EDs.

Since 2015, building on earlier ECVAM work on Good Cell Culture Practice (51), ECVAM has led the development of an OECD GD on Good *In Vitro* Method Practices (GIVIMP) for the development and implementation of *in vitro* methods for regulatory use in relation to human safety. This GD, published in 2018 (monograph ENV/JM/MONO(2018)19), aims at reducing the uncertainties with cell-based and tissue-based *in vitro* method-derived predictions, by applying all necessary good scientific, technical and quality practices from *in vitro* method development to *in vitro* method implementation for regulatory use.

A more-recent area of ECVAM activity concerns the development of *in vitro* methods and testing strategies for developmental neurotoxicity (DNT; (52)). ECVAM is currently contributing to an OECD GD for the application and interpretation of *in vitro* DNT assays and the definition of a tiered approach to testing and assessment. This was included in the OECD work plan in 2017 and is being led by the EC (through EFSA), Denmark and Germany.

ECVAM has also been active in the area of genotoxicity and carcinogenicity testing ((53−56); see also, Chapter 3.6). At the OECD level, this includes a contribution to the development of an IATA framework for non-genotoxic carcinogens.

4.2 Activities of ECVAM in the OECD Extended Advisory Group for Molecular Screening and Toxicogenomics

In addition to co-chairing the OECD Extended Advisory Group for Molecular Screening and Toxicogenomics, ECVAM has been involved in the development of generic guidance on AOPs (57), as well as individual AOPs. The latter include three of the first five AOPs that were endorsed by the OECD WNT and WPHA, and published in a new OECD Series on AOPs. ECVAM is also collaborating in the development and maintenance of the AOP Knowledge Base (AOP-KB), which is the central OECD hub for collecting, sharing and discussing knowledge around AOPs. In this context, ECVAM co-chairs the AOP-KB subgroup of the EAGMST, together with the US Environmental Protection Agency (EPA).

4.3 Activities of ECVAM in the OECD Working Party on Hazard Assessment

Since 2014, ECVAM has supported the OECD working group on combined exposures to multiple chemicals under the Working Party on Hazard Assessment (WPHA). Canada co-leads this activity with the OECD Secretariat, whereas the EU (through ECVAM) is leading a sub-activity on hazard assessment.

To support efforts of the OECD Member Countries to increase the use of alternative methods within IATA, and in particular, by developing respective guidance and tools, the IATA Case Studies Project was set up in 2015 under the OECD WPHA. The project is investigating the practical applicability of IATAs by discussing case studies ((58), see also, Chapter 5.4). To date, ECVAM has contributed two case studies, including a safety assessment workflow based on exposure considerations and non-animal methods (59, 60) and a case study on the grouping and read-across of nano-materials (61).

Within the OECD, ECVAM has also contributed to the development of IT tools as a member of the QSAR Toolbox Management Group, the eChemPortal Steering Committee (62) and the IUCLID User Group Expert Panel. These activities reflect the need to establish, at the international level, freely accessible tools for predictive toxicology and for exchanging information on chemical safety.

5. FUTURE OUTLOOK

While EU legislation on cosmetics and chemicals, the policies on endocrine disruptors and mixtures, and the need for internationally harmonised methods and approaches, will continue to be important drivers of ECVAM's work, some new policy initiatives are expected to provide further opportunities to expand the use of non-animal methods.

One of the difficulties in gaining acceptance for non-animal methods has been that they do not provide information that is directly applicable for classification and labelling purposes, because the classification criteria are mostly based on data generated by guideline animal methods, irrespective of their reliability and relevance. However, in 2016, an informal working group was set up under the UN Sub-Committee of experts on the Globally Harmonised System (GHS) to further explore the use of non-animal methods for classification. This review of the GHS will include *in vitro*, *in silico* and *in chemico* methods, as well as grouping and read-across, as a basis for hazard assessment. The ultimate goal is not only to show how non-animal methods can be used to satisfy existing classification criteria (e.g. for eye irritation and skin sensitisation), but ultimately, how the criteria themselves can be recast in terms of non-animal mechanistic data.

Another policy initiative is the so-called Non-Toxic Environment. This recognises that there are human health and environmental concerns that are not adequately addressed in the current regulatory framework, including age-related diseases, vulnerable populations, and the environmental impacts of persistent and mobile chemicals. It also recognises the need for sustainable product development, the substitution of chemicals of concern, and non-toxic material cycles. The Commission was tasked with developing a strategy for a Non-Toxic Environment in the seventh Environment Action Programme adopted by the Council and the European Parliament in 2013 (63). This policy represents an opportunity to introduce non-animal methods, because, for many of these human health and environmental concerns there are no regulatory requirements for testing and thus no standard animal tests to replace.

Finally, the ever-increasing availability of non-animal methods and approaches, many of which are not standardised, also presents a challenge in terms of the identification and practical validation of methods that are fit for multiple purposes (see also, Chapter 5.5). This is also linked to the evolution of regulatory acceptance criteria at both the EU and international levels, where the principle of MAD is key, but the interpretation of data has been restricted to guideline (and mostly animal) studies. While individual non-animal methods included in OECD TGs are covered by MAD, the combination of several *in vitro* and *in silico* methods in integrated testing strategies (see also, Chapter 5.4), which is needed for most of the toxicological endpoints, have so far only been reported in OECD Guidance Documents, which are not covered by MAD. To overcome some of these problems, and as follow-up to a 2016 ICATM workshop on the international regulatory applicability and acceptance of alternative non-animal approaches to skin sensitisation (64), ECVAM, together with ICCVAM and Health Canada, proposed a new project at OECD level on a Performance-based Test Guideline (PBTG) for DAs in the area of skin sensitisation. The resulting PBTG is expected to comprise DAs (rule-based combinations of methods) that provide the same level of information, or are more informative, than the traditional animal tests for human hazard identification and/or classification and labelling. The PBTG aims to substitute the need for animal testing for skin sensitisation. It will be on equal footing to existing *in vivo* TGs 406, 429, 442A and 442B, allowing for their replacement, depending on regulatory requirements in Member Countries. If the project is successful, a similar approach could be taken for other regulatory endpoints for which advanced alternative methods are available and optimal combinations of these methods have been established. More generally, this reflects a shift toward the evidence-based development of performance standards that can be applied, not only to single methods, but also to classes of methods and integrated approaches that provide similar information. This approach is now being actively pursued by EURL ECVAM (65).

REFERENCES

1. Balls, M. & Blaauboer, B. (Eds.). (1995), *Toxicology in Vitro: Vol. 9. The Validation of Replacement Alternative Methods*, pp. 789–869.
2. Alternatives to animal experiments: progress made and challenges ahead. In Balls, M. (Ed.), *ATLA: Vol. 30. Proceedings of the ECVAM Status Seminar 2002*, (2002). Suppl. 2, pp. 1–243.
3. EC. (1991). *Communication from the Commission to the Council and the European Parliament on the Establishment of a European Centre for the Validation of Alternative Methods. SEC (91) 1794, 29 June 1991.* Brussels, Belgium: European Commission.
4. EEC. (1986). Council Directive 86/609/EEC on the approximation of the laws, regulation and administrative provisions of the Member States regarding the protection of animals used for experimental and other scientific purposes. *Official Journal of the European Union* L358, 1–28.
5. Worth, A.P. & Balls, M. (2002). The principles of validation and the ECVAM validation process. *ATLA* 30(Suppl. 2), 15–21.
6. Balls, M. (1997). Defined structural and performance criteria would facilitate the validation and acceptance of alternative test procedures. *ATLA* 25, 484.
7. Spielmann, H. & Liebsch, M. (2002). Validation successes: chemicals. *ATLA* 30(Suppl. 2), 33–40.
8. Combes, R.D. (2002). The ECVAM workshops: a critical assessment of their impact on the development, validation and acceptance of alternative methods. *ATLA* 30(Suppl. 2), 151–165.
9. Halder, M., Hendriksen, C.F.M., Cussler, K. & Balls, M. (2002). ECVAM's contribution to the implementation of the Three Rs in the production and quality control of biologicals. *ATLA* 30, 93–108.
10. Clothier, R. (2002). ECVAM's collaborations with academia. *ATLA* 30(Suppl. 2), 175–183.
11. Sladowski, D. & Halder, M. (2002). ECVAM's activities in the EU candidate countries. *ATLA* 30(Suppl. 2), 203–205.
12. EC. (2001). *White Paper: Strategy for a Future Chemicals Policy*, 32pp. Brussels, Belgium: European Commission.
13. Worth, A.P. & Balls, M. (Eds.). (2002). *ATLA: Vol. 30. Alternative (Non-animal) Methods for Chemicals Testing: Current Status and Future Prospects. A Report Prepared by ECVAM and the ECVAM Group on Chemicals.* Suppl. 1, 1125pp.
14. EC. (2006). Regulation (EC) No 1907/2006 of the European Parliament and of the Council of 18 December 2006 concerning the Registration, Evaluation, Authorisation and Restriction of Chemicals (REACH), establishing a European Chemicals Agency, amending Directive 1999/45/EC and repealing Council Regulation (EEC) No 793/93 and Commission Regulation (EC) No 1488/94 as well as Council Directive 76/769/EEC and Commission Directives 91/155/EEC, 93/67/EEC, 93/105/EC and 2000/21/EC. *Official Journal of the European Union* L396, 1–849.
15. EU. (2010). Directive 2010/63/EU of the European Parliament and of the Council of 22 September 2010 on the protection of animals used for scientific purposes. *Official Journal of the European Union* L276, 33–79.

16. EC. (2008). Council Regulation (EC) No 440/2008 of 30 May 2008 laying down test methods pursuant to Regulation (EC) No 1907/2006 of the European Parliament and of the Council on the Registration, Evaluation, Authorisation and Restriction of Chemicals (REACH). *Official Journal of the European Union* **L142**, 1−739.

17. Halder, M. (2015). *Replacement, Reduction, Refinement of Animal Testing in the Quality Control of Human Vaccines*. JRC Report EUR 27646, 27pp.

18. Metz, B., Brunel, F., Chamberlin, C., *et al.* (2007). The potential of physicochemical and immunochemical assays to replace animal tests in the quality control of toxoid vaccines. The report and recommendations of ECVAM workshop 61. *ATLA* **35**, 323−331.

19. Hendriksen, C., Arciniega, J., Bruckner, L., *et al.* (2008). The consistency approach for the quality control of vaccines. *Biologicals* **36**, 73−77.

20. von Hunolstein, C., Gomez Miguel, M., Pezzella, C., *et al.* (2008). Evaluation of two serological methods for potency testing of whole cell pertussis vaccines. *Pharmeuropa Bio & Scientific Notes* **1**, 7−18.

21. Schutte, K., Szczepanska, A., Halder, M., *et al.* (2017). Modern science for better quality control of medicinal products "Towards global harmonization of 3Rs in biologicals": The report of an EPAA workshop. *Biologicals* **48**, 55−65.

22. EC. (2003). Directive 2003/15/EC of the European Parliament and of the Council of 27 February 2003 amending Council Directive 76/768/EEC on the approximation of the laws of the Member States relating to cosmetic products. *Official Journal of the European Union* **L66**, 26−35.

23. Eskes, C. & Zuang, V. (Eds.). (2005), *ATLA: Vol. 33. Alternative (Non-Animal) Methods for Cosmetics Testing: Current Status and Future Prospects*. Suppl. 1, 228pp.

24. Adler, S., Basketter, D., Creton, S., *et al.* (2011). Alternative (non-animal) methods for cosmetics testing: current status and future prospects. *Archives of Toxicology* **85**, 367−485.

25. EC. (2009). Regulation (EC) No 1223/2009 of the European Parliament and of the Council of 30 November 2009 on cosmetic products. *Official Journal of the European Union* **L342**(59), 151.

26. EU. (2016). Commission Regulation (EU) 2016/863 of 31 May 2016 amending Annexes VII and VIII to Regulation (EC) No 1907/2006 of the European Parliament and of the Council on the Registration, Evaluation, Authorisation and Restriction of Chemicals (REACH) as regards skin corrosion/irritation, serious eye damage/eye irritation and acute toxicity. *Official Journal of the European Union* **L144**, 27−31.

27. EU. (2016). Regulation (EU) 2016/1688 of 20 September 2016 amending Annex VII to Regulation (EC) No 1907/2006 of the European Parliament and of the Council on the Registration, Evaluation, Authorisation and Restriction of Chemicals (REACH) as regards skin sensitisation. *Official Journal of the European Union* **L255**, 14−16.

28. Eisenreich, S., Allanou, R., Aschberger, K., *et al.* (2008). *The European Chemicals Bureau: An Overview of 15 Years Experience in EU Chemicals Legislation*. JRC Report EUR 44584, 26pp.

29. ECHA. (2017). *Guidance on Information Requirements and Chemical Safety Assessment. Chapter R.7a: Endpoint Specific Guidance*. Version 6.0, 610pp. Helsinki, Finland: ECHA

30. Worth, A., Barroso, J.F., Bremer, S., *et al.* (2014). *Alternative Methods for Regulatory Toxicology − A State-of-the-art Review*. JRC Report EUR 26797, 470pp.

31. Kienzler, A., Bopp, S.K., van der Linden, S., *et al.* (2016). Regulatory assessment of chemical mixtures: requirements, current approaches and future perspectives. *Regulatory Toxicology and Pharmacology* **80**, 321−334.

32. Bopp, S., Berggren, E., Kienzler, A., *et al.* (2015). *Scientific Methodologies for the Assessment of Combined Effects of Chemicals - A Survey and Literature Review*. JRC Report EUR 27471, 64pp.

33. Munn, S., Worth, A., Lostia, A., *et al.* (2016). *Screening Methodology to Identify Potential Endocrine Disruptors According to Different Options in the Context of an Impact Assessment*. JRC Report EUR 27955, 54pp.

34. Bremer, S., Castello, P., Grignard, E., *et al.* (2012). Supporting the implementation of the EU Community Strategy on Endocrine Disrupters. The Mission of the Joint Research Centre. *ALTEX Proceedings* **1/12**, 109−114.

35. EC. (2015). *Communication from the Commission on the European Citizens' Initiative "Stop Vivisection"*. C (2015) 3773 final, 14pp. Brussels, Belgium: European Commission

36. Holley, T., Bowe, G., Campia, I., *et al.* (2016). *Accelerating Progress in the Replacement, Reduction and Refinement of Animal Testing Through Better Knowledge Sharing*. JRC Report EUR 28234, 64pp.

37. Zuang, V., Schäffer, M., Tuomainen, A.M., *et al.* (2013). *EURL ECVAM Progress Report on the Development, Validation and Regulatory Acceptance of Alternative Methods (2010−2013) − Prepared in the Framework of Directive 76/768/EEC and Regulation (EC) No 1223/2009 on Cosmetic Products*. JRC Report EUR 25981, 63pp.

38. Zuang, V., Desprez, B., Barroso, J.V., *et al.* (2014). *EURL ECVAM Status Report on the Development, Validation and Regulatory Acceptance of Alternative Methods and Approaches (2013−April 2014)*. JRC Report EUR 26702, 86pp.

39. Zuang, V., Desprez, B., Barroso, J.V., *et al.* (2014). *EURL ECVAM Status Report on the Development, Validation and Regulatory Acceptance of Alternative Methods and Approaches (2015)*. JRC Report EUR 27474, 114pp.

40. Zuang, V., Asturiol Bofill, D., Barroso, J.V., *et al.* (2016). *EURL ECVAM Status Report on the Development, Validation and Regulatory Acceptance of Alternative Methods and Approaches (2016)*. JRC Report EUR 28156, 90pp.

41. Zuang, V., Asturiol Bofill, D., Barroso, J.V., *et al.* (2017). *EURL ECVAM Status Report on the Development, Validation and Regulatory Acceptance of Alternative Methods and Approaches (2017)*. JRC Report EUR 28823, 116pp.

42. EURL ECVAM. (2014). *EURL ECVAM Recommendation on the Zebrafish Embryo Acute Toxicity Test Method (ZFET) for Acute Aquatic Toxicity Testing*. JRC Report EUR 26710, 37pp.

43. OECD. (2016). *Guidance Document on the Reporting of Defined Approaches and Individual Information Sources to be Used Within Integrated Approaches to Testing and Assessment (IATA) for Skin Sensitisation*. Series on Testing and Assessment No. 256, 24pp. Paris, France: OECD

44. OECD. (2016). *Guidance Document on the Reporting of Defined Approaches to be Used Within Integrated Approaches to Testing and Assessment.* Series on Testing & Assessment No. 255, 23pp. Paris, France: OECD

45. Balls, M., Berg, N., Bruner, L.H., *et al.* (1999). Eye Irritation Testing: The Way Forward. The Report and Recommendations of ECVAM Workshop 34. *ATLA* **27**, 53–77.

46. Scott, L., Eskes, C., Hoffmann, S., *et al.* (2010). A proposed eye irritation testing strategy to reduce and replace in vivo studies using Bottom-Up and Top-Down approaches. *Toxicology in Vitro* **24**, 1–9.

47. Coecke, S., Blaauboer, B.J., Elaut, G., *et al.* (2005). Toxicokinetics and metabolism. *ATLA* **33**(Suppl. 1), 147–175.

48. Coecke, S., Ahr, H., Blaauboer, B.J., *et al.* (2006). Metabolism: a bottleneck in in vitro toxicological test development. The report and recommendations of ECVAM workshop 54. *ATLA* **34**, 49–84.

49. Coecke, S., Pelkonen, O., Leite, S.B., *et al.* (2013). Toxicokinetics as a key to the integrated toxicity risk assessment based primarily on non-animal approaches. *Review. Toxicology in Vitro* **27**, 1570–1577.

50. EC. (1999). *Community Strategy for Endocrine Disrupters.* COM (99)706, 31pp. Brussels, Belgium: European Commission

51. Coecke, S., Balls, M., Bowe, G., *et al.* (2005). Guidance on good cell culture practice. A report of the second ECVAM task force on good cell culture practice. *ATLA* **33**, 261–287.

52. Bal-Price, A., Pistollato, F., Sachana, M., *et al.* (2018). Strategies to improve the regulatory assessment of developmental neurotoxicity (DNT) using in vitro methods. *Toxicology and Applied Pharmacology* **354**, 7–18.

53. Corvi, R., Albertini, S., Hartung, T., *et al.* (2008). ECVAM retrospective validation of in vitro micronucleus test (MNT). *Mutagenesis* **23**, 271–283.

54. Corvi, R., Aardema, M.J., Gribaldo, L., *et al.* (2012). ECVAM prevalidation study on in vitro cell transformation assays: general outline and conclusions of the study. *Mutation Research* **744**, 12–19.

55. Kirkland, D., Zeiger, E., Madia, F., *et al.* (2014). Can in vitro mammalian cell genotoxicity test results be used to complement positive results in the Ames test and help predict carcinogenic or in vivo genotoxic activity? II. Construction and analysis of a consolidated database. *Mutation Research* **775–776**, 69–80.

56. Corvi, R., Madia, F., Guyton, K.Z., *et al.* (2017). Moving forward in carcinogenicity assessment: Report of an EURL ECVAM/ESTIV workshop. *Toxicology in Vitro* **45**, 278–286.

57. OECD. (2017). *Guidance Document on Developing and Assessing Adverse Outcome Pathways.* Series on Testing and Assessment 184, 32pp. Paris, France: OECD

58. OECD. (2017). *Report on Considerations from Case Studies on Integrated Approaches for Testing and Assessment (IATA).* Series on Testing and Assessment No. 270, 44pp. Paris, France: OECD

59. OECD. (2017). *Chemical Safety Assessment Workflow Based on Exposure Considerations and Non-animal Methods.* Series on Testing & Assessment No. 275, 29pp. Paris, France: OECD

60. Berggren, E., White, A., Ouedraogo, G., *et al.* (2017). Ab initio chemical safety assessment: a workflow based on exposure considerations and non-animal methods. *Computational Toxicology* **4**, 31–44.

61. Worth, A.P., Aschberger, K., Asturiol Bofill, D., *et al.* (2017). *Evaluation of the Availability and Applicability of Computational Approaches in the Safety Assessment of Nanomaterials.* Final report of the Nanocomput project. JRC Report EUR 28617, 454pp.

62. Wittwehr, C. (2011). eChemPortal: Neuer Zugang zu Chemikalien-Daten. *Chemie in Unserer Zeit* **45**, 122–125.

63. EU. (2013). Decision No 1386/2013/EU of the European Parliament and of the Council of 20 November 2013 on a General Union Environment Action Programme to 2020 'Living well, within the limits of our planet'. *Official Journal of the European Union* **L354**, 171–200.

64. Casati, S., Aschberger, K., Barroso, J., *et al.* (2018). Standardisation of defined approaches for skin sensitisation testing to support regulatory use and international adoption: position of the International Cooperation on alternative test methods. *Archives of Toxicology* **92**, 611–617.

65. Whelan, M. & Eskes, C. (2016). Evolving the principles and practice of validation for new alternative approaches to toxicity testing. In C. Eskes & M. Whelan (Eds.), *Advances in Experimental Medicine and Biology* **856**. *Validation of Alternative Methods for Toxicity Testing,* pp. 387–399. Basel, Switzerland: Springer Verlag.

Chapter 2.11

The Center for Alternatives to Animal Testing in the USA and Europe

Alan Goldberg[1], Marcel Leist[2] and Thomas Hartung[1,2]
[1]*Johns Hopkins Bloomberg School of Public Health, Baltimore, MD, United States;* [2]*University of Konstanz, Konstanz, Germany*

SUMMARY

The Center for Alternatives to Animal Testing (CAAT) was founded in 1981. CAAT–USA is part of the Johns Hopkins University Bloomberg School of Public Health, Baltimore, now with a European branch (CAAT–Europe), located since 2010 at the University of Konstanz, Germany. This transatlantic organisation, with ties to all parts of the world, promotes humane science by supporting the creation, development, validation and use of alternatives to animals in research, product safety testing and education. CAAT seeks to effect change by working with scientists in industry, government and academia, to find new ways to replace animals with non-animal methods, reduce the numbers of animals necessary or refine methods to make them less painful or stressful to the animals involved. This is promoted by regular workshops organised by its transatlantic think tank for toxicology (t^4).

CAAT was initially funded by the US Cosmetic, Toiletries, and Fragrance Association (CTFA) with a $1M grant, but has since been supported by more than 50 companies and trade associations from various sectors, and philanthropic and public research funding. Over almost four decades, it expanded to all areas of animal use in industry, regulation and academia. Its work spans from proof-of-principle research into new alternatives funded competitively by various research funding bodies, to translational work of multi-stakeholder consensus processes, education and communication, as well as policy programmes, informing especially the US and EU legislative processes. Current focus areas with dedicated programmes include Microphysiological Systems, Pathway-based Toxicology (The Human Toxome), Good Cell Culture Practice, Evidence-based Toxicology, Green Toxicology, Refinement, *in silico* approaches, including Read-Across, and Thresholds of Toxicological Concern, as well as Integrated Testing Strategies.

1. CAAT–USA

The Johns Hopkins University Center for Alternatives to Animal Testing (CAAT) was founded in September 1981 (1). CAAT was initially funded by the Cosmetic, Toiletries, and Fragrance Association (CTFA, now called the Personal Care Product Council (PCPC), with a $1M grant. At that time, it was the single largest corporate-funded project at Johns Hopkins University. The focus of the project was to be on supporting the development of *in vitro* cell-based assays to replace animal tests for regulatory purposes. CAAT became the brand for which a new model was needed, concerning how to maintain independence while working with a trade association that reported to many different companies, some with differing agendas. An advisory board to CAAT was set up to advise the director and the university on the related issues to be confronted. CAAT, like all centres at the university, reports to a department and thus through the department to the office of the dean, Dean D.A. Henderson, at the time of its establishment.

CAAT's aim remains unchanged since 1997: *To be a leading force in the development and use of reduction, refinement, and replacement alternatives in research, testing, and education to protect and enhance the health of the public.*

The History of Alternative Test Methods in Toxicology. https://doi.org/10.1016/B978-0-12-813697-3.00014-7

The mission is to *promote and support research in the development of* in vitro *and other alternative techniques; serve as a forum to foster discussion among diverse groups leading to creative approaches to facilitate acceptance and implementation of alternatives; provide reliable information on the science, philosophy, and public policy of alternatives to academia, government, industry, and the general public; and educate and train in the application of alternatives.*

Outside of the pressures of regulating or being regulated, CAAT aims to be an engine of change in the safety sciences and other areas of animal use, overcoming the limitations of animal-based approaches and accelerating the uptake of new technologies by collaboration with all stakeholder groups.

2. CAAT–EUROPE

The Center for Alternatives to Animal Testing–Europe (CAAT–Europe), was inaugurated in March 2010 at the University of Konstanz, and is co-directed by Marcel Leist (representative of the University of Konstanz) and Thomas Hartung (representing the Johns Hopkins Bloomberg School of Public Health). CAAT–Europe coordinates international (European and transatlantic) activities, and and acts as an international expert and knowledge source for human-relevant methodologies for European authorities. It organises think tanks, workshops, information days, symposia, conference satellites and public-expert consultations, to: (a) identify current gaps in knowledge; (b) draw road-maps to overcome these gaps and other uncertainties related to the implementation of functional alternatives relevant to human physiology; (c) close the gaps between regulatory, academic and industrial safety sciences; and (d) bring the manifold of significant disciplines involved in modern consumer protection significantly into line with a meaningful hazard and risk assessment.

The board of CAAT–Europe is composed of 28 scientists representing the chemicals, pharmaceuticals, food and cosmetics industries, as well as public/NGO scientific organisations and authorities. The centre's unique principles of scientific independence and its role as facilitator of direct interactions between relevant parties is underscored by its singularity as a transatlantic information platform providing the sole independent scientific hub at the European Parliaments in Brussels and Strasbourg. Since 2014, CAAT–Europe has also served as an official external expertise service provider for the European Parliament in the area of 'Life sciences for human well-being'.

Since 2010, CAAT–Europe's activities have resulted in more than 50 peer-reviewed publications, involving more than 387 individual scientists representing academia (42%), industry (30%), regulatory authorities (22%) and relevant NGOs (6%). These publications have mostly resulted from more than 22 think tanks and workshops organised from 2010 to 2016. Moreover, more than 12 symposia have been organised all over Europe, and more than 15 information days for the Members of the European Parliament at the facilities of the European Parliaments in Brussels and Strasbourg.

3. THE CAAT PROGRAMMES

The CAAT programmes are multifaceted and initially focused on the Research Grants programme. The programmes that developed under the leadership of Alan Goldberg in the first 27 years of CAAT mostly continue today. In 2009, Thomas Hartung was appointed director of CAAT. Shortly after being appointed to head ECVAM in 2002, he became a CAAT board member, and numerous activities were shared. When accepting the position at Hopkins, Thomas Hartung asked Alan Goldberg to continue chairing the board and be a principal in the transatlantic think tank for toxicology (t^4) collaboration. This continued until November 2014, when Alan Goldberg chaired his last grant review at the board meeting and turned the chair over to James Freeman (ExxonMobil).

With the change in leadership in early 2009, CAAT expanded its programmes over the years: The core activities at the time included the Communication and Education programme and US policy programme. The immediate changes that took place in 2009 were the installation of a chair for Evidence-based Toxicology with an endowment from the Doerenkamp-Zbinden Foundation (DZF). With the support of an anonymous donor, the Evidence-based Toxicology Collaboration (EBTC) came to life in 2011, for which CAAT provides the secretariat, and was led until 2015 by Marty Stephens, who then handed over to Katya Tsaioun.

The creation of t^4 with the chairs for alternative methods in Konstanz, Germany, and Utrecht, The Netherlands, laid the ground for the creation of CAAT–Europe in 2010 (2), led by Marcel Leist and Thomas Hartung, as directors, and Mardas Daneshian, as CEO. t^4 organises workshops and commissions white papers, thus expanding the core activities of CAAT and making them transatlantic, as no alternative method will be used if only accepted on one side of the ocean.

In 2010, based on moving the centre into the School of Public Health in the course of 2009, laboratories were opened. They have prospered, enjoying funding from the FDA, the NIH, the Defense Threat Reduction Agency (DTRA) and the European Commission as their main supporters. The research serves as proof-of-principle of the methods being advocated. Most-recent examples include the creation of human mini-brains from induced pluripotent stem cells and automated read-across. Such competitive research gives CAAT credibility in understanding what science can deliver, which has brought a number of skilled students and researchers to the team, who are increasingly integrated into the core work of the center.

The generation change in CAAT was completed with the retirement of Alan Goldberg as chairman of the board in November 2014. This change in personnel and the accelerating change in the field led to the initiation of a strategy discussion to refocus CAAT's work: This included a meeting, where 12 representatives of the US agencies identified their needs and priorities for CAAT in 2014, an evaluation of the programme since 2009 by 10 panels formed by the board the same year, meeting without the presence of the CAAT staff, and a Board Retreat in 2015. Together with several staff retreats and many discussions with stakeholders, this led to the current strategy document. Key elements of the strategy are as follows: broadening the leadership of CAAT by creating a deputy director position; a modular approach, whereby different CAAT programmes have a director, an associated steering group of external experts and their own work programmes and budget; a focus on the implementation of alternative methods, which comprises integrated testing strategies and read-across and a focus on quality assurance, which includes Evidence-based Toxicology, validation and Good Cell Culture Practice.

This new structure assigns defined efforts for leading programmes to CAAT researchers, which then jointly form the CAAT leadership team and the leaders of the programmes. In the following sections, the major CAAT programmes are briefly summarised.

3.1 The Grants Programme

CAAT's first initiative was the establishment of a Grants Programme in the early 1980s. Several people on the board recommended that selected academics be contacted, to encourage them to submit grant applications. There was no guarantee that they would be supported, but they were encouraged to submit a one-page abstract on their proposed research. These abstracts were reviewed, then some individuals were asked to submit full applications. The odds of getting funding were between 35% and 50%. Writing a one-page abstract was not an onerous task for the great possibility of getting a grant. This model was well received, and the Grants Programme established the significance of the emerging field. Up to today, grant funding for more than 600 projects has totalled about 7 million dollars — not a huge sum for each project, but an important stimulus to the field. A main goal of CAAT grants is to provide the preliminary data necessary for larger grant applications. Since 2015, the programme has been led by CAAT deputy director, Helena Hogberg.

3.2 The Avon Programme Project

Avon provided funding for CAAT as part of the first CTFA grant, then continued to to fund the centre independently. After a few years, Avon, in the person of Yale Gressel, asked CAAT to take on a larger project — developing an *in vitro* assay to predict skin sensitisation. About eight laboratories working on various aspects of skin biology were invited to make presentations to their 'competitors and colleagues'. They were asked how they would approach the issue, and what aspects they saw as most important. Five individuals were invited to submit grant applications, with the provision that, if approved, up to three of the applications would be funded. The leaders of the funded projects would get together twice yearly in a roll-up-your-sleeves discussion about their progress and how to proceed further. The attendees at these 'lab' meetings were the participants, along with other experts from the university, government agencies and Avon. In essence, the corporate and government scientists wanted to know how to use the information generated, and the academics wanted to better understand the mechanisms involved. The project lasted nine years, and the science it generated formed the basis of our understanding of mechanisms of skin sensitisation. This project was very successful (3), and was characterised by the identification of many of the interleukins and cytokine pathways and the recognition that keratinocytes play an important role in sensitisation.

3.3 The Communications Programme

This programme, now led for many years by Michael Hughes, started with a newsletter, which over time became recognised as informative, interesting and well-respected. By the end of the 1990s, however, the cost of print and postage became prohibitive, so an addition to the CAAT website, *Altweb*, was developed as a collective portal for many organizations. It quickly became the premier website for news about alternatives. The two sites continue today — the main CAAT site highlights the centre's programmes and products, and *Altweb* acts as a portal for alternative websites worldwide. The programme now includes *Altweb*, with 18,000 individual visitors every month from more than 130 countries, the CAAT website (http://caat.jhsph.edu), the electronic *CAATwalk* newsletter with more than 8000 recipients, FaceBook with more than 12,000 fans, Twitter and work with journalists.

The journal, *ALTEX: Alternatives to Animal Experimentation*, published in Switzerland, is now closely associated with CAAT. Thomas Hartung became its American editor in 2009, and was followed by Joanne Zurlo in 2014 and Martin Stephens in 2017, and *ALTEX* became an International journal printed entirely in English, with a continuously rising Impact Factor. More-recently, *Applied In Vitro Toxicology* (*AIVT*) published its inaugural issue in March 2015, with Alan Goldberg as consulting editor.

3.4 Workshops and Technical Reports — The t⁴ Programme

When John Frazier was its associate director (1985—94), CAAT produced many technical reports, focused on limited topics and aimed at sharing the information broadly. In 1998, the US Environmental Protection Agency (EPA), Chemical Manufacturers Association (CMA) and Environmental Defense (ED) initiated the High Production Volume (HPV) Testing Program. To address the needs of this program, CAAT held several TestSmart workshops, which were well attended. After the initial focus on the HPV Program, a series of development neurotoxicity (DNT) workshops began, starting in 2005 with a collaboration between Alan Goldberg and Thomas Hartung, then at ECVAM. The DNT series continues today, and the eighth workshop was held in early 2017. CAAT—Europe is currently organising the fifth International conference in this series, for 2019.

One very important technical report was written by John Frazier in 1989, while acting as a consultant to the OECD (4). This single-author report identified the science necessary for a validation study and provided an important background piece to discussions about the principles of validation and their application, which took place in the early 1990s.

The support of the DZF from 2009 creation of the t⁴ programme coordinated by a programme coordinated by Thomas Hartung, Alan Goldberg, Marcel Leist and Bas Blaauboer. The concept of t⁴ is a collaboration of the three toxicology-oriented DZF chairs, and was created with the following aims:

- to analyse current tools and programmes and model/forecast the likely outcome with regard to safety and the economic burden (cost/benefit analyses);
- to compare different approaches on an international scale (especially transatlantic) and to support harmonisation;
- to further the concept of an evidence-based toxicology (EBT), following the role model of evidence-based medicine;
- to develop and assess the conceptual needs to enable the change of approaches (predictive toxicology, integrated testing, systems toxicology, organotypic and stem cell cultures); and
- to create and maintain information platforms (e.g. *AltWeb*, *ALTEX*, TestSmart workshops) to further the paradigm change in toxicology.

The programme has resulted in about 30 workshops up to now, with reports published in *ALTEX* and a dozen commissioned white papers.

A major activity of t⁴ was the production of a roadmap for animal-free systemic toxicity testing in 2011—2013. Alternative approaches have typically been developed as small initiatives, wherever there was an opportunity and desire for change. However, with the advent of the report on *Toxicity Testing in the 21st Century: A Vision and a Strategy* (Tox-21c; 5), it is widely perceived that actual paradigm change is now within reach.

Starting at Hopkins in early 2009, CAAT put forward a roadmap to implement the vision of Tox-21c — without a doubt the most important movement for change in regulatory science in many decades (6). Many of the challenges identified in this paper have been tackled by CAAT's work programme since then, such as Integrated Testing Strategies, Evidence-based Toxicology, new validation paradigms, and increasing the comfort of regulators to change. During the last six years, important steps were made in defining a roadmap from the other side, i.e. from the systemic toxicity information currently gathered by traditional animal tests. CAAT steered a truly transatlantic process, starting a 2011 report by the European Commission on the status of alternative methods. An independent review of this report with 19 experts from all over the world was carried out. Five white papers (three from the USA, two from Europe) then laid the basis for a CAAT consensus workshop with 35 experts, which resulted in a report published only 5 months later (7).

Shortly afterwards, CAAT teamed up with a dozen stakeholder groups to organise a 2-day forum in Brussels to discuss the roadmap. The event was hosted by CAAT—US and CAAT—Europe, ecopa, EUSAAT, the DZF, ESTIV, IVTIP, the Institute for In Vitro Sciences, Humane Society International and ToxCast (US EPA), together with cefic and Cosmetics Europe. This event also benefitted from the advisory comments of Eurogroup for Animals and ecopa, as well as from the contributions of the SEURAT-1 consortium, and the European Chemicals Agency (ECHA). About 150 colleagues joined for an intense discussion, and the roadmap was broadly endorsed. A similar stakeholder forum on this event was organised by CAAT on 30–31 May 2013 in Washington, D.C., hosted by the FDA Center for Food Safety and Advanced Nutrition and supported by the Hamner Institutes for Health Sciences, the Grocery Manufacturers Association, the US National Institute of Environmental Health Sciences, the Institute for In Vitro Sciences, the US Food and Drug Administration, the American Cleaning Institute, the Alternatives Research and Development Foundation, PETA International Science Consortium, Agilent, the American Society for Cellular and Computational Toxicology, the Physicians Committee for Responsible Medicine, CropLife America, CropLife Canada, the Human Toxicology Project Consortium, and the Humane Society of the United States. Along with an unknown number via the webcast, 140 people attended. Again, the discussions led to a broad endorsement of the suggested roadmap steps (8). Most recently, a workshop detailing further the roadmap for reproductive toxicity testing was held in Konstanz in 2017.

3.5 Education Programmes

Joanne Zurlo, who has been CAAT assistant director (1990–93), associate director (1993–2000) and senior scientist (from 2010), established an outreach and education programme with CAAT's science writer, Deborah Rudacille. Together, they worked with artistic designers to create the *CAATalyst* newsletter for middle and high school students. The final issue of *CAATalyst* was a comic book, *Adventures in Tier-Testing*, in which Dr In Vitro visited a cosmetic company to oversee the testing of a new acne cream. Another product of the outreach programme was the book, *Animals and Alternatives in Testing—History, Science and Ethics* (9), which was written to expose a non-scientific audience to the concept of the Three Rs. The education programme was coincident with the Baltimore City effort to stimulate science education.

CAAT's Academic Programmes, now led by Lena Smirnova, educates students and professionals in the research field about alternatives and humane science, helping them to gain a better understanding of the Three Rs and their role in improving the quality of science. CAAT has established a certified programme in humane sciences and toxicology policy in the Johns Hopkins Bloomberg School, and any individual who completes the curriculum can be awarded this certificate. The Humane Science and Toxicology Certificate Program is central to CAAT's academic mission, with a curriculum consisting of six courses, offered both in the classroom and online through the Johns Hopkins Bloomberg School of Public Health. CAAT has brought 90% of the certificated curriculum online, making it freely available worldwide. CAAT faculty also teach an online course entitled *Animals in Research: Law, Policy and Humane Sciences*, the objectives of which are to describe the principles that govern the use of laboratory animals in research; to identify the steps by which biomedical research involving animals is reviewed by Institutional Animal Care and Use Committees (IACUCs); to explain the guiding principles of humane science, including the Three Rs (Reduction, Refinement and Replacement), and to assess the ways in which the application of humane science principles in biomedical research can lead to more-robust scientific methodology and results.

A new Master of Science and Public Health (MSPH) in Toxicology includes 13 90-minute lectures, each on *Toxicology for the 21st Century* and on *Evidence-based Toxicology*. *Toxicology for the 21st Century* provides students with perspectives on current paradigm changes in regulatory toxicology. The course on *Evidence-based Toxicology* provides students with fundamental knowledge of Evidence-based Medicine, which was a revolution in the objective and transparent condensation of information in the health-care sciences. The tools of systematic reviews, meta-analysis, quality scoring of studies, risk-of-bias analysis and various approaches to quality assurance, such as validation and Good Practices, are introduced. Lecturers steering the US EBTC have been recruited to record the respective lectures. These lecture series will shortly be made publicly available.

CAAT Academy (https://www.caat-academy.org/) was established in 2016 in Europe, under the leadership of Francois Busquet, to increase the use of validated alternative methods by providing hands-on training. In a nutshell, a variety of technical experts are gathered over two days to the benefit of a small group (maximum 15) in a laboratory. After some preliminary lectures, the participants manipulate and/or walk through the different methods or technologies. This is an opportunity to closely interact with experts on data interpretation for regulatory purposes and to accumulate know-how and confidence with the new tools.

3.6 The Refinement Programme

From the very beginning of the Center, the Refinement R has been very important to CAAT. Intermittent support was obtained from several sponsors, and Refinement research was funded by a grant mechanism. CAAT now funds research at institutions worldwide that was initiated by animal technicians and postdoctoral fellows in comparative medicine groups, to solve very specific animal welfare issue, at up to $6000 (for 1 year). Projects that were funded and were successful were presented at the PRIM&R annual meetings. At the request of the pharmaceutical companies supporting CAAT and with help of the Klingenstein Foundation, a Refinement programme, led by Joanne Zurlo, was added in 2011. CAAT is an affiliate member of the American Association for Laboratory Animal Science (AALAS) and participates in its annual meeting with an exhibit booth and speakers. A series of Refinement workshops continues, recently focusing on social housing of laboratory animals, and CAAT gives out its Science-based Refinement awards. In 2017, the programme is now led by Kathrin Herrmann.

3.7 US and EU Policy Programmes

Paul Locke, an attorney and public health professional, joined the CAAT faculty in 2001 and initiated the Policy Programme in 2007. This programme is aimed at educating policy makers and legislators about the need for alternatives to the use of animals in toxicity and safety testing and in biomedical research, and has grown rapidly. An important aspect has been its outreach to the Animal Law Community. Strong ties have been established with the Lewis and Clark Center for Animal Legal Studies, the Animal Legal Defense Fund, and the Animal Law Section of the Maryland Bar. The programme also maintains important strategic relationships with the National Academy of Sciences Institute for Laboratory Animal Research (ILAR) and the American Consortium on EU Studies (ACES).

In 2012, a European policy programme was created under the leadership of Francois Busquet, based in Brussels, Belgium, to promote the implementation of human-relevant methodologies in legal texts and guidelines. This foresees direct interaction with parliamentarians, the organisation of workshops and symposia in the European Parliament (in Brussels and Strasbourg) and participation in all relevant events at the Parliament. CAAT's Policy programme intends to serve as a voice of humane science to policy makers, to create a legislative and policy culture that values the lives of animals, to serve as information hub for policy makers on the availability and feasibility of alternative approaches and to bring policy makers into contact with scientists that have enhanced the field of Toxicology for the 21st century. The purpose of CAAT–Europe's Policy Program is to educate legislators and politicians on the availability of new methods and to weaken the reluctance to move away from animal testing, by showing the scientific and technological value of the alternatives as a new economy and a source for jobs and growth.

Since its creation, CAAT has participated in 14 workshops at the European Parliament (several of them organised by CAAT itself), with policy makers, regulatory bodies and representatives from industry, animal welfare and consumer organisations. Because of the action of the CAAT–Europe Policy bureau in Brussels, strong collaborations with the diverse stakeholders have been established, and it is already considered to be an honest broker.

4. FROM A SYMPOSIUM SERIES TO WORLD CONGRESSES

In May 1982, CAAT held its first symposium, entitled *Product Safety Evaluation*, and further symposia were held about every 18 months, focusing on specific topics aimed at advancing the *in vitro* field. The 11 volumes of the In Vitro Toxicology symposium series, published by Mary Ann Liebert, Inc., New York, are available on the CAAT website.

In 1990, Alan Goldberg met and visited with Bert van Zutphen at the University of Utrecht, The Netherlands, and suggested that they should work together on a *World Congress on Alternatives and Animal Use in the Life Sciences*. The First World Congress took place in Baltimore in 1993, with more than 600 attendees. Bert van Zutphen invited Michael Balls, from ECVAM, to join him in organising Second World Congress, held in Utrecht in 1996, then to plan the Third World Congress, which was in Bologna, Italy, in 1996, with Andrew Rowan as co-chairman. This established a pattern for subsequent world congresses, now typically with more than 1000 attendees. Thomas Hartung organised the Seventh World Congress with Hermann Koeter in Rome, Italy, in 2009. The 10th World Congress was held in Seattle in August 2017, with Joanne Zurlo of the CAAT team as co-host.

Andrew Rowan, who organised the 2002 conference in New Orleans, initiated a slightly more formal approach, by creating the Alternatives Congress Trust, which is now responsible for future congresses and guarantees their continuation. At the World Congress in Japan (2007), CAAT celebrated its 25th anniversary. Alan Goldberg gave a presentation on *The Science of Alternatives: 25 Years and Tomorrow* (10), which presented a timeline of events related to the use of the rodent in biomedical research and the development of alternatives and *in vitro* approaches in toxicology, by looking at each issue and its 'initial truths' from 1981 and contrasting it with the 'current realities' of 2007. The article featured many photographs of individuals involved at the time. Other detailed timelines devoted to the Three Rs in toxicity testing have also been published (9, 11), and two websites associated with CAAT provide endless amounts of historical information (http://altweb.jhsph.edu/, http://caat.jhsph.edu).

A news series of PanAmerican conferences was started in Baltimore in 2016. The 2018 conference, to be held in Rio de Janeiro, Brazil, is currently being prepared, and a third conference is foreseen for 2010 in Canada.

5. TOXICOLOGY TESTING IN THE 21ST CENTURY – THE HUMAN TOXOME PROJECT

The T-21c report (5) had numerous inputs from CAAT staff and board members (more than 50% of its authors were either current or past CAAT grantees or board members). Thomas Hartung presented to the committee, and Alan Goldberg was one of the external reviewers. While the final report was in press, CAAT's board retreat in Tucson, AZ, considered how the report would affect academic scientists, regulators and corporate scientists. This publication was, and is, a major advancement in *in vitro* toxicology, alternatives and risk assessment. It created major new research approaches and opportunities.

With the Human Toxome Project (http://humantoxome.com; (12)), funded as an NIH Transformative Research grant for 2011 to 2017, CAAT contributed to developing the concepts and the means for deducing, validating and sharing molecular pathways of toxicity (PoT) to implement the vision of toxicity testing for the 21st century. Using the test case of oestrogenic endocrine disruption, the responses of MCF-7 human breast cancer cells were phenotyped by transcriptomics and mass-spectrometry-based metabolomics. The bioinformatics tools for PoT deduction represented a core deliverable. A number of challenges for quality and standardisation of cell systems, omics technologies and bioinformatics have been addressed. In parallel, concepts for the annotation, validation and sharing of PoT information, as well as their link to adverse outcomes, were developed. A reasonably comprehensive public database of PoT, the Human Toxome Knowledge-base, as an ultimate goal, could become a point of reference for toxicological research and regulatory test strategies. The Human Toxome collaboration is led by Andre Kleensang, who took over from Mounir Bouhifd in 2016.

The European flagship project, EUToxRisk, sponsored by the European Commission with €30 million, includes both CAAT-USA and CAAT-Europe in prominent roles, alongside more than 35 other European partners. The project is co-ordinated by Bob van de Water, Leiden, The Netherlands. Several elements of the Human Toxome project and CAAT's read-across program are being pursued there.

6. THE EVIDENCE-BASED TOXICOLOGY COLLABORATION

Emerging technologies and numerous initiatives are being created worldwide, to promote their use to assess toxicity. To assist in the culture change and paradigm shift that CAAT advocates, it is important to establish a mutually beneficial dialogue among stakeholders in the current system. This dialogue will focus on quality assurance of the novel tools. Traditionally, this was attempted by formal validation. Starting in 2004 at ECVAM, the idea of leveraging approaches from Evidence-based Medicine (EBM), an approach, which had been pioneered primarily by the Cochrane Collaboration, to complement this process was spearheaded, leading to a first conference in Como, Italy, in 2007. CAAT's toxicity testing symposia touched on this issue, which was taken up in detail at a CAAT-organised conference, *21st Century Validation for 21st Century Tools*, in July 2010. Based on that conference, a steering group was formed that included representation from CAAT, the EPA, the FDA, the National Toxicology Program, the American Chemistry Council, CropLife America, the pharmaceutical industry, the Humane Society of the US, the Institute for In Vitro Sciences and ILSI/HESI. The group has embraced the concept of Evidence-based Toxicology (EBT) as a substitute for traditional validation (13) and views the development of this concept as a prime opportunity to collaborate toward change in regulatory toxicology. This group of stakeholders has set up a private–public partnership, the Evidence-based Toxicology Collaboration (EBTC) involving agencies and industry, to promote quality assurance and the implementation of new approaches. EBTC was inaugurated in March 2011 as a satellite activity to the 50th Society of Toxicology conference in Washington, DC.

The primary interest of the EBTC is in assessing the performance of toxicological test methods and addressing questions about the safety of substances to human health and the environment. The EBTC's formation was timely, as there is now a growing interest in applying systematic reviews in toxicology (14), which would be facilitated by a growing recognition that new test assessment approaches are needed.

Initially, the EBTC's activities were conducted by a secretariat in coordination with the US and European Steering Committees. However, it soon became apparent that its governance needed to be united under one roof, to ensure efficiency, unite international stakeholders and retain its focus. Therefore, a Governance Work Group was formed that has written EBTC Operating Guidelines and has worked on selecting the members of a board of trustees. The first board meeting was held in Baltimore in 2015. The EBTC aims to ensure stakeholder balance on the board and its scientific advisory committee, in terms of geographic representation and the various sectors: government, academia, industries and non-government organisations (NGOs).

A European counterpart of the US EBTC was launched in 2012, in conjunction with EUROTOX 2012. The EBTC has grown into an internationally-recognised private—public partnership, with a website designed to become a publicly available repository for guidance and reference documents in EBT (similar to the Cochrane library for EBM). CAAT provides a secretariat for the central coordination of the US and EU EBTC activities.

The EBTC held a workshop on *Evidence-based Toxicology for the 21st Century: Opportunities and Challenges*, in Research Triangle Park, NC, in January 2012. The presentations largely reflected two EBTC priorities: to apply evidence-based methods to assessing the performance of emerging pathway-based testing methods consistent with the 2007 T-21c report and to adopt a governance structure and work processes to move that effort forward. The workshop served to clarify evidence-based approaches and to provide food for thought on substantive and administrative activities for the EBTC. Priority activities include conducting pilot studies to demonstrate the value of evidence-based approaches to toxicology as well as conducting educational outreach on these approaches. This workshop report was later published (15).

Since then, the EBTC has organised symposia at the International Congress of Toxicology held in 2013 in Seoul, South Korea, and at various EUROTOX and Society of Toxicology meetings. A workshop on *The Emergence of Systematic Review and Related Evidence-based Approaches in Toxicology* took place at Johns Hopkins in 2014, which brought together Cochrane Collaboration experts, the US and European regulators, academia, government institutions, industry and NGOs, in discussion of the applications of systematic review as a core tool of evidence-based toxicology for risk assessment in relation to chemicals, food ingredients and pharmaceuticals. More-recent accomplishments have included papers on assessing methodological and reporting quality (16), and general guidance on conducting systematic reviews (14, 17). As an example, a systematic review on the performance of the Zebrafish embryotoxicity test will shortly be available.

7. THE GREEN TOXICOLOGY COLLABORATION

The most important addition in 2013 was the Green Toxicology programme, started with the EPA and the chemical industry. The basic idea is to use alternative methods to help to abandon unsafe molecules at very early stages of product development, so that they never require animal testing. Alternative methods, usually created for regulatory purposes due to their lower costs and duration, lend themselves to this use, which, notably, does not require formal validation. So far, eight conferences and symposia have been organised, and the programme, led by Alexandra Maertens (18, 19), now moving toward dedicated education, offers web-based lecture programmes especially for chemists, to familiarise them with the opportunities of modern toxicology based on alternative methods.

8. THE READ-ACROSS PRACTICE COLLABORATION

In 2014, CAAT started a read-across programme (20). Read-across aims to use test data for similar chemicals to assess the potential toxic properties of a not-tested compound. This can avoid the need for animal tests. In fact, the largest animal-consuming programme in history, the European REACH legislation, sees that about 70% of submissions have a read-across component. The key problem here is that experience on how to conduct read-across properly, and how to handle its uncertainties, is very limited. The read-across programme is therefore currently completing a Good Read-Across Practice guidance, with its first parts published in 2016 (21, 22) and discussed in stakeholder forums in Washington and Brussels in 2016. This programme has the largest potential for effective avoidance of the use of animals. A strong focus is currently on the regulatory acceptability of read-across, supported by parallel work on automated read-across (23).

9. THE GOOD CELL CULTURE PRACTICE COLLABORATION

In 2015, CAAT followed earlier work between 1996 and 2005, which led to guidance on quality assurance of cell culture studies via Good Cell Culture Practice (GCCP), to take into account new technologies, which have revolutionised cell culture, namely, stem cell culture and organ-on-a-chip technologies (24). Two workshops took place in 2015 (25, 26), and a GCCP Collaboration is being formed to develop further guidance on GCCP ('GCCP 2.0') and promote its use.

ACKNOWLEDGEMENTS

A History of The Johns Hopkins Center for Alternatives to Animal Testing (1) by Alan Goldberg, published by MaryAnn Liebert, provides considerably more detail and personal stories than space allows for in this chapter. Some of the text for the chapter come from that article, with the permission of the publisher. There are so many people who made CAAT special. Their advice and friendship made CAAT what it is.

REFERENCES

1. Goldberg, A.M. (2015). A history of the Johns Hopkins Center for Alternatives to Animal Testing (CAAT): The first 28 years (1981–2009). *Applied In Vitro Toxicology* **1**, 99–108.
2. Daneshian, M., Leist, M. & Hartung, T. (2010). Center for alternatives to animal testing – Europe (CAAT-EU): a transatlantic bridge for the paradigm shift in toxicology. *ALTEX* **27**, 63–69.
3. Elmets, C. (1996). The AVON Program Project. A report of progress. *In Vitro Toxicology* **9**, 223.
4. Frazier, J. (1990). Scientific criteria for validation of in vitro toxicity tests. In *Environment Monograph No. 36*, 62pp. Paris, France: OECD.
5. National Research Council. (2007). *Toxicity Testing in the 21st Century: A Vision and a Strategy*, 216pp. Washington, DC, USA: The National Academies Press.
6. Hartung, T. (2009). A toxicology for the 21st century: Mapping the road ahead. *Toxicological Sciences* **109**, 18–23.
7. Basketter, D.A., Clewell, H., Kimber, I., *et al.* (2012). A roadmap for the development of alternative (non-animal) methods for systemic toxicity testing. *ALTEX* **29**, 3–89.
8. Leist, M., Hasiwa, N., Rovida, C., *et al.* (2014). Consensus report on the future of animal-free systemic toxicity testing. *ALTEX* **31**, 341–356.
9. Zurlo, J., Rudacille, D. & Goldberg, A.M. (1994). *Animals and Alternatives in Testing – History, Science and Ethics*, 86pp. New York, NY, USA: Mary Ann Liebert, Inc.
10. Goldberg, A.M. (2008). The science of alternatives: 25 years and tomorrow. In *Proceedings of the 6th World Congress on Alternatives & Animal Use in the Life Sciences, 2007, Tokyo, Japan*, pp. 29–36. AATEX 14, Special Issue.
11. Stephens, M. & Mak, N. (2014). The 3Rs in toxicity testing – from Russell and Burch to 21st century toxicology. In D. Allen, & M. Waters (Eds.), *Reducing, Refining and Replacing the Use of Animals in Toxicity Testing, Issues in Toxicology*, pp. 1–43. London, UK: Royal Society of Chemistry.
12. Bouhifd, M., Andersen, M.E., Baghdikian, C., *et al.* (2015). The Human Toxome Project. *ALTEX* **32**, 112–124.
13. Hartung, T. (2010). Evidence based toxicology – the toolbox of validation for the 21st century. *ALTEX* **27**, 241–251.
14. Stephens, M.L., Betts, K., Beck, N.B., *et al.* (2016). The emergence of systematic review in toxicology. *Toxicological Sciences* **152**, 10–16.
15. Stephens, M.L., Andersen, M., Becker, R.A., *et al.* (2013). Evidence-based toxicology for the 21st century: Opportunities and challenges. *ALTEX* **30**, 74–104.
16. Samuel, G.O., Hoffmann, S., Wright, R., *et al.* (2016). Guidance on assessing the methodological and reporting quality of toxicologically relevant studies: a scoping review. *Environment International* **92–93**, 630–646.
17. Hoffmann, S., de Vries, R.B.M., Stephens, M.L., *et al.* (2017). A primer on systematic reviews in toxicology. *Archives of Toxicology* **91**, 2551–2575.
18. Maertens, A., Anastas, N., Spence, P.J., *et al.* (2014). Green Toxicology. *ALTEX* **31**, 243–249.
19. Maertens, A. & Hartung, T. (2018). Green toxicology – know early about and avoid toxic product liabilities. *Toxicological Sciences* **161**, 285–289.
20. Patlewicz, G., Ball, N., Becker, R.A., *et al.* (2014). Read-across approaches - misconceptions, promises and challenges ahead. *ALTEX* **31**, 387–396.
21. Ball, N., Cronin, M.T.D., Shen, J., *et al.* (2016). Toward Good Read-Across Practice (GRAP) guidance. *ALTEX* **33**, 149–166.
22. Zhu, H., Bouhifd, M., Kleinstreuer, N., *et al.* (2016). Supporting read-across using biological data. *ALTEX* **33**, 167–182.
23. Hartung, T. (2016). Making big sense from big data in toxicology by read-across. *ALTEX* **33**, 83–93.
24. Pamies, D. & Hartung, T. (2017). 21st century cell culture for 21st century toxicology. *Chemical Research in Toxicology* **30**, 43–52.
25. Pamies, D., Bal-Price, A., Simeonov, A., *et al.* (2017). Good cell culture practice for stem cells and stem-cell-derived models. *ALTEX* **34**, 95–132.
26. Pamies, D., Ball-Price, A., Chesne, C., *et al.* (2018 Apr 13). Good cell culture practice for human primary and stem cell-derived models and organoids. *ALTEX*. https://doi.org/10.14573/altex.1710081 [Epub ahead of print] in press.

Chapter 2.12

USA: ICCVAM and NICEATM

Warren Casey[1] and Anna Lowit[2]

[1]*National Institute of Environmental Health Sciences, Durham, NC, United States;* [2]*Environmental Protection Agency, Office of Pesticide Products, Arlington, VA, United States*

SUMMARY

The Interagency Coordinating Committee on the Validation of Alternative Methods (ICCVAM) and the National Toxicology Program's Interagency Center for the Evaluation of Alternative Toxicological Methods (NICEATM) are the primary organisations within the US government responsible for coordinating interagency evaluation of new approach methodologies for toxicological testing. From 1997 to 2013, ICCVAM established guidance on the validation of alternative methods, evaluated alternative methods for regulatory use, and made formal recommendations to federal agencies on a number of test methods. A new direction for the committee was set in 2013, emphasising the importance of federal agency engagement over the entire validation process. The reinvention of ICCVAM culminated with the 2018 publication of *A Strategic Roadmap for Establishing New Approaches to Evaluate the Safety of Chemicals and Medical Products in the United States*, which provides a conceptual framework that promotes a focus on human health, understanding end-user needs and transparent implementation plans.

1. GENESIS OF ALTERNATIVE PROGRAMMES IN THE UNITED STATES

The establishment of the US National Toxicology Program (NTP) in 1978 represented the first effort by the USA to coordinate the development, validation and implementation of new technologies for toxicity testing across federal agencies (1); Table 1. The NTP is a cooperative effort between the US Food and Drug Administration (FDA), the Centers for Disease Control and Prevention (CDCs) and the US National Institute of Environmental Health Sciences (NIEHS), the programme's headquarters, with the Director of the NIEHS serving concurrently as the Director of the NTP.

The *National Institutes of Health (NIH) Revitalization Act of 1993* was the first legislation in the USA to address the development and utilisation of non-animal testing approaches (2). The Act directed the NIEHS to establish an interagency committee to develop recommendations relating to the validation and acceptance of new and revised testing methods that would replace, reduce or refine the use of animals for biomedical research and toxicity testing. In addition, the Act directed the NIEHS to establish a centre 'to develop and validate assays and protocols, including alternative methods that can reduce or eliminate the use of animals in acute or chronic safety testing'. In response to this directive, the Interagency Coordinating Committee on the Validation of Alternative Methods (ICCVAM) was established in 1994 as an *ad hoc* committee to develop an interagency process for achieving the regulatory acceptance of alternative testing methods (3). In 1997, ICCVAM became a standing committee to evaluate new test methods of interest to federal agencies and to coordinate cross-agency dialogue on issues regarding test method development, validation, acceptance and international harmonisation (3). The NTP Interagency Center for the Evaluation of Alternative Toxicological Methods (NICEATM) was established within the NIEHS in 1998, to provide operational support for ICCVAM and to organise committee-related activities, such as technical evaluations, peer reviews, data analysis and workshops for test methods of interest to federal agencies (4).

The *ICCVAM Authorization Act of 2000* (5) established ICCVAM as a permanent committee 'to establish, wherever feasible, guidelines, recommendations, and regulations that promote the regulatory acceptance of new or revised scientifically valid toxicological tests that protect human and animal health and the environment, while reducing, refining, or

The History of Alternative Test Methods in Toxicology. https://doi.org/10.1016/B978-0-12-813697-3.00015-9

TABLE 1 Summary Timeline

1966	Animal Welfare Act
1978	The US National Toxicology Program is established
1993	NIH Revitalization Act, ICCVAM is established as an *ad hoc* committee
1997	ICCVAM is established as a standing committee
2000	ICCVAM Authorization Act establishes ICCVAM as a permanent committee
2002	Animal Welfare Act amended to exclude coverage of rats, mice and birds
2007	NAS Report on Toxicology Testing in the 21st century
2008	Tox21 Collaboration formalised: NTP, NCATS, EPA NCCT (FDA joins in 2010)
2009	ICATM established
2013	ICCVAM is 'reinvented', NICEATM under new leadership
2014	ICCVAM describes New Path Forward and begins work on Strategic Roadmap
2018	ICCVAM publishes 'A Strategic Roadmap for Establishing New Approaches to Evaluate the Safety of Chemicals and Medical Products in the United States'

replacing animal tests and ensuring human safety and product effectiveness'. The following are the purposes of ICCVAM according to the Act:

1. Increase the efficiency and effectiveness of federal agency test method review.
2. Eliminate unnecessary duplicative efforts and share experiences between federal regulatory agencies.
3. Optimise the utilisation of scientific expertise outside the federal government.
4. Ensure that new and revised test methods are validated to meet the needs of federal agencies.
5. Replace, reduce or refine the use of animals in testing, where feasible.

The Committee comprises the heads of 16 US federal regulatory and research agencies that use or generate toxicological information (Table 2). The *ICCVAM Authorization Act* directs ICCVAM to carry out the following duties:

1. Coordinate the technical review and evaluation of new, revised or alternative test methods.
2. Foster interagency and international harmonisation of test protocols that encourage replacing, reducing and refining animal test methods.
3. Assist with and provide guidance on validation criteria and processes.
4. Promote the acceptance of scientifically valid test methods.
5. Promote awareness of accepted test methods.
6. Submit ICCVAM test method recommendations to appropriate US federal agencies.
7. Consider requests from the public to review and evaluate new, revised or alternative test methods that have evidence of scientific validity.
8. Make ICCVAM's final test recommendations available to the public.
9. Prepare biennial reports on ICCVAM progress and accomplishments under the Act and make them available to the public.

The *ICCVAM Authorization Act* also established a Scientific Advisory Committee, now designated the Scientific Advisory Committee on Alternative Toxicological Methods (SACATM), to advise ICCVAM and NICEATM with regard to ICCVAM's activities. SACATM is composed of representatives from various types of organisations specified in the Act, including certain industry sectors, the animal protection community, state governments, academia and test method developers, with individual members appointed by the NIEHS Director.

2. ORGANISATIONAL STRUCTURE AND LEADERSHIP OF NICEATM AND ICCVAM

As noted earlier, ICCVAM is a committee of representatives from 16 federal agencies. Leadership of the committee has typically been provided by two co-chairs, with elections held every 2 years and no limit on the number of terms held by an

TABLE 2 ICCVAM Agencies

Agency for Toxic Substances and Disease Registry
National Cancer Institute
National Institute for Occupational Safety and Health
National Institute of Environmental Health Sciences
National Institute of Standards and Technology
National Institutes of Health
National Library of Medicine
Occupational Safety and Health Administration
Consumer Product Safety Commission
Department of Agriculture
Department of Defense
Department of Energy
Department of the Interior
Department of Transportation
Environmental Protection Agency
Food and Drug Administration

TABLE 3 Key Personnel

NIEHS and NTP Directors
- 2009—Present, Linda S. Birnbaum, PhD
- 2005—07, David A. Schwartz, MD, NIEHS and NTP Director
- 1991—2005, Kenneth Olden, PhD, NIEHS and NTP Director

NICEATM Directors
- 2013—Present, Warren Casey, PhD
- 1997—2012, William Stokes, DVM

NICEATM Deputy Directors
- 2015—Present, Nicole Kleinstreuer, PhD
- 2010—13, Warren Casey, PhD
- 2005—08, Ray Tice, PhD

ICCVAM Co-Chairs
- 2018—Present, Emily Reinke, US DoD
- 2013—Present, Anna Lowit, PhD, US EPA
- 2013—17, Abby Jacobs, PhD, US FDA
- 2011—13, Joanna Matheson, PhD, CPSC
- 2007—2012, Jodie Kulpa-Eddy, DVM, USDA
- 2001—09, Marilyn Wind, PhD, CPSC
- 2001—06, Len Schechtman, PhD, US FDA
- 1997—2001, William Stokes, DVM, NIEHS
- 1997—2001, Richard Hill, MD, PhD, US EPA

individual. Importantly, ICCVAM has no legal authority and therefore cannot 'require' an agency or institution to adopt new approach methodologies (NAMs). In fact, the *ICCVAM Authorization Act* specifically states that *Nothing in this Act shall prevent a Federal agency from retaining final authority for incorporating the test methods recommended by the ICCVAM in the manner determined to be appropriate by such Federal agency or regulatory body.* The committee has no direct (discretionary) funding; all its activities are supported by NICEATM, a branch of the NTP Division within the NIEHS. NICEATM is staffed by two federal employees who serve as Director and Deputy Director, with administrative and scientific support provided via a contract with Integrated Laboratory Systems Inc (Table 3).

3. REGULATORY LANDSCAPE IN THE UNITED STATES

The *Animal Welfare Act* (AWA; (6)) is the only federal law in the USA that regulates the treatment of animals in research, naming the US Department of Agriculture Animal and Plant Health Inspection Service (USDA APHIS) as responsible for its enforcement. The law was passed in 1966, primarily in response to public outcry over the poor treatment of domesticated animals by commercial breeders and dealers. The scope of the AWA expanded over the years to cover 'all warm-blooded animals used in testing, experimentation, exhibition, as pets or sold as pets'. However, in 2002, the Act was amended to specifically exclude the species most commonly used in research and toxicity testing, namely, birds, rats and mice (7). Importantly, because these species are not considered 'animals' under the AWA, there is limited legal basis for mandating accountability of the number of animals used or the type of procedures conducted in research or toxicity testing. Additionally, the US differs from the EU and most other countries in that there is no legal requirement to use a non-animal method if one is available, leaving the decision to the discretion of company conducting the test.

Toxicological testing requirements in the USA are complex and not always prescriptive, which contributes to the difficulty of validating NAMs to meet the needs of multiple agencies. Even within a single agency, testing requirements can vary significantly. For example, the US Environmental Protection Agency (EPA) Office of Pesticide Products (OPP) administers the Federal Insecticide, Fungicide and Rodenticide Act (FIFRA; (8)),which requires specific testing of agricultural chemicals, whereas the EPA Office of Pollution Prevention and Toxics (OPPT) oversees the registration of chemicals under the Toxic Substances Control Act and the Pollution Prevention Act (TSCA; (9)), which does not delineate specific testing requirements. Some federal agencies (e.g. the Consumer Product Safety Commission (CPSC)) specify testing requirements but do not receive test data or results, whereas others (e.g. the Occupational Safety and Health Administration (OSHA)) require products to be 'properly labelled' with regard to safety hazards but do not specify how the determination is made. Even when common testing requirements are identified (e.g. for acute oral lethality), the purpose of the test and the use of data can be different from agency to agency, and even within the same agency. Another obstacle is presented by the lack of harmonisation among US agencies with regard to systems used for the classification and labelling of chemicals, with the United Nations Globally Harmonized System (GHS), the EPA Classification system and variations of each of them currently in use.

In 2016, the *Frank R. Lautenberg Chemical Safety for the 21st Century Act* (10) amended the TSCA and called for the EPA to 'develop a strategic plan to promote the development and implementation of alternative test methods and strategies to reduce, refine, or replace vertebrate animal testing and provide information of equivalent or better scientific quality and relevance for assessing risks of injury to health or the environment'. The plan was published in June 2018 (Document EPA-740-R1-8004).

4. KEY CONTRIBUTIONS, ACTIVITIES AND MILESTONES

4.1 The Early Years: 1997—2013

The primary activities of ICCVAM during its first 17 years were focused on establishing a paradigm for the review of validation studies, reviewing methods for the refinement and reduction of animal use for toxicity testing of chemicals and opportunities related to refining the testing of biological products (i.e. vaccines), as this type of testing requires a disproportionate number of animals for safety testing compared with other product types. Formal recommendations were made to federal agencies on a number of test methods. These methods are listed on the NTP website (http://ntp.niehs.nih.gov/go/regaccept), with the most significant contributions described in the following section.

Shortly after its establishment as a standing committee, ICCVAM published documents to provide test developers with guidance on obtaining ICCVAM endorsement for their alternative methods: *Validation and Regulatory Acceptance of Toxicological Test Methods: A Report of the ad hoc Interagency Coordinating Committee on the Validation of Alternative Methods* (3) and *Evaluation of the Validation Status of Alternative Toxicological Methods: Guidelines for Submission to ICCVAM* (11). The principles outlined in these documents served as the basis for all subsequent ICCVAM evaluations and carried forward in developing international criteria outlined in OECD Guidance Document (GD) 34, *Guidance Document on the Validation and International Acceptance of New or Updated Test Methods for Hazard Assessment*, published in 2005 (12).

The US EPA established a technical task force to revise the Up-Down Procedure (UDP) for acute oral lethality testing, and in 1999 asked ICCVAM to conduct an independent peer review of the revised protocol, which used fewer animals. ICCVAM complied and subsequently made recommendations to US agencies that the revised UDP, OECD Test Guideline (TG) 425 (13) was acceptable as an alternative to the traditional LD50 test for assessing acute oral toxicity. ICCVAM, in partnership with the EPA and the International Life Sciences Institute (ILSI), held a training workshop on acute toxicity testing methods in 2002. The workshop provided practical information and case studies to facilitate the understanding and implementation of the UDP and other *in vivo* and *in vitro* alternative methods for acute toxicity.

In 1998, NICEATM convened an independent peer review panel to review the validity of the Local Lymph Node Assay (LLNA) as an alternative to the Buehler test and the guinea-pig maximisation test for assessing the allergic contact dermatitis hazard potentials of chemicals. ICCVAM reviewed the validation material and peer panel report, and in 1999 recommended the LLNA to US agencies as an alternative for guinea-pig tests (14). The LLNA was adopted by the OECD as TG 429 in 2002 and by the US EPA as OPPTS 870.2600 in 2003. In 2008, ICCVAM developed LLNA performance standards describing essential test method components, a minimum list of reference chemicals, and accuracy and reliability values. The performance standards were used by ICCVAM to evaluate and recommend a number of LLNA variants, namely updated and reduced LLNA protocols in 2009 (requiring 20% and 40% fewer animals, respectively), LLNA: DA and BrdU-ELISA in 2010 (nonradioisotopic LLNA test methods) and LLNA for potency categorisation of skin sensitisers in 2011 (protocol refinement and reduction of animal use). ICCVAM, in partnership with the ILSI Health and Environmental Sciences Institute (HESI) Alternatives to Animal Testing Technical Committee, organised a training workshop for the LLNA in 2001. The primary objective of the workshop was to train regulatory scientists and industry toxicologists on how to perform the LLNA and interpret data in accordance with regulatory testing requirements.

The first non-animal alternative method reviewed and recommended by ICCVAM was CORROSITEX (InVitro International, Inc.), an *in vitro* test for the identification of potential dermal corrosives. CORROSITEX was accepted as an alternative to a procedure specified in the US Department of Transportation (DOT) Hazardous Materials Regulations (DOT-SP 10,904) for DOT packing group classification of corrosive materials and was adopted by the OECD as TG 435 in 2006 (15). At the request of the EPA, ICCVAM established performance standards for *in vitro* skin corrosion test methods. These standards, which were based on ICCVAM evaluations of *in vitro* methods to identify potential dermal corrosives, can be used to evaluate the usefulness and limitations of other test methods that are based on similar scientific principles that measure or predict the same biological or toxic effect (16). Subsequently, ICCVAM and NICEATM drafted proposed updates to OECD TGs for *in vitro* methods for identifying skin corrosives (OECD TGs 430 (17) and 431 (18)). These updates, based on the ICCVAM performance standards, were adopted by the OECD in 2013. The US DOT's Pipeline and Hazardous Materials Safety Administration revised its hazardous materials regulations to include acceptance of the *in vitro* methods described in the OECD TGs.

In 2003, the EPA nominated four *in vitro* methods for evaluation by ICCVAM: the Bovine Corneal Opacity and Permeability (BCOP) test, the Isolated Chicken Eye (ICE) test, Hen's Egg Test-Chorioallantoic Membrane assay (HET-CAM) and the isolated rabbit eye (IRE) test. ICCVAM prepared the Test Method Evaluation Report (19) and recommended the BCOP and ICE tests to US agencies as screening tests to identify substances as ocular corrosives and severe irritants for use in a tiered approach. In 2009, the BCOP test was adopted as OECD TG 437 (20) and the ICE test as TG 438 (21).

Although some progress was being made, the pace and direction of ICCVAM's activities drew criticism from the animal welfare community and from several members of Congress who had sponsored the original ICCVAM legislation. As a result, language in the fiscal year 2007 Senate Appropriations Report required ICCVAM to create a five-year plan to address the research, development, translation and validation of alternative assays for integration into the federal agency testing programmes. The resulting NICEATM-ICCVAM Five-Year Plan, issued in 2008, included the promotion of training on the use of alternative test methods as a major objective. Consequently, two Best Practices Workshops were held in 2011 to help create awareness and encourage the use of NAMs (22). Over 70 scientists from industry, academia, research and regulatory agencies and animal welfare organisations gathered at the NIH in Bethesda for each workshop.

In 2009, the EU, Canada, Japan and the USA signed a Memorandum of Cooperation (MoC), forming the International Cooperation on Alternative Test Methods (ICATM) to promote enhanced cooperation, collaboration and communication among their respective validation organisations: the European Union Reference Laboratory for Alternatives to Animal Testing (EURL ECVAM), Health Canada, the Japanese Center for the Validation of Alternative Methods (JaCVAM) and ICCVAM. An updated agreement, adding the Korean Center for the Validation of Alternative Methods (KoCVAM) to the ICATM agreement, was signed in March 2011. Since 2015, China and Brazil have also been participating in ICATM activities as observers.

In September 2010, NICEATM, ICCVAM and their ICATM partners held an international workshop on alternative methods that can reduce, refine and replace animals for vaccine potency and safety testing. The workshop, which was attended by nearly 200 scientists representing relevant stakeholder organisations from 13 countries, reviewed the state of the science of alternative methods that are currently available for this purpose and developed recommendations for priority research needed to further advance alternative methods.

One of the highest priority implementation activities was the organisation of an international workshop on alternative methods for rabies vaccine potency testing. In October 2011, NICEATM, ICCVAM and their international partners convened a workshop on alternative methods for rabies vaccine potency testing, focused on the following three areas: (a) reduction and refinement opportunities for the *in vivo* mouse challenge test; (b) validation status, data gaps and implementation strategies for serological antibody quantification methods; and (c) validation status, data gaps and implementation strategies for *in vitro* antigen quantification methods. The workshop proceedings were published in 2012 (23).

Acting on high-priority recommendations from the September 2010 vaccine workshop, a workshop on *Leptospira* vaccines was held in 2012, bringing together over 80 international scientific experts from government, industry and academia to review recent advances in science and technology, in addition to available methods and approaches for *Leptospira* vaccine potency testing. The workshop proceedings were published in 2013 (24).

4.2 A New Direction: 2013–2018

Early on, ICCVAM was widely viewed as productive and having impact, when most efforts involved establishing the foundational processes for the submission, review and regulatory acceptance of alternative toxicological methods. However, the US Congress, the public and animal welfare groups eventually began to raise concerns regarding the lack of tangible progress by ICCVAM. Expectations for real reductions in animal use were not being realised, leading the Director of the NIEHS to implement substantive change in NICEATM's leadership (25) and to challenge ICCVAM to develop a new strategic vision better aligned with that described in the 2007 National Academy of Sciences report on *Toxicity Testing in the 21st Century* (26). In turn, NICEATM would expand its scope and concentrate its resources on providing bioinformatic and computational toxicology support to the interagency Tox21 projects (see also Chapter 2.13), positioning ICCVAM to address how data from these new methods could be integrated into the existing regulatory framework. ICCVAM developed a draft document, entitled *A New Path Forward: ICCVAM and NICEATM*, which presented ICCVAM's areas of priority and scientific focus for immediate resource investment (over 3–5 years), plans for improved communications with stakeholders and the public, and interest in exploring new paradigms for the validation and utilisation of alternative toxicological methods (27). By 2017, ICCVAM had achieved all of the following goals identified in the 'New Path Forward' document:

1. The USDA–APHIS decreased the number of hamsters used in *Leptospira* vaccine potency testing by 30%;
2. The US EPA issued guidance to waive acute dermal toxicity testing for pesticide formulations (28);
3. Battery-based approaches involving *in silico*, *in chemico* and *in vitro* tests to assess the skin sensitising potential of chemicals were evaluated, and collaborations with international partners were initiated, to support ongoing development and the validation of *in vitro* skin sensitisation test methods (29–32)
4. Annual 'public forums' were established to provide updates on agency Three Rs activities and to facilitate in-person dialogue between stakeholders and agency representatives.

During this period, the committee would also begin work on a more-comprehensive long-term strategic plan to address the many challenges of replacing long-standing toxicity tests that relied on animal use. The concept of developing a strategic roadmap (hereafter referred to as the Roadmap) to establish new approaches for toxicity testing in the USA was proposed and endorsed at the 2015 SACATM meeting and further developed at the 2016 SACATM meeting. Acting on this endorsement, over 90 federal scientists from 16 agencies and multiple interagency workgroups convened in 2017 at the NIH to discuss and develop the key elements of a new strategy for toxicity testing that would improve human relevance and reduce the use of animals. A strategic roadmap would help establish the use of these new approaches by providing a conceptual framework to support the development, evaluation and utilisation of NAMs, and to facilitate communication and collaboration within and between government agencies, stakeholders and international partners.

An important first step in developing the Roadmap was a retrospective evaluation aimed at understanding and addressing the shortcomings of ICCVAM's historical approach to validation, which noted the following:

1. In the past, the development of alternative methods was often initiated by researchers and test method developers with little input from the end-users, namely, federal agencies and regulated industries. Failure to understand regulatory needs, and particularly the various contexts of use, produced methods that did not adequately meet the testing requirements of the end-users. Consequently, these methods were either not accepted by federal agencies or accepted by the agencies but not used by the regulated community. The likelihood of regulatory acceptance and industry adoption would be greatly increased if NAMs were developed 'with the end in mind', to ensure fitness for purpose. Achieving this objective requires end-users to be actively engaged during the research and development process. Likewise, it is

critical that federal agencies provide clear guidance on their information needs, context of use and willingness to accept NAMs in place of traditional animal-based tests.

2. Previous validation efforts coordinated by ICCVAM typically adhered to the principles described in OECD GD 34 (12), which provides guidance on the design and conduct of validation studies, including the assessment of reliability, reproducibility and relevance. Conforming to GD34 was intended to improve the expediency and efficiency of regulatory acceptance and incorporation of new methods into OECD TGs. While GD34 allows a great deal of flexibility via a 'modular approach' to validation, this flexibility was not usually applied to ICCVAM-coordinated validation studies, contributing greatly to the expense and duration of these studies. In addition, GD34, published in 2005 on the basis of principles formulated in the OECD Solna workshop of 1996 (33), does not fully address all considerations required for the effective evaluation of many modern technologies and approaches. Although GD34 will continue to serve as the default validation standard for the near future, the timely incorporation of 21st century science into modern risk assessment and hazard identification will require new approaches for establishing confidence in NAMs, which incorporate the overarching principles described in GD34, but in a more flexible and efficient manner.

3. Historically, most validation studies were coordinated by a central organisation (i.e. NICEATM). In retrospect, it may be more appropriate for other organisations or agencies to coordinate the evaluation of NAMs. Moving forward, the USA needs to develop an approach for establishing confidence in NAMs that is better suited to capitalise on its vast, but highly decentralised, resources.

In January, 2018, ICCVAM published *A Strategic Roadmap for Establishing New Approaches to Evaluate the Safety of Chemicals and Medical Products in the United States* (34). The Roadmap was developed to guide the application of new technologies, such as high-throughput screening, tissue chips and computational models, to the toxicity testing of chemicals and medical products. It describes three strategic goals required for progress as follows:

1. Connecting new test method developers with end-users.
2. Promoting flexible approaches for establishing confidence in new methods.
3. Helping ensure the adoption of new methods by federal agencies and regulated industries once validated.

This strategic Roadmap is a resource to guide US federal agencies and stakeholders seeking to adopt new approaches to safety and risk assessment of chemicals and medical products that improve human relevance and replace or reduce the use of animals. ICCVAM workgroups will develop detailed implementation plans to address Roadmap goals, tailored to specific toxicological endpoints of concern. These implementation plans will include the following four key elements: (a) definition of testing needs; (b) identification of any available alternative tests and computer models; (c) a plan to develop integrated approaches to testing and assessment and defined approaches for interpreting data; and (d) a plan to address both scientific and non-scientific challenges, including regulatory challenges, such as international harmonisation. Progress will be tracked on the ICCVAM website and publically reported at least twice a year at the ICCVAM public forum and SACATM meetings.

Although there are many benefits associated with achieving these goals, the primary objective of the Roadmap is to protect and improve public health through the use of more human-relevant approaches to safety testing. This differs significantly from most other international efforts, particularly those in the EU, where ethical considerations are driving most of the previous and ongoing Three Rs efforts. Ultimately, focusing on human-relevance will obviate the need for testing in animals while also reducing the cost of product development and registration. However, there is also an immediate need to move away from some animal testing requirements based on ethical concerns alone (e.g. oral and inhalation acute lethality, dermal and ocular irritation, *Leptospirosis* and rabies vaccine testing). These methods represent more-tractable targets for the replacement of animal tests than the repeat-dose sub/chronic-studies used to assess multiple complex endpoints and will provide valuable experience for exploring new processes and navigating the many obstacles necessary for replacing animal-based tests.

5. CONCLUSIONS

ICCVAM and NICEATM have played an important role in activities related to the development of NAMs in the USA and internationally through interactions with ICATM partners and the OECD. The operating model for how these organisations operate and interact with each other and external stakeholders has evolved considerably since 2013, leading to significant advances in activities approaches that reduce or eliminate the use of animals for toxicity testing. Publication of the US Roadmap document represents the culmination of a multi-year effort conducted by 16 federal agencies and interagency workgroups and establishes a new framework for the future development and implementation of NAMs.

REFERENCES

1. NIEHS. (1978). *Notice of Establishment: The National Toxicology Program.* FRN 43-221. November 15, 1978. Research Triangle Park, NC, USA: NIEHS.
2. United States Code. (1993). *National Institutes of Health Revitalization Act of 1993. Public Law 103−143.* Washington, DC, USA: US Government Printing Office.
3. ICCVAM. (1997). *Validation and Regulatory Acceptance of Toxicological Test Methods: A Report of the Ad hoc Interagency Coordinating Committee on the Validation of Alternative Methods.* NIH Publication No. 97.3981, 105pp. Research Triangle Park, NC, USA: NIEHS.
4. NIEHS. (1997). *Notice of Meeting to Discuss the Procedures and Activities of the National Toxicology Program (NTP) Center for the Evaluation of Alternative Toxicological Methods and the Interagency Coordinating Committee on the Validation of Alternative Methods (ICCVAM).* Washington, DC, USA: Government Printing Office. FRN 62−207. October 27, 1997.
5. United States Congress. (2000). *The ICCVAM Authorization Act of 2000.* Washington, DC, USA: Government Printing Office. Public Law 106−545. December 19, 2000.
6. United States Congress. (1966). *Laboratory Animal Welfare Act of 1966.* Washington, DC, USA: Government Printing Office. Public Law 89−544. August 24, 1966.
7. United States Congress. (2002). *Farm Security and Rural Investment Act.* Washington, DC, USA: Government Printing Office. Public Law 107−171. January 23, 2002.
8. United States Congress. (1910). *The Federal Insecticide, Fungicide, and Rodenticide Act (FIFRA).* Washington, DC, USA: US Government Printing Office, 8. Public Law 61−152. April 26, 1910.
9. United States Congress. (1976). *The Toxic Substances Control Act (TSCA).* Washington, DC, USA: US Government Printing Office. Public Law 94−469. October 11, 1976.
10. United States Congress. (2016). *Frank R. Lautenberg Chemical Safety for the 21st Century Act.* Washington, DC, USA: US Government Printing Office. Public Law 114−182. June 22, 2016.
11. ICCVAM. (1999). *Evaluation of the Validation Status of Toxicological Methods: General Guidelines for Submissions to ICCVAM,* 43pp. Research Triangle Park, NC, USA: NIEHS. NIH Publication No. 99-4496.
12. OECD. (2005). Guidance document on the validation and international acceptance of new or updated test methods for hazard assessment. In *Series on Testing and Assessment No. 34,* 96pp. Paris, France: OECD.
13. OECD. (2008). *OECD TG 425: Acute Oral Toxicity: Up-and-Down Procedure,* 27pp. Paris, France: OECD.
14. ICCVAM. (1999). *The Murine Local Lymph Node Assay: A Test Method for Assessing the Allergic Contact Dermatitis Potential of Chemicals/Compounds.* NIH Publication No. 99-4494, 211pp. Research Triangle Park, NC, USA: NIEHS.
15. OECD. (2006). *OECD TG 435: In Vitro Membrane Barrier Test Method for Skin Corrosion,* 15pp. Paris, France: OECD.
16. ICCVAM. (2004). *Recommended Performance Standards for In Vitro Test Methods for Skin Corrosion.* NIH Publication No. 04-4510, 100pp. Research Triangle Park, NC, USA: NIEHS.
17. OECD. (2004). *OECD TG 430: In Vitro Skin Corrosion: Transcutaneous electrical Resistance Test (TER),* 20pp. Paris, France: OECD.
18. OECD. (2004). *OECD TG 431: In Vitro Skin Corrosion: Human Skin Model Test,* 8pp. Paris, France: OECD.
19. ICCVAM. (2010). *Test Method Evaluation Report: Current Validation Status of In Vitro Test Methods Proposed for Identifying Eye Injury Hazard Potential of Chemicals and Products.* NIH Publication No. 10-7553, 1324pp. Research Triangle Park, NC, USA: NIEHS.
20. OECD. (2009). *OECD TG 437: Bovine Corneal Opacity and Permeability Test Method for Identifying Ocular Corrosives and Severe Irritants,* 18pp. Paris, France: OECD.
21. OECD. (2017). *OECD TG 438: Isolated Chicken Eye Test Method for Identifying i) Chemicals Inducing Serious Eye Damage and ii) Chemicals not Requiring Classification for Eye Irritation or Serious Eye Damage,* 20pp. Paris, France: OECD.
22. ICCVAM. (2012). *Biennial Progress Report 2010−2011.* NIH Publication No. 12-7873, 104pp. Research Triangle Park, NC, USA: NIEHS.
23. Stokes, W., McFarland, R., Kulpa-Eddy, J., *et al.* (2012). Report on the international workshop on alternative methods for human and veterinary rabies vaccine testing: State of the science and planning the way forward. *Biologicals* **40**, 369−381.
24. Stokes, W., Srinivas, G., McFarland, R., *et al.* (2013). Report on the international workshop on alternative methods for Leptospira vaccine potency testing: State of the science and the way forward. *Biologicals* **41**, 279−294.
25. Birnbaum, L.S. (2013). 15 years out: Reinventing ICCVAM. *Environmental Health Perspectives* **121**, a40.
26. NRC. (2007). *Toxicity Testing in the 21st Century: A Vision and a Strategy,* 216pp. Washington, DC: The National Academies Press.
27. Casey, W., Jacobs, A., Maull, E., *et al.* (2015). A new path forward: Interagency coordinating committee on the validation of alternative methods (ICCVAM) and national toxicology program's interagency center for the evaluation of alternative toxicological methods (NICEATM). *Journal of the American Association for Laboratory Animal Science* **54**, 170−173.
28. EPA. (November 9, 2016). *Guidance for Waiving Acute Dermal Toxicity Tests for Pesticide Formulations & Supporting Retrospective Analysis,* 12pp. Washington, DC, USA: US EPA.
29. Casati, S., Aschberger, K., Barroso, J., *et al.* (2017). Standardisation of defined approaches for skin sensitisation testing to support regulatory use and international adoption: position of the International Cooperation on Alternative Test Methods. *Archives of Toxicology* **92**, 611−671.
30. Strickland, J., Zang, Q., Paris, M., *et al.* (2017). Multivariate models for prediction of human skin sensitization hazard. *Journal of Applied Toxicology* **37**, 347−360.
31. Zang, Q., Paris, M., Lehmann, D.M., *et al.* (2017). Prediction of skin sensitization potency using machine learning approaches. *Journal of Applied Toxicology* **37**, 792−805.

32. OECD. (2016). Guidance Document on the Reporting of Defined Approaches and Individual Information Sources to be used within Integrated Approaches to Testing and Assessment (IATA) for Skin Sensitisation. No. 256. In *Series on Testing and Assessment*, 24pp. Paris, France: OECD.

33. OECD. (2009). *Final Report of the OECD Workshop on "Harmonization of Validation and Acceptance Criteria for Alternative Toxicological Test Methods"* (Solna Report). ENV/MC/CHEM/TG(96)9, 53pp. Paris, France: OECD.

34. ICCVAM. (2018). *A Strategic Roadmap for Establishing New Approaches to Evaluate the Safety of Chemicals and Medical Products in the United States*, 13pp. Research Triangle Park, NC, USA: NIEHS.

Chapter 2.13

US Vision for Toxicity Testing in the 21st Century

Robert J. Kavlock[1], Christopher P. Austin[2] and Raymond R. Tice[3]

[1]Washington, DC, United States; [2]National Center for Advancing Translational Sciences, Bethesda, MD, United States; [3]RTice Consulting, Hillsborough, NC, United States

SUMMARY

In response to a growing recognition over the past couple of decades that the field of toxicology needed to transition from a largely descriptive science to one based on the mechanisms of chemical effects in living systems, a partnership among several US government agencies (initially the Environmental Protection Agency, the National Toxicology Program and the NIH Chemical Genomics Center, later joined by the Food and Drug Administration) emerged in the early 21st century. This partnership, which was formally established in 2007 and came to be called Tox21, was based on the complementary expertise of the member agencies and was committed to advancing the science in a transparent manner, with open access to all methodologies and results, and with community involvement in science generation and analysis. The consortium represents a unique collaboration across the US federal government, and in its relatively short existence has had a significant impact on moving the field of toxicology to more mechanism-based *in vitro* approaches. This chapter reviews the history of the consortium, its major objectives and accomplishments, and identifies new strategic directions that are being formulated to address gaps in technology and knowledge.

1. THE NTP VISION AND ROADMAP

The US National Toxicology Program (NTP) is an interagency programme located within the National Institute of Environmental Health Sciences (NIEHS) in Research Triangle Park, North Carolina (NC). Established in 1978, its mission is to evaluate agents of public health concern and to provide the resulting information to government agencies, the scientific and medical communities and the general public. In 2004, the NTP released a Vision Statement (1) to support the evolution of toxicology from a largely observational science at the level of disease-specific models to a predominantly predictive science focused on target-specific, mechanism-based biological observations. To implement this vision, NTP developed a Roadmap (1) that placed an increased emphasis on the use of alternative assays for targeting key pathways, molecular events or processes linked to disease. The Roadmap included the development of a high-throughput capability for mechanistic targets and an evaluation of the use of non-mammalian animal models. In response to the Roadmap, the NTP established in 2005 a High Throughput Screening (HTS) programme and subsequently, the Biomolecular Screening Branch to manage the programme.

2. THE EPA FRAMEWORK FOR A COMPTOX RESEARCH PROGRAM

The US Environmental Protection Agency (EPA) has a long history of applying computational methods to chemical hazard assessment, as exemplified by efforts to develop quantitative structure activity relationship (QSAR) models for fish toxicity (2). Recognising the potential for the application of emerging molecular tools to probe biological processes, in 2003, the EPA Office of Research and Development released a Framework for a Computational Toxicology Research Program (3). It defined computational toxicology as the application of mathematical and computer models and molecular biological approaches to improve the Agency's prioritisation and risk assessments of chemicals. This framework identified three strategic objectives as follows: (a) to improve linkages across the source-to-outcome continuum; (b) to develop approaches for prioritising chemicals for subsequent screening and testing; and (c) to produce better methods and predictive models for quantitative risk assessment. Success would ultimately be judged by the ability to produce faster, cheaper and less-uncertain risk assessments. Importantly, it introduced the fields of systems biology and the promise of high throughput screening (HTS) as a means of understanding the potential toxicity pathways for thousands of data-poor chemicals under the EPA's jurisdiction. By following this path, questions of 'when and how' to test specific chemicals for hazard and risk character-isation could be addressed. In 2005, the EPA established the National Center for Computational Toxicology (NCCT) with the charge of integrating advances in biology, biotechnology, chemistry and computer science to identify biological path-ways at risk to disruption from chemical exposure.

3. THE NIH MOLECULAR LIBRARIES PROGRAM

Just as toxicity testing of environmental chemicals was historically performed in animals, discovery of drugs for thera-peutic purposes utilised animal models almost exclusively until the 1990s, when the advent of molecular cloning and cell culture made possible the target-based and cell-based screening of chemicals for activities relevant to disease. During the 1990s, tremendous increases in chemical libraries and assays with sensitivities amenable to miniaturisation further drove parallel processing to 96-, 384- or 1536-microwell plate formats, among others, and created the concept of HTS. 'High throughput' is a relative term, but it is generally defined as the testing of 10,000 to 100,000 compounds per day, accomplished with mechanisation that ranges from manually operated workstations to fully automated robotic systems (4).

HTS, medicinal chemistry, cheminformatics and molecular modelling for drug discovery was developed and practiced almost exclusively within the pharmaceutical industry until the early 2000s. At that time, completion of the Human Genome Project led to the discovery of tens of thousands of novel genes of unknown function (5). This led to a series of genome-scale initiatives at the National Human Genome Research Institute (NHGRI) to generate publicly available tools and technologies that would catalyse discovery of the functions and therapeutic potentials of all human genes. The largest of these was the Molecular Libraries Initiative (MLI; (6)), created under the aegis of the NIH Roadmap for Medical Research (7).

The MLI was a multifaceted programme that adapted the assay, HTS, and chemical technologies initially developed in the pharmaceutical industry for the creation of pharmacological probes to explore novel gene and cell functions. The first component of the MLI to be created was the NIH Chemical Genomics Center (NCGC), housed within the intramural research program of the NHGRI. The NCGC's focus was on technologies that would allow exploration of novel target space and ultimately establish general principles of small molecule-target interactions. One of the first such technologies developed was quantitative high throughput screening (qHTS), which, for the first-time, permitted the testing of tens to hundreds of thousands of compounds for biological activity in concentration–response assays, typically over 5 orders of magnitude (8).

4. THE NATIONAL ACADEMY OF SCIENCES AND THE FUTURE OF TOXICITY TESTING

In 2004, the National Academy of Sciences (NAS) was asked to develop a long-range vision for toxicity testing and a strategic plan for implementing that vision. The subsequent National Research Council (NRC) final report, *Toxicity Testing in the 21st Century: A Vision and a Strategy* (9), articulated a future system that could: (a) provide broad coverage of chemicals and outcomes; (b) reduce the cost of time and testing; (c) use fewer laboratory animals; and (d) develop a more robust scientific basis for assessing the health effects of environmental agents. The ensuing process described in the report included chemical characterisation related to exposure pathways, toxicity testing based on characterising toxicity pathways using human-relevant biological assays followed by targeted testing and dose–response modelling and finally placing the information into appropriate human context. In response, in 2009, the EPA released a report (10) establishing a strategic plan based on the principles of the NRC report that outline a multi-year effort comprised of screening and prioritisation efforts, the incorporation of toxicity pathways in risk assessment and, importantly, institutional transition, so that necessary human capital resources for implementation would exist. One rather unanticipated result of the 2007 vision was the realisation that several government agencies (the NIEHS, the NHGRI and the EPA) working together on the strategy would greatly advance the vision, so they agreed to form the Tox21 partnership to coordinate resources and expertise (see the following section).

Momentum for implementation of the new approach gained further support as the NAS went on to issue reports on the future of exposure science (11) and on the integration of advances in exposure science and toxicity testing (12). In the latter report, the NAS highlighted priority-setting, chemical assessment, site-specific assessment and assessments of new chemicals as ripe for benefit from the application of the emerging tools of 21st century science.

5. THE EPA'S TOXCAST PROGRAM

With the establishment of the NCCT in 2005, efforts at the EPA began in earnest to implement the new toxicity testing strategies. A unique aspect of the NCCT was its initial 5-year charter, after which progress would be judged relative to a continued investment in the area. The sunset clause provided motivation for a focused effort to adopt existing biological assays used in pharmaceutical drug development (13), rather than trying to develop new methods that might be more appropriate to the study of environmental chemicals. Hence, the ToxCast (toxicity forecaster) programme was launched that took approximately 300 well-studied chemicals (virtually all food-use pesticides that had a wealth of toxicological studies available through the EPA pesticide registration programme) and tested them in wide variety of molecular screening platforms (14). This proof-of-concept programme, while pointing out the complexity of designing a research approach to implement the new strategy, provided sufficient evidence of progress to merit continued investment in computational toxicology. As a result, the programme went on to expand the chemical testing library to several thousand chemicals (15, 16). One clear result of the screening is that, unlike pharmaceutical chemicals, environmental chemicals are generally non-specific in terms of the biological pathways that are perturbed by exposure to them, making at times problematic the determination of the key toxicity pathways responsible for an adverse health outcome. While a number of limitations of this massive screening approach became evident (e.g. non-volatile, dimethyl sulphoxide-soluble chemicals only, general lack of xenobiotic metabolism), it did form the basis for pivoting the EPA endocrine disruption screening program for oestrogenic potential from a largely animal-based approach to one using a battery of *in vitro* assays (17, 18). This was the first formal adoption by the regulatory side of the EPA of the new computational toxicology tools, although they were used earlier in the emergency response to the Deep Water Horizon spill in the Gulf of Mexico to screen the proposed surfactants for biological activity (19).

6. THE TOX21 MEMORANDUM OF UNDERSTANDING

In 2008, in response to the NRC report on *Toxicity Testing in the 21st Century, a Vision and a Strategy* (9), Collins *et al.* (20) outlined a collaboration between the NIEHS/NTP, the EPA's NCCT and the NHGRI's NCGC to develop a vision and devise an implementation strategy to shift the assessment of chemical hazards from traditional experimental animal toxicology studies to target-specific, mechanism-based biological observations, largely obtained by using *in vitro* assays. The Tox21 partner agencies agreed to collaborate to: (a) research, develop, validate and translate innovative compound testing methods to characterise toxicity pathways; (b) identify compounds, assays, informatic analyses and targeted testing needed to support development of the new methods; (c) identify patterns of compound-induced biological response to characterise toxicity pathways, facilitate cross-species extrapolation and model low-dose extrapolation; (d) prioritise compounds for more-extensive toxicological evaluation; (e) develop predictive models for biological response in humans; and (f) make all the data publicly available. To support the goals of Tox21, four working groups — Compound Selection, Assays and Pathways, Informatics and Targeted Testing — were established. In mid-2010, the US Food and Drug Administration (FDA) joined the Tox21 partnership.

7. TOX21 PHASE I: PROOF OF PRINCIPLE (2005–10)

In 2005, the NTP entered into a formal relationship with the NCGC, to screen compounds for toxicologically relevant effects by using their qHTS approach. Designated as a proof-of-principle effort, the NTP provided 1408 compounds and identified several commercially available assays for consideration (e.g. Promega CellTiter Glo cell viability assay, Promega Caspase Glo 3/7, 8 and 9 assays) to evaluate assay performance, methods of assay protocol optimisation and the extent to which protocols could be varied without compromising the results. The qHTS data generated were also used to develop appropriate statistical analysis procedures to allow for the automated evaluation of thousands of qHTS concentration curves to identify active, inactive and inconclusive compounds in each assay. The first project used the CellTiter Glo cell viability assay to evaluate the extent of cytotoxicity induced in 13 cell types (9 human, 2 rat, 2 mouse; (21)). Shortly after the NTP provided the compounds, the NCCT provided a set of 1462 compounds; this library included compounds screened in ToxCast Phase I, as well as others of interest to the EPA. Ultimately, in Phase I, which ended in 2010, the NTP and/or

EPA compound sets were screened in 140 qHTS assays representing 77 predominantly cell-based reporter gene endpoints; all the data were made public via PubChem (22).

Phase I provided valuable experience in the use of qHTS approaches for the toxicity screening of environmental compounds. While this approach was promising, limitations were also identified (23). Through Small Business Innovative Research grants and contracts, research collaborations and communications with commercial assay suppliers, the development of *in vitro* assays compatible with qHTS requirements was increased. Furthermore, to advance the screening capabilities, a public nomination process for assays to be considered for inclusion was developed.

8. TOX21 PHASE II: EXPANDED COMPOUND SCREENING (2011–PRESENT)

Developing a comprehensive compound library was deemed critical to the ultimate ability of Tox21 to develop relevant prioritisation schemes and to identify patterns of toxicities for different classes of compounds. The NTP, the EPA and the NCGC all contributed about one-third each to the formation of what became known as the Tox21 10K compound library. The library was announced in December 2011 (24) and had 8193 unique compounds (25). It included multiple samples of many compounds, providing another measure of compound and assay variability. To evaluate within-run reproducibility, a set of 88 broadly bioactive compounds was included in duplicate on each 1536-well assay plate. Each qHTS assay at the NCGC (now NCATS) is screened in triplicate, with compounds in a different well location during each run, to better evaluate assay reliability and to increase the ability to distinguish between weak active and inactive compounds. To address compound identity and purity, to confirm the stock solution concentration (generally 20 mM) and to determine compound stability in dimethyl sulphoxide (DMSO) under the storage conditions used, quality control analysis of the entire library was conducted by using a tiered approach and made publicly available (26). In March 2011, the Tox21 partners dedicated a new robotics facility at the NCGC to be used for the dedicated testing of the 10K library (27).

Taking the Phase I experience and the results of a comprehensive analysis of disease-associated cellular pathways (e.g. Ref. (28)) into account, the Phase II strategy was to initially focus on measuring the induction of stress-response pathways (29) and interactions with nuclear receptors. The selection of stress-response pathway assays (e.g. apoptosis, antioxidant response, cytotoxicity, DNA damage, endoplasmic reticulum stress-response, heat shock, inflammatory response mitochondrial damage) was based on the premise that compounds that induce one or more stress-response pathways are more likely to exhibit *in vivo* toxicity than those that do not. The human nuclear receptor assays (e.g. androgen; aryl hydrocarbon; oestrogen-α; farnesoid X; glucocorticoid; liver X; peroxisome proliferator-α, -δ, and -γ; progesterone; pregnane X; retinoid X; thyroid-β; vitamin D) were selected because of the key roles they play in endocrine and metabolism pathways.

Also, a collaborative effort was initiated to evaluate the inter-individual differential sensitivities of 1086 different human lymphoblastoid cell lines representing nine human groupings to 179 toxicants by using the Promega CellTiter Glo cell viability assay to assess cytotoxicity. This study identified several genetic factors that contributed to differential sensitivity among the population (30). Importantly, the data generated in this project were used to establish a crowd sourcing challenge managed by Sage Bionetworks (31). A subsequent data challenge used Tox21 data to build models to predict toxicity assay responses based on chemical structure (32).

The limitations of Phase II included the following: chemical space limited to DMSO-soluble non-volatile compounds; biological space limited to single or at most two assays; the use of mostly transformed cell populations; the lack of xenobiotic biotransformation; only short-term exposure protocols; lack of tools to analyse and interpret 'big' data and the use of single compounds as opposed to mixtures.

9. TOX21 PHASE III: IMPROVING ON BIOLOGICAL COVERAGE AND RELEVANCE (2013–PRESENT)

To potentially overcome the Phase II limitations, in 2013 the Tox21 partners began an effort designated to improve on biological coverage and relevance. Efforts included the following:

- A focus on more physiologically relevant *in vitro* cell systems. This effort included the NTP providing libraries of ∼90 compounds to interested scientists, for *in vitro* functional endpoint testing, by using human-induced pluripotent stem cell (iPSC)-derived differentiated cell populations, with a focus on neuronal endpoints (33) and cardiomyocytes (34).
- Developing approaches for retrofitting the HTS assays with xenobiotic metabolism (35) and characterising the utility of HepaRG cells in 2-D and 3-D models (36) that incorporate xenobiotic metabolism and allow for longer-term exposure.
- The increased characterisation of the utility of alternative animal models (e.g. zebrafish, *Caenorhabditis elegans*) for toxicological evaluations (37–40).

- The development and implementation of a high throughput transcriptomics platforms for human, rat, mouse, zebrafish and *C. elegans* (41, 42).
- The increased use of computational models and virtual projects to predict metabolism/toxicity and to extrapolate from *in vitro* data to *in vivo* conditions (43–53).

10. ACCELERATING THE PACE OF CHEMICAL RISK ASSESSMENTS

To promote the adoption of what has become known as 'New Approach Methodologies' (NAMs) internationally, the EPA convened a group of regulatory scientists representing the United States, Canada, Europe, Australia and Asia to discuss desires and barriers to their use in regulatory decision-making at a workshop entitled *Accelerating the Pace of Chemical Risk Assessments (APCRA*; (54)). The participants noted that the different regulatory needs for chemical risk assessments needed individual attention. In some regulatory settings, specific testing is required for decision-making, and the use of NAMs is simply not an option. Here, legislative changes may be needed. Another significant barrier was the current practice of comparing NAM results with those from laboratory animal studies. It is improbable that NAMs will replace these laboratory animal studies at a one-to-one level, and this notion needs to be dispelled. Indeed, the use of animal tests as the gold standard needs to be reconsidered, given the increasing body of evidence from epidemiological studies that question their predictiveness and their limited coverage of significant adverse health outcomes, as well as their reliability (55). Another barrier is the lack of understanding and confidence in applying these NAMs, which requires increased engagement, coordination and education for decision-makers and the general public. The more-consistent and more-transparent characterisation of NAMs will also increase confidence and encourage their acceptance for use in a regulatory setting. A key opportunity for progress includes working together globally to increase data sharing and to do so through a shared data platform such as the OECD's eChemPortal that can be accessed and updated from multiple sources. Improved access to data and data sharing are likely to be the most imperative first steps to improving chemical risk assessment. Finally, a number of other barriers to implementation exist, including moving data acquisition on NAMs from the research laboratory to commercial facilities that can be accessed by the regulated industry, obtaining more examples of small successes to build confidence, accelerating the *in vitro* to *in vivo* extrapolation of test results to place NAM results in the proper perspective, achieving international agreement on NAM protocols, examining how NAMs can be used in the classification of hazard (an important element of many regulatory programmes), understanding the significance of negative results, demonstrating that qualitative risk assessments based on NAMs can have utility, and understanding the relative uncertainties and variabilities present in NAMs relative to traditional toxicological studies. To overcome these barriers, a number of case studies were identified in the areas of exposure evaluation, assessing data poor chemicals, comparing points of departure from NAM studies with traditional risk assessments, and analysing specific chemical classes such as the per- and polyfluorinated alkyl substances (PFAS). These efforts are now under way as evidenced by the second meeting of the APCRA that was hosted by the European Chemicals Agency in Helsinki in October 2017 (56).

11. CONCLUSIONS

One of the key promises of Tox21 and ToxCast was that all data generated by these programmes would be made publicly available and this promise continues to be kept. The ToxCast data set is freely available (57), and by the end of 2017, 159 Tox21 data sets have been posted on the EPA Dashboard (58) and in PubChem (59). These data sets, which contain in excess of 80 million data points, provide a unique community resource, both in terms of the number of compounds screened and in the diversity of assays being used for making activity calls and for relating those calls to 'truth' based on existing human and animal data. The determination of which approach is most appropriate depends on *a priori* knowledge of the assay in question, the purpose of the study and the structure of the data. These collections of data are being used to create a diagram of the biological network that responds to chemical perturbations that will be linked to toxicological effects in animals and humans (60). A PubMed search of articles published by the end of 2017 that include 'ToxCast' or 'Tox21' as keywords indicated 225 publications authored by scientists within the Tox21 community, as well as within the broader world-wide scientific community, indicating the extent to which these data are being analysed. In addition to making all the data publicly available, all the Tox21 partners have established websites to provide the scientific community with resources and tools for understanding and evaluating the assays and the resulting data (61–63).

Although good progress has been made in laying the groundwork to enable us to answer the question of whether these programmes can fulfil the expectations to transform toxicity testing, the area that requires the most work is that of targeted testing. This term encompasses designing and carrying out confirmatory assays for a given biological outcome in different (i.e. orthogonal) *in vitro* assays; incorporating engineered human tissue models; confirming a response in a whole organism such as *C. elegans*, zebrafish or rodents; and employing methods for extrapolating from *in vitro* concentration to *in vivo* dose levels. Perhaps the most important type of targeted testing that must be accomplished is to compare the output of Tox21 with what we know from existing databases of animal and human toxicology. Although predictive models of phenotypic outcomes will require considerable effort to evaluate their reliability and relevance to support regulatory action, the technologies employed in the Tox21/ToxCast programmes are actively being investigated for application to the prioritisation of chemicals in testing programmes by the EPA. For example, in the EDSP21 program (64, 65), the short-term goal is to use the technologies to prioritise chemicals for nomination for screening in the current EDSP assay battery, whereas the intermediate and long-term goals target the incorporation and ultimate replacement of the current assays with *in silico* and molecular-based high throughput assays.

We fully appreciate that the Tox21/ToxCast approaches faced some very difficult issues: 'perfect' assays do not exist, as all assays are subject to some limitations; coverage of all chemicals of interest is incomplete (e.g. volatiles); an HTS for measuring the free concentration of a compound *in vitro* is not yet available; xenobiotic metabolism is lacking in virtually all *in vitro* assays; interactions between cells are poorly captured; distinguishing between statistical and biological significance is difficult; extrapolating from *in vitro* concentration to *in vivo* dose or blood levels is not straightforward; identifying when a perturbation to a gene or pathway would lead to an adverse effect *in vivo* is difficult; and achieving routine regulatory acceptance of the developed prediction models is to be achieved at some time in the future. However, we are making progress in integrating data from diverse technologies and endpoints into what is effectively a systems biology approach to toxicology. This can only be accomplished when comprehensive knowledge is obtained with broad coverage of chemical and biological/toxicological space. The efforts described thus far reflect the initial stage of an exceedingly complicated effort, one that will likely take decades to fully achieve its goals. However, even at this stage, the information obtained has gained considerable attention and discussion by the international scientific community and, we believe, foretells the future of toxicology.

ACKNOWLEDGEMENTS

The US Tox21/ToxCast efforts are a prime example of what teams of dedicated scientists working together can accomplish. It is impossible to credit everyone who has significantly contributed to these projects, but they would never have happened without the active support of Drs John Bucher (Associate Director, NTP), Linda Birnbaum (Director, NTP and NIEHS), Paul Gilman (former head of ORD/EPA), and Francis Collins (former Director NCATS, current Director NIH). We also complement the current leadership of the Tox21 and ToxCast programmes, as they continue to evolve the science and advance the original goals.

REFERENCES

1. NTP. (2004). *Toxicology in the 21st Century: The Role of the National Toxicology Program Vision Statement and Roadmap*, 4pp. Research Triangle Park, NC, USA: NIEHS.
2. Veith, G.D. (2004). On the nature, evolution and future of quantitative structure-activity relationships (QSAR) in toxicology. *SAR and QSAR in Environmental Research* **15**, 323−330.
3. EPA. (2003). *A Framework for a Computational Toxicology Research Program*. EPA/600/R-03/065, 56pp. Washington, DC, USA: US EPA.
4. Inglese, J., Johnson, R.L., Simeonov, A., *et al.* (2007). High-throughput screening assays for the identification of chemical probes. *Nature Chemical Biology* **3**, 466−479.
5. Collins, F.S., Morgan, M. & Patrinos, A. (2003). The human genome project: Lessons from large-scale biology. *Science, New York* **300**, 286−290.
6. Austin, C.P., Brady, L.S., Insel, T.R., *et al.* (2004). NIH molecular libraries initiative. *Science, New York* **306**, 1138−1139.
7. Zerhouni, E. (2003). The NIH roadmap. *Science, New York* **302**, 63−72.
8. Inglese, J., Auld, D.S., Jadhav, A., *et al.* (2006). Quantitative high-throughput screening: A titration-based approach that efficiently identifies biological activities in large chemical libraries. *Proceedings of the National Academy of Science of the USA* **103**, 11473−11478.
9. NRC. (2007). *Toxicity Testing in the 21st Century: A Vision and a Strategy*, 216pp. Washington, DC, USA: The National Academies Press.
10. EPA. (2009). *The US Environmental Protection Agency's Strategic Plan for Evaluating the Toxicity of Chemicals*. EPA/100/K-09/001, 35pp. Washington, DC, USA: US EPA.
11. NRC. (2012). *Exposure Science in the 21st Century*, 210pp. Washington, DC, USA: The National Academies Press.
12. NRC. (2017). *Using 21st Century Science to Improve Risk-related Evaluations*, 200pp. Washington, DC, USA: The National Academies Press.
13. Houck, K.A. & Kavlock, R.J. (2008). Understanding mechanisms of toxicity: insights from drug discovery research. *Toxicology and Applied Pharmacology* **227**, 63−78.
14. Dix, D.J., Houck, K.A., Martin, M.T., *et al.* (2007). The ToxCast program for prioritizing toxicity testing of environmental chemicals. *Toxicological Sciences* **95**, 5−12.
15. Kavlock, R., Chandler, K., Houck, K., *et al.* (2012). Update on EPA's ToxCast program: Providing high throughput decision support tools for chemical risk management. *Chemical Research in Toxicology* **25**, 1287−1302.

16. Richard, A.M., Judson, R.S., Houck, K.A., *et al.* (2016). ToxCast chemical landscape: Paving the road to 21st century toxicology. *Chemical Research in Toxicology* **29**, 1225−1251.
17. Browne, P., Judson, R.S., Casey, W.M., *et al.* (2015). Screening chemicals for estrogen receptor bioactivity using a computational model. *Environmental Science and Technology* **49**, 8804−8814.
18. Browne, P., Judson, R.S., Casey, W.M., *et al.* (2017). Correction to screening chemicals for estrogen receptor bioactivity using a computational model. *Environmental Science and Technology* **51**, 9415.
19. Judson, R.S., Martin, M.T., Reif, D.M., *et al.* (2010). Analysis of eight oil spill dispersants using rapid, in vitro tests for endocrine and other biological activity. *Environmental Science and Technology* **44**, 5979−5985.
20. Collins, F.S., Gray, G.M. & Bucher, J.R. (2008). Toxicology: Transforming environmental health protection. *Science, New York* **319**, 906−907.
21. Xia, M., Huang, R., Witt, K.L., *et al.* (2008). Compound cytotoxicity profiling using quantitative high-throughput screening. *Environmental Health Perspectives* **116**, 284−291.
22. Tice, R.R., Austin, C.P., Kavlock, R.J., *et al.* (2013). Improving the human hazard characterization of chemicals: A Tox21 update. *Environmental Health Perspectives* **121**, 756−765.
23. NCATS. (2018). *High-throughput Screening Assay Guidance Criteria.* Available at https://ncats.nih.gov/preclinical/drugdev/assay.
24. NIEHS. (2011). *US Tox21 to Begin Screening 10,000 Chemicals. Press Release 7 Dec 2011.* Available at https://www.niehs.nih.gov/news/newsroom/releases/2011/december07/index.cfm.
25. EPA. (2018). *TOX21S: Tox21 Chemical Inventory for High-throughput Screening Structure-index File.* Available at https://comptox.epa.gov/dashboard/chemical_lists/tox21sl.
26. NCATS. (2018). *Chemical Browser Hosting the Tox21 10K Library Compound Structures and Annotations.* Available at https://tripod.nih.gov/tox21.
27. Attene-Ramos, M.S., Miller, N., Huang, R., *et al.* (2013). The Tox21 robotic platform for assessment of environmental chemicals − from vision to reality. *Drug Discovery Today* **1**, 716−723.
28. Gohlke, J.M., Thomas, R., Zhang, Y., *et al.* (2009). Genetic and environmental pathways to complex diseases. *BMC Systems Biology* **3**, 46.
29. Simmons, S.O., Fan, C.-Y. & Ramabhadran, R. (2009). Cellular stress response pathway system as a sentinel ensemble in toxicological screening. *Toxicological Sciences* **111**, 202−225.
30. Abdo, N., Xia, M., Brown, C.C., *et al.* (2015). Population-based in vitro hazard and concentration-response assessment of chemicals: The 1000 genomes high throughput screening study. *Environmental Health Perspectives* **123**, 458−466.
31. Eduati, F., Mangravite, L., Wang, T., *et al.* (2015). Prediction of human population responses to toxic compounds by a collaborative competition. *Nature Biotechnology* **33**, 933−940.
32. Huang, R. & Xia, M. (2017). Editorial: Tox21 challenge to build predictive models of nuclear receptor and stress response pathways as mediated by exposure to environmental toxicants and drugs. *Frontiers in Environmental Science* **5**, 3.
33. Ryan, K.R., Sirenko, O., Parham, F., *et al.* (2016). Neurite outgrowth in human induced pluripotent stem cell-derived neurons as a high throughput screen for developmental neurotoxicity. *NeuroToxicology* **53**, 271−281.
34. Sirenko, O., Grimm, F.A., Ryan, K.R., *et al.* (2017). *In vitro* cardiotoxicity assessment of environmental chemicals using an organotypic human induced pluripotent stem cell-derived model. *Toxicology and Applied Pharmacology* **322**, 60−74.
35. EPA. (2017). *Announcing the Transform Toxicity Testing Challenge Stage Two Winners.* Available at https://www.epa.gov/innovation/announcing-transform-toxicity-testing-challenge-stage-two-winners.
36. Ramaiahgari, S.C., Waidyanatha, S. & Dixon, D. (2017). Three-dimensional (3D) HepaRG spheroid model with physiologically relevant xenobiotic metabolism competence and hepatocyte functionality for liver toxicity screening. *Toxicological Sciences* **159**, 124−136.
37. Padilla, S., Corum, D., Padnos, B., *et al.* (2012). Zebrafish developmental screening of the ToxCast™ Phase I chemical library. *Reproductive Toxicology* **33**, 174−187.
38. Truong, L., Reif, D.M., St Mary, L., *et al.* (2014). Multidimensional in vivo hazard assessment using zebrafish. *Toxicological Sciences* **137**, 212−233.
39. Boyd, W.A., Smith, M.V., Co, C.A., *et al.* (2016). Developmental effects of the ToxCast™ Phase I and Phase II chemicals in *Caenorhabditis elegans* and corresponding responses in zebrafish, rats, and rabbits. *Environmental Health Perspectives* **124**, 586−593.
40. NTP. (2018). *SEAZIT: Systematic Evaluation of the Application of Zebrafish in Toxicology.* Available at https://ntp.niehs.nih.gov/go/seazit.
41. NTP. (2018). *S1500 gene set Strategy.* Available at https://ntp.niehs.nih.gov/go/S1500.
42. Shah, I., Harrill, J., Setzer, R.W., *et al.* (2018). Predicting chemical mechanisms of action using high-throughput transcriptomic data. In *Abstract, 57th Annual Meeting of the Society of Toxicology, San Antonio, March 11−15*.
43. Sipes, N.S., Martin, M.T., Reif, D.M., *et al.* (2011). Predictive models of prenatal developmental toxicity from ToxCast high-throughput screening data. *Toxicological Sciences* **124**, 109−127.
44. Martin, M.T., Knudsen, T.B., Reif, D.M., *et al.* (2011). Predictive model of rat reproductive toxicity from ToxCast high throughput screening. *Biology of Reproduction* **85**, 327−339.
45. Kleinstreuer, N.C., Reif, D.M., Sipes, N.S., *et al.* (2011). Environmental impact on vascular development predicted by high-throughput screening. *Environmental Health Perspectives* **119**, 1596−1603.
46. Sun, H., Veith, H., Xia, M., *et al.* (2012). Prediction of cytochrome P450 profiles of environmental chemicals with QSAR models built from drug-like molecules. *Molecular Informatics* **31**, 783−792.
47. Kleinstreuer, N.C., Dix, D.J., Houck, K.A., *et al.* (2013). In vitro perturbations of targets in cancer hallmark processes predict rodent chemical carcinogenesis. *Toxicological Sciences* **131**, 40−55.

48. Huang, R., Xia, M., Sakamuru, S., *et al.* (2016). Modelling the Tox21 10 K chemical profiles for *in vivo* toxicity prediction and mechanism characterization. *Nature Communications* **7**, 10425.
49. EPA. (2018). *Virtual Tissue Models: Predicting How Chemicals Impact Development.* Available at https://www.epa.gov/chemical-research/virtual-tissue-models-predicting-how-chemicals-impact-development.
50. Rotroff, D.M., Wetmore, B.A., Dix, D.J., *et al.* (2010). Incorporating human dosimetry and exposure into high-throughput in vitro toxicity screening. *Toxicological Sciences* **117**, 348–358.
51. Wetmore, B.A., Wambaugh, J.F., Ferguson, S.S., *et al.* (2013). Relative impact of incorporating pharmacokinetics on predicting in vivo hazard and mode of action from high-throughput in vitro toxicity assays. *Toxicological Sciences* **132**, 327–346.
52. Wetmore, B.A., Allen, B., Clewell, H.J., 3rd, *et al.* (2014). Incorporating population variability and susceptible subpopulations into dosimetry for high-throughput toxicity testing. *Toxicological Sciences* **142**, 210–224.
53. Wetmore, B.A., Wambaugh, J.F., Allen, B., *et al.* (2015). Incorporating high-throughput exposure predictions with dosimetry-adjusted in vitro bioactivity to inform chemical toxicity testing. *Toxicological Sciences* **148**, 121–136.
54. Kavlock, R. (2016). Practitioner insights: Bringing new methods for chemical safety into the regulatory toolbox; It is time to get serious. *BNA Daily Environment Report 223 DEN B-1*, 1–3.
55. Birnbaum, L.S., Burke, T.A. & Jones, J.J. (2016). Informing 21st-century risk assessments with 21st-century science. *Environmental Health Perspectives* **124**, A60–A63.
56. Gwinn, M.R., Bahadori, T., Rasenberg, M., *et al.* (2018). Accelerating the pace of chemical risk assessment workshop: Advancing progress in the use of new alternative methods for regulatory support. In *Abstract, 57th Annual Meeting of the Society of Toxicology, San Antonio, March 11–15.*
57. EPA. (2018). *Toxicity Forecasting: Advancing the Next Generation of Chemical Evaluation.* Available at https://www.epa.gov/chemical-research/toxicity-forecasting.
58. EPA. (2018). *ToxCast Dashboard.* Available at https://www.epa.gov/chemical-research/toxcast-dashboard.
59. PubChem. (2017). *Tox21-designated Data Sets.* Available at https://www.ncbi.nlm.nih.gov/pcassay?term=%22Tox21%22.
60. Huang, R., Grishagin, I., Wang, Y., *et al.* (2018). The NCATS BioPlanet — an integrated platform for exploring the universe of cellular signaling pathways for toxicology, systems biology, and chemical genomics. *Molecular Systems Biology* (submitted).
61. NTP. (2018). *NTP Tox21 Toolbox.* Available at https://ntp.niehs.nih.gov/results/tox21/tbox.
62. NTP. (2018). *Chemical Effects in Biological Systems (CEBS).* Available at https://www.niehs.nih.gov/research/resources/databases/cebs/index.cfm.
63. NCATS. (2018). *Toxicology in the 21st Century.* Available at https://ncats.nih.gov/tox21.
64. EPA. (2011). *Endocrine Disruptor Screening Program for the 21st Century: (EDSP21 Work Plan). The Incorporation of In Silico Models and In Vitro High Throughput Assays in the Endocrine Disruptor Screening Program (EDSP) for Prioritization and Screening. Summary Overview*, 6pp. Washington, DC, USA: US EPA.
65. EPA. (2013). *Endocrine Disruptor Screening Program (EDSP) Comprehensive Management Plans.* Available at https://www.epa.gov/endocrine-disruption/endocrine-disruptor-screening-program-edsp-comprehensive-management-plans.

Chapter 2.14

USA: Contributions From the Institute for *In Vitro* Sciences and the Animal Protection Community

Rodger D. Curren[1], Erin H. Hill[1] and Martin L. Stephens[2]

[1]*Institute for In Vitro Sciences, Gaithersburg, MD, United States;* [2]*Johns Hopkins Bloomberg School of Public Health, Baltimore, MD, United States*

SUMMARY

In the United States, non-governmental organisations have played a major role over the last 30 or more years in moving *in vitro* toxicology from modest beginnings to routine use by many companies in their internal product stewardship and development programmes, as well as in many regulatory applications. The Institute for In Vitro Sciences is an example of a non-profit, science-based organisation, whose laboratories have consistently participated in major international and US validation programmes, resulting in the acceptance of many non-animal assays by regulatory agencies. Its Education and Outreach programmes have promoted and facilitated the use of these scientifically-validated assays throughout the world. US animal protection organisations have promoted this move away from animal testing in many ways, including mobilising consumers, lobbying legislators and regulators, and supporting Three Rs efforts financially.

1. INTRODUCTION

In this chapter, we discuss the contributions of non-governmental organisations (NGOs) in the United States toward the advancement of alternative methods in toxicology. We first discuss the activities of a science-based NGO, the Institute for In Vitro Sciences (IIVS), which has played an important role in moving the field forward. Next, we will review the contributions of US animal protection NGOs, widely known for certain activities in support of the move away from animal testing, such as critiquing these methods and encouraging consumers to purchase products not tested on animals. Together, IIVS and the animal protection NGOs have effectively provided the scientific and ethical arguments that have supported the continued ascendance of *in vitro* toxicology in the USA.

2. THE INSTITUTE FOR *IN VITRO* SCIENCES

Despite the progress of *in vitro* toxicology in the 1980s and early 1990s, it was clear by the mid-1990s that the field of alternatives in the USA was still far from being an established option for toxicological safety assessments. Considerable research and educational activities seemed likely to be required before government regulators — and even many industrial toxicologists — were fully convinced that non-animal methods could provide useful information about the safety for humans of new products and ingredients. It appeared that an organisation which could devote time and effort to activities, such as teaching *in vitro* methods, holding workshops to facilitate the exchange of new research findings, and providing a forum for animal protection organisations, government and industry to safely discuss their concerns, could facilitate further progress. Thus, the idea to establish the IIVS as a non-profit organisation was conceived.

In March 1997, three principals, Erin Hill, John Harbell and Rodger Curren, established IIVS as a non-profit, charitable organisation (also known as a 501(c) (3) organisation, a reference to the relevant US tax code). The organisation's purpose, as stated in the IIVS Articles of Incorporation and approved by the US Internal Revenue Service, was as follows:

1. To prevent cruelty to animals by reducing or eliminating the use of animals in biological research and experimentation through education, training and the development, promotion and performance of non-animal research and analysis.
2. To educate, train and lecture the public sector and the private sector in the use of non-animal research and analysis, and to publish the results of non-animal research and experimentation to establish the validity and reliability of the methods of biomedical research and experimentation.
3. To lessen the burdens of government, including, without limitation, the National Institute of Health, in connection with developing methods of biomedical research and experimentation.
4. To encourage the acceptance by the scientific community of valid and reliable methods of biomedical research and experimentation.

Since that time, the mission has been codified more succinctly, as *to increase the use and acceptance of non-animal testing worldwide*.

2.1 Early Support for IIVS

The concept of a non-profit institute founded not only to help promote the idea of non-animal testing, but to also actually conduct the non-animal toxicity assays in-house, was quickly supported by both industry and animal protection organisations. Substantial financial contributions were received from Colgate-Palmolive Company, The Gillette Company, Johnson & Johnson, Kimberly-Clark Corporation and the Procter & Gamble Company (P&G), and representatives from these companies became the core of the IIVS Science Advisory Panel. These members were challenged to inform IIVS of what they felt were the important unfulfilled tasks that IIVS should address to ensure that *in vitro* toxicology tests would become acceptable alternatives to the animal tests required by the regulatory agencies. Soon afterwards, several animal protection organisations, e.g. People for the Ethical Treatment of Animals (PETA), New England Anti-Vivisection Society (NEAVS), International Foundation for Ethical Research (IFER), Doris Day Animal League (DDAL) and the Coalition for Consumer Information on Cosmetics (CCIC), made additional financial contributions that helped ensure IIVS's early success. This also signalled the beginning of closer cooperation between animal welfare and industry, with IIVS as the catalyst. A common goal of both types of organisations was the advancement of *in vitro* testing methods, and IIVS was crucial to the achievement of these goals, as it worked as an independent, unbiased entity to promote the evaluation and use of the new methods. This shared goal is expressed in the IIVS tagline, *Advancing Science and Animal Welfare Together*. Both animal protection and industry also agreed that IIVS's focus on three key concepts, namely, Science, Education and Outreach, was the way toward success.

In addition to financial support described earlier, IIVS benefited to an immense degree from scientific collaborations with the European Center for the Validation of Alternative Methods (ECVAM) and the Federal German Centre for Documentation and Evaluation of Alternative Methods to Animal Experiments (ZEBET). The relationship with ECVAM, and its Head, Professor Michael Balls, was especially important, as it allowed IIVS to participate in European alternatives activites, which were the most active and productive in the world at that time.

2.2 Science Programmes at IIVS

The IIVS Science programmes were designed to support progress through: (a) extensive use and subsequent publication of *in vitro* data for acute toxicity assays; (b) assistance to companies by developing and utilising *in vitro* assays for specific toxicological questions; and (c) participation in *in vivo/in vitro* validation exercises at the national and international levels.

2.2.1 Prevalidation and Validation Studies

From the outset, scientists at IIVS understood that prevalidation (1) and validation (2) endeavours would be key components of the scientific information that would lead regulatory bodies to the acceptance of non-animal toxicological test methods for safety evaluations. Thus, a major portion of the IIVS scientific strategy was organisation and participation in multi-laboratory prevalidation and validation studies which were conducted in collaboration with the ECVAM, ZEBET, the US National Toxicology Program Interagency Center for the Evaluation of Alternative Toxicological Methods (NICEATM) and various industry or trade association partners. This included studies on *in vitro* cytotoxicity tests for acute toxicity, including the 3T3 and NHEK tests (3); the EpiOcular, Bovine Cornea Opacity and Permeability (BCOP) and Cytosensor Microphysiometer test methods for eye irritancy (4, 5); an *in vitro* ocular testing strategy for the EPA Office of Pesticide Programs assessment of anti-microbial cleaning products (6); the EpiDerm test and optimised methods for skin irritation (7, 8); the Corrositex test for skin corrosion (9); the KeratinoSens and LuSens assays for skin sensitisation; and the Embryonic Stem Cell test for embryotoxicity.

In alignment with its demand for high scientific standards in the organisation and conduct of major validation studies (10–12), IIVS was an early and strong voice for the application of Good Laboratory Practices (GLPs) in *in vitro* studies, especially in large-scale validation studies. In 1998, IIVS and ECVAM co-organised a workshop entitled *The Principles of Good Laboratory Practice: Application to In Vitro Toxicology Studies* (13), which laid out a new way forward for the conduct of *in vitro* toxicology studies. Prior to this ground-breaking meeting, it was generally thought that imposing GLP standards on *in vitro* validation studies would be impossible. However, after careful examination of how GLPs (originally designed to apply specifically to animal studies) could be intelligently applied to *in vitro* studies, the participants at the workshop agreed on recommendations that would positively, and continuously, affect the future progress of the *in vitro* toxicology field.

2.2.2 Collaborations Led to Some 'Firsts' for IIVS

Some of IIVS' earliest efforts in optimising *in vitro* toxicology assays were were with the BCOP assay (14), in which test materials are applied directly to the corneas of cow eyes obtained from abattoirs. However, as the BCOP assay could possibly be considered an animal test, because animal tissue was used, although it was from normally discarded material whose collection did not involve additional pain or suffering, a number of companies hesitated to use the assay, fearing reprisals from the animal protection community. To resolve this issue, IIVS scientists went directly to PETA to explain the situation and to determine whether PETA would oppose this use of normally discarded animal material. After cordial and detailed discussions, PETA published a letter stating that *PETA accepts the BCOP test as an interim test for measuring eye irritation until sufficient non-animal models are developed and validated*. After this assurance, many companies proceeded to adopt the BCOP methodology, thereby eliminating their dependence on the animal eye irritation test. This was one of the first examples in which IIVS, animal protection and industry worked together to progress the use of *in vitro* toxicology models and the subsequent elimination of suffering for many laboratory animals.

Collaborations with various industrial companies have helped IIVS to develop and evaluate new methods for eye irritation that benefit companies around the world. For example, P&G transferred to IIVS, for further use and evaluation, a methodology – developed in P&G laboratories – involving the use of the Silicon Microphysiometer (15) to predict eye irritation (16). The results obtained using the instrument were quite encouraging, and IIVS was asked to write a detailed Background Review Document (BRD) on its performance for ECVAM. After review of the BRD (5), the ECVAM Scientific Advisory Committee (ESAC) stated that the Silicon Microphysiometer (now called Cytosensor (17)) was capable of accurately determining the non-irritating effects of certain classes of chemicals, without the use of additional animal tests (6). Thus a test developed by the industry, and with the assistance of IIVS, became the first non-animal test to be certified as a stand-alone method for the identification of non-eye irritants within defined chemical classes.

A further example of the working together of industry, animal protection and IIVS to obtain success with *in vitro* methods is the approach that led to a non-animal testing strategy for eye irritation to register anti-microbial cleaning products (AMCPs) with the US Environmental Protection Agency (EPA). AMCPs are an interesting class of products that consist of household and industrial cleaners that make the claim that they are anti-microbial (i.e. they kill bacteria and viruses). Most of these products have been safely used for many years, without the anti-microbial claim and animal testing. However, once the anti-microbial claim was made, by US law the products become classified as pesticides and were subject to the EPA's animal testing requirements before they could be registered. In 2003, representatives of animal protection sitting on the EPA's Pesticide Program Dialog Committee suggested that the agency should allow these products to be registered without additional animal tests because of their history of safe use. The EPA agreed that this could be considered, and IIVS organised a consortium of AMCP manufactures and a consulting group (The Accord Group, Washington, DC) to provide evidence that the *in vitro* tests being used by the manufacturers were adequate. Seven companies, namely, The Clorox Company, Colgate-Palmolive, The Dial Corporation, EcoLabs, JohnsonDiversey, Inc., S.C. Johnson & Son and P&G, shared their existing data and contributed to the production of new data (without conducting new animal tests), which IIVS used to create a BRD outlining a non-animal eye irritation testing strategy. After review of the data package, the EPA issued an interim policy allowing the use of this non-animal approach for the registration of AMCPs. Review of the registration submissions submitted under the interim policy led to a permanent policy in 2015 (7), the first non-animal approach to a registration requirement that had been accepted by the EPA.

Collaborations have also led to the development of *in vitro* toxicology assays that assist industry in making safety decisions for new products in situations where the traditional animal testing approach is prohibited by law. Such is the case where the European Cosmetics Legislation (*Regulation (EC) No 1223/2009 of the European Parliament and of the Council of 30 November 2009 on cosmetic products*) prohibits the conduct of an animal test for genotoxicity. This is problematic, because the existing *in vitro* genotoxicity assays are known to be highly over-predictive (18). To address this problem, P&G asked IIVS to use its expertise with 3-D human tissue models to develop a genetic toxicology assay involving reconstructed human skin (EpiDerm, MatTek Corporation, Ashland, MA). IIVS successfully developed the assay (19), then transferred the protocol to P&G scientists and other laboratories. Subsequently, Cosmetics Europe, the European trade association for the personal care and cosmetics industry, financed a multi-year, multi-laboratory, validation programme (20), which has culminated in the Reconstructed Skin Micronucleus (RSMN) Assay, now, in 2018, being proposed for regulatory acceptance. The RSMN is the first *in vitro* assay developed specifically to meet the animal testing prohibitions of the EU Cosmetics Directive for a genetic toxicology endpoint.

2.2.3 The Co-founding of a Scientific Society

For several years, IIVS scientists recognised that Europe led the way in having scientific societies specifically dedicated to *in vitro* toxicology. The USA had none, so, in 2010, IIVS's current president, Erin Hill, in conjunction with Kristie Sullivan from Physician's Committee for Responsible Medicine (PCRM), founded the American Society for Cellular and Computational Toxicology (ASCCT). Over the last eight years, ASCCT has grown to having nearly 300 members. These numbers reflect the impressive growth of *in vitro* toxicology in the USA over the same period, and fully justify the investments that IIVS has made to promote *in vitro* alternatives.

2.3 Educational and Outreach Programmes at IIVS

Education and Outreach initiatives transform IIVS's technical expertise with *in vitro* methods into increased use and acceptance by industry and regulatory agencies. In the 1990s, many scientists from industry and government had a limited understanding of what *in vitro* methods existed and their use in making safety determinations. To bring this information to a wide audience, IIVS created the *Practical Methods for In Vitro Toxicology* hands-on training course (now in its 21st year). The programme is a combination of lecture and laboratory exercises and has been attended by many scientists from US industry, government, animal protection organisations and contract laboratories. Also, more than 250 students from more than a dozen other countries have been trained.

Because the Practical Methods course was consistently oversubscribed, IIVS began to offer smaller, specialised laboratory courses throughout the year, and in addition, developed an international programme to provide instruction on-site at government and academic laboratories. To date, nearly 1000 scientists have attended these trainings at multiple locations worldwide. IIVS's success in this area was acknowledged in 2014, in co-sharing the first Lush prize for training, specifically *for their vital work on training researchers in non-animal methods from Brazil to Japan* (21).

Around the world, non-animal test methods accepted by regulatory agencies are almost always optional, rather than required. Thus, many companies still perform the animal test when given the option. When queried as to why a company would choose the animal model instead of an accepted *in vitro* method, the answer is often twofold, as follows: (a) the time to approve a safety dossier with non-animal data takes longer than one containing animal data; and (b) if the company has to conduct the animal test to register in at least one country, it is more efficient and cost-effective to submit the same data to all the agencies concerned.

To overcome the first hurdle, IIVS provides training directly to reviewers within regulatory agencies, not only in the USA, but also in Europe, Brazil, China, Russia and Vietnam. Knowledge of the biological basis of the method, combined with in-depth data analysis, equips regulators with the information they need to confidently and efficiently make decisions based on the submitted *in vitro* data. The second hurdle highlights the detrimental result of lack of international harmonisation. In response to this, IIVS focuses training in countries such as China, where animal testing is required for the registration and post-market surveillance of cosmetics (22). In 2014, IIVS signed a Memorandum of Understanding, revised and expanded in 2017, with the China Food and Drug Administration (CFDA), to assist them in adopting non-animal tests for the registration of cosmetics. A key component of this agreement is in-depth hands-on training for provincial regulators. This training not only results in proficient laboratories, but also builds capacity for the CFDA to conduct testing — a stated requirement by Chinese regulators. An early indicator of the success of this collaborative effort is the 2016 announcement of acceptance of data for the *in vitro* 3T3 Neutral Red Uptake Phototoxicity Assay by the CFDA.

2.4 Conclusions

During the last 20 years, considerable progress has been made in the uptake of non-animal safety testing methods for both corporate product stewardship and for regulatory use. IIVS has played a critical role in this transition, due to its science programmes, coupled with education and outreach. Collaborations among regulators, industry and animal protection groups have been an important driver of change, and it is hoped that further international collaborations will succeed in harmonising the use of non-animal testing methods throughout the world.

3. US ANIMAL PROTECTION ORGANISATIONS

In this section, we discuss the contributions that animal protection organisations based in the USA have made to advancing non-animal methods in toxicology. Although many of these organisations are active internationally as well as domestically, we focus primarily on efforts within the USA itself. Our discussion is focused on the different types of relevant activities carried out by these organisations (lobbying, funding, etc.) rather than on the individual organisations themselves. Where we mention particular animal groups or staff members, these are intended to serve as examples. Our overarching theme is that the US-based animal protection community has made significant and diverse contributions to advancing alternative methods and approaches within toxicity testing.

3.1 Criticising Animal Testing

Animal-based toxicity tests were prime targets for animal protection organisations throughout the second half of the twentieth century. The Draize Eye Irritancy Test, the LD50 Test and others were easily depicted as crude, cruel and increasingly out of step with the scientific advances of the post-World War II era. They were especially vulnerable to criticism when applied to cosmetics, where the costs to the animals seemed disproportionate to the benefits to consumers.

By the late 1970s, it became commonplace for animal groups to have public education materials criticising these testing practices. However, by itself, the distribution of these materials did not pose a major threat to the *status quo*. Then, in 1980, came what arguably remains the best example of animal protection organisations' criticism of then-current practices in toxicity testing. Henry Spira of Animal Rights International (ARI) took out a full-page advertisement in the *New York Times* on behalf of a coalition of hundreds of animal protection organisations, including the Humane Society of the United States (HSUS), the American Society for the Prevention of Cruelty to Animals (ASPCA), the Massachusetts SPCA and the Animal Cruelty Society in Chicago. The advertisements' headline-like text asked *How many rabbits does Revlon blind for beauty's sake?* and was accompanied by an image of a rabbit in a laboratory setting. As a result of subsequent negotiations, Revlon funded research at Rockefeller University to seek an alternative to the Draize test, and the cosmetics industry trade association funded the establishment of the Center for Alternatives to Animal Testing (CAAT) at Johns Hopkins University, in Baltimore (23).

Animal protection critiques that drew on the scientific literature, such as Weil and Scala's report on the irreproducibility of the Draize eye and skin irritation tests (24), and Zbinden and Flury-Roversi's report on the LD50 Test (25), showed the scientific vulnerabilities of these tests and added to the sense of urgency for their replacement.

3.2 Encouraging Consumer Action

Although toxicity tests are used widely across industries, the cosmetics industry has been particularly vulnerable to criticism on humane grounds, as Spira's campaign showed. Animal protection organisations took advantage of this vulnerability by encouraging consumers to boycott cosmetics companies that tested their products on animals and to patronise companies that avoided this practice. A small but increasing number of cosmetics companies began marketing 'cruelty-free' products. However, it was not always clear what this and similar designations actually meant in practice. In 1996, several animal groups formed the CCIC to standardise the definition of 'not tested on animals' to encourage progressive cosmetics companies to adhere to this definition and to encourage consumers to patronise those companies. More than 800 companies are currently on the CCIC list, some of which have negotiated with the CCIC to use the Leaping Bunny logo on their products to flag their participation in the programme.

3.3 Funding Alternatives Research and Development

Funding research on alternative methods is an obvious means of facilitating progress in limiting the use and suffering of animals in testing. Some animal protection organisations, including PETA, have provided targeted funding for alternatives to animal testing, mostly for research, but also for validation studies, equipment, workshops, training for regulators, and support to the general efforts of alternatives centres. Some other animal groups established affiliated organisations dedicated to funding and otherwise promoting alternative methods. In 1985, NEAVS launched the IFER, now associated with the National Anti-Vivisection Society (NAVS), to fund non-animal research, and in 1989, the American Anti-Vivisection Society (AAVS) created what is now named the Alternatives Research and Development Foundation (ARDF), which provides similar funding (26).

3.4 Honouring Individual Scientists

Several animal protection organizations in the USA and elsewhere have established awards for scientists who have made outstanding contributions to advancing alternative methods. For example, at each *World Congress on Alternatives and Animal Use in the Life Sciences*, the HSUS bestows the Russell and Burch Award. Similarly, ARDF confers The William & Eleanor Cave Award to honour achievements in advancing alternatives to the traditional use of animals in testing, research or education. This award is now presented biennially at the annual ASCCT meeting. Such awards, both of which include honoraria, are intended to recognise scientists for their contributions, encourage other scientists to make similar efforts and demonstrate the awarding organisation's commitment to alternative methods.

3.5 Lobbying for Government Action

Lobbying government officials has been a key activity of many US-based animal protection organisations. These groups can mobilise their members to contact their elected representatives in local, state and federal governments, and can also hire in-house lobbyists to advance their cause directly with Government officials. While legislative advances often result from the interplay of various factors, it is clear that animal groups have made significant contributions within the animal testing arena. For example, lobbying by animal protection organisations (e.g. Humane Society Legislative Fund (HSLF), PCRM and others) was critical to the passage of the 2000 *ICCVAM Authorization Act* and the 2016 *Frank R. Lautenberg Chemical Safety for the 21st Century Act* (27), both of which advanced alternatives to animal testing. In practice, when animal protectionists and other stakeholders (e.g. industry) are advocating for the same legislation, the case for its adoption is strengthened.

Lobbying can also take other forms. For example, in 1998, the EPA launched the High Production Volume (HPV) Challenge Program, which called upon the industry to voluntarily make available existing or newly-generated toxicity data for chemicals produced in high volume. This raised the spectre of a massive amount of new animal testing. PETA, along with several other animal protection organisations, successfully worked to secure alternative-friendly provisions in the programme (27).

3.6 Influencing from within — Participating in Influential Scientific Bodies

In the USA, animal groups on the one hand and corporations and federal agencies on the other initially regarded each other with some suspicion and ill will. This antagonism diminished over time. One consequence of this was that representatives from animal protection organisations began to be invited to join influential multi-stakeholder forums that already included representatives from other sectors, such as industry and academia. Perhaps the biggest breakthrough in this regard came in 2002 at the OECD, which runs a highly influential programme that issues consensus test guidelines accepted by all its Member Countries. Animal welfare groups noted that environmental and business representatives participated in the OECD's test guideline meetings as formally recognised advisory bodies. They approached the OECD to see if they could participate as well, and were advised to form a coalition and apply. Several animal protection organisations from the USA, the EU and Asia formed such a group, which was then permitted to attend the relevant meetings. The resulting group, the International Council on Animal Protection in OECD Programmes (ICAPO) has been a voice for alternative-friendly practices within the OECD's Test Guidelines Programme and related activities.

Another example of 'influencing from within' concerns the US National Academies of Science (NAS), to which the federal government turns for advice on key scientific issues. The advice is given via reports from committees appointed and hosted by the NAS but whose members are drawn mostly from outside institutions, especially universities. In 2003, the EPA asked the NAS to prepare a report on the future of toxicity testing. Among the individuals appointed to the committee was Martin Stephens, a scientist then at the HSUS, an appointment that would have been highly unlikely a decade or two earlier, and a reflection of the current positive role that animal protection scientists play in advancing *in vitro* toxicology. This was the committee that went on to write the highly influential report, *Toxicity Testing in the 21st Century, A Vision and a Strategy* (29).

3.7 Participating in Joint Efforts with Other Stakeholders

Over time, US-based animal groups increasingly partnered with progressive individuals and entities in government, industry and academia to advance alternative testing methods. The example of the co-founding of the ASCCT by PCRM and IIVS has already been mentioned. Other examples of these joint efforts include the cofounding of the AltTox website (http://alttox.org) by the HSUS and P&G, and the organisation and funding of the triennial *World Congresses on Alternatives and Animal Use in the Life Sciences* by multiple animal groups and other stakeholders.

3.8 Making the Case to Scientists

By the early 1980s, companies marketing cosmetics and other consumer products realised that they needed to do something in response to pressure from campaigners and consumers concerned about animal testing. Some companies may have been willing to simply cease animal testing, full stop, but most of the others wanted some other way to address product safety. Animal groups helped make the case that the Three Rs approach, especially *Replacement*, was the way forward. They succeeded, in part, because of their own scientists, who quietly made the case to fellow scientists in industry, government and academia. Animal protection scientists did this through presentations and writings, and involvement in multi-stakeholder activities, as well as in simple face-to-face interactions that helped to erode some of the antagonism that each side had for the other. Andrew Rowan of the HSUS (and formerly of FRAME and Tufts University) was a pioneer in this regard.

3.9 Other Three Rs-Related Activities

In addition to the activities mentioned earlier, US-based animal protection organisations have also advanced alternative testing methods and approaches in other ways, some more subtle and indirect than others. A few of these contributions will serve as examples.

The Animal Welfare Institute (AWI) helped finance the distribution in the USA of Russell and Burch's seminal book on the Three Rs (30), following its publication in the UK in 1959. AWI also was involved in organising and contributing to the publication (in 1977) of the first 'establishment' book in the USA to discuss 'alternatives' — the National Research Council's *The Future of Animals, Cells, Models and Systems in Research, Development, Education and Testing* (31).

Throughout the 1960s, 1970s and 1980s, William Russell and Rex Burch, the originators of the Three Rs concept, were regarded as historical figures. After the publication of their 1959 book, they moved on to other pursuits and were unaware of developments in the very field they had inspired. By 1990, prominent leaders in the alternatives community did not know whether or not Russell or Burch were still living. It was that year that the HSUS was able to locate them, with help from the Universities Federation for Animal Welfare (UFAW), which had sponsored the work that resulted in the 1959 book. HSUS was seeking Russell and Burch's approval to name the organisation's alternatives award in their honour. They agreed and were reunited with each other in 1993 for the first time since the publication of their book, at a meeting with an HSUS representative (facilitated by UFAW). Russell (32) went on to be an inspiring presence at the first three *World Congresses on Alternatives and Animal Use in the Life Sciences* (and other venues), as well as being a thoughtful commentator on the alternatives field.

3.10 Conclusions

Our activity-focused approach serves to illustrate the diverse ways that the US-based animal protection organisations have advanced alternative testing methods. Those seeking a fuller understanding of the contributions of particular groups should consult the websites of those organisations.

We believe that, in the USA, the animal protection community has been a major driving force in the uptake and application of the Three Rs approach to animal testing. The approach operationalised an ethic of caring and of limiting both the suffering and numbers of animals used in testing, all within a readily useable and understood framework for change. Animal protection organisations pushed the envelope by making animal testing a public issue and giving consumers a role to play in advancing change. Through lobbying, funding and other activities, these groups promoted the Russell and Burch framework (especially *Replacement*), elevating what had been a rather obscure approach and putting it on a firmer foundation.

Animal groups marshalled scientific criticism of the *status quo* and highlighted the power of non-animal approaches. In doing so, they helped usher in the era of 21st century toxicology, with its emphasis on the development of human relevant, *in vitro* and computational approaches, often automated via high-throughput, robotics-assisted platforms. The 2007 NRC report on 21st century toxicology (29) *envisions a not-so-distant future in which virtually all routine toxicity testing would be conducted in human cells or cell lines* in vitro … *using high-throughput tests…* (33). That this transition from animal tests to *in vitro* tests is well under way is remarkable from a number of perspectives, not least of which is that the animal protection community has helped lay the foundation for major change in an animal-based enterprise that involves mostly rats and mice. To be sure, dogs, rabbits, non-human primates and a few other species that more-readily evoke public sympathy are used in testing, but not nearly in the numbers at which rodents are used.

ACKNOWLEDGEMENTS

The authors would like to thank Drs Jonathan Balcombe, Paul Locke, Andrew Rowan, Kenneth Shapiro, Bernard Unti, and Quanshun Zhang, for their assistance in the preparation of this chapter.

REFERENCES

1. Curren, R., Southee, J., Spielmann, H., *et al.* (1995). The role of prevalidation in the development, validation and acceptance of alternative methods. *ATLA* **23**, 211−217.
2. Goldberg, A.M., Frazier, J.M., Brusick, D., *et al.* (1993). Framework for validation and implementation of *in vitro* toxicity tests: Report of the Validation and Technology Transfer Committee of the Johns Hopkins Center for Alternatives to Animal Testing. *In Vitro Toxicology* **6**, 47−55.
3. Prieto, P., Cole, T., Curren, R., *et al.* (2013). Assessment of the predictive capacity of the 3T3 Neutral Red Uptake cytotoxicity test method to identify substances not classified for acute oral toxicity (LD50>2000 mg/kg): Results of an ECVAM validation study. *Regulatory Toxicology and Pharmacology* **65**, 344−365.
4. Curren, R.D., Sizemore, A., Nash, J., *et al.* (2008). *Background Review Document of Existing Methods for Eye Irritation Testing: Silicon Microphysiometer and Cytosensor Microphysiometer.* External report to ECVAM, Contract No. CCR.IHCP.C431305.X, 212pp. Ispra, Italy: EC Joint Research Centre.
5. Kreysa, J. (2009). *Statement on the Scientific Validity Of Cytotoxicity/Cell Function Based In vitro Assays for Eye Irritation Testing*, 6pp. Ispra, Italy: EC Joint Research Centre.
6. EPA. (2015). *Use of an Alternative Testing Framework for Classification of Eye Irritation Potential of EPA Pesticide Products*, 39pp. Washington, DC, USA: EPA Office of Pesticide Programs.
7. Spielmann, H., Hoffmann, S., Liebsch, M., *et al.* (2007). The ECVAM international validation study on *in vitro* tests for acute skin irritation: Report on the validity of the EPISKIN and EpiDerm assays and on the Skin Integrity Function Test. *ATLA* **35**, 559−601.
8. Zuang, V., Balls, M., Botham, P.A., *et al.* (2002). Follow-up to the ECVAM prevalidation study on *in vitro* tests for acute skin irritation. ECVAM Skin Irritation Task Force Report 2. *ATLA* **30**, 109−129.
9. Fentem, J.H., Archer, G.E., Balls, M., *et al.* (1998). The ECVAM international validation study on *in vitro* tests for skin corrosivity. 2. Results and evaluation by the management team. *Toxicology in Vitro* **12**, 483−524.
10. Bruner, L., Carr, G., Chamberlain, M., *et al.* (1996). No prediction model, no validation study. *ATLA* **24**, 139−142.
11. Bruner, L.H., Carr, G.J., Curren, R.D., *et al.* (1998). Validation of alternative methods for toxicity testing. *Environmental Health Perspectives* **106**(Suppl. 2), 477−484.
12. Curren, R., Bruner, L., Goldberg, A., *et al.* (1998). Validation and acute toxicity testing 13th meeting of the Scientific Group on Methodologies for the Safety Evaluation of Chemicals (SGOMSEC). *Environmental Health Perspectives* **106**(Suppl. 2), 419−425.
13. Cooper-Hannan, R., Harbell, J.W., Coecke, S., *et al.* (1999). The principles of Good Laboratory Practice: Application to *in vitro* toxicology studies. *ATLA* **27**, 539−577.
14. Gautheron, P., Dukic, M., Alix, D., *et al.* (1992). Bovine corneal opacity and permeability test: an *In vitro* assay of ocular irritancy. *Fundamental and Applied Toxicology* **18**, 442−449.
15. McConnell, H.M., Owicki, J.C., Parce, J.W., *et al.* (1992). The cytosensor microphysiometer: biological applications of silicon technology. *Science, New York* **257**, 1906−1912.
16. Bruner, L.H., Miller, K.R., Owicki, J.C., *et al.* (1991). Testing ocular irritancy *in vitro* with the silicon microphysiometer. *Toxicology in Vitro* **5**, 277−284.
17. Nash, J.R., Mun, G., Raabe, H.A., *et al.* (2014). Using the cytosensor microphysiometer to assess ocular toxicity. *Current Protocols in Toxicology* **61**, 1.13.1−1.13.11.
18. Kirkland, D., Aardema, M., Muller, L., *et al.* (2006). Evaluation of the ability of a battery of three *in vitro* genotoxicity tests to discriminate rodent carcinogens and non-carcinogens. II. Further analysis of mammalian cell results, relative predictivity and tumour profiles. *Mutation Research* **608**, 29−42.
19. Curren, R.D., Mun, G., Gibson, D.P., *et al.* (2006). Development of a method for assessing micronucleus induction in a 3D human skin model (EpiDerm). *Mutation Research* **607**, 19−204.

20. Pfuhler, S., Fautz, R., Ouedraogo, G., *et al.* (2014). The Cosmetics Europe strategy for animal-free genotoxicity testing: project status up-date. *Toxicology in Vitro* **28**, 18–23.

21. Anon. (2013). 2012 Lush training prize winner: The Institute for *In Vitro* Sciences (IIVS), USA. *ATLA* **41**, 513–514.

22. Curren, R. & Jones, B. (2012). China is taking steps toward alternatives to animal testing. *ATLA* **40**, 1–2.

23. Rowan, A.N. (1984). *Of Mice, Models, and Men*, 323pp. Albany, NY, USA: SUNY Press.

24. Weil, C.S. & Scala, R.A. (1971). Study of intra- and interlaboratory variability in the results of rabbit eye and skin irritation tests. *Toxicology and Applied Pharmacology* **19**, 276–360.

25. Zbinden, G. & Flury-Rovers, M. (1981). Significance of the LD50-test for the toxicological evaluation of chemical substances. *Archives of Toxicology* **47**, 77–99.

26. Stephens, M. & Mak, N. (2013). History of the 3Rs in Toxicity Testing: From Russell and Burch to 21st Century Toxicology. In D.G. Allen, & M.D. Waters (Eds.), *Reducing, Refining and Replacing the Use of Animals in Toxicity Testing* **19**(1) 1–43. London, UK: Royal Society of Chemistry.

27. US Congress. (2016). *Frank R. Lautenberg Chemical Safety for the 21st Century Act.* Public Law 114 182 June 22, 2016, 67pp. Washington, DC, USA: US Congress.

28. Bishop, P.L., Manuppello, J.R., Willett, C.E., *et al.* (2012). Animal use and lessons learned in the U.S. High Production Volume Chemicals Challenge Program. *Environmental Health Perspectives* **120**, 1631–1639.

29. NRC. (2007). *Toxicity Testing in the 21st Century: A Vision and a Strategy*, 216pp. Washington, DC, USA: The National Academies Press.

30. Russell, W.M.S. & Burch, R.L. (1959). *The Principles of Humane Experimental Technique*, 238pp. London, UK: Methuen.

31. NRC. (1977). *The Future of Animals, Cells Models, and Systems in Research Development Education and Testing*, 351pp. Washington, DC, USA: National Academy of Sciences.

32. Stephens, M.L. (2006). Remembering William Russell. *ATLA* **34**, 474–476.

33. Andersen, M.E. & Krewski, D. (2009). Toxicity testing in the 21st century: Bringing the vision to life. *Toxicological Sciences* **107**, 324–330.

Chapter 2.15

Involvement of the Organisation for Economic Cooperation and Development

Michael Balls[1], Andrew P. Worth[2] and Robert D. Combes[3]

[1]University of Nottingham, Nottingham, United Kingdom; [2]Joint Research Centre, European Commission, Ispra, Italy; [3]Independent Consultant, Norwich, United Kingdom

SUMMARY

In the early 1980s, the Organisation for Economic Cooperation and Development (OECD) began to publish test guidelines (TGs) on how *in vivo* toxicity tests should be conducted in laboratory animals, although where and when such TGs should be applied was the responsibility of national and regional regulatory authorities. The first TGs for non-animal tests involved *in vitro* methods for genotoxicity, but, by the mid-1990s, alternative tests for other types of toxicity began to be validated and proposed for regulatory acceptance. The OECD published guidance on the development of TGs and on the validation and acceptance of new or updated methods for hazard assessment, and by the mid-1990s, TGs for validated individual non-animal tests began to be published. Later, guidance was published on the development, validation and acceptance of Quantitative Structure—Activity Relationship models and integrated testing strategies.

1. EARLY DAYS

The international harmonisation of regulatory toxicity testing originated in the early 1980s, to avoid the costs of duplicative testing and to facilitate international trade in chemicals. Given the importance of these goals, it was inevitable that the Organisation for Economic Cooperation and Development (OECD) would come to play an essential and pivotal role in the acceptance and application of test methods. This was achieved by introducing the OECD *Guidelines for the Testing of Chemicals* in 1981 (Table 1-A (T1-A)), which, alongside the Principles of Good Laboratory Practice, were intended to promote the mutual acceptance of test data in regulatory toxicology (T1-B).

However, it took time for this to happen, not least because the OECD had to work by consensus among the National Coordinators of the Test Guidelines (TGs) Programme, as the representatives of the organisation's Member Countries. It was clear that many regulatory toxicologists were content to rely on the animal TGs, and even as late as the *2nd World Congress on Alternatives and Animal Use in the Life Sciences* (Utrecht, 1996), a regulator from the US FDA said that there were 'few incentives … to use scientific data from an alternative method in support of the safety substantiation for a new product', and that 'government scientists have a low comfort level with new methods, due to uncertainty about the incorporation of new data vs traditional standards' (1).

Against this background, it was academic scientists and animal welfare organisations, together with a few industry and government scientists, who recognised that the barriers to the acceptance and use of alternative methods could only be overcome if it could be shown that the data they provided were at least as reliable and relevant as those produced by the 'traditional' methods.

TABLE 1 Organisation for Economic Cooperation and Development (OECD) Documents

A	Guidelines for the Testing of Chemicals (1981).
B	Decision of the Council Concerning the Mutual Acceptance of Data in the Assessment of Chemicals (1981). C(81)30/FINAL.
C	Draft Record of the Second Meeting of National Co-ordinators of the Test Guidelines Programme, Environment Directorate (1991). ENV/MC/CHEM/TG/M(91)1, 13pp. Record available only via the OECD archives.
D	Guidance Document for the Development of OECD Guidelines for Testing Chemicals (1993). Re-published in 1995 as OECD Environment Monograph 76, 27pp. Revised and Re-published in 2006 as Series on Testing and Assessment No. 1, 33pp.
E	Final Report of the OECD Workshop on Harmonization of Validation and Acceptance Criteria for Alternative Toxicological Test Methods (1996). ENV/MC/CHEM/TG(96)9, 46pp.
F	Draft Guidance Document on the Development, Validation and Regulatory Acceptance of New and Updated Internationally Acceptable Test Methods in Hazard Assessment (2001). OECD Environment, Health and Safety Publications Series on Testing and Assessment, No. 34, 43pp.
G	Report of the OECD Conference on Validation and Regulatory Acceptance of New and Updated Methods in Hazard Assessment, held in Stockholm, Sweden, on 6–8 March 2002. ENV/JM/TG/M(2002)2/ADD1.
H	Guidance Document on the Validation and International Acceptance of New or Updated Test Methods for Hazard Assessment (2005). OECD Environment, Health and Safety Publications Series on Testing and Assessment No. 34, 67pp.
I	US EPA/EC Joint Project on the Evaluation of (Quantitative) Structure Activity Relationships (1994). OECD Environment Monograph No. 88, GD(94)28, 81pp.
J	Report of the OECD Workshop on Quantitative Structure Activity Relationships (QSARS) in Aquatic Effects Assessment (1992). OECD Environment Monograph No. 58, GD(92)168, 100 pp.
K	Guidance Document for Aquatic Effects Assessment (1995). OECD Environment Monograph No. 92, GD(95)18, 118 pp. ENV/MC/CHEM/TG.
L	Application of Structure-Activity Relationships to the Estimation of Properties Important in Exposure Assessment (1993). OECD Environment Monograph No. 67, GD(93)125, 67 pp.
M	Structure-Activity Relationships for Biodegradation (1993). OECD Environment Monograph No. 68, GD(93)126, 105pp.
N	Report from the Expert Group on (Q)SARs on the validation of (Q)SARs (2004). Series on Testing and Assessment No. 49. ENV/JM/MONO(2004)24, 154pp.
O	Guidance Document on the Validation of (Quantitative) Structure-Activity Relationships [(Q)SAR] Models (2007). Series on Testing and Assessment No. 69. ENV/JM/MONO(2007)2, 154pp.
P	Guidance Document on the Reporting of Defined Approaches to be Used within Integrated Approaches to Testing and Assessment (2016). Series on Testing and Assessment No. 255. ENV/JM/MONO(2016)28, 23pp.
Q	Report on the Regulatory Uses and Applications in OECD Member Countries of (Quantitative) Structure-Activity Relationship [(Q)SAR] models in the Assessment of New and Existing Chemicals, 2007. ENV/JM/MONO(2006)25, 79pp.
R	Guidance Document for the Use of Adverse Outcome Pathways in Developing Integrated Approaches to Testing and Assessment (IATA) (2016). Series on Testing and Assessment No. 260. ENV/JM/MONO(2016)67, 25pp.
S	Report on Considerations from Case Studies on Integrated Approaches for Testing and Assessment (IATA). First Review Cycle (2015). Case Studies on Grouping Methods as a Part of IATA. Series on Testing and Assessment No. 250. ENV/JM/MONO(2016)48, 29pp.
T	Guidance Document on Integrated Approaches to Testing and Assessment for Skin Irritation and Corrosion (2014). Series on Testing and Assessment No. 203. ENV/JM/MONO(2014)19, 64pp.
U	Guidance Document on an Integrated Approach on Testing and Assessment (IATA) for Serious Eye Damage and Eye Irritation (2017). Series on Testing and Assessment No. 263. ENV/JM/MONO(2017)15, 90pp.
V	The Adverse Outcome Pathway for Skin Sensitisation Initiated by Covalent Binding to Proteins Part 1: Scientific Evidence (2012). Series on Testing and Assessment No. 168. ENV/JM/MONO(2012)10, Part 1, 105pp.
W	Guidance Document on the Reporting of Defined Approaches and Individual Information Sources to be Used Within Integrated Approaches to Testing and Assessment (IATA) for Skin Sensitisation (2016). Series on Testing and Assessment No. 256. ENV/JM/MONO(2016)29, 24pp.
X	Report on Consideration from Case Studies on Integrated Approaches for Testing and Assessment (IATA) (2016). 29 pp. - First Review Cycle (2015). Series on Testing and Assessment No. 250. ENV/JM/MONO(2016)48, 29pp.
Y	Workshop Report on OECD Countries Activities Regarding Testing, Assessment and Management of Endocrine Disrupters (2012). Series on Testing and Assessment No. 256. ENV/JM/MONO(2012)2, 83pp.
Z	Guidance Document on Standardised Test Guidelines for Evaluating Chemicals for Endocrine Disruption (2012). Series on Testing and Assessment No. 150. ENV/JM/MONO(2012)22ENV/JM/MONO(2016)29, 524pp.

Some crucial developments took place in the late 1980s and early 1990s. John Frazier, from the Center for Alternatives to Animal Testing (CAAT), was invited to produce a report on validation for the OECD (2), and in 1990, CAAT and ERGATT organised a workshop on the principles of validation at Amden, Switzerland (Amden I; 3). Shortly afterwards, ERGATT and DGXI of the European Commission (EC) organised a second workshop at Vouliagmeni, Greece, on promotion of the regulatory acceptance of validated non-animal procedures (3). This workshop was attended by, among others, Hugo Van Looy of the OECD's Environment Directorate, and Herman Koëter, then at TNO-CIVO Toxicology and Nutrition Institute, Zeist, The Netherlands.

2. THE EMERGENCE OF GUIDANCE AND THE FIRST ALTERNATIVE TEST GUIDELINES

At the second meeting of National Coordinators of the TGs Programme, held in Paris on 17—18 September 1991 (T1-C), some important decisions were made about alternatives: 'The Secretariat did not present an overview of what was happening in respect of development of alternatives on the international scene. It just drew attention to recent publications by FRAME' (3, 4) 'that dealt with problems of validation and acceptance by regulatory authorities of alternative tests.' Questions asked were: 'how could OECD play a more active role?' and 'was there a need for a more formal mechanism?' The meeting asked the Secretariat to 'make proposals for OECD initiatives and for stronger OECD involvement in monitoring and stimulation of the development of alternative methods including validation of promising methods'.

As a result, in 1993, the OECD published a *Guidance Document for the Development of Guidelines for Testing Chemicals* (T1-D), which stipulated that new animal or alternative tests should undergo an independent evaluation programme. At about this time, European Centre for the Validation of Alternative Methods (ECVAM), which had been established by the European Commission in 1991, became effective, and at the ECVAM Opening Symposium in 1994, Koëter, now at the OECD Environmental Health and Safety Division, emphasised the need for collaboration, to reach consensus on validation criteria and strategies for incorporating alternative tests into hazard and risk assessment procedures (5). To this end, the National Coordinators of the TGs Programme agreed that having a workshop would be the best approach, and a steering committee met in Stockholm, Sweden, early in 1995, which involved CAAT, ECVAM and CFN (the Swedish Board for Laboratory Animals), among others, to plan a workshop to be held in Solna, Sweden.

The Solna *OECD Workshop on Harmonization of Validation and Acceptance Criteria for Alternative Toxicological Test Methods* took place on 22—24 January 1996, in line with the insistence of the National Coordinators that existing approaches to validation, including those of CAAT, ECVAM, FRAME and Center for Documentation and Evaluation of Alternative Methods to Animal Experiments (ZEBET), should be used as the basis for an internationally acceptable approach, rather than the development of yet another concept. This aim was achieved at the workshop (T1-E), and in September 1996, the National Coordinators endorsed the validation and acceptance criteria put forward at Solna and agreed that a guidance document (GD) should be produced, in line with the 'Solna principles'. These principles were fully in line with those agreed at Amden I (3) and Vouliagmeni (4), and, in 1995, at ECVAM Workshop 5 on practical aspects of validation (Amden II; 6).

The development of a *Guidance Document on the Validation and International Acceptance of New or Updated Test Methods for Hazard Assessment* started in 1998 as a follow-up to the Solna workshop. A crucial step was the Secretariat's consultation with a selected number of internationally recognised experts in June 1998, which eventually resulted in the circulation of a draft GD to Member Countries and other stakeholders in September 2001 (T1-F). This led to a proposal to hold an OECD conference in Stockholm in March 2002, to develop, and achieve consensus on, practical guidance on principles and processes for the validation and acceptance of animal and non-animal test methods for regulatory hazard assessment purposes.

At the Stockholm Conference, 40 specific recommendations were made on how the draft GD could be improved and extended (T1-G). The main issues were the validation of Quantitative Structure—Activity Relationships (QSARs), data interpretation procedures, the use of human and existing data, retrospective validation, and the development of TGs from validated protocols. Further consultations with experts took place, and a revised version of the GD was published in August 2005 (T1-H).

While all these developments were taking place, the OECD Secretariat had consulted widely with many experts and agencies, but the roles of ECVAM and ICCVAM, after its establishment in 1997, were particularly important, as were the extended secondments to Paris of Errol Zeiger (US NIEHS), Dorothy Canter (USA), Alan Goldberg (CAAT) and Manfred Liebsch (ZEBET).

Liebsch was to play an important role in the drafting of the EC test method and OECD TG for the first *in vitro* method to be successfully validated, the 3T3 Neutral Red Uptake (NRU) test for phototoxicity (7). The validation study was sponsored by the EC and COLIPA, and it is worth noting that the test did not replace an *in vivo* animal test, as no such test existed. Also the test items evaluated in the study had been selected by experts on both animal and human phototoxicity, at ECVAM Workshop 2 (8).

The EC was under pressure from some of its Member States to accept validated *in vitro* tests for regulatory purposes, and, as reviewed by Spielmann and Liebsch (9), the phototoxicity test was accepted by the EC in 1998. However, acceptance at the OECD level was delayed by the complexity of the OECD's TG procedures, so the test was unilaterally accepted by the EU Member States in 2000 and published in Annex V of *Directive 67/548/EEC* on the classification, packaging and labelling of dangerous substances. A draft proposal for the test, as TG 432, was accepted by the National Coordinators of the TGs Programme in 2002.

3. QUANTITATIVE STRUCTURE–ACTIVITY RELATIONSHIPS

OECD activities on QSARs started in the early 1990s, following a 1989 OECD workshop on notification schemes for new chemicals. One of the workshop recommendations was to evaluate the predictive power of the QSAR models being used at the time by the US EPA in the context of the Pre-Manufacturing Notification programme. This would be accomplished by comparing the QSAR predictions with independent data obtained in the context of the European Community's new chemicals programme (managed at the time by the JRC's European Chemicals Bureau). The results of this study, which were a unique and unprecedented exercise, were published in 1994 as OECD Environment Monograph 88 (T1-I).

During the early 1990s, the OECD undertook further efforts to assess QSAR methodologies, including: (a) a workshop in 1990 on the use of QSARs in the assessment of aquatic effects (T1-J), which led to a GD (T1-K); (b) guidance on the estimation of properties important in exposure assessment (T1-L); and (c) guidance on the estimation of biodegradation (T1-M).

In the early 2000s, the *Guidance Document on the Validation and International Acceptance of New or Updated Test Methods for Hazard Assessment* (T1-H) made reference to the need to apply established validation principles to QSAR models, but did not elaborate a validation framework. A set of validation principles was developed during an ICCA-LRI workshop held in 2002 in the Portuguese coastal town of Setubal (10–12). The so-called 'Setubal principles' were based on the ECVAM principles for test development (13) and some early ECVAM publications on the validation of computational methods (14, 15).

In November 2002, the 34th Joint Meeting of the Chemical Committee and the Working Party on Chemicals, Pesticides and Biotechnology held a Special Session to review the Setubal workshop recommendations, as well as information submitted by member countries and other organisations. The Special Session pointed out the need for transparency in QSAR models and clear procedures for validation and applicability evaluation. As a follow-up, the OECD Expert Group on (Q)SARs was established in the early 2003, to evaluate the utility and applicability of the Setubal principles. Based on the work of this group, the Setubal principles were adopted, with a few modifications, as the 'OECD principles for (Q)SAR validation for regulatory purposes' (T1-N) at the 37th Joint Meeting of the Chemicals Committee and Working Party on Chemicals, Pesticides and Biotechnology in November 2004.

The need for practical guidance on how to apply the QSAR validation principles was subsequently fulfilled by the JRC (European Chemicals Bureau), which developed a preliminary GD in consultation with a QSAR Working Group of European Member State nominees (16). This laid the foundation for the eventual OECD GD (T1-O), as well as regulatory guidance by EU regulatory bodies such as ECHA (17) and EFSA (18).

Unlike TGs, individual QSAR models do not fall under the Mutual Acceptance of Data (MAD) system, which ensures mutual acceptance of test results (but not necessarily regulatory conclusions derived from test results) between Member and Partner countries. Thus, while guidance on how to characterise, validate and report QSAR models has been accepted at the OECD level and is applied by certain regulatory bodies within OECD countries, there is no formal adoption procedure for QSAR models and no official inventory of 'accepted models'. This reflects the fact that QSARs are generally used to provide pieces of information that contribute to an overall weight of evidence within regulatory assessments, rather than as direct replacements for standard (animal) tests.

The experience in developing principles and reporting standards for QSARs has led to similar guidance for so-called 'defined approaches' (DAs) (T1-P). Furthermore, in 2017, the EU (JRC ECVAM) and USA (EPA) initiated an OECD project to develop guidance on the characterisation, validation and reporting of mathematically-based models, including physiologically-based kinetic and dynamic models.

In November 2004, the OECD Member Countries decided that the focus of OECD QSAR work should shift to the regulatory application of QSAR models. Subsequently, in August 2006, the OECD published a case study report (T1-Q), which compiled current and prospective regulatory applications in 11 OECD Member Countries. Since then, there have been two major initiatives: (a) the development of the OECD QSAR Toolbox (first released in March 2008) as a freely available software tool for estimating chemical properties using QSARs and other 'profilers' and for filling data gaps by grouping and read-across; and (b) the sharing of experience on the practical use of QSARs and other non-testing methods in the context of Integrated Approaches to Testing and Assessment (IATA; see below).

4. INTEGRATED TESTING STRATEGIES

The OECD has coined the term 'Integrated Approach to Testing and Assessment (IATA)' to refer to any integrated approach based on multiple data streams. According to guidance published in 2016 (T1-R), an IATA is defined as:

An approach based on multiple information sources used for the hazard identification, hazard characterisation and/or safety assessment of chemicals. An IATA integrates and weights all relevant existing evidence and guides the targeted generation of new data, where required, to inform regulatory decision-making regarding potential hazard and/or risk. Within an IATA, data from various information sources (i.e. physicochemical properties, in silico models, grouping and read-across approaches, in vitro methods, in vivo tests and human data) are evaluated and integrated to draw conclusions on the hazard and/or risk of chemicals.

OECD activities on IATA (T1-S) are motivated by the recognition that use of standardised methods such as TGs will not, in themselves, meet legislative mandates that require increased numbers of chemical assessments to be undertaken without a concomitant increase in the use of animals and resources. Instead, TG methods need to be supplemented by the use of non-guideline methods in the context of IATA.

Most of the current OECD activities were initiated in the late 2000s and 2010s, and have included the following activities: (a) the development of guidance on QSAR validation (see above); (b) the development of the OECD QSAR Toolbox (see above); (c) the development of guidance on grouping and filling data gaps by read-across; (d) the development of Adverse Outcome Pathways (AOPs) and a web-based platform for disseminating AOP-related information (AOP Knowledge Base) under the EAGMST; (e) the development of guidance on the use of AOPs within IATA (T1-R); (f) sharing information and experiences on the development and application of IATA within the IATA Case Studies Project (initiated in 2015); and (g) the reporting of DAs to be used within IATA (T1-P).

Much of this work has been carried out by OECD groups outside the TGs Programme, by more-recently established groups such as the Task Force (now Working Party) on Hazard Assessment and the Extended Advisory Group for Molecular Screening and Toxicogenomics (EAGMST). It is also important to note that while the various outputs promote harmonisation efforts between Member and Partner countries, IATA are not (currently) subject to MAD.

The first endpoint-related IATA to be accepted at OECD level was for skin irritation/corrosion and for eye irritation/ severe eye damage. Initially, these IATA took the form of tiered testing strategies, which were included as appendices to the relevant OECD TGs (TGs 414 and 415). Their inclusion as appendices meant that the testing strategies were not subject to MAD. It was subsequently decided to elaborate and update these tiered strategies, removing them from the TGs and publishing them as separate GDs. The guidance on IATA for the hazard identification and classification of skin irritation/ corrosion was adopted by the WNT in 2014 (T1-T), whereas guidance on IATA for eye irritation/severe eye damage was adopted in 2017 (T1-U).

The next milestone is expected the regulatory acceptance of DAs for the hazard identification and classification of skin sensitisation. This is because the mechanistic basis of this endpoint is well established (T1-V), and there have been many efforts to develop computational models and tests for the individual key events within the skin sensitisation AOP (T1-W). For the early key events (haptenation, keratinocyte and dendritic cell activation), relevant *in chemico* or *in vitro* tests have been formally validated and gained regulatory acceptance as OECD TG 442C (OECD 2015), TG 442D (OECD 2015) and TG 442E (OECD 2016). For later key events (T-cell activation and proliferation), *in vitro* tests are either lacking or not yet validated.

As a step toward accepted DAs for skin sensitisation, the EU (JRC ECVAM), USA (ICCVAM) and Canada (Health Canada) started project in 2017, to develop a Performance-based TG (PBTG) for DAs suitable for the assessment of skin sensitisation. The resulting PBTG is expected to comprise a series of DAs, including examples where the data integration is based on computational approaches that are considered suitable replacements for the standard animal test (the local lymph node assay).

For the systemic toxicities, IATA have not yet been accepted at OECD, although steps are underway. For example, ongoing projects are developing assessment frameworks for non-genotoxic carcinogens and for developmental neurotoxicity. In addition, the OECD's Working Party on Hazard Assessment (WPHA) has established an IATA Case Studies Project to share experiences in developing and applying IATA but not to formally adopt any particular assessment strategies (T1-X).

5. THE CURRENT SITUATION

Current OECD activities aimed at harmonising regulatory assessments and promoting the Three Rs are carried out within the TGs Programme and in more-recently established programmes, as described above. A list of currently adopted TGs based on non-animal methods is given in Table 2.

In addition to the work on TGs, computational models and IATA, other activities have played an important role, which cannot be described in detail here. These include: (a) the development of methods (including TGs) and GDs for the regulatory assessment of nanomaterials (via the Working Party on Manufactured Nanomaterials; WPMN); (b) the development of methodologies for the assessment of endocrine disrupting properties (via the Endocrine Disruptors Testing and Assessment Advisory Group [EDTA], the Validation Management Group on Non-Animal Methods (VMG NA) and the Validation Management Group on Ecotoxicity [VMG Eco]); (c) the development of guidelines for assessing the combined effects of chemicals (mixtures); and (d) the development of IT tools for recording chemical information, such as IUCLID and OECD Harmonised Templates, internet-based tools for disseminating information on chemical properties, such as eChemPortal (19), and the AOP Knowledge base (20), as well as computational prediction tools such as the OECD QSAR Toolbox (21).

Reviews of OECD activities are given elsewhere; in particular, Gourmelon and Delrue (22) provide an overview of the TGs programme, with emphasis on the importance of validation and experiences gained in the validation of test methods at the OECD. Rasmussen *et al.* reviewed OECD work on nanomaterials (23), and OECD work on methodology for endocrine disruptors was summarised in 2012 (T1-Y). Activities on endocrine disruptors have included the production of a Detailed Review Paper on the use of an exogenous source of biotransformation enzymes in new tests for endocrine disrupters (24) and the development of guidance on how to interpret the results of the endocrine-related TGs (T1-Z; update ongoing in 2017).

6. CONCLUDING REMARKS

With the original aim of avoiding the costs of duplicative testing and facilitating international trade in chemicals, the OECD has become the major global player in the international harmonisation of regulatory toxicity testing. The cornerstone of these efforts has been the TGs programme. In more recent years, scientific and technological developments have led the OECD to establish additional collaborative and harmonisation activities concerned with the regulatory use of 'new approach methodologies' such as computational models and integrated testing strategies. To date, only individual TGs have fallen under the MAD agreement, with newer approaches (e.g. QSAR models, testing strategies) being harmonised to the extent possible (e.g. in terms of reporting standards), but without being subject to MAD. This approach has provided a means of adapting to the rapidly evolving state of the science, while developing a broader understanding of, and trust in, the new methodologies. However, it is also posing a challenge as the traditional distinction between test methods and so-called non-testing methods becomes increasingly blurred. State-of-the-art computational approaches are increasingly being developed to analyse and interpret multiple data streams, which are themselves derived from new technologies. As a result, it is not uncommon to find a multitude of solutions being proposed for a given regulatory question (for example, the classification of skin sensitisers or the identification of endocrine disruptors). The challenge of reconciling flexibility with acceptability cannot be avoided, and will ultimately need to be tackled on a number of fronts, taking into account a range of scientific, practical and social considerations.

TABLE 2 The Organisation for Economic Cooperation and Development (OECD) Test Guideline (TG) Status of *In Vitro* and *Ex Vivo* Non-Animal Methods for Toxicity Testing

TG No.	Year Adopted	Year Updated	Title
319A	2018		Intrinsic Clearance using Cryopreserved Rainbow Trout Hepatocytes (RT-HEP)
319B	2018		Intrinsic Clearance using Rainbow Trout Liver S9 Subcellular Fraction (RT-S9)
428	2004		Skin Absorption: *In Vitro* Method
430	2004	2015	Skin Sensitisation: Rat Skin Transcutaneous Electrical Resistance (TER) Test
431	2004	2015 2016	Skin Corrosion: Reconstructed Human Epidermis (RHE) Test: Episkin SCT, Epiderm SCT, SkinEthic RHE SCT, epiCS SCT (formerly EST-1000); Vitrolife-Skin
432	2004		Phototoxicity: 3T3 Neutral Red Uptake (NRU) Test
			Application of 3T3 NRU Phototoxicity Test to UV Filter Chemicals
435	2006	2015	Skin Corrosion: In Vitro Membrane Barrier Test Method: CORROSITEX
437	2009	2013	Eye Irritation: Bovine Corneal Opacity Permeability (BCOP) Test
438	2009	2013 2015 2018	Eye Irritation: Isolated Chicken Eye (ICE) Test
439	2010	2015	Skin Irritation: Reconstructed Human Epidermis Test Method: Episkin SIT, Epiderm SIT, SkinEthic RHE SIT, LabCyte EPI-MODEL24 SIT
442C	2015		Skin Sensitisation: Direct Peptide Reactivity Assay (DPRA)
442D	2015	2018	Skin Sensitisation: ARE-Nrf2 Luciferase Test Method: KeratinoSens
442E	2016		Skin Sensitisation: Human Cell Line Activation Test (h-CLAT)
442E	2017		Skin Sensitisation: U937 Test (U-SENS)
455	2012	2015 2016	Oestrogenic Activity: Performance-Based Test Guideline for Stably Transfected Human Receptor-Alpha Transcriptional Activation Assays for Detection of Oestrogenic Agonist-Activity of Chemicals
456	2011		Steroidogenesis: H295R assay
457	2012		Oestrogenic Activity: BG1Luc ER TA Test Method For Estrogen Agonists and Antagonists
458	2016		Androgenic Activity: Stably Transfected Human Androgen Receptor Transcriptional Activation Assay (ARTA) for Detection of Androgenic Agonist and Antagonist Activity of Chemicals
460	2012		Eye Irritation: Fluorescein Leakage (Barrier Function)
471	1997		Mutagenicity: Bacterial Reverse Mutation (Ames) Test
473	1983	2014 2016	Mutagenicity: *In Vitro* Mammalian Chromosomal Aberration Test
476	1997	2015 2016	Mutagenicity: *In Vitro* Mammalian Cell Gene Mutation Tests Using The Hprt and Xprt Genes
487	2010	2014 2016	Mutagenicity: *In Vitro* Mammalian Cell Micronucleus Test
490	2015	2016	Mutagenicity: *In Vitro* Mammalian Cell Gene Mutation Test using the Thymidine Kinase Gene
491	2015		Eye Irritation: Short Time Exposure (STE) In Vitro Test Method for Identifying Chemicals not Requiring Classification for Eye Irritation or Serious Eye Damage
492	2017	2018	Eye Irritation: Reconstructed Human Cornea-like Epithelium (RhCE) Test Method for Identifying Chemicals not Requiring Classification and Labelling for Eye Irritation or Serious Eye Damage
493	2015		Oestrogenic Activity: Performance-Based Test Guideline for Human Recombinant Estrogen Receptor (hrER) In Vitro Assays to Detect Chemicals with ER Binding Affinity
DRAFT	2012		Eye Irritation: Cytosensor Microphysiometer
DRAFT	2016		Skin Sensitisation: IL-8 Luc Assay
DRAFT	2016		Phototoxicity: Reactive Oxygen Species (ROS) Assay (Non-biological Method)

REFERENCES

1. Connor, A.M. (1997). Barriers to regulatory acceptance. In L.F.M. van Zutphen, & M (Eds.), *Animal Alternatives, Welfare and Ethics*, pp. 1173–1181. Amsterdam, The Netherlands: Elsevier.
2. Frazier, J. (1990). Scientific Criteria for Validation of in vitro Toxicity Tests. In *Environment Monograph* **36**, 62 pp. Paris, France: OECD.
3. Balls, M., Blaauboer, B., Brusick, D., *et al.* (1990). Report and recommendations of the CAAT/ERGATT workshop on the validation of toxicity test procedures. *ATLA* **18**, 313–337.
4. Balls, M., Botham, P., Cordier, A., *et al.* (1990). Report and recommendations of an international workshop on promotion of the regulatory acceptance of validated non-animal toxicity test procedures. *ATLA* **18**, 339–344.
5. Koëter, H.B.W.M. (1995). Validation: a highly charged concept. *Toxicology in Vitro* **9**, 851–856.
6. Balls, M., Blaauboer, B.J., Fentem, J.H., *et al.* (1995). Practical aspects of the validation of toxicity test procedures. The report and recommendations of ECVAM Workshop 5. *ATLA* **23**, 129–147.
7. Spielmann, H., Balls, M., Dupuis, J., *et al.* (1998). A study on UV filter chemicals from Annex VII of the European Union Directive 76/768/EEC, in the in vitro 3T3 NRU phototoxicity test. *ATLA* **26**, 679–708.
8. Spielmann, H., Lovell, W.W., Hölzle, E., *et al.* (1994). In vitro phototoxicity testing. The report and recommendations of ECVAM Workshop 2. *ATLA* **22**, 314–348.
9. Spielmann, H. & Liebsch, M. (2002). Validation successes: chemicals. *ATLA* **30**(Suppl. 2), 33–40.
10. Cronin, M.T.D., Jaworska, J.S., Walker, J.D., *et al.* (2003). Use of QSARs in international decision-making frameworks to predict health effects of chemical substances. *Environmental Health Perspectives* **111**, 1391–1401.
11. Eriksson, L., Jaworska, J.S., Worth, A.P., *et al.* (2003). Methods for reliability and uncertainty assessment and for applicability evaluations of classification- and regression-based QSARs. *Environmental Health Perspectives* **111**, 1361–1375.
12. Jaworska, J.S., Comber, M., Auer, C., *et al.* (2003). Summary of a workshop on regulatory acceptance of (Q)SARs for human health and environmental endpoints. *Environmental Health Perspectives* **111**, 1358–1360.
13. Balls, M. & Karcher, W. (1995). The validation of alternative test methods. *ATLA* **23**, 884–886.
14. Dearden, J.C., Barratt, M.D., Benigni, R., *et al.* (1997). The development and validation of expert systems for predicting toxicity. The report and recommendations of an ECVAM/ECB workshop (ECVAM workshop 24). *ATLA* **25**, 223–252.
15. Worth, A.P., Barratt, M.D. & Houston, J.B. (1998). The validation of computational prediction techniques. *ATLA* **26**, 241–247.
16. Worth, A.P., Bassan, A., Gallegos, A., *et al.* (2005). *The Characterisation of (Quantitative) Structure-Activity Relationships: Preliminary Guidance*. JRC Report EUR 21866 EN, 95pp.
17. ECHA. (2011). *Guidance on Information Requirements and Chemical Safety Assessment, Chapter R.5 : Adaptation of Information Requirements*, 28pp. Helsinki, Finland: ECHA.
18. EFSA. (2016). Guidance on the establishment of the residue definition for dietary risk assessment. *EFSA Journal* **14**(4549), 129.
19. Wittwehr, C. (2011). eChemPortal: Neuer Zugang zu Chemikalien-Daten. *Chemie in Unserer Zeit* **45**, 122–125.
20. Delrue, N., Sachana, M., Sakuratani, Y., *et al.* (2016). The adverse outcome pathway concept: A basis for developing regulatory decision-making tools. *ATLA* **44**, 417–429.
21. Diderich, R. (2010). Tools for category formation and read-across: Overview of the OECD (Q)SAR application toolbox. In M.T.D. Cronin, & J.C. Madden (Eds.), *In Silico Toxicology: Principles and Applications*, pp. 385–407. Cambridge, UK: The Royal Society of Chemistry.
22. Gourmelon, A. & Delrue, N. (2016). Validation in support of internationally harmonised OECD test guidelines for assessing the safety of chemicals. In C. Eskes, & M. Whelan (Eds.), *Advances in Experimental Medicine and Biology: Vol. 856. Validation of Alternative Methods for Toxicity Testing*, pp. 9–32. Basel, Switzerland: Springer Verlag.
23. Rasmussen, K., González, M., Kearns, P., *et al.* (2016). Review of achievements of the OECD Working Party on Manufactured Nanomaterials' Testing and Assessment Programme. From exploratory testing to test guidelines. *Regulatory Toxicology and Pharmacology* **74**, 147–160.
24. Jacobs, M.N., Janssens, W., Bernauer, U., *et al.* (2008). The use of metabolising systems for in vitro testing of endocrine disruptors — a detailed review paper. *Current Drug Metabolism* **9**, 796–826.

Section 3

Important Issues Related to Types of Application

Chapter 3.1

Animal-Free Cosmetics in Europe

Vera Rogiers

Vrije Universiteit Brussel, Brussels, Belgium

SUMMARY

Because of ethical, scientific and economic considerations, the EU cosmetic legislation evolved over the years toward the abolition of animal testing for cosmetics and their ingredients. It all started with the introduction of the Three Rs concept of Russell and Burch, and eventually resulted in a testing and marketing ban, irrespective of the availability of alternative non-animal tests. These decisions had significant implications on the risk assessment process for cosmetic products. This chapter provides an overview of the current safety evaluation and existing alternative methods for cosmetics in Europe, as well as some key events related to EU cosmetic legislation.

1. PIVOTAL EVENTS DETERMINING THE ACTUAL EU COSMETICS LEGISLATION

To understand how the animal-free safety testing challenge for cosmetics and their ingredients evolved in Europe, it is necessary to go back in history and follow up the various factors involved. In Fig. 1, a timeline is given, which summarises most of these major events.

1.1 Overview of Events as a Function of Time

It all started in 1959, with the publication of a groundbreaking book by two scientists, William Russell and Rex Burch, on the concept of humanity in the sense of "humane-ness" versus inhumanity in the context of animal experimentation (1). The so-called Three Rs concept was born, incorporating *Replacement* of animal use in experimental research and testing as much as possible according to evolving new technology. However, when animals would be still needed, a *Reduction* strategy was advocated, namely, to use the strict minimum of animals necessary for the particular experiment and to do this under the most stringent humane conditions (*Refinement*). When this book was launched, nobody could predict what a huge impact it would have — worldwide and particularly in Europe — on society and on legislation, with an emphasis on cosmetics. An abridged version of *The Principles of Humane Experimental Technique* is available, which updated, simplified and clarified the original version, to make it more accessible to a wider audience (2).

In 1976, the Member States of the European Economic Community (EEC) harmonised their cosmetics legislation, not only to better protect the consumer, but also to improve the free circulation of products among the EEC Member States (3). The outcome was *Directive 76/768/EEC* (4), which led to the formation of a Scientific Committee on Cosmetology (SCC) in 1979. The name of this advisory group of independent scientists has changed frequently over time, and its current name is Scientific Committee on Consumer Safety (SCCS). Its composition has also been revised several times. This independent Committee generates scientific opinions on the safety of cosmetic ingredients, and the SCCS *Notes of Guidance* are available for free downloading (5). They contain a wealth of toxicological information on the so-called Annex substances (preservatives, colourants, UV-filters, hair dyes). These opinions are cited worldwide, and although they are advisory, over the years they have almost gained the status of being legislatively binding.

In Europe, most legislative frameworks are vertical, meaning that they apply to a specific product category (e.g. cosmetics, drugs, food additives, chemicals). However, *Directive 86/609/EEC on the protection of experimental*

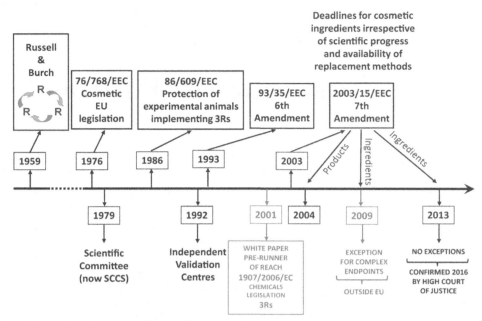

FIGURE 1   Evolving EU cosmetic legislation and factors affecting it. Different colours are used to indicate the changes from science-driven (in blue (black in print versions)) toward non-science-supported changes (from orange (light grey in print versions) to red (grey in print versions)).

animals used for experimental and other scientific purposes (6) was horizontal, and was supposed to be implemented over time in the different legislative frameworks. It was clearly science-based and inspired by the Three Rs concept.

This piece of legislation was at the basis of the creation of ECVAM, the European Centre for the Validation of Alternative Methods (ECVAM), now named the European Union Reference Laboratory for Alternatives to Animal Testing (EURL ECVAM; (7)). It is a relatively independent centre for the validation of alternative methods. ECVAM's original mission was to look worldwide for available Three Rs alternative methods, and to see whether they met the agreed validation criteria set before (relevance, reliability, reproducibility, with a well-defined purpose and with the results applied via prediction models to issues of toxicological concern). Its tasks were extended in the provisions of *Directive 2010/63/ EU* (8), which updated and replaced the 1986 Directive, and in which a more active role of the EU Member States and the EU Commission became mandatory. EURL ECVAM's mandate now covers the entire life cycle of alternative methods, from the development of a test, via its validation to its regulatory acceptance, international recognition and application. EURL ECVAM makes recommendations on the validity of a test method, including its limitations and proper scientific use, possible regulatory applicability, and possible follow up activities in view of addressing knowledge gaps.

The EU initiative to create a dedicated centre for alternatives was followed by several equivalent initiatives in other parts of the world, including the creation of the Interagency Coordinating Committee on the Validation of Alternative Methods (ICCVAM) in the USA in 1997, in Canada the Canadian Council on Animal Care (CCAC) in 2001 and the Japanese Center for the Validation of Alternative Methods (JaCVAM) in 2005. Along with more-recent centres, they are involved in the International Cooperation on Alternative Test Methods (ICATM), which has a positive impact on harmonisation in different parts of the world.

A further milestone in the European cosmetic landscape was the *Sixth Amendment of the Cosmetics Directive* (9), which drastically modified the policy behind the Directive and turned it into risk-based legislation aiming at a high level of consumer protection. The main changes made were that the following would now be required: (a) notification of any cosmetic product marketed in the EU, making effective in-market control possible; (b) the production of an inventory of ingredients by the Commission, with the help of the industry; (c) the introduction of an International Nomenclature of Cosmetic Ingredients (INCI) and labelling of the qualitative composition on the packaging; (d) the labelling of the product's function, where relevant; (e) the obligation, for every cosmetic product on the EU market, to compile a technical information file (TIF), containing a mandatory safety assessment of the product and proof of the claims made for the product; (f) the introduction of a clear industrial responsibility via a responsible person (RP) for every cosmetic product brought onto the EU market; and (g) ban on animal testing of ingredients, whenever validated alternative methods are available. This ban was postponed twice (10, 11), and the final implementation date was eventually fixed as 30 June 2002.

In the meantime, a White Paper, the forerunner of the legislation on chemicals, i.e. REACH (Registration, Evaluation, Authorisation and Restriction of Chemicals) system (12), was introduced, which involved the implementation of a Three Rs strategy. Chemicals placed on the EU market, including cosmetic ingredients, need to be registered as required by REACH, accompanied by a human and environmental safety assessment, the latter being the most important piece of environmental legislation for cosmetic ingredients.

Shortly after the introduction of REACH, the *Seventh Amendment* became available (13), which, in contrast to all earlier legislation and unique for the EU, established a prohibition to test finished cosmetic products and cosmetic ingredients on animals (the testing ban), and a prohibition to market in the EU finished cosmetic products and ingredients included in cosmetic products, which had been tested on animals (the marketing ban). These bans were linked to two fixed deadlines, 11 March 2009 and 11 March 2013, respectively, irrespective of the availability of alternative non-animal tests. Exceptions were made for repeated-dose toxicity tests, reproductive toxicity and toxicokinetics. For these, testing was allowed until the 2013 date, but only when it was performed outside the EU. Also a strict hazard-based ban of so-called CMR-substances (carcinogenicity, mutagenicity and toxic for reproduction substances) was introduced, irrespective of their safety in cosmetic products.

A new *EU Regulation, EC N° 1223/2009,* on cosmetic products was implemented (14) and replaced, from July 2013 onwards, *Directive 76/768/EEC* and its many amendments. Basically, no substantial changes with respect to animal testing were introduced, and the testing and marketing bans remained unaltered. Only the legal format was changed, which made any taken decision directly applicable in all the EU Member States. An electronic Cosmetic Product Notification Portal (CPNP) system also became available, which is intended to make effective in-market control possible.

1.2 Final Outcome

The aim of the *6th Amendment*, to use the Three Rs strategy to protect experimental animals, was welcomed by all parties, including those involved in academia, animal welfare, the industry and regulatory bodies. Europe was already playing a leading role in developing and implementing alternative methods as innovation tools for the future.

It is important to mention that despite the *6th Amendment*, there was still a general consensus among those concerned with the EU legislation for the different product categories (e.g. biocides, chemicals, cosmetics, food additives and pharmaceuticals) on how to increase safety. This was also the case among the laws and legislative bodies in other parts of the world. This was to change drastically.

Indeed, from the 1980s onwards, many factors had an increasing impact on the ongoing discussions for changing legislation and having a more-stringent application of the Three Rs principles. These included: (a) the pressure and lobbying from non-governmental organisations (NGOs), which were steadily growing; their actions were initiated by members fighting for a better environmental protection and those involved in animal welfare; (b) the exaggerated promises made by scientists, companies and politicians, which did not provide a realistic picture of the real status of alternative methods and the time frame necessary for new realisations (c) the frequent use by the responsible authorities of the "easy way out" by applying the precautionary principle and not taking the necessary safety responsibility; (d) the failure of the majority of the people involved in the debates about experimental animal use to understanding the huge difference between the concepts "hazard" and "risk"; this paradigm had already been introduced by Paracelsus (1496–1541) and is still the firm foundation of the toxicological sciences; and (e) the tendency of the general public to see things in black and white: "*We have more than enough alternative methods; we do not need animal models anymore; science has advanced so far that we can replace all animal methods by innovative new technology; animal models do not represent at all the human situation; we have more than enough cosmetics and cosmetic ingredients; we do not need cosmetics; regulatory bodies are not willing to adapt our legislation ...*"

This multitude of factors led to a turning point, forcing political decisions which were unfortunately no longer science-driven and which were brought forward as "incentives to change". The ongoing pressure was very huge, and can be best illustrated by the European Citizens "Stop Vivisection" Initiative, supported by 1.17 million signatures, in favour of using *Directive 2010/63/EU* to insist on the compulsory use of human data instead of data from experimental animals (15). So, 10 years after the science-driven *6th Amendment* came the political decision of the 2003 *7th Amendment*, following two postponements of the marketing ban to the discontent of the legislators (16). The impact on the cosmetic industry was great, in that only replacement alternatives could be used for cosmetic purposes – there would be no Three Rs approach, but only One R could be applied. In addition, only *validated* alternatives for cosmetic ingredients could be used for regulatory purposes.

Four deadlines became installed: (a) 11/09/2004 for finished cosmetic products; (b) an immediate ban when an alternative was available; (c) 11/03/2009 for a testing and marketing ban for cosmetic ingredients; and (d) 11/03/2013 as a testing and marketing ban for more-complex endpoints, being essential for risk assessment (repeated-dose toxicity, developmental toxicity and toxicokinetics).

There were several warnings by various EU scientific committees and associations about the imbalance between science and legislation, but with no positive outcome.

Today, *Regulation 1223/2009*/EC is the official cosmetic legislation in all the EU Member States. The same principles apply, as in *Directive 76/768/EEC*, namely, that cosmetics must be safe for the consumer and that safety is based on safe ingredients. However, what is totally different is the obligatory demonstration of safety through risk assessment, by using *only validated animal-free alternatives*. These changes introduce a never-seen-before dissent with respect to the methodology needed to guarantee the safety of cosmetics and their ingredients. The new EU cosmetic legislation in fact disrupts the science-based principle that was clearly present earlier, when the Three Rs principles were applied. Key replacement alternatives, needed for quantitative risk assessment, that can replace the animal studies that are necessary to determine the no observable adverse effect level (NOAEL) of a new compound (mostly derived from repeated-dose toxicity or reproductive toxicity studies), are not yet available and are not present in the pipeline for official validation (17). The final outcome is that no new cosmetic ingredients have been developed in Europe since the coming into force of the 2013 deadline, although new preservatives and UV-filters are greatly needed. Of course, new cosmetic products are launched on the EU market at a comparable frequency to what went before, but these do not contain innovative new ingredients. They are new formulations of already-existing cosmetic ingredients.

The question can be posed as to whether these invasive legislative changes have saved a lot of animals. From the last official EU numbers on experimental animal use, cosmetics represent only 0.24% of the animals used per year for experimental purposes. This figure, however, is an underestimate, as cosmetic ingredients were often tested as chemicals or food ingredients by the corresponding ingredient manufacturers. As different rules now apply for the risk assessment process in the cosmetic legislation in comparison with the other consumer products legislations, this is no longer possible.

2. THE SAFETY EVALUATION OF COSMETICS IN THE EU

The safety of cosmetic products is supported through the quantitative risk assessment of their ingredients, backed by physicochemical, microbiological and stability data on the final product, together with acute (if available) and local toxicity data.

In Europe, two channels for safety evaluation are in operation (Fig. 2). The first one is situated at the EU level, under DG SANTE through the SCCS (5). As mentioned above, the SCCS performs a safety evaluation of those substances for which some concern exists with respect to human health. These are the Annex ingredients, composed of two negative and three positive lists. Annex II lists prohibited ingredients, which are mostly pharmaceutical substances, and Annex III lists forbidden substances, with some exceptions subject to restrictions in concentration and application conditions. Annex III contains all the tested and permitted hair dyes (with restrictions). Annexes IV, V and VI contain the permitted colouring agents, preservatives and UV-filters, respectively. The second safety channel consists of risk assessment carried out at the industrial level by an independent safety assessor, who must have the necessary educational background as foreseen in *Regulation 1223/2009*. Indeed, all ingredients used in a cosmetic product, actives as well as non-actives, have to be taken into consideration during the safety evaluation of the finished product. Risk characterisation of the ingredients is composed of hazard identification, dose-response assessment and exposure assessment, as described in the SCCS *Notes of Guidance* (5). All the information gained must be made available in the product information file (PIF). This consists of two major parts: Part A with the information on the ingredients and the finished product, and Part B with the safety assessment by the Responsible Person (RP) through the safety assessor.

As mentioned earlier, the animal testing and marketing bans represent major challenges in the safety evaluation of new cosmetic ingredients, as validated alternatives exist for local toxicity and short-term exposure, but not for long-term exposure. For repeated-dose toxicity (sub-acute, sub-chronic and chronic toxicity), carcinogenicity, developmental toxicity and the major part of toxicokinetics, no validated replacement alternatives are yet available (17). Unfortunately, the *in vivo* tests involved not only consume high numbers of animals, but they are also crucial in the risk assessment methodology that is applied today for most other consumer products. Usually, the margin of safety (MoS) of the ingredients is calculated on the basis of their systemic exposure dose (SED) and systemic NOAEL (NOAELsyst), derived from long-term studies, such as repeated-dose toxicity and reproductive toxicity/teratogenicity (18). As established by the World Health Organisation, the MoS (NOAEL divided by SED) should be higher or equal to 100. The default value of 100 represents 10×10, where one 10 stands for interspecies extrapolation (from animal to man) and the other 10 for

SAFETY ASSESSMENT OF COSMETIC INGREDIENTS

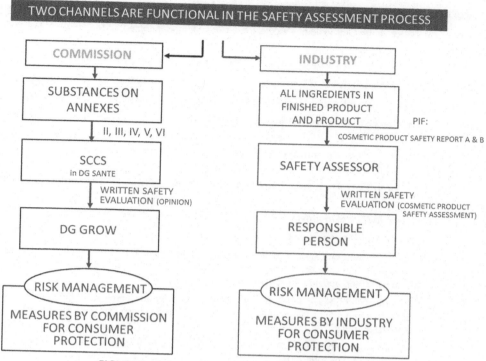

FIGURE 2   Safety evaluation of cosmetic ingredients in the EU.

intraspecies differences (differences in age, gender, body weight, ethnicity, etc.). Both numbers can be further sub-divided into toxicokinetic and toxicodynamic factors (18). The situation for cosmetics, allowing only validated replacement alternatives, is difficult, as essential alternative methods or strategies are missing. Some new methodologies are under development, but when these become available, their validation will take time and resources. It is not yet fully clear whether and how the results obtained under the REACH legislation for chemicals can be incorporated into cosmetic safety testing (12). Some alternative methods proposed for chemical evaluation may not be suitable for the quantitative risk assessment of cosmetic ingredients. In this context, some practical interpretation of article 18 on animal testing in *Regulation 1223/2009* on cosmetics was given by the European Commission (19).

3. CURRENT STATUS OF VALIDATED ALTERNATIVE METHODS FOR COSMETIC INGREDIENTS

3.1 Acute Toxicity

Validated alternatives for acute toxicity testing exist for the oral route (fixed-dose method; acute toxic class method; up-and-down procedure; Table 1:1—3 [T1:1—3]), the inhalation route (fixed-dose method; acute toxic class method; T1:4—5), and the dermal route (draft for fixed-dose method; T1:6), but these are all *Refinement* and *Reduction animal* tests and thus are not suitable for cosmetic ingredients testing.

In 2013, EURL ECVAM published a recommendation on the *in vitro* 3T3 Neutral Red Uptake test for the identification of substances not requiring classification for acute oral toxicity to be used in a weight-of-evidence (WoE) approach or integrated testing strategy (ITS) for supporting hazard identification and safety assessment at the level of oral LD50 >2000 mg/kg body weight, potentially supporting conclusions on the absence of acute oral toxicity of industrial chemicals (20).

In vitro cytotoxicity test methods for estimating the starting doses for acute oral systemic toxicity tests were already validated and adopted in 2010.

TABLE 1 OECD Test Guidelines (TGs) and Related Publications

1.	OECD 420: TG for Acute Oral Toxicity - Fixed Dose Method; adopted 17 July 1992, last updated 8 February 2002.
2.	OECD 423: TG for Acute Oral toxicity – Acute Toxic Class Method; adopted 22 March 1996, last updated 8 February 2002.
3.	OECD 425: TG for Acute Oral Toxicity – Up-and-Down-Procedure; adopted 16 October 2008.
4.	OECD 433: TG for Acute Inhalation Toxicity – Fixed Concentration Procedure; adopted 9 October 2017.
5.	OECD 436: TG for Acute Inhalation Toxicity – Acute Toxic Class (ATC) Method; adopted 8 September 2009.
6.	OECD 434: Draft proposal for a new TG for Acute Dermal Toxicity – Fixed Dose Procedure; 1st version, 14 May 2004.
7.	OECD 430: TG for *In Vitro* Skin Corrosion – Transcutaneous Electrical Resistance Test (TER); adopted 13 April 2004, updated 26 July 2013.
8.	OECD 431: TG for *In Vitro* Skin Corrosion Reconstructed Human Epidermis (RHE) Test Method; adopted 29 July 2016.
9.	OECD 439: TG for *In Vitro* Skin Irritation – Reconstructed Human *Epidermis* Test Method; adopted 23 July 2010.
10.	OECD 405: TG for Acute Eye Irritation/Corrosion; adopted 12 May 1981, last updated 9 October 2017.
11.	OECD 437: TG for Bovine Corneal Opacity and Permeability Test Method for Identifying (1) Chemicals Inducing Serious Eye Damage and (2) Chemicals Not Requiring Classification for Eye Irritation and Serious Eye Damage; adopted 7 September 2009, updated 9 October 2017.
12.	OECD 438: TG for Isolated Chicken Eye Test Method for Identifying: (a) Chemicals Inducing Serious Eye Damage; and (b) Chemicals Not Requiring Classification for Eye Irritation and Serious Eye Damage; adopted 7 September 2009, updated 9 October 2017.
13.	OECD 460: TG for Fluorescein Leakage Test Method for Identifying Ocular Corrosives and Severe Irritants; adopted 2 October 2012, updated 9 October 2017.
14.	OECD 491: TG for Short Time Exposure *In vitro* Test Method for Identifying: i) Chemicals Inducing Serious Eye Damage, and ii) Chemicals Not Requiring Classification for Eye Irritation or Serious Eye Damage; adopted 28 July 2015; updated 9 October 2017.
15.	OECD 492: TG for Reconstructed human Cornea-like Epithelium (RhCE) test method for identifying chemicals not requiring classification and labelling for eye irritation or serious eye damage; adopted 28 July 2015, updated 9 October 2017.
16.	OECD 2012A: Proposal for a template and guidance on developing and assessing the completeness of Adverse Outcome Pathways; made in 2012.
17.	OECD 2012B: The Adverse Outcome Pathway for skin sensitisation initiated by covalent binding to protein, part I: scientific evidence. Series on testing and assessment No. 168, 2012.
18.	OECD 442C: TG for *In Chemico* Skin Sensitisation – Direct Peptide Reactivity Assay (DPRA); adopted 4 February 2015.
19.	OECD 442D: TG for ARE-Nrf2 Luciferase Test Method; adopted 5 February 2015.
20.	OECD 442E: TG for *In Vitro* Skin Sensitisation; adopted 9 October 2017.
21.	OECD 429: TG Skin Sensitisation – Local Lymph Node Assay; adopted 23 July 2010.
22.	OECD 442A: TG for Skin Sensitisation – Local Lymph Node Assay: DA; adopted 23 July 2010.
23.	OECD 442B: TG for Skin Sensitisation – Local Lymph Node Assay: BrdU-ELISA; adopted 23 July 2010.
24.	OECD 432: TG for *In Vitro* 3T3 NRU phototoxicity test; adopted 23 November 2004.
25.	OECD 428: TG for Skin Absorption: *In vitro* method; adopted 23 November 2004.
26.	OECD 471: TG for Bacterial Reverse Mutation Test; adopted 26 May 1983, last updated 21 July 1997.
27.	OECD 476: TG for *In Vitro* Mammalian Cell Gene Mutation Test; adopted 4 April 1984, last updated 21 July 1997.
28.	OECD 487: TG for *In Vitro* Mammalian Cell Micronucleus Test (MNvit); approved 23 July 2010.

TABLE 1 OECD Test Guidelines (TGs) and Related Publications—cont'd

29.	OECD 473: TG for *In Vitro* Mammalian Chromosomal Aberration Test; adopted 26 May 1983, last updated 21 July 1997.
30.	OECD 495: Draft TG for *In Vitro Syrian Hamster Embryo (SHE) Cell Transformation Assay*; draft approved February 2013; unclassified 22 May 2015, ENV/JM/MONO(2015)18.
31.	OECD 455: TG for Performance-based Test for Stably Transfected Transactivation in Vitro Assays to Detect Estrogen Receptor Agonists and Antagonists; adopted 8 September 2016.
32.	OECD 457: TG for BG1Luc Estrogen Receptor Transactivation Test Method for Identifying Estrogen Receptor Agonists and Antagonists; adopted 2 October 2012.
33.	OECD 458: TG for Stably Transfected Human Androgen Receptor Transcriptional Activation Assay for Detection of Androgenic Agonist and Antagonist Activity of Chemicals; adopted 29 July 2016.
34.	OECD 493: TG for Performance-Based Test Guideline for Human Recombinant Estrogen Receptor (hrER) *In vitro* Assays to Detect Chemicals with ER Binding Affinity; adopted: 28 July 2015.
35.	OECD 456 H295R Steroidogenesis Assay; adopted 28 July 2011.

3.2 Skin Corrosion

Five validated replacement alternatives exist for skin corrosion testing: one is the transcutaneous electrical resistance (TER) test for measuring electrical resistance in rat skin (T1:7) and four tests are based on reconstructed human epidermal (RHE) equivalents, namely, Episkin, EpiDerm, SkinEthic and EpiCS (T1:8). In addition, Corrositex is accepted in the USA.

3.3 Skin Irritation

Three validated *Replacement* tests that can be applied to cosmetics and their ingredients are available, namely, the EpiSkin, modified EpiDerm and SkinEthic RHE tests (T1:9). A similar Japanese test, named LabCyte RPI-MODEL 24 SIT, is accepted in Japan.

3.4 Eye Irritation and Corrosion

The *in vivo* Draize eye test (T1:10) cannot yet be completely replaced by *in vitro* methodology. It has, however, undergone a number of refinements, but it still is an *in vivo* test. The Bovine Cornea Opacity Permeability (BCOP) test (T1:11) and the Isolated Chicken Eye (ICE) test (T1:12) are validated *in vitro* screening tests for eye corrosion. They can be used to identify both: (a) chemicals which induce serious eye damage; and (b) chemicals not requiring classification for eye irritation or serious eye damage. Other screening *in vitro* tests which can provide supportive evidence are the Isolated Rabbit Eye (IRE) test and the Hen's Egg Test-Chorio Allantoic Membrane (HET-CAM). Also, the Fluorescein Leakage Test (FLT; T1:13), the Short Time Exposure test (STE; T1:14) and the EpiOcular test (EIT; T1:15) have been validated. Up to now, the EIT is the only validated human-based reconstructed tissue model for eye irritation testing. For the Cytosensor Microphysiometer (CM) test, only a draft proposal guideline is available.

3.5 Skin Sensitisation

In vivo skin sensitisation testing cannot yet be fully replaced by validated *in vitro* alternative tests or strategies, although important progress has recently been made via an Adverse Outcome Pathway (AOP) approach (T1:16—17; (21)), which aims to develop mechanism-based alternative methods. However, a number of useful *in vitro* alternative methods have been validated: (a) the Direct Peptide Reactivity Assay (DPRA; T1:18) for measuring binding to proteins, which is an essential step in skin sensitisation induction; (b) KeratinoSens, which shows activation of keratinocytes (T1:19); (c) the hCLAT (THP-1 Human Cell Line Activation) test (T1:20) and U-Sens (earlier named the MUSST, Myeloid U-937 Skin Sensitisation Test), which both measure the upregulation of dendritic cell activation. Also, the IL-8 LucAssay, using the stable reporter cell line THP-G8, was recently adopted (T1:20). Although the refined murine Local Lymph Node Assay

(LLNA; T1:21) is a very useful test, applied for testing chemicals under the chemicals REACH legislation, it still is an animal test and is not suitable for cosmetic purposes. A validated Reduced LLNA (rLLNA) and two non-radioactive tests are also available (T1:22, 23).

3.6 Skin Phototoxicity

The 3T3 Neutral Red Uptake Phototoxicity Test (3T3 NRU PT) is a validated *Replacement* alternative, which makes use of 3T3 fibroblasts in culture (T1:24). Positives can eventually be followed up by repeating the test with reconstructed human skin. A negative response in the latter overrules the positive response in the former.

3.7 Repeated-Dose Toxicity

Large numbers of animals are used for sub-acute, sub-chronic and chronic toxicity testing, for which no validated alternative methods are available. There is little prospect of their replacement in the near future, although developments with human stem cells and organs-on-a-chip could eventually provide some solutions (17).

3.8 Toxicokinetics

Absorption, Distribution, Metabolism and Excretion (ADME) are very important for quantitative risk assessment, but progress has been limited with respect to validated *Replacement* alternatives. A validated *in vitro* test is available for dermal absorption (T1:25), which is important for calculating the SED of a given compound that is topically applied. The test uses Franz-cells, and for cosmetic ingredients, it can be performed with human or pig skin. Specific guidance on performing this *in vitro* test on cosmetic ingredients is provided in the SCCS *Notes of Guidance* (5).

3.9 Reproductive Toxicity

Three validated alternatives have been developed for embryotoxicity, namely, the Whole Embryo Culture (WEC) test, the MicroMass test (MM) and Embryotoxic Stem Cell Test (EST), but they have not been taken up in the legislation because they do not cover all the complex mechanisms involved in reproductive toxicity (22).

3.10 Mutagenicity/Genotoxicity Testing

Three endpoints are considered here: for mutagenicity at the gene level, for chromosomal breakage and/or re-arrangements (clastogenicity), and for numerical chromosomal aberrations (aneugenicity). The standard *in vitro* three-test battery is composed of: (a) a bacterial reverse mutation test (the Ames test; T1:26); (b) an *in vitro* mammalian cell gene mutation test (T1:27); or (c) an *in vitro* micronucleus test (T1:28) or an *in vitro* mammalian chromosomal aberration test (T1:29). For cosmetic ingredients, only a two-test battery is applied, composed of tests (a) and (c), because of the high number of false positives. Methods have also been developed for the follow-up of false positives, such as the *in vitro* micronucleus test or the Comet assay in reconstructed human skin. Also, reporter gene assays have been published, which show a high sensitivity and specificity. For example, ToxTracker has been successfully combined with Vitotox (23). The risk of false positive results can also be reduced on mechanistic grounds, by using HepaRG cells in culture and determining the transcriptomics fingerprint with and without exposure to the suspected compound (24).

3.11 Carcinogenicity

Replacing *in vivo* carcinogenicity testing will involve great difficulties and complexities. An *in vitro* Cell Transformation Assay (CTA) has been proposed, based on morphological alterations and disorganised patterns of colony growth in various rodent cell lines (T1:30). It is thought to be able to identify genotoxic and non-genotoxic carcinogens.

3.12 Endocrine Disrupting Activity

The SCCS has not considered endocrine disruption to be a separate toxicity endpoint, as possible effects can be detected by systemic toxicity tests. *In vitro* tests that measure interactions with oestrogen and androgen receptors have been developed (T1:31−35).

4. CONCLUSIONS

It is clear that, today, we do not yet have the required *in vitro* methodology to adequately respond to *EU Cosmetics Regulation 1223/2009*. A number of validated *Replacement* alternatives exist, in particular, for the hazard identification of acute local toxicity, but not for quantitative risk assessment. No adequate *in vitro* test proposals exist today for repeated-dose toxicity testing and reproductive toxicity. Both are essential for the quantitative risk assessment of new ingredients. As a result, it has not been possible to develop any new cosmetic ingredients in Europe during the last three years. In certain areas, e.g. preservatives, the situation has become critical.

It would have been much wiser, if, as now in other parts of the world, the Three Rs concept had been actively promoted, but only applied rigorously when validated alternative methods and strategies for a certain endpoint actually became scientifically available. It is my sincere belief that the legislation should follow the science — not *vice versa*!

New strategies need to be built up, not merely to replace *in vivo* tests, test by test, but rather to develop integrated testing schemes which take advantage of the combination of mechanistic tests and new emerging technologies, involving human cells and tissues wherever possible.

REFERENCES

1. Russell, W.M.S. & Burch, R.L. (1959). *The Principles of Humane Experimental Technique*, 238pp. London, UK: Methuen.
2. Balls, M. (2009). *The Three Rs and the Humanity Criterion*, 131pp. Nottingham, UK: FRAME.
3. Chave, J. (2016). *Celebrating 40 years of EU cosmetics legislation, 1976–2016*, 1p. Brussels, Belgium: Cosmetics Europe — The Personal Care Association.
4. EEC. (1976). Council Directive 76/768/EEC of 27 July 1976 on the approximation of the laws of the Member States relating to cosmetic products, 169pp. In *Official Journal of the European Communities* **L262**, 169–200.
5. SCCS. (2015). *The SCCS notes of guidance for the testing of cosmetic substances and their safety evaluation, 9th Revision, 145pp. SCCS/1564/15. Adopted at the 11th SCCS plenary meeting of 29 September 2015*. Brussels, Belgium: European Commission.
6. EEC. (1986). Council Directive 86/609/EEC of 24 November 1986 on the approximation of laws, regulations and administrative provisions of the Member States regarding the protection of animals used for experimental and other scientific purposes. *Official Journal of the European Communities* **L358**, 1–28.
7. EURL ECVAM. (2018). *The European Union Reference Laboratory for alternatives to animal testing (EURL ECVAM)*. Available at: https://eurl-ecvam.jrc.ec.europa.eu.
8. EU. (2010). Directive 2010/63/EU of the European Parliament and of the Council of 22 September 2010 on the protection of animals used for scientific purposes. *Official Journal of the European Union* **L276**, 33–79.
9. EEC. (1993). Council Directive 93/35/EEC of 14 June 1993 amending for the sixth time Directive 76/768/EEC on the approximation of the laws of the Member States relating to cosmetic products. *Official Journal of the European Communities* **L151**, 32–37.
10. EC. (1997). Commission Directive 97/18/EC of 17 April 1997 postponing the date after which animal tests are prohibited for ingredients or combinations of ingredients of cosmetic products. *Official Journal of the European Communities* **L114**, 43–44.
11. EC. (2000). Commission Directive 2000/41/EC of 19 June 2000 postponing for a second time the date after which animal tests are prohibited for ingredients or combinations of ingredients of cosmetic products. *Official Journal of the European Communities* **L145**, 25–26.
12. EC. (2006). Regulation (EC) No 1907/2006 of the European Parliament and of the Council of 18 December 2006 concerning the Registration, Evaluation, Authorisation and Restriction of Chemicals (REACH), establishing a European Chemicals Agency, amending Directive 1999/45/EC and repealing Council Regulation (EEC) No 793/93 and Commission Regulation (EC) No 1488/94 as well as Council Directive 76/769/EEC and Commission Directives 91/155/EEC, 93/67/EEC, 93/105/EC and 2000/21/EC. *Official Journal of the European Union* **L396**, 1–849.
13. EC. (2003). Directive 2003/15/EC of the European Parliament and of the Council of 27 February 2003 amending Council Directive 76/768/EEC on the approximation of the laws of the Member States relating to cosmetic products. *Official Journal of the European Union* **L066**, 26–35.
14. EC. (2009). Regulation (EC) No 1223/2009 of the European Parliament and of the Council of 30 November 2009 on cosmetic products (recast). *Official Journal of the European Union* **L342**, 59–209.
15. EC. (2015). *European Commission press release No. IP/15/5094, of 3 June 2015*.
16. EC. (1992). Council Directive 92/32/EEC of 30 April 1992 amending for the seventh time Directive 67/548/EEC on the approximation of the laws, Regulations and administrative provisions relating to the classification, packaging and labelling of dangerous substances. *Official Journal of the European Communities* **L154**, 1–29.
17. Zuang, V., Asturiol Bofill, D., Barroso, J.V., *et al.* (2017). EURL ECVAM Status Report on the Development, Validation and Regulatory Acceptance of Alternative Methods and Approaches (2017). *JRC Report EUR* **28823**, 116.
18. Rogiers, V. & Pauwels, M. (2006). Good science must be the key factor in the development and use of alternative methods for safety assessment of cosmetics. *ALTEX* **23**, 346–352.
19. EC. (2015). *Documentation in the product information file in relation to article 18 of Regulation EC 1223/2009 on cosmetics*. Brussels, Belgium: DG SANCO, 13/SANCO/COS/COSCOM/19.

20. EURL ECVAM. (2013). EURL ECVAM recommendation on the 3T3 neutral red uptake cytotoxicity assay for acute oral toxicity testing. *JRC Report EUR* **25946**, 46.

21. Vinken, M., Landesmann, B., Goumenou, M., *et al.* (2013). Development of an adverse outcome pathway from drug-mediated bile salt export pump inhibition to cholestatic liver injury. *Toxicological Sciences* **136**, 97–106.

22. Marx-Stoelting, P., Adriaens, E., Ahr, H.J., *et al.* (2009). A review of the implementation of the embryonic stem cell test (EST). The report and recommendations of an ECVAM/ReProTect Workshop. *ATLA* **37**, 313–328.

23. Ates, G., Favyts, D., Hendriks, G., *et al.* (2016). The Vitotox and ToxTracker assays: A two-test combination for quick and reliable assessment of genotoxic hazards. *Mutation Research – Genetics Toxicology and Environmental Mutagenesis* **810**, 13–21.

24. Ates, G. (2017). *Gene expression analysis in human cells as cornerstone of an integrated testing strategy in genetic toxicology* (Doctor of Pharmaceutical Sciences thesis). Brussels, Belgium: Vrije Universiteit Brussel.

Chapter 3.2

Safety Assessment of Pharmaceuticals

J Gerry Kenna and Rebecca Ram

Safer Medicines Trust, Kingsbridge, United Kingdom

SUMMARY

Non-clinical animal toxicity studies continue to be used routinely to evaluate the safety of pharmaceuticals, and are mandated by regulatory guidelines, but they have important limitations. Their use in early drug discovery, when there is abundant chemical choice, is not practical, and they are unable to detect many clinically significant human toxicities (most notably, idiosyncratic human adverse drug reactions). *In vitro* methods that use human cells, and assess mechanistically relevant endpoints, have the potential to address these limitations. Useful *in vitro* assays for genotoxicity, skin sensitisation and eye irritancy have already been developed, and have been incorporated into regulatory guidelines. Exciting progress has also been made in the development of useful *in vitro* human cardiotoxicity and drug-induced liver injury (DILI) assays. It will now be important to ensure that the utility of these assays, for the prediction of human cardiotoxicity and DILI, is accepted by the scientific community and that they gain regulatory acceptance.

1. INTRODUCTION

Non-clinical safety studies on new candidate drugs are undertaken prior to, and alongside, human clinical trials to identify and eliminate compounds that can cause significant harm to humans, thereby affording protection for them during clinical trials. Such studies are conducted according to internationally agreed regulatory guidelines, and include the evaluation of repeated dose systemic toxicity (which can affect single or multiple organ systems), carcinogenicity, irritancy, reproductive toxicity and developmental toxicity and skin sensitisation in both rodent and non-rodent species, most often, in dogs (1).

Once approval, based on pre-clinical test results, has been obtained, the human testing of new drugs and devices can begin. It is conducted in four phases (2). Each phase is considered separately, and the data provided have to be submitted to and evaluated by the respective regulatory agency before continuing to the next phase. Phase I studies assess the safety of a drug or device, including short-term effects, after the administration of escalating dose-levels. It takes several months, and typically involves 20—100 healthy volunteers. Phase II studies are intended to evaluate the efficacy of a drug or device and last from several months to 2 years, usually involving several hundred patients. Randomised trial designs are often used, where one group of patients receives the drug, and a second group receives a placebo. Often, neither the patients nor the researchers know who has received the drug, until the experimental part of the study has ended. Phase III trials involve randomised and blind testing in hundreds to thousands of patients, and can last for several years. The data provide more details of how well the drug helps patients. Approval at this stage permits the company concerned to seek marketing authorisation.

During all the above clinical trials, patients are continuously and closely monitored for signs of side effects, and can immediately be withdrawn from the study if necessary. In addition, they have the right to terminate their participation at any time, for any reason.

There is increasing interest, particularly on the part of regulatory bodies, on achieving first administration to humans of new drugs at an earlier stage than Phase I. This is referred to as Phase 0/microdosing and consists of applying microdose amounts of the drug, several orders of magnitude lower than the expected therapeutic threshold, for an effect. The amounts

The History of Alternative Test Methods in Toxicology. https://doi.org/10.1016/B978-0-12-813697-3.00020-2

administered are insufficient to elicit toxicity, while being sufficiently large to be detected by sensitive analytical methods, and behaving in similar ways in terms of distribution and excretion to those with the higher doses in Phase I, II and III. This is discussed in detail in Chapter 3.8.

Phase IV studies, often called Post Marketing Surveillance Trials, may be conducted after a drug or device has been approved for use by consumers. There are several objectives at this stage, including: (a) comparison of the drug or device with others already on the market; (b) monitoring the long-term effectiveness of the drug or device and its impact on a patient's quality of life; and (c) determining the cost-effectiveness of the therapy relative to other traditional and new therapies. Phase IV studies can result in the removal of a drug or device from the market, or the placing of restrictions on its use, depending on findings during the study.

The use of animal toxicity studies to assess human drug safety assumes that such studies are able to detect clinically concerning adverse drug reactions (ADRs) that will arise in humans. However, the relevance to human drug safety of the data provided by animal toxicity studies remains unclear, and this continues to be a highly controversial topic. In large part, this problem has arisen because most of the relevant data have not been made readily accessible in the public domain.

Bailey *et al.* conducted an extensive comparison between animal toxicity findings in multiple species and ADRs reported in humans, for more than 3000 licensed pharmaceuticals (3–5). They used a proprietary database developed by Instem Scientific Limited (the Safety Intelligence Programme), which compiled data obtained from a wide variety of public domain sources and was not restricted to human ADRs observed during clinical trials. Their analysis revealed that the animal toxicity findings did not provide useful predictions of the reported human ADRs that were caused by the drugs (3–5).

Further retrospective analyses have explored the potential value to humans of animal toxicity findings. For example, in a 2012 Dutch study of 93 serious human ADRs, only 19% were identified as having a 'true positive' outcome in corresponding animal toxicity studies (6). Markedly poorer concordance between other human and animal adverse effects has been revealed by other studies, especially for liver and skin toxicities (7). More recently, a translational database was used to compare data between animal safety studies and human Phase I clinical trials for 182 candidate drugs (8). In this study, the negative predictive value of the animal data for human drug safety in clinical Phase I trials was high (>80%). However, the positive human predictive value of the animal data was poor (<50%) and the analysis did not address human ADRs, which could have occurred in later clinical studies of the drugs (8).

It is clear that human clinical adverse effects can and do occur during Phase I and other clinical trials. Recent examples include life-threatening human toxicities that occurred during Phase I trials on the fatty acid amide hydrolase inhibitor, BIA 10−2474, in France in 2016 (9), in which one volunteer died, and on the CD28 superantagonist antibody, TGN1412, in the UK in 2006 (10). In addition, a lack of concordance has been reported between the five most common central nervous system-related human adverse events observed in Phase I clinical trials (headache, nausea, dizziness, fatigue/somnolence, and pain) and the standard multi-parameter neuro-functional assessments (Functional Observational Battery/Irwin test; 11).

A key limitation of the drug safety data, that can be obtained from studies undertaken in animals and in clinical trials, is that many pharmaceuticals cause ADRs infrequently in humans (typical incidence = <1:1000), and only in certain susceptible individuals. Idiosyncratic ADRs pose a major problem, because they are caused by many hundreds of widely prescribed drugs, and they can cause severe and potentially life-threatening human organ toxicities, of which the most frequent are drug-induced liver injury (DILI), cardiac and cardiovascular toxicities, immune-mediated hypersensitivities and haematologic and skin reactions (12). Because of this, idiosyncratic ADRs are important causes of failed drug registration, cautionary and restrictive labelling, and even the withdrawal from use of previously licensed drugs. Idiosyncratic ADRs cannot be detected in conventional animal toxicity studies. Furthermore, they may only become evident when many human patients have been treated with the drug for prolonged time intervals, so they are often detected for the first time only in Phase III trials, or even after drug registration.

In addition to their inability to detect idiosyncratic ADRs and other important human toxicities, animal studies have further key limitations. They require substantial amounts of test compound and are relatively expensive, so they are undertaken only on relatively few test compounds. Also, animal studies deliver results slowly, over the course of many weeks or months. In contrast, the routine compound design/make/test assess cycle that is used to support drug discovery has a much shorter time-frame (generally 2 weeks). Therefore, animal toxicity studies cannot be used to influence compound design and selection during the phases of drug discovery when there is an abundant choice of candidate compounds. This is why many potential candidate drugs exhibit toxicities in animal safety studies, which prevent their further progression (13).

The many limitations of animal toxicity studies, plus the desire to minimise and replace animal procedures, have stimulated investigations of the underlying mechanisms of toxicity. The insights provided by such studies have made possible the development of a wide variety of non-animal test methods, some of which are highlighted in the following sections. These include non-animal *in vitro* and *in silico* approaches that are more-suitable for assessment of human ADRs than animal toxicity studies, and clinical biomarker methods, which permit the improved detection of ADRs in humans.

2. NON-ANIMAL TOXICITY METHODS

2.1 Genetic Toxicology

This topic is discussed in detail in Chapter 3.6 on *Carcinogenicity and Reproductive Toxicity*. Readers are encouraged to read this chapter, which contains a more thorough review of the key issues.

Cancer is a multi-step process, which involves initiation, promotion and progression. For most carcinogenic chemicals, a key initiating event is interaction with, or damage to, DNA, a process known as genotoxicity. The presence of the DNA damage induces DNA repair, which can be error-free or error-prone. The former is undertaken by a process known as excision repair, in which the damage is removed and the missing DNA is restored by DNA polymerase activity. With the latter, mistakes occur during attempts to restore the damaged DNA to its native structure. Therefore, the consequences of DNA damage can be complex, and may result either in no detectable errors (i.e. when repair is complete) or in mistakes which lead to gene mutations, changes to chromosome structure (clastogenicity) or altered chromosome number (aneugenicity and polyploidy). If these mistakes lead to a replicable change in base sequence in genes that influence tumour development, carcinogenesis can be an eventual outcome.

Some chemicals can cause effects that emulate genotoxic ones but via mechanisms that indirectly lead to DNA damage. These are termed epigenetic effects (or non-genotoxic carcinogens). One example would be an effect on the DNA repair enzymes system, which makes the system more error-prone. Such chemicals should not be labelled as genotoxins. Similarly, the promotion of tumour formation is caused by chemicals that act via a variety of mechanisms not involving DNA damage, and these are distinct from genotoxins.

Recommendations on suitable test methods have been issued by the Organisation for Economic Cooperation and Development (OECD) and other international expert panels of scientists, most notably, the International Conference on Harmonisation of Technical Requirements for Registration of Pharmaceuticals for Human Use (ICH). These have been incorporated within guidelines issued by regulatory agencies, which include the US Food and Drug Administration (FDA; 14) and the European Medicines Agency (EMA; 15).

Deleterious genotoxic effects caused by chemicals can be evaluated by using cell-based assays. However, no single cell-based method is able to detect all of the mechanisms by which genotoxicity can arise, so a tiered assay cascade is used. Initial evaluations are undertaken, by using an *in vitro* reverse gene mutation method (the Ames test), which was first described in the early 1970s (16). Numerous compounds are not themselves genotoxic but are metabolised to genotoxic products.

Most of the enzymes which catalyse compound biotransformation are not present in the bacterial cells used in the Ames assay but are present in liver tissue. Therefore, to allow for compound biotransformation, the Ames assay is conducted in the presence of a liver S9 fraction, which contains many different microsomal and cytosolic xenobiotic metabolising enzymes.

This approach permits the detection of the majority of genotoxic rodent and human carcinogens at relatively low cost and high throughput. However, it has many inherent limitations, which include a relatively high frequency of false positives (17). Therefore, additional studies are also needed. These focus on the evaluation of chromosomal damage in mammalian cells, which typically is first undertaken *in vitro* and may then be repeated *in vivo* by undertaking studies in animals. *In vivo* chromosomal damage tests are considered important because they can take account of potentially important additional factors, such as absorption, distribution, metabolism and excretion, and because some compounds are mutagenic *in vivo* but not *in vitro*. However, a clear limitation of *in vivo* studies in animals is that they evaluate genotoxicity caused by parent compounds or metabolites formed in animals but not genotoxicity that might be caused by metabolites whose formation is catalysed by enzymes present only in humans.

The genotoxicity assays that are required to comply with regulatory guidance have been widely used and are considered to provide reproducible and reliable data. They are able to identify compounds that might cause cancer in animals or humans, via genotoxic mechanisms, with high sensitivity. However, alternative approaches have been described, which provide improved sensitivity and specificity. For example, the 'GreenScreen HC' reporter gene assay is undertaken in a human lymphoblastoid cell line (18) and more recently, the Blue Screen (BS-AF; 19), which uses a human TK6 white cell line and human S9 fraction. Both have been reported to detect genotoxic chemicals with high sensitivity and specificity. Therefore, it can be expected that the recommended assay battery will evolve in the future, as more, widespread acceptance, uptake and experience are acquired for these and other test methods.

A further limitation of the current genotoxicity assay battery is that it does not detect all of the mechanisms by which chemicals may cause cancer. Notable omissions include tumour promotion, nuclear hormone receptor-mediated effects, inflammation or tissue-specific cell toxicity that triggers inflammatory responses. Therefore, follow-on evaluations of non-genotoxic carcinogenicity are also undertaken *in vivo* in rodents (20). A major limitation of *in vivo* carcinogenicity studies is that they evaluate effects in rodents which may or may not be relevant to humans, and that the test compound doses used in the studies are much higher than the doses to which humans could possibly be exposed. Therefore, the relevance to humans of the data provided by the studies is highly questionable. Consequently, the development of non-animal methods that can detect non-genotoxic carcinogenicity with high sensitivity and specificity, and could replace rodent carcinogenicity bioassays, is an important unmet need and objective (21).

2.2 Cardiovascular Toxicity

Toxicities which affect the cardiovascular system (i.e. the heart, blood vessels and blood constituents) are a relatively frequent finding during the non-clinical safety testing of candidate drugs in animals, and are an important cause of human ADRs detected during clinical trials or post-licensing (22). Cardiovascular toxicities can cause serious, or even life-threatening, illness. Therefore, they are an important cause of non-clinical and clinical drug attrition during clinical drug development, withdrawal of licensed drugs and cautionary drug labelling (22). Cardiovascular toxicities are caused by both cardiovascular and non-cardiovascular pharmaceuticals, with many different modes of action, which include anthracyclines and other cancer chemotherapeutics (23).

Toxicity affecting cardiac function has been a focus of particular attention in recent decades, when it was recognised that some drugs may cause rare, but life-threatening, human ventricular arrhythmia via delayed cardiac repolarisation (torsades de pointes, TdP) (24). The human *Ether-à-go-go-*Related Gene (hERG) potassium channel, which is expressed on cardiomyocytes, plays a key role in cardiac repolarisation, and drugs that caused TdP have been shown to inhibit hERG activity (25). To permit the early identification of this potential problem, and to reduce attrition at late clinical stages due to TdP risk, an ICH Expert Safety Working Group recommended the clinical evaluation of drug effects on cardiac electrophysiology in human volunteers. Their recommendations were incorporated within regulatory guidance issued in 2005 by the US Food and Drug Administration (FDA) and other regulatory agencies (26). In addition, a non-clinical strategy for detecting and minimising hERG inhibition by drugs was developed by the ICH, and issued by regulatory agencies (27). A key component of the strategy is the quantification of the effects of drugs on hERG activity in cardiac cells *in vitro*.

The need to develop *in vitro* methods that could quantify hERG inhibition by drugs prompted the development and commercial provision of cell lines that express HERG, which are suitable for use in high-volume electrophysiology studies. In addition, high throughput patch-clamp platforms have also been produced, as have structure-based computational models, that have enabled the design of compounds with reduced likelihood of inhibiting hERG (28). Furthermore, significant effort has been expended on data analysis and interpretation. This revealed that evaluation of the safety risk posed by hERG inhibition is reduced markedly, when *in vivo* drug exposure is also considered (29). Moreover, it has become clear that a strategy for the reduction of cardiotoxicity risk, which focuses primarily on hERG inhibition, has significant limitations. This is because other cardiac ion channels also play important roles in influencing myocardial conductivity and contractility. Also, drugs may cause cardiotoxicity via additional mechanisms, notably, via the impairment of contractility and cardiac cell viability (28).

To address these challenges, the Comprehensive *in vitro* Proarrhythmia Assay (CiPA) initiative has been established and is currently underway. The initiative aims to develop and validate an *in silico–in vitro* approach, which can provide improved prediction of human drug cardiotoxicity potential. In addition to hERG inhibition, the CiPA initiative is evaluating the effects of drugs on other cardiac ion channels, contractility and cell structure. These studies are being greatly aided by the availability of cardiomyocyte-like human cells, generated via induced pluripotent stem cell technology (28).

2.3 Hepatotoxicity

Liver toxicity occurs relatively frequently during the non-clinical safety testing of drugs in animals, and is an important cause of compound attrition prior to clinical trials (13). In addition, numerous drugs cause liver toxicity in humans but not in animal toxicity studies. In general, such 'human-specific' DILI arises infrequently ('idiosyncratically') and only in certain susceptible individuals, hence it is not recognised until late in clinical trials or after drug registration (30). Human idiosyncratic DILI can result in severe liver damage, including acute liver failure, and therefore is a leading cause of failed clinical development and failed licensing. Furthermore, many hundreds of licensed drugs cause idiosyncratic DILI, and in many cases this has resulted in cautionary labelling (31).

DILI arises via complex mechanisms, which include both compound-related adverse effects on liver cells and patient-related susceptibility factors (32). Drug-induced acute liver failure, which is the most clinically concerning consequence of DILI, appears to arise following the activation of stress responses within hepatocytes plus the activation of innate and adaptive immune responses (30).

Regulatory agencies have recognised the need to reduce the number of licensed drugs that cause human DILI. Guidance on methods to detect and manage patients who develop drug-associated liver dysfunction during clinical trials was issued in 2009 by the FDA (31). This guidance is used when deciding whether to license new drugs, whether cautionary DILI labelling is required and/or whether routine monitoring of DILI-related clinical chemistry should be conducted in patients treated with licensed drugs. The recommended approach for the detection of human liver dysfunction is quantification in serum of the enzyme, alanine aminotransferase (ALT), which is released from damaged hepatocytes, plus total bilirubin, which is cleared very efficiently from the bloodstream into bile in individuals with healthy livers. A threefold elevation in serum ALT above the upper limit of the normal reference range, plus a twofold elevation in serum bilirubin, is considered to indicate liver injury. The consideration and exclusion of other plausible causes of liver dysfunction (e.g. concurrent viral infection, extra-hepatic obstruction, pre-existing liver injury prior to drug treatment) is required to establish likely DILI causality. Even a few cases of otherwise unexplained liver dysfunction, which arise in patients treated with a new investigational drug, are considered to raise concern (31). Drugs given cautionary labels by the FDA, or for which regular monitoring of liver function is required, are at substantial commercial disadvantage. Therefore, the guidance has high-lighted the need for the pharmaceutical industry to develop methods that can reliably predict and detect human DILI prior to the commencement of clinical trials.

A wide variety of different approaches have been described, which permit the *in vitro* evaluation of mechanisms relevant to DILI and, in principle, could be used as predictive screens. Assays that quantify individual compound-related DILI-initiating mechanisms have attracted particular interest. The mechanisms evaluated include the formation of chemically reactive metabolites, metabolite-mediated cell cytotoxicity, mitochondrial impairment and inhibition of the hepatic Bile Salt Export Pump (BSEP; 32, 33). In addition, some investigators have evaluated toxicity to isolated hepatocytes from humans or animal species (34), or to human liver spheroids, which contain hepatocytes plus other liver cell types, and can be exposed to test compounds for many days (35). All of the currently published data demonstrate that assays which focus on individual DILI-initiating mechanisms yield low DILI sensitivity (<50%) and modest DILI specificity – i.e. numerous drugs which do not cause DILI exhibit activity in the assays (e.g. 32, 35). The DILI specificity of assays can be markedly improved by incorporating *in vivo* drug exposure data when interpreting assay data. The simplest way in which this can be achieved is by calculating the ratio between *in vivo* plasma drug exposure and *in vitro* assay potency (i.e. C_{max}/EC_{50}; (35), (36)). However, the use of more-complex and physiologically-relevant *in vivo* drug exposure simulation models (e.g. by the use of proprietary DILIsym software) has been shown to provide marked additional value (37).

High DILI sensitivity (>70%) was achieved when toxicity studies were undertaken for several days *in vitro* by using liver spheroids (35) or when data provided by multiple mechanistically relevant assays were combined. Useful combinations include reactive metabolite formation plus cell cytotoxicity (38); BSEP inhibition plus mitochondrial injury (33) and reactive metabolite formation plus cell toxicity, BSEP inhibition and mitochondrial injury (32, 36).

The data provided by these *in vitro* methods are far more predictive of human DILI than data provided by conventional animal safety studies. Therefore, the routine use of these approaches during non-clinical drug safety evaluations has the potential to reduce markedly the incidence of late project attrition, failed registration, drug withdrawal and cautionary labelling, which continue to be caused by unexpected human DILI.

2.4 Skin Sensitisation

The key mechanisms by which drugs and other chemicals can cause skin sensitisation have been elucidated, and this information has been summarised in an Adverse Outcome Pathway (AOP), which was recently accepted by the OECD (39). The AOP identifies three key events, each of which can be evaluated by using *in silico* or *in vitro* methods. The first key event, the Molecular Initiating Event (MIE), is chemical reactivity with skin proteins, which can be predicted by using *in silico* tools, and evaluated by using the *in vitro* Direct Peptide Reactivity Assay (DPRA; OECD Test Guideline [TG] 442C; 40). The second key event is the inflammatory activation of keratinocytes, as well as gene expression associated with specific cell signalling pathways. This is measured by the *in vitro* KeratinoSens assay (OECD TG 442D), which detects activation of the Keap1-Nrf2-ARE pathway by reactive electrophilic xenobiotics (41). The third and final key event is dendritic cell activation, which is evaluated by using the Human Cell Line Activation Test (h-CLAT, OECD TG 442E). The h-CLAT test uses a human monocytic leukaemia cell line (THP-1) to quantify changes in two cell surface markers, CD86 and CD54 (42).

The development of the skin sensitisation test cascade, which has been accepted at the international OECD level, involved considerable optimisation work. This included the successful demonstration of the sensitivity and specificity of the *in vitro* methods when compared with extensive *in vivo* skin sensitisation data, which previously had been obtained by using the guinea-pig maximisation test (GPMT; OECD TG 406) and the Local Lymph Node Assay (LLNA; OECD TG 429). The GPMT involves administering an initial test dose of chemical to animals, followed by a period of 10–14 days to allow an immune response to develop, and then the administration of a second 'challenge' dose. The LLNA requires the administration of the test chemical to the ears of mice, then the evaluation of the weight of the auricular lymph nodes.

The acceptance of the skin sensitisation AOP has encouraged research on many other AOPs (43).

2.5 Eye Irritancy

Non-clinical eye irritation studies are conducted to assess the ocular tolerability of pharmaceuticals, and are carried out when they are considered relevant to the route of administration or potential localised adverse effects. For example, the EMA guideline states that for ocular tolerance, the level of testing required depends on the extent to which the eyes will be exposed to the product, i.e. a specific ophthalmic product versus a product (e.g. a cosmetic liquid or lotion) developed for other purposes, which may come into contact with the eyes accidentally (44).

The currently approved reference model is the Draize eye irritation test, which measures changes in the eye surface following topical application of the test substance to eyes of rabbits, and which has changed little since it was first described in 1944 (OECD TG 405; 45). Because of its severity, and the possibility that the test compound may be corrosive, the OECD guideline emphasises a stepwise strategy, progressing through the use of 1–3 rabbits, as required, to determine the eye irritation properties. The method remains one of the most controversial *in vivo* animal toxicity tests, due to concerns about both its scientific validity and animal welfare, and it has been the focus of replacement research for more than 3 decades.

A variety of *in vitro* methods, which can partially replace the rabbit Draize test, and which can be combined as required to form an integrated testing strategy (ITS), by using either bottom-up or top-down approaches, have been validated scientifically and accepted at the OECD level. The Bovine Corneal Opacity and Permeability (BCOP) assay (OECD TG 437), and the Isolated Chicken Eye (ICE) assay (OECD TG 438) involve the use of eyes obtained from slaughterhouses. The Fluorescein Leakage Test uses a canine kidney cell line (MDCK) to identify ocular corrosives and severe irritants (OECD TG 460). Other methods, which have been approved for identifying chemicals not requiring classification and labelling for eye irritation or serious eye damage, are the short-time rabbit corneal cell exposure test (OECD TG 491) and the reconstructed human cornea-like epithelium (RhCE) assay (OECD TG 492).

Extensive comparisons between data from these *in vitro* methods and *in vivo* data from the Draize test have been undertaken, as has the mining of vast quantities of existing *in vivo* and *in vitro* eye irritation data (46). This includes large-scale efforts to combine the results of several databases (47–49). This work revealed extensive duplicative *in vivo* testing of compounds, with the same chemicals being tested in rabbits as many as 90 times (50), highlighting the urgent need to fully replace the Draize test as soon as possible.

The current regulatory guidelines on eye irritancy (44) emphasise that combinations of *in vitro* methods should be used whenever possible, with justification required for use of *in vivo* methods. In addition, all available weight-of-evidence data must be taken into account before considering new *in vivo* studies, and ocular toxicity should be included in a general toxicity assessment, to avoid further standalone tests. Critically, the guidelines also state that non-validated, as well as validated OECD *in vitro* methods, should be considered on a case-by-case basis, with regard to the specific context of use. This is also reflected in the ICH guideline on non-clinical safety studies required prior to human clinical trials and the marketing authorisation of pharmaceuticals (51).

Drugs that are administered via the ocular route may enter the systemic circulation and therefore have the potential to cause systemic adverse effects. This topic has recently been reviewed by Faroukh *et al.* (52), who have emphasised that children are at a much higher risk of systemic drug side effects following ocular dosing than adults are. This is because the drug dose in eye drops is not weight-adjusted, and also, there are physiological differences (for example, in liver function) between children and adults that can affect drug clearance.

2.6 Reproductive and Developmental Toxicity

The clinical draft guideline for the reproductive toxicity testing of pharmaceuticals (53) specifies that any testing strategy should address the anticipated use of the drug with regard to reproductive potential and disease severity. Reproductive and developmental toxicity is one of the most complex areas of testing because individual tests can require very high numbers of animals, and a number of assays are carried out to address different endpoints in parents and in offspring. For example, fertility and embryonic-foetal development tests are generally conducted in rodents and rabbits (e.g. Prenatal Developmental Test, OECD TG 414), but the results of other toxicity studies to assess fertility (e.g. long-term repeated dose testing) may use dogs, minipigs or non-human primates. Recently, it was agreed that the long-used two-generation reproductive test (OECD TG 416) has only a limited impact on the overall study outcome. The extended one-generation reproductive toxicity study (EOGRTS; OECD TG 443) is the preferred approach because it uses approximately half the number of animals when compared with the two-generation test (1400 rats per test versus 2600).

Several strategies have been recommended, which reduce live animal use and, in some scenarios, defer the requirement to use a second species as part of an integrated testing strategy. The EMA guidelines include reference pharmaceutical compound lists, which inform the design and use of alternative testing strategies. In 2002, three *in vitro* test methods were endorsed by the ECVAM Scientific Advisory Committee (ESAC) as scientifically validated for use. These are the embryonic stem cell test for embryotoxicity (which uses two cell lines), the micromass embryotoxicity assay and the whole rat embryo embryotoxicity assay.

These methods do not replace the requirement for *in vivo* animal tests. However, when used as part of an integrated testing strategy, they can contribute to a reduction in live animal testing. Animal use can also be minimised or avoided by consideration of data obtained previously with chemically similar, or pharmacologically similar compounds.

The ReProtect project, which ran from 2004 to 2009, resulted in the development of a number of additional *in vitro* assays, which address different endpoints within the reproductive cycle (54). Various other projects are ongoing, to develop new *in vitro* and *in silico* models for reproductive and developmental toxicity. For example, The Virtual Embryo Project, established by the US EPA's National Center for Computational Toxicology (NCCT), aims to predict chemical effects on the developing embryo by establishing a number of high throughput models that address key functions such as blood vessel and thyroid formation (55).

3. CONCLUSIONS

The current routine use of *in vitro* methods in many areas of toxicity testing provides a clear demonstration that such methods can be used to facilitate human toxicity risk assessments. They also provide an extremely useful illustration of key issues that need to be addressed, when developing and implementing useful non-animal safety assessment methods. These can be summarised as follows:

1. *In vitro* methods which evaluate mechanistically-relevant processes need to be selected.
2. The methods must be shown to deliver data which are sufficiently robust and reproducible when generated in multiple laboratories.
3. The data provided by the methods must be able to discriminate between drugs that cause relevant human toxicity and drugs which do not, with high specificity and sensitivity. It can be generally expected that effective data interpretation will take account of both *in vitro* assay potency and *in vivo* drug exposure.
4. Scientific consensus on the usefulness of the assay results, and how best to interpret them, needs to achieved. This will require publications in peer-reviewed scientific journals plus the formation of expert groups sponsored by international agencies (e.g. the OECD, the ICH). The development of relevant AOPs can inform and support this process.
5. Suitable regulatory guidance needs to be developed and issued.

Extremely impressive progress on skin sensitisation has been achieved, and it will be important to ensure that the assay battery developed, which is based on the definition of the AOP, is used routinely, in place of the more conventional animal sensitisation studies. Pro-active effort will be essential to ensure that this happens. The skin sensitisation AOP can also act as a useful 'blueprint' for other AOPs in development.

The continued use of Draize rabbit eye testing for the assessment of eye irritancy, even though numerous validated *in vitro* methods are available, highlights the need to focus on the following additional important aspects: (a) increased awareness and recognition of non-animal toxicity test methods which are available currently and have been suitably validated; (b) the updating of regulations and guidance documents, so that they mandate the use of suitably validated and 'fit-for-purpose' non-animal methods; and (c) the identification of knowledge and data gaps that need to be addressed by developing and validating additional methods.

Substantial progress has already been made in developing methods that appear to be suitable for the evaluation of drug-induced human cardiotoxicity and DILI. The predictive value of the currently available approaches is promising, especially when compared with the markedly inferior performance of animal safety studies. This highlights that it would be inappropriate to attempt to validate the non-animal methods assays by comparing the data they provide with toxicities observed in animals. In the future, to ensure that the value of the non-animal methods is accepted by the scientific community, it will be important that the most suitable methods are selected and shown to deliver reproducible data in multiple laboratories. Unless these goals can be achieved, it is unreasonable to expect that they will be incorporated within the new non-animal regulatory guidance that will be urgently required to enable efficient development of safe new pharmaceuticals.

Very recently, the need to improve the efficiency of drug discovery has been highlighted in a report (56) issued in the UK by the BioIndustry Association and the Medicines Discovery Catapult, which is an independent not-for-profit company that was formed to bring together industry, academia, charities, technologists and other key stakeholders. The report concludes that 'humanising' the process of drug discovery and testing is the most important way to ease the 'productivity crisis' in pharmaceutical research. Change *is* possible, as demonstrated by the abandonment of acute (single high dose) animal toxicity studies during pharmaceutical safety assessment. A thorough evaluation of the impact of acute animal toxicity studies revealed that these did not provide useful information when undertaken during drug development, so they were not needed and could be discontinued (57).

Furthermore, once effective non-animal drug safety regulatory guidance has been issued and adopted, it will be possible to evaluate whether conventional animal toxicity studies provide significant additional predictive value concerning human safety. This could pave a way to challenge, and ultimately replace, the current animal toxicity paradigm for drug safety evaluation. Further, background information can be found in refs. 58–60.

REFERENCES

1. Baldrick, P. (2017). Getting a molecule into the clinic: Nonclinical testing and starting dose considerations. *Regulatory Toxicology and Pharmacology* **89**, 95–100.
2. Anon. (2018). *Overview of Clinical Trials*, 1p. Boston, MA, USA: CenterWatch. Available at: https://www.centerwatch.com/clinical-trials/overview.aspx.
3. Bailey, J., Thew, M. & Balls, M. (2013). An analysis of the use of dogs in predicting human toxicology and drug safety. *ATLA* **41**, 335–350.
4. Bailey, J., Thew, M. & Balls, M. (2014). An analysis of the use of animal models in predicting human toxicology and drug safety. *ATLA* **42**, 181–199.
5. Bailey, J., Thew, M. & Balls, M. (2015). Predicting human drug toxicity and safety via animal tests: can any one species predict drug toxicity in any other, and do monkeys help? *ATLA* **43**, 393–403.
6. van Meer, P., Kooijman, M., Gispen-de Wied, C., *et al.* (2012). The ability of animal studies to detect serious post marketing adverse events is limited. *Regulatory Toxicology and Pharmacology* **64**, 345–349.
7. Greaves, P., Williams, A. & Eve, M. (2004). First dose of potential new medicines to humans: how animals help. *Nature Reviews Drug Discovery* **3**, 226–236.
8. Monticello, T.M., Jones, T.W., Dambach, D.M., *et al.* (2017). Current nonclinical testing paradigm enables safe entry to First-In-Human clinical trials: The IQ consortium nonclinical to clinical translational database. *Toxicology and Applied Pharmacology* **334**, 100–109.
9. Kaur, R., Sidhu, P. & Singh, S. (2016). What failed BIA 10–2474 Phase I clinical trial? Global speculations and recommendations for future Phase I trials. *Journal of Pharmacology and Pharmacotherapeutics* **7**, 120–126.
10. Hünig, T. (2012). The storm has cleared: lessons from the CD28 superagonist TGN1412 trial. *Nature Reviews Immunology* **12**, 317–318.
11. Mead, A.N., Amouzadeh, H.R., Chapman, K., *et al.* (2016). Assessing the predictive value of the rodent neurofunctional assessment for commonly reported adverse events in phase I clinical trials. *Regulatory Toxicology and Pharmacology* **80**, 348–357.
12. Alderton, W., Holder, J., Lock, R., *et al.* (2014). Reducing attrition through early assessment of drug safety, pp.373–377. In, *Drugs of the Future: Vol. 39. Highlights from the Society of Medicines Research Symposium, held on March 13th, 2014.*
13. Waring, M.J., Arrowsmith, J., Leach, A.R., *et al.* (2015). An analysis of the attrition of drug candidates from four major pharmaceutical companies. *Nature Reviews Drug Discovery* **14**, 475–486.
14. ICH. (2012). *S2(R1) Genotoxicity Testing and Data Interpretation for Pharmaceuticals Intended for Human Use*, 35pp. Silver Spring, MD, USA: US FDA.
15. EMA. (2012). *ICH Guideline S2 (R1) on Genotoxicity Testing and Data Interpretation for Pharmaceuticals Intended for Human Use*, 28pp. London, UK: European Medicines Agency.
16. Ames, B.N., Durston, W.E., Yamasaki, E., *et al.* (1973). Carcinogens are mutagens: a simple test system combining liver homogenates for activation and bacteria for detection. *Proceedings of the National Academy of Sciences of the USA* **70**, 2281–2285.
17. Tweats, D.J., Scott, A.D., Westmoreland, C., *et al.* (2007). Determination of genetic toxicity and potential carcinogenicity in vitro—challenges post the Seventh Amendment to the European Cosmetics Directive. *Mutagenesis* **22**, 5–13.
18. Hastwell, P.W., Webster, T.W., Tate, M., *et al.* (2009). Analysis of 75 marketed pharmaceuticals using the GADD45a-GFP 'GreenScreen HC' genotoxicity assay. *Mutagenesis* **24**, 455–463.
19. XCellR8. (2017). *Genotoxicity Testing. Test Code CT-037. Blue Screen Animal Free (BS-AF)*, 2pp. Cheshire, UK.
20. EMA. (1998). *ICH Topic S1B Carcinogenicity: Testing for Carcinogenicity of Pharmaceuticals. Note for Guidance on Carcinogenicity: Testing for Carcinogenicity Of Pharmaceuticals (CPMP/ICH/299/95)*, 8pp. London, UK: European Medicines Agency.

21. Corvi, R., Madia, F., Guyton, K.Z., *et al.* (2017). Moving forward in carcinogenicity assessment: Report of an EURL ECVAM/STIV workshop. *Toxicology in Vitro* **45**, 278−286.
22. Laverty, H., Benson, C., Cartwright, E., *et al.* (2011). How can we improve our understanding of cardiovascular safety liabilities to develop safer medicines? *British Journal of Pharmacology* **163**, 675−693.
23. Curigliano, G., Cardinale, D., Suter, T., *et al.* (2012). Cardiovascular toxicity induced by chemotherapy, targeted agents and radiotherapy: ESMO Clinical Practice Guidelines. *Annals of Oncology* **23**(Suppl. 7), 155−166.
24. Yap, Y.G. & Camm, A.J. (2003). Drug-induced QT prolongation and torsades de pointes. *Heart* **89**, 1363−1372.
25. Roden, D.M. (2004). Drug-Induced prolongation of the QT Interval. *New England Journal of Medicine* **350**, 1013−1022.
26. ICH. (2005). *E14 Clinical Evaluation of QT/QTc Interval Prolongation and Proarrhythmic Potential for Non-antiarrhythmic Drugs*, 20pp. Silver Spring, MD, USA: US FDA.
27. ICH. (2005). *S7B Nonclinical Evaluation of the Potential for Delayed Ventricular Repolarization (QT Interval Prolongation) by Human Pharmaceuticals*, 13pp. Silver Spring, MD, USA: US FDA.
28. Gintant, G., Sager, P.T. & Stockbridge, N. (2016). Evolution of strategies to improve preclinical cardiac safety testing. *Nature Reviews Drug Discovery* **15**, 457−471.
29. Redfern, W.S., Carlsson, L. & Davis, A.S. (2003). Relationships between preclinical cardiac electrophysiology, clinical QT interval prolongation and torsade de pointes for a broad range of drugs: evidence for a provisional safety margin in drug development. *Cardiovascular Research* **58**, 32−45.
30. Mosedale, M. & Watkins, P.B. (2017). Drug-induced Liver Injury: Advances in Mechanistic Understanding that Will Inform Risk Management. *Clinical Pharmacology & Therapeutics* **101**, 469−480.
31. FDA. (2009). *Drug-induced liver injury: Premarketing clinical evaluation*, 28pp. Silver Spring, MD, USA: US FDA.
32. Thompson, R.A., Isin, E.M., Li, Y., *et al.* (2012). In vitro approach to assess the potential for risk of idiosyncratic adverse reactions caused by candidate drugs. *Chemical Research in Toxicology* **25**, 1616−1632.
33. Aleo, M.D., Luo, Y., Swiss, R., *et al.* (2014). Human drug-induced liver injury severity is highly associated with dual inhibitin of liver mitochondrial function and bile salt export pump. *Hepatology* **60**, 1015−1022.
34. Garside, H., Marcoe, K.F., Chesnut-Speelman, J., *et al.* (2014). Evaluation of the use of imaging parameters for the detection of compound-induced hepatotoxicity in 384-well cultures of HepG2 cells and cryopreserved primary human hepatocytes. *Toxicology in Vitro* **28**, 171−181.
35. Proctor, W.R., Foster, A.J., Vogt, J., *et al.* (2017). Utility of spherical human liver microtissues for prediction of clinical drug-induced liver injury. *Archives of Toxicology* **91**, 2849−2863.
36. Kenna, J.G., Stahl, S.H., Eakins, J.A., *et al.* (2015). Multiple compound-related adverse properties contribute to liver injury caused by endothelin receptor antagonists. *Journal of Pharmacology and Experimental Therapeutics* **352**, 281−290.
37. Woodhead, J.L., Watkins, P.B., Howell, B.A., *et al.* (2017). The role of quantitative systems pharmacology modelling in the prediction and explanation of idiosyncratic drug-induced liver injury. *Drug Metabolism and Pharmacokinetics* **32**, 40−45.
38. Sakatis, M.Z., Reese, M.J., Harrell, A.W., *et al.* (2012). Preclinical strategy to reduce clinical hepatotoxicity using in vitro bioactivation data for >200 compounds. *Chemical Research in Toxicology* **25**, 2067−2082.
39. OECD. (2014). *The Adverse Outcome Pathway for Skin Sensitisation Initiated by Covalent Binding to Proteins*. Series on Testing and Assessment No. 168, 105pp. Paris, France: OECD.
40. Gerberick, F., Vassallo, J., Bailey, R., *et al.* (2004). Development of a peptide reactivity assay for screening contact allergens. *Toxicological Sciences* **8**, 332−343.
41. Emter, R., Ellis, G. & Natsch, A. (2010). Performance of a novel keratinocyte-based reporter cell line to screen skin sensitizers in vitro. *Toxicology and Applied Pharmacology* **245**, 281−290.
42. Ashikaga, T., Yoshida, Y., Hirota, M., *et al.* (2006). Development of an in vitro skin sensitization test using human cell lines: the human CellLine Activation Test (h-CLAT). I. Optimization of the h-CLAT protocol. *Toxicology in Vitro* **5**, 767−773.
43. OECD. (2018). *Adverse Outcome Pathway Knowledge Base (AOP-KB)*, 1p. Paris, France: OECD.
44. EMA. (2015). *Guideline on non-clinical Local Tolerance Testing of Medicinal Products*, 9pp. London, UK: European Medicines Agency.
45. Draize, J.H., Woodard, G. & Calvery, H.O. (1944). Methods for the study of irritation and toxicity of substances applied topically to the skin and mucous membranes. *Journal of Pharmacology and Experimental Therapeutics* **82**, 377−390.
46. Hartung, T., Bruner, L., Curren, R., *et al.* (2010). First alternative method validated by a retrospective weight-of-evidence approach to replace the Draize eye test for the identification of non-irritant substances for a defined applicability domain. *ALTEX* **27**, 43−51.
47. Adriaens, E., Barroso, J., Eskes, C., *et al.* (2014). Retrospective analysis of the Draize test for serious eye damage/eye irritation: importance of understanding the in vivo endpoints under UN GHS/EU CLP for the development and evaluation of in vitro test methods. *Archives of Toxicology* **88**, 701−723.
48. Spielmann, H., Liebsch, M., Kalweit, S., *et al.* (1996). Results of a validation study in Germany on two in vitro alternatives to the Draize eye irritation test, HET-CAM test and the 3T3 NRU cytotoxicity test. *ATLA* **24**, 741−858.
49. Bagley, D.M., Botham, P.A., Gardner, J.R., *et al.* (1992). Eye irritation: reference chemicals data bank. *Toxicology in Vitro* **6**, 487−491.
50. Luechtefeld, T., Maertens, A., Russo, D.P., *et al.* (2016). Analysis of Draize eye irritation testing and its prediction by mining publicly available 2008-2014 REACH data. *ALTEX* **33**, 123−134.
51. EMA. (2009). *ICH Guideline M3(R2) on Non-clinical Safety Studies for the Conduct of Human Clinical Trials and Marketing Authorisation for Pharmaceuticals*, 26pp. London, UK: European Medicines Agency.

52. Farkouh, A., Frigo, P. & Czejka, M. (2016). Systemic side effects of eye drops: A pharmacokinetic perspective. *Clinical Ophthalmology* **10**, 2433−2441.

53. EMA. (2017). *ICH S5 (R3) Guideline on Reproductive Toxicology: Detection of Toxicity to Reproduction for Human Pharmaceuticals*, 63pp. London, UK: European Medicines Agency.

54. Lorenzetti, S., Altieri, I., Arabi, S., *et al.* (2011). Innovative non-animal testing strategies for reproductive toxicology: the contribution of Italian partners within the EU project ReProTect. *Annali dell'Istituto Superiore di Sanita* **47**, 429−444.

55. EPA. (2018). *Virtual Tissue Models: Predicting How Chemicals Impact Development*, 1p. Washington, DC, USA: EPA.

56. Medicines Discovery Catapult. (2018). *State of the Discovery Nation 2018 and the Role of the Medicines Discovery Cataput*, 36pp. Alderley Edge, Cheshire, UK: Medicines Discovery Catapult.

57. Robinson, S., Delongeas, J.L., Donald, E., *et al.* (2008). A European pharmaceutical company initiative challenging the regulatory requirement for acute toxicity studies in pharmaceutical drug development. *Regulatory Toxicology and Pharmacology* **50**, 345−352.

58. Regev, A. (2014). Drug-induced liver injury and drug development: industry perspective. *Seminars in Liver Disease* **34**, 27−39.

59. Chen, M., Vijay, V., Shi, Q., *et al.* (2011). FDA-approved drug labelling for the study of drug-induced liver injury. *Drug Discovery Today* **16**, 697−703.

60. Thompson, R.A., Isin, E.M., Li, Y., *et al.* (2011). Risk assessment and mitigation strategies for reactive metabolites in drug discovery and development. *Chemico-biological Interactions* **192**, 65−71.

Chapter 3.3

Chemicals and Pesticides: A Long Way to Go

John Doe[1] and Philip Botham[2]

[1]Parker Doe LLP, Stockport, United Kingdom; [2]Product Safety, Syngenta, Jealott's Hill, United Kingdom

SUMMARY

The development of alternative models to assess the toxicity of chemicals has been under way since the 1980s, spurred on by the time taken, the cost and the number of animals, which must be used in compliance with regulatory requirements. There has been progress in the development of a tiered testing strategy to predict the outcome of laboratory animal-based tests for compound selection, but to date, progress has been limited in gaining regulatory acceptance for alternative tests. Alternative tests and testing strategies for acute local toxicity, sensitisation and acute systemic toxicity are becoming more accepted. However, while non-animal methodology for repeat-dose toxicity and carcinogenicity is developing, its progress and acceptance will require a change in philosophy, as well as in technology. A way forward would be to use an exposure-based tiered approach, but the current emphasis in the European Union legislation on classification and labelling, as the basis for risk management is hindering progress toward the replacement of animals in safety assessment.

1. INTRODUCTION

The development of alternative models to assess the toxicity of chemicals has been under way since the 1980s (1). The first areas to be explored were skin and eye irritation. At that time, there was disquiet over the use of tests for irritation in rabbit eyes, the so-called Draize test, and it was considered that, of all the toxicological effects chemicals could have, damage to the eye or skin was likely to be caused by a few relatively simple modes of action, and hence would be the most amenable to replacement by alternative toxicology tests.

At the same time as these early efforts to develop alternative methods, the routinely-used laboratory animal procedures were being standardised and adopted as OECD Health Effects Test Guidelines (TGs). These guidelines became the framework for regulatory systems for chemicals and agrochemicals around the world (2). They represented a great step forward in the reduction of the use of animals because one study design was accepted all over the world, so testing did not need to be repeated with minor variations to meet the requirements of different regulatory authorities. The OECD TGs standardised were widely adopted during the 1990s.

The full set of studies required to register a pesticide is extensive, covering acute toxicity, repeat-dose toxicity, reproductive and developmental toxicity and carcinogenicity. A full evaluation requires the use of 8000 to 9000 animals and takes over 3 years to perform, not to mention the considerable financial cost (3).

Three factors, namely, the time taken, the cost and the number of animals used, have spurred efforts to develop alternatives (4). In addition, the development of legislation for general chemical use has created the pressure to test many chemicals already in use, an estimated 95% of which have not been subjected to the full examination. It would be unrealistic to try to fully test every one of the estimated 50,000 chemicals thought to be in use (5). There are not enough laboratories able to do the work, and the thought of using the 400 million animals, which would be required, is most disturbing.

The History of Alternative Test Methods in Toxicology. https://doi.org/10.1016/B978-0-12-813697-3.00021-4

TABLE 1 Current Adopted Non-Animal Organisation for Economic Cooperation and Development (OECD) Test Guidelines by Toxicological Endpoint

Acute Local Toxicity	Acute Systemic Toxicity	Sensitisation	Mutagenicity	
430, 431, 435 Skin corrosivity		442C *In chemico* skin sensitisation 442D *In vitro* skin sensitisation 442E *In vitro* skin sensitisation	471 Bacterial mutation 480 *Saccharomyces cerevisiae*, gene mutation 481 *Saccharomyces cerevisiae*, miotic recombination	
439 Skin irritation			476, 490 Mammalian mutation	
437, 438, 460, 491, 492 Severe eye irritation			473, 476, 487 Cytogenetics/micronucleus	
432 Phototoxicity			482 UDS	
			479 SCE	
Repeat-Dose Toxicity	**Carcinogenicity**	**Developmental and Reproductive Toxicity**		**ADME/Kinetics**
		455, 457, 493 Oestrogenic agonists/antagonists 458 Androgenic agonists/antagonists		428 Dermal absorption
		456 Steroidogenesis		

Many companies in the agrochemicals sector have followed the lead of the pharmaceuticals sector, by developing a tiered testing strategy to predict the outcome of the battery of laboratory animal-based tests, to select the compounds, which have optimal efficacy, and the best safety profiles. It was hoped that these tests could be used as replacements for the laboratory animal-based methods, but to date, progress has been limited in gaining regulatory acceptance for alternatives. Table 1 lists the non-animal studies, which had been accepted the OECD by mid-2017 in the different areas of toxicology, for which there are OECD animal-based studies (see also Chapter 2.15). A cursory inspection reveals that there is a long way to go before animals will no longer be used to assess the toxicity of pesticides and other chemicals.

In this chapter, the progress in each of these areas is reviewed.

2. ACUTE SYSTEMIC TOXICITY

The assessment of acute systemic toxicity has primarily focused on lethality as the endpoint of concern. The lethal dose 50 (LD50) was the first numerical expression of toxicity to be used. It was a concept borrowed from assays for biological effects, when the potencies of different materials need to be compared. In concept, the dose of agent is varied from that which causes no effect to a dose causing a 100% effect. The mid-point of the dose-response curve is then calculated as the ED50. This concept was used to help answer the question: how toxic is compound x when compared with compound y. The LD50 was determined by giving doses of the agent to groups of rats or mice, then observing them for a period of up to 14 days to determine how many died. Once a sufficient range of responses between no lethality and 100% lethality had been determined, the LD50 could be calculated. The LD50 then determined whether the substance would be labelled as very toxic, toxic, harmful or non-toxic, in accordance with accepted toxicity classification and labelling criteria (6).

The animal methods have been refined over the years, to move away from the accurate determination of the LD50 to determining into which of these toxicity categories a substance should be placed (7). This has reduced both the number of animals used, and the number which suffer severe toxicity. It has also permitted the development of *in vitro* models, which can be less precise than would be required to predict a numerical LD50 value. *In vitro* assays based on cytotoxicity have also been developed, based on the rationale that the same processes, which cause a cell to be non-viable, also cause an animal to be non-viable.

In practice, this has turned out to be a reasonable assumption, and cytotoxicity assays, such as the Neutral Red Uptake (NRU) assay (8), provide good predictions of lethality. The assays show a better correlation for predicting toxicity than they do for predicting non-toxicity because there are some causes of lethality, which act on systems that are found only in whole animals, e.g. the cardiovascular and neurological systems. As a consequence, there is a reluctance to accept a negative result *in vitro* as a demonstration of lack of toxicity. In practice, these assays are used as part of a tiered approach, where substances, which do not show toxicity, are subsequently tested in animals (9). This has reduced the overall number of animals used, and it has also reduced the number of animals experiencing severe toxicity. However, none of these methods has yet been adopted as an OECD TG.

3. ACUTE LOCAL TOXICITY

The combination of public concern over instilling irritant materials into rabbit eyes and their relatively less-complex biology compared with the human eye led to methods to assess acute local toxicity being among the first alternatives to be investigated. Oliver and his co-workers developed methods to assess skin corrosivity, based on assessing the integrity of the dermis as measured by electrical conductivity (1). However, this method could not predict skin irritancy. Therefore, combinations of cytotoxicity and dermal barriers were developed, based on the theory that irritation was caused by substances penetrating the skin and causing local cytotoxicity, which led to inflammation.

A parallel path was followed for assessing eye irritancy, and methods have been accepted for both skin irritancy and eye irritancy by OECD Member Countries (10, 11). These methods are used mainly as part of a tiered testing strategy (12), but again, results indicating irritancy are more readily accepted as definitive than those indicating a lack of irritancy.

4. SENSITISATION

The Magnusson and Kligman maximisation test (13) in guinea pigs involves the injection of the test substance in Freund's Complete Adjuvant, a mineral oil containing killed mycobacteria. This stimulates the immune system by inducing inflammation but often leads to severe wounds on the backs of the guinea pigs. It was also difficult to obtain an estimate of sensitisation potency from this assay.

Concerns for animal welfare, and doubts about the utility of the results of the guinea pig test, led to the development of the local lymph node assay (LLNA) by Kimber and his colleagues (14). In this assay, the test substance is applied to the ears of mice, then, after an interval of 5–7 days, the mice are killed and the draining lymph nodes are removed and examined. Proliferation of lymphocytes is taken as evidence of sensitisation.

The work of Kimber *et al.*, in understanding the mechanism of sensitisation, led to the development of *in vitro* alternatives. Three sequential components are modelled: absorption of the substance across the skin; reactivity of the substance with protein; and the ability of the substance to release cytokines to stimulate sensitisation (15). The individual components have been put together into defined approaches (DA), for example, using algorithms based on Bayesian networks (16). These DAs are able to predict the sensitising potential of a substance with reasonable accuracy. The individual test method components of the DA have been accepted as OECD TGs (2). DAs can be used either on their own or as component parts of Integrated Approaches to Testing and Assessment (IATA; see also Chapter 5.4). Work is ongoing at the OECD to develop a performance-based test guideline (PBTG) for the DAs themselves (see also Chapter 2.10).

5. REPEAT-DOSE TOXICITY

Repeat-dose systemic toxicity is the most difficult area of toxicology for which to develop alternatives, because the range of possible adverse effects is so broad. A laboratory animal contains all the systems and organs that can be adversely affected, whereas *in vitro* systems usually model a part of one system or organ. The quest to develop alternatives to the full battery of animal-based assays has nevertheless been pursued vigorously, with some success. However, this has largely been in the areas of reduction and refinement, rather than complete replacement.

5.1 Typical Data Set

The typical repeat-dose testing data set for a pesticide comprises a 90-day study in rats, a two-year study in rats combined with a carcinogenicity assay, a 90-day study in dogs and a one-year study in dogs. These 90-day studies are designed to mimic the intermediate length of exposure experienced by those who may be spraying a compound or ingesting food containing a residue over a period of a few weeks. A two-year study is designed to mimic the experience of someone ingesting food over an extended period of years. Two species are used to take account of the possibility that one species may be markedly less sensitive than humans.

5.2 The Need for Dog Studies

In both the rat and the dog, the 90-day studies are preceded by studies of shorter duration (4–6 weeks). These studies were originally designed to aid dose-setting for the longer-term studies, and they focused on body weight and clinical condition. In practice, it is rare for a new manifestation of toxicity to appear in the longer studies, which would not have been seen in the dose-setting study, and, recently, the animals from the dose-setting studies have been the subject of a full evaluation. These studies have become the main provider of information on which decisions are taken to proceed or halt the development of a new substance.

The use of both the 90-day and one-year dog study was questioned in the early 2000s (3). It was noted that the no observed effect levels (NOELs) rarely decreased in the one-year study, and no new toxic effects were seen. As a consequence, the one-year dog study has ceased to be a requirement in many regulatory schemes for pesticides (17).

The use of short-term studies to predict the outcome of long-term studies is based on the same concept as the Adverse Outcome Pathway (AOP) approach to safety assessment. If a substance causes a biological effect, this effect may have adverse consequences. The adverse consequences may not be apparent after shorter-term exposure, but the initiating biological effect (Molecular Initiating Event), or effects, will be. Short-term *in vivo,* or *in vitro,* methods have been developed to investigate a wide range of target organs and modes of action, including toxicity to the liver, kidney, nervous system and endocrine system. These methods can identify potential toxic activity, and they are most useful when investigating a series of structurally related compounds.

5.3 Using Batteries of Short-Term Tests

The idea emerged that a battery of these assays could be used to predict repeat-dose toxicity. However, there are two issues that must be addressed. First, each assay addresses a single mode of action, and can only answer the specific question: 'Does this compound affect this target?' However, repeat-dose toxicity testing addresses the wider question of 'What adverse effects can this compound cause?' This poses a problem for the idea of using *in vitro* approaches, as it would require a large number of assays. The second issue lies in answering the question: 'At what doses would the adverse effects occur?' This requires extrapolating from *in vitro* concentrations to *in vivo* doses, which is complicated.

There are two main ways to address these questions. In the US, the Environmental Protection Agency (EPA) has developed the ToxCast Program (18; see also Chapter 2.13). This is based on 700 high-throughput assays and 300 signalling pathway assays, which aim to cover most possible adverse effects. So far, 1800 chemicals with *in vivo* data have been put through the battery of tests, and algorithms have been developed to correlate the *in vitro* data with the *in vivo* data. The battery also contains some basic absorption and metabolism assays, which can be used to calculate the external dose, which would generate an internal concentration of chemical, which correlates to the active concentration in the relevant *in vitro* assay (4).

The other major initiative has been the SEURAT-1 project in Europe (19). SEURAT-1 was a multicentre international project based on the guiding principle of adopting a toxicological mode-of-action framework to describe how substances may adversely affect human health. SEURAT-1 is mainly focused on the liver, as this is the organ most commonly affected in toxicology studies. The project has been followed up by EU-ToxRisk21 (20), which is extending its reach to include other organs/systems (e.g. lung, kidney and nervous system), as well as the liver.

Thomas *et al.* (21) outlined an approach aimed at incorporating the outcomes from both approaches. They suggested that chemicals could be considered to be in three broad categories:

1. Non-specific toxicity: chemicals which cause disruption of biological processes whenever they come into contact with them at sufficiently high concentrations; these can be identified as causing cytotoxicity at low doses in a range of *in vitro* assays.
2. Specific toxicity: chemicals which have effects on specific biological processes because they inhibit enzymes or bind to receptors; they can be identified by being active at low concentrations in the specific assays in the battery.
3. Non-toxic: chemicals which have no cytotoxicity or specific toxicity, which can be identified by only having effects at high doses in a range of *in vitro* assays.

Once a chemical has been through the initial broad battery of assays, the results will be used to determine whether a more-targeted investigation is required to refine the range of effects and to determine the likely *in vivo* safe dose. This could include targeted *in vivo* studies.

6. CARCINOGENICITY AND MUTAGENICITY

6.1 Genotoxic Carcinogens

Some of the first alternative assays to be developed, in the 1970s, were the so-called short-term tests for carcinogenicity (see also Chapter 3.6). The Ames test (22) was the first such assay to be developed, and to be adopted by the OECD, and by regulatory authorities. It was based on the idea that cancer is essentially a result of a mutation or mutations, which allow cells to escape from regulation of cell division and to proliferate. At first, there was a very good correlation between carcinogenicity and the results of these assays, as most of the known carcinogens had been identified by epidemiological studies in humans. However, as long-term bioassays in rodents started to be used to identify carcinogens, there was only poor correlation between the results of the short-term tests and carcinogenicity (23). This is explained by the fact that the short-term tests for carcinogenicity were, in reality, tests for mutagenicity and that mutagenicity was only one of the modes of action, which could lead to cancer.

6.2 Non-Genotoxic Carcinogens

It was noted in the 1990s (24) that approximately half of the long-term cancer bioassays gave rise to an increased incidence of tumours, even for compounds which were not genotoxic. The relevance of these findings to humans was questioned. There were concerns over the use of high doses in these studies, with the top dose set to be as high as can be tolerated for the duration of the study, namely, the Maximum Tolerated Dose (MTD; 25). The relevance of these findings was investigated by trying to determine the mode of action by which the chemicals had caused cancer in the laboratory animals. It was discovered that the tumours seemed to be the result of prolonged toxicity, leading to cell division to replace damaged cells, or prolonged stimulation of pathways, leading to the generation of more cells. Some of the mechanisms were specific to rodents and had no relevance to humans, while others might be relevant to humans but only after prolonged, high dosing (26).

It became important to try to predict potential carcinogenicity in the development of agrochemicals, because chemicals which showed evidence of carcinogenicity were subjected to restricted use by the regulatory authorities. The major site for the development of tumours in long-term bioassays is the liver, and there have been a number projects that attempted to predict non-genotoxic liver carcinogens (27). The goal has been to develop short-term assays for non-genotoxic carcinogens, to place alongside the mutagenicity assays for genotoxic carcinogens, but this has proved to be difficult to achieve in practice. Several modes of action have been identified as risk factors for non-genotoxic carcinogenicity, but the ability to discriminate between chemicals, which would produce tumours and those which would not, has proved to be very difficult to achieve.

6.3 Carcinogenesis and Risk Assessment

Modern theories of carcinogenesis (28) can shed light on why the above difficulty has been encountered. Genotoxic carcinogenicity is seen as an accumulation of mutations over a period of time, in cells which have divided. Some of the mutations make the cells non-viable, while others allow the cells to survive and escape from control mechanisms. Most of these cells are eliminated, but some survive. Any agent which causes mutations or which leads to increased cell division has the potential to result in cancer.

Non-genotoxic carcinogens cause an increase in cell division as a result of frank toxicity or a change in a homoeostatic mechanism, which leads to increased activity in an organ or system. The probability that cancer will result depends on the duration of treatment and the dose level, but because carcinogenesis is a multi-step process, there is considerable variability between individuals in the induction of cancer, even within the same mode of action.

Non-genotoxic carcinogenicity is now being regarded as one possible outcome from prolonged toxicity, and not as a special property of a chemical. This is reflected in the way risk assessment is carried out for non-genotoxic carcinogens. Instead of various low-dose extrapolation techniques that are applied to genotoxic carcinogens (assuming the absence of a low-dose threshold, based on the theory that a single genotoxic event could cause cancer), most schemes apply a margin of exposure from a NOEL of the toxicity which leads to cancer (29, 30). It is therefore unlikely that reliable *in vitro* assays for non-genotoxic carcinogenesis will ever be developed, but they are not needed, as long as there are assays that can reliably identify and quantify repeat-dose toxicity.

7. DEVELOPMENTAL AND REPRODUCTIVE TOXICITY

Reproductive toxicity, the impairment of fertility, can be considered to be repeat-dose toxicity with a functional endpoint. Indeed, histopathology is generally more sensitive than measuring fertility in rats, because rats have a significant functional reserve, in, for example, sperm number and activity. So far, no *in vitro* assays have been specifically targeted at fertility. However, there are many assays for assessing oestrogenic and androgenic stimulation and inhibition as a mode of causing disruption to fertility (31). Assays are also available for assessing the inhibition of steroidogenesis (31).

There have been several attempts to devise assays for developmental toxicity, especially for teratogenicity (see also Chapter 3.6). The whole embryo culture test (32) is an *ex vivo* system that uses rat or mouse embryos in culture with the test substance. However, the limited period of embryogenesis in this assay restricts the range of malformations that can be induced and may render the testing system unsuitable for compounds that are likely to exert their major toxicological effects late in gestation. Other assays use non-mammalian systems such as *Hydra*, flatworms, zebra fish and *Xenopus* (33). These systems have been used as pre-screens, but none has reached the stage where they have been adopted by the OECD.

8. METABOLISM AND KINETICS

A major issue with the development of *in vitro* alternatives has been the extrapolation from *in vitro* to *in vivo*. The first concern is to be certain that the correct substance is being evaluated in the *in vitro* assay. Many chemicals are metabolised once they have been absorbed. This can make them more toxic or less toxic, giving rise to concern for false negatives and for false positives if the non-metabolised (parent) chemical is used in the *in vitro* assay. The first approach to address this issue was equipping the test system with some metabolic capacity, such as the S9 fraction of liver enzymes, as was originally developed for the Ames test (22). This overcame some of the difficulty, but not all chemicals are metabolised by the non-microsomal soluble enzymes in the S9 fraction. In addition, the S9 mix can interfere with some *in vitro* assays, by reducing chemical uptake into the indicator cells.

The second approach has been to use modelling or *in vitro* or *in vivo* systems to understand the biotransformation of the chemical and to apply the appropriate metabolite to the *in vitro* assay. This approach is preferable but requires knowledge of the chemical, which makes it less suitable for general screening, but would make it suitable for second-tier studies. Once a potential adverse effect has been identified *in vitro*, the next step is to estimate the safe dose in humans for risk assessment. The experience of the pharmaceutical sector in studying drug kinetics has been drawn on to develop *in vitro* and *in silico* models.

In the pharmaceutical sector, the models are used to predict the concentration at the intended site of action resulting from therapeutic dosing by the oral, inhalation, dermal or other routes. In the agrochemical and general chemical sector, the calculation is done in reverse; the threshold concentration in the *in vitro* assay is taken as the starting point, and the oral, dermal or inhalation exposure required to reach that concentration is calculated. There are *in vitro* assays for dermal and oral absorption and for biotransformation. The data obtained with these assays can be used as inputs to physiologically, based biokinetic (PBK) algorithms, which can carry out the necessary calculations for *in vitro* to *in vivo* extrapolation (4).

9. THE WAY FORWARD

A four-phase process has been suggested (34) for the transition from animal study-based assessment to non-animal-based assessment:

Phase 1: Animal Studies — definitive safety assessments require the results of animal studies. Non-animal studies are used for prediction and explanation.

Phase 2: Animal Studies with Non-animal-based Study Waiving — definitive safety assessments made by using animal studies, but some studies will not be required if non-animal data indicate they are not needed.

Phase 3: Non-animal studies with Animal Studies in Exceptional Circumstances — definitive safety assessments will be made by using non-animal data, but some animal studies will be necessary to address uncertainty.

Phase 4: Non-Animal Studies — definitive safety assessments will be made by using non-animal data, and no animal data will be required/allowed.

Both the agrochemical and general chemical sectors currently are in Phase 2. What will be required to reach Phase 3? The European Chemicals Agency (ECHA) has defined its criteria for accepting new methodology. The results must be: (a) suitable for classification; (b) suitable for risk assessment; (c) cover the same parameters as existing assays; and (d) have a fully documented scientific explanation (35). These can be interpreted as being able to identify the same breadth of hazards as the traditional methods and to be able to estimate safe exposure levels. The current methodologies for acute local toxicity, sensitisation and acute systemic toxicity are at the stage where this is possible. Repeat-dose toxicity and carcinogenicity are nearing the stage where this should be possible, but its progress will require a change in philosophy and acceptance, as well as in technology. The current philosophy can be summarised as 'Do all the toxicology studies then think about the exposure, as anything less is second best or even unacceptable'. The new philosophy needs to be 'Think about the problem that needs to be addressed, and then select sources of information which will have the most value'.

This means bringing in exposure into the design of the safety assessment programme, asking a closed question 'Is this situation safe?' rather than the open question 'What adverse effects can this chemical have under any circumstances?' (36). It also means that the current emphasis in the EU on the regulatory classification of chemicals, based on studies that require maximum dosing in animal studies, is hindering progress toward the replacement of animals in safety assessment.

REFERENCES

1. Oliver, G.J.A., Pemberton, M.A. & Rhodes, C. (1986). An *in vitro* skin corrosivity test - modifications and validation. *Food and Chemical Toxicology* **24**, 507–512.
2. OECD. (2018). *OECD Guidelines for the Testing of Chemicals.* Available at: http://www.oecd.org/chemicalsafety/testing/oecdguidelinesforthetestingofchemicals.htm.
3. Doe, J.E., Boobis, A.R., Blacker, A., et al. (2006). A tiered approach to systemic toxicity testing for agricultural chemical safety assessment. *Critical Reviews in Toxicology* **36**, 37–68.
4. Rotroff, D., Wetmore, B., Dix, D., et al. (2010). Incorporating human dosimetry and exposure into high-throughput *in vitro* toxicity screening. *Toxicological Sciences* **117**, 348–358.
5. Fischetti, M. (2010). The great chemical unknown: a graphical view of limited lab testing. *Scientific American* **303**, 92.
6. ECHA. (2017). *Guidance on the Application of the CLP Criteria. Guidance to Regulation (EC) No 1272/2008 on Classification, Labelling and Packaging (CLP) of Substances and Mixtures, Version 5.0,* 647pp. Helsinki, Finland: ECHA.
7. OECD. (2008). *OECD TG 425: Acute Oral Toxicity: Up-and-down Procedure,* 27pp. Paris, France: OECD.
8. Kinsner-Ovaskainen, A., Bulgheroni, A., Hartung, T., et al. (2009). ECVAM's ongoing activities in the area of acute oral toxicity. *Toxicology in Vitro* **23**, 1535–1540.
9. OECD. (2010). Guidance Document on Using Cytotoxicity Tests to Estimate Starting Doses for Acute Oral Systemic Toxicity Tests on the Reporting of Defined Approaches to be Used Within Integrated Approaches to Testing and Assessment. In *Series on Testing and Assessment No. 129,* 54pp. Paris, France: OECD.
10. OECD. (2015). *OECD TG No. 439 In Vitro Skin Irritation: Reconstructed Human Epidermis Test Method,* 21pp. Paris, France: OECD
11. OECD. (2015). *OECD TG No. 491: Short Time Exposure In Vitro Test Method for Identifying i) Chemicals Inducing Serious Eye Damage and ii) Chemicals not Requiring Classification for Eye Irritation or Serious Eye Damage,* 14pp. Paris, France: OECD.
12. Gallegos Saliner, A. & Worth, A. (2007). *Testing Strategies for the Prediction of Skin and Eye Irritation and Corrosion for Regulatory Purposes.* JRC Report EUR 22881, 46pp.
13. Magnusson, B. & Kligman, A.M. (1969). The identification of contact allergens by animal assay. The guinea pig maximization test. *Journal of Investigative Dermatology* **52**, 268–276.
14. Kimber, I., Dearman, R.J., Scholes, E.W., et al. (1994). The local lymph node assay: developments and applications. *Toxicology* **93**, 13–31.
15. Casati, S., Worth, A., Amcoff, P., et al. (2013). *EURL ECVAM Strategy for Replacement of Animal Testing for Skin Sensitisation Hazard Identification and Classification.* JRC Report EUR 25816, 30pp.
16. Jaworska, J. (2016). Integrated testing strategies for skin sensitization hazard and potency assessment—state of the art and challenges. *Cosmetics* **3**, 16.
17. NC3Rs. (2015). *The One-year Dog Study in Agrochemical Testing: Time for a Global Change,* 1p. London, UK: NC3Rs. Available at: https://www.nc3rs.org.uk/news/one-year-dog-study-agrochemical-testing-time-global-change.
18. EPA. (2017). *Toxicity Forecasting—Advancing the Next Generation of Chemical Evaluation,* 1p. Washington, DC, USA: US EPA. Available at: https://www.epa.gov/chemical-research/toxicity-forecasting.
19. SEURAT-1. (2016). *Towards the Replacement of In Vivo Repeated Dose Systemic Toxicity Testing,* 1p. Available at: http://www.seurat-1.eu.
20. EU-ToxRisk. (2017). *An Integrated European 'Flagship' Programme Driving Mechanism-based Toxicity Testing and Risk Assessment for the 21st Century,* 1p. Available at: http://www.eu-toxrisk.eu.
21. Thomas, R.S., Philbert, M.A., Auerbach, S.S., et al. (2013). Incorporating new technologies into toxicity testing and risk assessment: moving from 21st century vision to a data-driven framework. *Toxicological Sciences* **136**, 4–18.
22. Ames, B.N. (1979). Identifying environmental chemicals causing mutations and cancer. *Science, New York* **204**, 587–593.
23. Ames, B.N. & Gold, L.W. (1990). Chemical carcinogenesis: Too many rodent carcinogens? *Proceedings of the National Academy of Sciences* **87**, 7272–7276.
24. Gold, L., Slone, T. & Bernstein, L. (1989). Summary of carcinogenic potency and positivity for 492 rodent carcinogens in the Carcinogenic Potency Database. *Environmental Health Perspectives* **79**, 259–272.
25. Slikker, W., Jr., Andersen, M.E., Bogdanffy, M.S., et al. (2004). Dose-dependent transitions in mechanisms of toxicity. *Toxicology and Applied Pharmacology* **201**, 203–225.

26. Pastoor, T. & Stevens, J. (2005). Historical perspective of the cancer bioassay. *Scandinavian Journal of Work, Environment & Health* **31**(Suppl. 1), 129—140.

27. Vinken, A., Doktorova, T., Ellinger-Ziegelbauer, H., *et al.* (2008). The carcinoGENOMICS project: Critical selection of model compounds for the development of omics-based *in vitro* carcinogenicity screening assays. *Mutation Research* **659**, 202—210.

28. Tomasetti, C., Li, L. & Vogelstein, B. (2017). Stem cell divisions, somatic mutations, cancer aetiology, and cancer prevention. *Science, New York* **355**, 1330—1334.

29. EPA. (2014). *Framework for Human Health Risk Assessment to Inform Decision Making, EPA/100/R-14/001*, 76pp. Washington, DC, USA: US EPA.

30. CoC. (2012). *A Guidance Statement From the Committee on Carcinogenicity of Chemicals in Food, Consumer Products and the Environment (COC) - A Strategy for the Risk Assessment of Chemical Carcinogens. COC/G1 — Version 4*, 17pp. London, UK: Committee on Carcinogenicity of Chemicals in Food, Consumer Products and the Environment, Public Health England.

31. OECD. (2012). *Conceptual Framework for Testing and Assessment of Endocrine Disruptors (as revised in 2012)*, 5pp. Paris, France: OECD.

32. Webster, W.S., Brown-Woodman, P.D. & Ritchie, H. (1997). A review of the contribution of whole embryo culture to the determination of hazard and risk in teratogenicity testing. *International Journal of Developmental Biology* **41**, 329—335.

33. Schumann, J. (2010). Teratogen screening: State of the art. *Avicenna Journal of Medical Biotechnology* **2**, 115—121.

34. Burden, N., Doe, J., Gellatly, N., *et al.* (2017). Steps towards the international regulatory acceptance of non-animal methodology in safety assessment. *Regulatory Toxicology and Pharmacology* **89**, 50—56.

35. Knight, D. (2015). Regulatory & Scientific Acceptance of Non-Animal Approaches: The Regulatory Processes Involved in Acceptance of Non-Animal Tests. *Chemical Watch Webinar*, 10 June 2015. Available at: http://www.piscltd.org.uk/wp-content/uploads/2015/06/Regulatory-acceptance-webinar-slides.pdf.

36. Pastoor, T.P., Bachman, A.N., Bell, D.R., *et al.* (2014). A 21st century roadmap for human health risk assessment. *Critical Reviews in Toxicology* **44**, 1—5.

Chapter 3.4

Alternative Approaches for the Assessment of Chemicals in Food

Alexandre Feigenbaum[1] and Andrew P. Worth[2]

[1]FCM, Rishon Lezyion, Israel; [2]Joint Research Centre, European Commission, Ispra, Italy

SUMMARY

This chapter provides an overview of the Threshold of Toxicological Concern (TTC) concept and the ways in which it has been applied, or proposed for application, in the EU-wide risk assessment of chemicals in food. The basis of the TTC approach is described in relation to key historical developments, including policy and research initiatives.

1. INTRODUCTION

The Threshold of Toxicological Concern (TTC) approach is a risk assessment methodology that can be used to assess substances of unknown toxicity present at low levels in the diet. It is based on empirical evidence that for non-cancer effects, there are thresholds below which toxicity does not occur, whereas for cancer effects, the likelihood of tumours is zero to very small at very low exposure levels. Thus, for chemicals of unknown toxicity, human exposure thresholds can be established, below which there is a low probability of adverse effects on health. Accordingly, a range of human exposure thresholds (TTC values) have been developed for both cancer and non-cancer endpoints, on the basis of historical data from extensive toxicological testing in animals. The TTC approach requires only knowledge of the chemical structure of the substance of interest, in addition to information on human exposure. As no new animal testing is required, the TTC approach can be regarded as an alternative (non-animal) approach to risk assessment.

The TTC approach has gained acceptance in situations where toxicity data are not available and cannot easily be acquired (such as impurities, reaction products and trace contaminants in food, feed and water), where evaluation of a large number of compounds with low exposure levels is required (such as flavouring substances), in the prioritisation of large numbers of compounds (such as non-plastic food contact materials), where resources are limited (e.g. contaminants in surface water) or when a rapid safety assessment is needed (such as in chemical food safety incidents). The TTC approach is not accepted in situations where toxicity data are required (e.g. for active ingredients of pesticides).

The presence of chemicals in food raises special considerations in relation to the use of alternative methods. Food obviously includes a complex mixture of naturally occurring chemicals, intentionally added ones and contaminants. Some of these chemicals undergo a complex series of transformations in the journey from 'field to fork'. In addition, food commodities are processed and cooked, so the product is modified after purchase (as with tobacco products; see Chapter 3.5). Furthermore, although these chemicals are typically present at low levels in food, humans are repeatedly exposed to them over a lifetime. For these reasons, information on repeat-dose toxicity, genotoxicity and carcinogenicity are more relevant than acute toxicity. Indeed, where information requirements exist (for authorised substances, such as flavourings), these are the types of information that are typically required. However, in many cases, it is practically impossible to test all the chemicals found in food, and this has created an opportunity to establish a risk assessment approach (i.e. TTC) that makes the best use of existing data, without animal testing.

The History of Alternative Test Methods in Toxicology. https://doi.org/10.1016/B978-0-12-813697-3.00022-6

The TTC approach has also been considered for other applications, including personal and household care products, cosmetics, industrial chemicals and pharmaceutical impurities, with varying degrees of uptake (reviewed by Ref. (1)). In this chapter, we focus on the historical development of the TTC approach and its application in the food safety area, where the approach originated.

2. HISTORICAL DEVELOPMENT OF THE TTC APPROACH

The origins of threshold approaches can be traced back to 1967, when John Frawley (2) at the US Food and Drug Administration (FDA) analysed a distribution of No Effect Levels from chronic rodent studies in a database of 132 chemicals (excluding heavy metals and pesticides) and proposed a safe dietary level of 0.1 ppm (0.1 mg/kg food or drink). This established the principle that the trends found in databases of evaluated substances can be extrapolated to non-evaluated substances. It also led to the idea that it is possible to categorise chemicals into those of low and high concern.

In the 1970s, efforts were under way at the FDA to classify food flavourings (3) and other chemicals in food, according to their chemical structures. This resulted in the well-known Cramer decision tree (after Greg Cramer *et al.* (4)), comprising three structural classes for the classification of non-cancer effects (Table 1). The decision tree categorises a chemical into one of the three Cramer classes, based on the answers to a series of 33 questions relating mostly to chemical structure.

Subsequently, FDA scientists (5) concluded that carcinogenicity was the most sensitive endpoint and analysed the carcinogenic potencies of 343 chemicals from the 'Gold' database (named after the original developer, Lois Gold, also known as the Carcinogenic Potency Database, CPDB; (6)). Based on a probabilistic analysis of potency (TD50) values in the database, and assuming a linear non-threshold dose–response relationship, Alan Rulis generated a distribution of Virtual Safe Dose (VSD) values. These were dietary exposure levels corresponding to a one-in-a-million excess lifetime tumour risk (this value was a policy choice, the upper bound level of 'acceptable risk').

In 1991, in a seminal study, Ashby and Tennant correlated chemical structures with mutagenic and carcinogenic effects (7). Their investigation of 301 chemicals (154 alerting and 147 non-alerting) which had been tested in the US National Toxicology Program (NTP), led to several important findings: (a) structural alerts for DNA reactivity (mutagenicity) were based on chemical electrophilicity; (b) most of the rodent carcinogens were among the 154 structurally alerting chemicals; (c) most of the structurally alerting chemicals were mutagenic; and (d) among the 147 non-alerting chemicals, less than 5% were mutagenic.

The CPDB was updated to 709 chemicals by Mitchell Cheeseman *et al.* (8). By analysing the cancer potency data for these chemicals, they identified structural classes associated with high-potency carcinogens (N-nitroso-compounds, benzidine-structures and three other structural classes), and on this basis recommended their exclusion from the Threshold of Regulation (TOR) approach.

A further evaluation of the CPDB was carried out by Ian Munro and the Canadian Centre for Toxicology (9). Using potency data for four different subsets of carcinogens, Munro found that the type of data subset and the statistical approach to low-dose extrapolation were significant factors in determining the probability of excessive lifetime cancer risk. However, the percentage of new substances assumed to be carcinogens had the most impact.

On the basis of these analyses, the FDA introduced the TOR of 0.5 ppb for food contact materials (10). Using the FDA default values for a combined food and drink intake of 3 kg/d per person and 60 kg body weight (bw), the level of 0.5 ppb (µg/kg) food (corresponding to a daily exposure of 0.025 µg/kg bw/d or 1.5 µg/person) was considered to be a very conservative estimate, even if the substance was later identified to be a carcinogen. However, the TOR approach was not

TABLE 1 Cramer Structural Classes for Non-Cancer Endpoints

Cramer Class	Definition
I (low concern)	Substances with simple chemical structures and for which efficient modes of metabolism exist, suggesting a low order of oral toxicity.
II (intermediate concern)	Substances which possess structures that are less innocuous than class I substances but do not contain structural features suggestive of toxicity like those substances in class III.
III (high concern)	Substances with chemical structures that permit no strong initial presumption of safety or may even suggest significant toxicity or have reactive functional groups.

TABLE 2 Overview of Structural Classes for Cancer and Non-Cancer Endpoints (following EFSA and WHO, 2016 (16))

	TTC in µg/person/day	TTC in µg/kg bw/day*
High-potency carcinogens[a] Substances known or predicted to bioaccumulate[b] Steroids[c] Substances which are not in the Cramer or Munro databases[d]	TTC approach not applicable. Perform a substance-specific evaluation.	
Substances with alert for genotoxicity	0.15	0.0025
Organophosphates and carbamates	18	0.3
Cramer Class III	90	1.5
Cramer Class II	540	9
Cramer Class I	1800	30

*Based on the historical assumption of an adult body weight of 60 kg.
[a]Aflatoxin-like, azoxy (RN = N⁺(O⁻)R) and N-nitroso (RR'N−N = O) compounds; benzidines; hydrazines.
[b]Polyhalogenated dibenzodioxins, dibenzofurans and biphenyls; heavy metals.
[c]Substances which have not been tested for their endocrine properties, other than steroids, can be evaluated using the TTC approach.
[d]Inorganic substances, organometallics, proteins, nanomaterials, radioactive substances, mixtures of substances containing unknown chemical structures.

applicable to compounds known to be carcinogens, which are not permitted in food according to the 'Delaney Clause' (after Congressman James Delaney) of the Food, Drugs, and Cosmetic Act.

In the 1990s, further developments focused on the development of threshold values for non-cancer effects. Munro *et al.* (11) evaluated a dataset of 613 substances with 2941 No Observed Adverse Effect Level (NOAEL) values, representing a broad range of chemicals. They recorded information from the most sensitive species, sex and toxicological endpoints, to identify the most conservative NOAEL value for each substance. The substances were divided into three chemical classes, based on their chemical structure, by using the Cramer decision tree (4). The cumulative distributions of NOAELs for the compounds in each Cramer structural class were plotted, and a log-normal distribution was fitted in each case. The fifth percentile value of each distribution was calculated and converted to a corresponding human intake. The resulting TTC values are given in Table 2.

Since 1997, a tiered approach incorporating these TTC values has been used for the safety evaluation of flavouring substances by the Joint FAO/WHO Expert Committee on Food Additives (JECFA; (12)).

Subsequent work by Robert Kroes and an ILSI Europe Expert Group (13, 14) extended the JECFA approach. Kroes introduced, as a first step, the exclusion of high-potency genotoxic substances (aflatoxin-like compounds, N-nitroso compounds, azoxy compounds) and the identification of structural alerts for high-potency carcinogenicity and genotoxicity. A generic threshold of 0.15 µg/person/day (0.0025 µg/kg bw/day) for potentially genotoxic compounds was applied.

The next step considers non-genotoxic substances (lacking structural alerts for genotoxicity), in a sequence of steps related to their structure and estimated intake. For organophosphates and carbamates (alerts for neurotoxicity), a TTC of 18 µg/kg bw/day was proposed, whereas for substances belonging to Cramer classes I, II and III, TTC levels of 90, 540 and 1800 µg/person/day were proposed based on the work of Munro *et al.* ((11); Table 2).

3. REGULATORY AND SCIENTIFIC DEVELOPMENTS IN THE FOOD AREA

3.1 The EFSA Scientific Committee's Opinion on the TTC Approach

In July 2012, EFSA took an important step by publishing an opinion on the relevance, reliability and applicability of the TTC approach for dietary risk assessment (15). In December 2014, EFSA and the WHO organised a stakeholder public hearing and a workshop, to provide recommendations on how to improve the existing TTC approach. The final report was published in 2016 (16). These developments led to some important refinements and recommendations, including improvements to the Cramer decision tree questions (16), the use of dietary exposure calculations for infants and children (17), and the treatment of less than lifetime exposure scenarios. A decision scheme based on (16) is given in Table 3.

TABLE 3 Decision scheme for the application of the TTC approach (following EFSA and WHO, 2016 [16])

Step	Question	If YES	If NO
0	Does the substance have a known structure and are exposure data available?	Go to Step 1	TTC approach cannot be applied. Chemical-specific risk assessment required
1	Is the substance a member of an exclusion category?	TTC approach cannot be applied. Chemical-specific risk assessment required	Go to Step 2
2	Are there structural alerts for genotoxicity data?	Go to Step 3	Go to Step 4 for non-genotoxic considerations
3	Does estimated intake exceed TTC of 0.0025 mg/kg bw per day?	TTC approach cannot be applied. Chemical-specific risk assessment required	Substance not expected to be a safety concern - low probability that lifetime cancer risk exceeds 1 in 10^6
4	Is the compound an organophosphate or carbamate?	Go to Step 5	Go to Step 6
5	Does estimated intake exceed TTC of 0.3 µg/kg bw per day?	Chemical-specific risk assessment required.	Substance not expected to be a safety concern
6	Is the compound in Cramer class III?	Go to Step 7	Go to Step 8
7	Does estimated intake exceed TTC of 1.5 µg/kg bw per day?	Chemical-specific risk assessment required.	Substance not expected to be a safety concern
8	Is the compound in Cramer class II?	Go to Step 9	Go to Step 10
9	Does estimated intake exceed TTC of 9 µg/kg bw per day?	Chemical-specific risk assessment required.	Substance not expected to be a safety concern
10	Does estimated intake exceed TTC of 30 µg/kg bw per day?	Chemical-specific risk assessment required	Substance not expected to be a safety concern

3.2 Flavouring Substances Already on the EU Market

An EU-harmonised approach to the evaluation of flavouring substances was first laid down in *Regulation (EC) No 2232/96* (18), for a Community Procedure for flavouring substances used, or intended for use, in or on foodstuffs. In view of the large number of these substances (more than 2500; (19)), they were classified into 34 chemical Flavouring Groups of structurally related substances with similar metabolic and biological behaviour (18, 20). For the purpose of Flavouring Group Evaluations (FGEs), read-across was permitted, so that toxicity data available for some substances could be extrapolated to other members of the same group (21). Dietary exposure to flavourings was estimated and compared with the corresponding TTC thresholds. No toxicity data were required, when the substance could be predicted to be metabolised to innocuous compounds and when the estimated daily intake of the substance was lower than its TTC. However, toxicity data were requested for substances with structural alerts. EFSA has evaluated 2067 of around 2500 flavouring substances used in the European Union. In 2010, further data were needed to finalise the evaluations for 400 substances.

3.3 New Flavouring Substances

EFSA's guidance on the risk assessment of new flavourings (22), prior to their authorisation for use in the EU, has been in force since September 2012. The successful experience from the previous grouping approach was taken over, with data requirements depending on the exposure compared with the TTC threshold of the flavouring substance.

3.4 Food Contact Materials: Intentionally and Non-Intentionally Added Substances

Food Contact Materials (FCM) contain a variety of Intentionally Added Substances (IAS) and Non-Intentionally Added Substances (NIAS), which may migrate into food. While IAS are added for a specific technical purpose, NIAS are impurities of authorised starting substances, as well as reaction and degradation products formed during the manufacture and use of the material. While IAS are evaluated by EFSA and regulated at the EU level (23), the safety assessment of NIAS is not harmonised and is left to the responsibility of the industry (24).

In 2016, EFSA published an opinion entitled *Recent developments in the risk assessment of chemicals in food and their potential impact on the safety assessment of substances used in food contact materials* (25). In the version of the Guidance valid at that time for applications for new FCM substances, exposure was evaluated from migration data by using conventional assumptions. The higher the migration, the greater the amount of toxicity data required.

The 2016 opinion referred to new risk assessment tools. One major area revisited was consumer exposure, which could be assessed by using EFSA's Comprehensive European Food Consumption Database and figures set by the WHO for infants. The opinion also opened the door to the use of TTC thresholds and read-across, especially for NIAS.

Surprisingly, in 2017, none of these new approaches were introduced in the update of the old FCM guidance for the evaluation of additives and monomers (intentionally added). The word 'exposure' is hardly mentioned, whereas 'TTC' and 'threshold' are not mentioned at all in this updated guidance. In the introduction, however, it is mentioned that the 2016 opinion is a scientific reference to be considered for the safety evaluation of nanomaterials and of NIAS that may migrate from FCM.

According to the EU legislation (26), NIAS must be assessed *in accordance with internationally recognised scientific principles on risk assessment*. Apparently, there is no agreement yet on these 'recognised principles'. Looking to the future, the use of exposure considerations and the TTC approach represents a scientifically robust opportunity.

3.5 Contaminants in the Food Chain

An example of the regulatory use of the TTC approach for contaminants is illustrated by the evaluation of *Alternaria* toxins (produced by fungi that attack crops). These were divided into five different classes, based on their chemical structures. As there were few to no data on the toxicity of several substances, application of the TTC approach (27) led to the conclusion that genotoxicity data should be generated (28).

3.6 Pesticides and Their Metabolites

In practice, the consumer is exposed not only to pesticide active substance residues but also to a range of metabolites for which limited toxicity information is usually available. In 2012, the EFSA Panel on Plant Protection Products and the Residues (PPR Panel) developed an Opinion on non-testing approaches, including TTC, to evaluate the toxicological relevance of such metabolites in dietary risk assessment (29). The TTC values recommended by EFSA (15) for genotoxic and toxic compounds (Table 2) were found to be sufficiently conservative for chronic exposure. Assessment schemes for chronic and acute dietary risk assessment of pesticide metabolites, involving the use of the TTC approach combined with QSAR and read-across, were proposed. Tentative TTC values for acute exposure were also established. It was anticipated that, on many occasions, further testing would be needed to reach a firm conclusion on the toxicological relevance of the metabolites. However, the benefit of applying the approach is that it will permit the prioritisation of metabolites for subsequent testing.

Building on its Opinion, EFSA subsequently published guidance on the assessment of pesticide residues (30), which describes a stepwise and weight-of-evidence approach based on toxicological and metabolism data, as well as the use of non-testing methods (QSAR, read-across, TTC). In this guidance, the TTC approach serves to complement, rather than supersede, the use of substance-specific toxicological data.

3.7 Residues of Pharmacologically Active Substances in Food

In 2013, the EFSA Panel on Contaminants in the Food Chain (CONTAM) established guidance on the principles and methods to be taken into account when establishing Reference Points for Action for non-allowed pharmacologically active substances present in food of animal origin (31). CONTAM considered that the TTC approach, with the use of Cramer classes, was not applicable for deriving Toxicological Screening Values (TSVs) for two reasons: (a) some groups of substances (e.g. steroids) are excluded from the TTC approach (15); and (b) the traditional TTC database only contains a small number of pharmacologically active substances.

Therefore, to derive TSV values, CONTAM used a distribution of 167 Acceptable Daily Intake (ADI) values of pharmacologically active substances collected by the European Medicines Agency (EMA). The corresponding TSV values are given in Table 4 (31).

TABLE 4 Assignment of Toxicological Screening Values for Non-allowed Pharmacologically Active Substances in Food (31)

	Can Genotoxicity Be Excluded?	Does the Substance Act Pharmacologically on the Nervous or Reproductive System and/or Is It a Corticoid?	Toxicological Screening Value (TSV) (µg/kg bw per day)
Group I	NO		0.0025
Group II	YES	YES	0.0042
Group III	YES	NO	0.65

The TTC approach has also been applied to pharmaceutical substances found as contaminants in treated wastewater used for the irrigation of root crops (32, 33).

3.8 The Polemics of TTC

3.8.1 The Perception of TTC as 'an Industry-Driven Approach'

The strongest criticisms of the TTC approach, and particularly EFSA's role in developing it, have come from Pesticide Action Network Europe (PAN Europe), who stated (34):

A new PAN Europe report reveals that 10 out of 13 members of the EFSA working group on TTC have a conflict of interest. TTC is an industry-driven approach and these members have been developing or promoting this method in the past jointly with industry. The interlinking of these people shows they are operating as a network.

While the second author of the current chapter was 'not evaluated', it was claimed that 'there is a strange connection with the JRC, EFSA and Nestlé on QSAR and TTC' on the grounds that the three institutions co-authored a paper (35). This statement was followed by a series of highly personal attacks against prominent EFSA scientists. An opinion piece was published with some other organisations (36), which presented very weak scientific arguments.

3.8.2 Endocrine Disruptors and Non-Monotonic Dose–Response Relationships

One of the criticisms of the TTC approach is that it does not take into account the potential low-dose effects of endocrine-active substances (34). According to the low-dose hypothesis, endocrine-active substances or endocrine disruptors may cause adverse effects at low doses but not necessarily at all higher doses.

To date, no scientific consensus has been reached on the existence of this low-dose phenomenon (37, 38). Both the EFSA Scientific Committee (15) and the PPR Panel (29) considered that the applicability of the TTC approach should be re-evaluated, when there is consensus on how to assess endocrine disruptor activity and once an EU-wide approach for defining and assessing endocrine disrupters has been finalised.

4. SCIENTIFIC AND TECHNICAL DEVELOPMENTS

There has been growing scientific interest in the further development of the TTC approach, which can be attributed in part to an increasing consideration by regulatory bodies such as EFSA (15) and the EU's non-food scientific committees (39).

As described above, the TTC values for different endpoints were derived on a probabilistic basis by using purpose-built data sets. Therefore, the coverage, quality and treatment of the underlying data have an impact on the resulting TTC values. For this reason, there have been numerous attempts to expand the coverage, improve the quality and enhance the consistency and transparency of data treatment in the TTC databases. Scientific developments have also focused on improving the classifiers used to identify genotoxic carcinogens and non-genotoxic chemicals, on developing QSAR models for repeat-dose toxicity and carcinogenicity, and on developing software tools to implement these predictive approaches.

The pace of these developments, which has resulted in the increasing availability of diverse methods and tools, has led to calls for the establishment of regulatory guidelines to prevent TTC from 'dis-harmonisation' (40).

4.1 Improvement of TTC Databases and Their Use to Refine TTC Values

4.1.1 Carcinogens

An electronic version of the CPDB was first made publicly available by EFSA (41), facilitating further analyses of the data. The current (July 2017) version of the CPDB contains 1547 chemicals (positive and negative carcinogenicity results) and is publicly accessible from the US National Institutes of Health.

It has been argued that the original TTC value for cancer was derived by using toxicological data and making assumptions that no longer reflect the state-of-the-science (42). With a view to addressing the concerns, the CPDB is currently being expanded and curated in a project funded by the European Chemical Industry Council Long-Range Initiative (CEFIC LRI).

4.1.2 Non-Carcinogens With Repeat-Dose Toxicity

The original TTC database was an appendix to a Munro's paper (11), and an electronic version of the Munro database was first made publicly available by EFSA (41).

A considerable development was later made by Chihae Yang and collaborators in the context of the EU-funded COSMOS project. To explore the applicability of the TTC approach to cosmetics (43, 44), the COSMOS TTC database contained 552 cosmetics-related chemicals. This database was then combined with an updated version of the Munro database to provide an expansion of chemical space (966 substances). The combined COSMOS-Munro TTC database is the largest quality controlled TTC database to have been made publicly available.

Even though the different TTC databases were designed to include chemicals having specific use categories (food additives, food contaminants, cosmetics, industrial chemicals), chemoinformatic analyses of the coverage of structural features and physicochemical properties have elucidated similarities and differences in the chemical space covered between different types of chemicals, such as food-related and cosmetics-related substances (45, 46).

4.1.3 Challenges to the Munro Threshold Values

There have been several challenges to the Munro threshold values, especially for Cramer Class III (47). The argument is that the threshold for Class III was originally determined with carbamates and organophosphates included in this class. Later, these substances were moved into separate classes leading several authors, including Munro himself (48), to recalculate the Class III threshold and propose revised threshold values up to 600 μg/day (48−50). These proposals have not been adopted by EFSA or the WHO, as a major modification of the TTC threshold values would reduce the conservatism of the TTC approach.

A number of studies have evaluated the reliability (adequacy of protection) of the TTC thresholds, where reliability is defined as the percentage of substances having an ADI larger than their TTC values in a given database. In a study on 845 FCM substances, comparison of the TDI values with TTC values revealed that the TTC values were protective for (lower than) 96% of the TDIs based on chemical-specific assessments (51). Similarly, in a study on 328 pesticides that had been fully evaluated, the current Class III threshold of 90 μg/person per day was found to provide a reliability of 97.5% (52). These types of study have also identified specific substances that have been 'underevaluated' by the TTC approach (43, 51−54). The accumulation of such examples has allowed common structural features to be identified and thus to flag the chemical structures which may be 'underevaluated' by use of the TTC approach. However, these proposed refinements of the Cramer tree have yet to gain widespread acceptance.

4.2 Defining Endpoint-Specific TTC Values

Attempts have been made to determine endpoint-specific TTC values, and in particular, for reproductive and development toxicity endpoints. van Ravenzwaay et al. (55) used a database built by using REACH and industry (BASF) data, without allocating the substances to Cramer classes. The calculated endpoint-specific TTC values are the range of 100 μg/person per day for developmental toxicity, depending slightly on the tested animal species (rats or rabbits). These findings are consistent with previous findings, which support the view that reproductive and development toxicity effects are covered by the Munro threshold for Cramer Class III (e.g. Refs. (56, 57)).

4.3 Development of New Structural Alerts and Prediction Models

4.3.1 Carcinogens

A failure to identify high-potency carcinogens and genotoxic substances will lead to false negatives (underestimated toxicity) and a non-conservative evaluation. Therefore, with the aim of increasing the sensitivity (minimising the false negative rate) of the TTC approach, the EFSA PPR Panel proposed the application of a suite of computational methods, involving structural alerts, QSAR and read-across, as a complement to the TTC approach in the assessment scheme for pesticide-metabolite exposure (29). Since the original publication of structural alerts by Ashby and Tennant (7), research efforts have focused on the development of new approaches (alerts and QSARs) for predicting DNA-reactivity (58), genotoxicity and carcinogenicity (59, 60) and repeat-dose toxicity (61).

4.3.2 Non-Carcinogens With Repeat-Dose Toxicity

The EFSA Scientific Committee (15) recommended that the Cramer classification scheme should be revised in the short term, to make it easier to understand and to use. In the longer term, it recommended the development of new structure-based classification schemes that are more discriminating between substances with different toxic potencies. An EFSA-sponsored project showed the potential use of multivariate statistical methods to uncover new structural features that may be useful in setting human exposure thresholds (41). Subsequent work in the COSMOS project developed structural features for liver toxicants (45, 62) and for chemicals acting by various mechanisms, including mitochondrial toxicity (63) and phospholipidosis (64). In addition to structural alerts, QSAR models have been developed to predict the potency of repeat-dose effects directly (e.g. Ref. (65)).

4.3.3 Introduction of Biokinetics

There have also been attempts to amend the Cramer decision tree by introducing the consideration of metabolism. In practice, questions on metabolism were already included in several questions of the Cramer decision tree. The relevant questions were slightly reformulated following the EFSA-WHO workshop (16).

A current project funded by Cosmetics Europe is seeking to further refine the TTC approach, by introducing the concept of an internal TTC (as opposed to external exposure limits), and to explore the utility of QSAR and biokinetic modelling to establish internal TTC values (66). If successful, this will provide a more-sophisticated means of assessing various sources of uncertainty in extrapolation.

4.4 Computational Tools for TTC Analysis

While the Cramer classification tree undoubtedly served to improve consistency between the toxicological evaluations made by different experts, its original paper-based application presupposed a degree of expert judgement and subjectivity. Therefore, following a recommendation made in a JRC workshop (67), the JRC commissioned the development of Toxtree, a software to facilitate the consistent application of the Cramer scheme. Toxtree was made freely downloadable from the JRC website and subsequently from Sourceforge. This was the first time a computational implementation of the Cramer tree had been put in the public domain. Subsequently, several additional TTC-relevant rulebases were added, including the Cramer rulebase with extensions (five extra rules to correct for some false negative classifications) and the decision tree of Kroes *et al.* (13). The Toxtree implementation of the Cramer scheme has been evaluated in several studies (53, 68) and has also been compared with the later implementation in the OECD QSAR Toolbox (69, 70).

In addition to these structure-based classification tools, models for predicting the potency of repeat-dose effects (i.e. NOAELs, LOAELs) have been developed and made freely available in the VEGA software suite (65).

5. CONCLUSIONS

The current TTC approach, based on the assessment of both cancer and non-cancer endpoints, is based on around 50 years of experience and is widely considered to be protective of human health for low-level exposure scenarios. The approach integrates data from hundreds of chemicals on which extensive information is available on chemical structure, metabolism and toxicity. With developments in science and technology, many refinements to the TTC approach have been proposed in the scientific literature. These refinements are based on the establishment of larger and better curated toxicological databases, improved knowledge on the relationship between toxicity and chemical features and physicochemical properties.

For the most part, however, these refinements have not translated into regulatory practice. A possible reason for this is that the TTC approach is applied differently in different sectors, and there is no mechanism at the international level to evaluate and harmonise these variants of the TTC approach. A useful step toward harmonisation was made by the FDA, EFSA and the WHO. In the future, a comprehensive and systematic analysis of the underlying uncertainties will permit a more-transparent elucidation of the differences between different implementations of the TTC approach. This is the focus of a project initiated in 2017 by ILSI Europe. Furthermore, there is considerable opportunity to further integrate QSARs (71–73) and mechanistic *in vitro* tests (74) into the TTC approach. Ultimately, an international organisation will be needed to 'champion' these harmonisation efforts.

At the time of publication (late 2018), EFSA was completing a guidance document on the TTC approach, as a follow-up to its 2012 Opinion.

REFERENCES

1. Hartung, T. (2017). Thresholds of toxicological concern – setting a threshold for testing below which there is little concern. *ALTEX* **34**, 331–351.
2. Frawley, J.P. (1967). Scientific evidence and common sense as a basis for food-packaging regulations. *Food and Cosmetics Toxicology* **5**, 293–308.
3. Oser, B.L. & Hall, R.L. (1977). Criteria employed by the expert panel of FEMA for the GRAS evaluation of flavouring substances. *Food and Cosmetics Toxicology* **15**, 457–466.
4. Cramer, G.M., Ford, R.A. & Hall, R.L. (1978). Estimation of toxic hazard – a decision tree approach. *Food and Cosmetics Toxicology* **16**, 255–276.
5. Machuga, E.J., Pauli, G.H. & Rulis, A.M. (1992). A threshold of regulation policy for food-contact articles. *Food Control* **34**, 180–182.
6. Gold, L.S., Sawyer, C.B., Magaw, R., *et al.* (1984). A carcinogenic potency database of the standardized results of animal bioassays. *Environmental Health Perspectives* **58**, 9–319.
7. Ashby, J. & Tennant, R.W. (1991). Definitive relationships among chemical structure, carcinogenicity and mutagenicity for 301 chemicals tested by the U.S. NTP. *Mutation Research* **257**, 229–306.
8. Cheeseman, M.A., Machuga, E.J. & Bailey, A.B. (1999). A tiered approach to threshold of regulation. *Food and Chemical Toxicology* **37**, 387–412.
9. Munro, I.C. (1990). Safety assessment procedures for indirect food additives: an overview. Report of a workshop. *Regulatory Toxicology and Pharmacology* **12**, 2–12.
10. FDA. (1995). Food additives: Threshold of regulation for substances used in food-contact articles; final rule. *Federal Register* **60**, 36582–36596.
11. Munro, I.C., Ford, R.A., Kennepohl, E., *et al.* (1996). Correlation of structural class with no-observed-effect levels: A proposal for establishing a threshold of concern. *Food and Chemical Toxicology* **34**, 829–867.
12. WHO. (1997). *Evaluation of Certain Food Additives and Contaminants. Forty-sixth Report of the Joint FAO/WHO Expert Committee on Food Additives*. WHO Technical Report Series, No. 868, 69pp. Geneva, Switzerland: WHO.
13. Kroes, R., Renwick, A.G., Cheeseman, M.A., *et al.* (2004). Structure-based thresholds of toxicological concern (TTC): Guidance for application to substances present at low levels in the diet. *Food and Chemical Toxicology* **42**, 65–83.
14. Kroes, R., Renwick, A.G., Feron, V., *et al.* (2007). Application of the threshold of toxicological concern (TTC) to the safety evaluation of cosmetic ingredients. *Food and Chemical Toxicology* **45**, 2533–2562.
15. EFSA. (2012). Scientific opinion on exploring options for providing advice about possible human health risks based on the concept of threshold of toxicological concern (TTC). *EFSA Journal* **10**(2750), 103.
16. EFSA & WHO. (2016). Review of the threshold of toxicological concern (TTC) approach and development of new TTC decision tree. *EFSA Supporting Publication* **13**(1006), 50.
17. EFSA. (2017). Guidance on the risk assessment of substances present in food intended for infants below 16 weeks of age. *EFSA Journal* **15**(4849), 58.
18. EC. (1996). Regulation (EC) No 2232/96 of the European Parliament and of the Council of 28 October 1996 laying down a Community Procedure for flavouring substances used or intended for use in or on foodstuffs. *Official Journal of the European Communities* **L299**, 1–4.
19. EU. (2012). Commission Implementing Regulation (EU) No 872/2012 of 1 October 2012 adopting the list of flavouring substances provided for by Regulation (EC) No 2232/96 of the European Parliament and of the Council, introducing it in Annex I to Regulation (EC) No 1334/2008 of the European Parliament and of the Council and repealing Commission Regulation (EC) No 1565/2000 and Commission Decision 1999/217/EC. *Official Journal of the European Union* **L267**, 120–125.
20. SCF. (1999). *Opinion on a Programme for the Evaluation of Flavouring Substances (Expressed on 2 December 1999). Scientific Committee for Food*. SCF/CS/FLAV/TASK/11 Final 6/12/1999, 10pp. Luxembourg: European Commission.
21. Engel, K.-H., Feigenbaum, A., Lhuguenot, J.-C., *et al.* (2012). Food contact materials, flavouring substances and smoke flavourings, 8pp. *EFSA Journal* **10**, s1007
22. EFSA. (2010). Guidance on the data required for the risk assessment of flavourings to be used in or on foods. *EFSA Journal* **8**(1623), 53.
23. SCF. (2001). *Guidelines of the Scientific Committee on Food for the Presentation of an Application for Safety Assessment of a Substance to be Used in Food Contact Materials Prior to Its Authorisation. Scientific Committee on Food*. SCF/CS/PLEN/GEN/100 Final, 6pp. Luxembourg: European Commission.
24. EFSA. (2012). Report of ESCO WG on non-plastic Food Contact Materials. *EFSA Supporting Publication* **139**, 63.

25. EFSA. (2016). Recent developments in the risk assessment of chemicals in food and their potential impact on the safety assessment of substances used in food contact materials. *EFSA Journal* **14**(4357), 28.

26. EU. (2011). Commission Regulation (EU) No 10/2011 of 14 January 2011 on plastic materials and articles intended to come into contact with food. *Official Journal of the European Union* **L12/1**, 15.1.2011.

27. Alexander, J., Benford, D., Boobis, A., *et al.* (2012). Risk assessment of contaminants in food and feed, 12pp *EFSA Journal* **10**, s1004.

28. EFSA. (2011). Scientific Opinion on the risks for animal and public health related to the presence of *Alternaria* toxins in feed and food. *EFSA Journal* **9**(2407), 97.

29. EFSA. (2012). Scientific Opinion on evaluation of the toxicological relevance of pesticide metabolites for dietary risk assessment. *EFSA Journal* **10**(2799), 187.

30. EFSA. (2016). Guidance on the establishment of the residue definition for dietary risk assessment. *EFSA Journal* **14**(4549), 129.

31. EFSA. (2013). Guidance on methodological principles and scientific methods to be taken into account when establishing Reference Points for Action (RPAs) for non-allowed pharmacologically active substances present in food of animal origin. *EFSA Journal* **11**(3195), 24.

32. Malchi, T., Maor, Y., Tadmor, G., *et al.* (2014). Irrigation of root vegetables with treated wastewater: evaluating uptake of pharmaceuticals and the associated human health risks. *Environmental Science & Technology* **48**, 9325–9333.

33. Riemenschneider, C., Al-Raggad, M., Moeder, M., *et al.* (2016). Pharmaceuticals, their metabolites, and other polar pollutants in field-grown vegetables irrigated with treated municipal wastewater. *Journal of Agricultural and Food Chemistry* **64**, 5784–5792.

34. PAN Europe. (2011). *A toxic Mixture? Industry Bias Found in EFSA Working Group on Risk Assessment for Toxic Chemicals*, 28pp. Brussels, Belgium: Pesticide Action Network Europe.

35. Lo Piparo, E., Worth, A., Manibusan, M., *et al.* (2011). Use of computational tools in the field of food safety. *Regulatory Toxicology and Pharmacology* **60**, 354–362.

36. Buonsante, V.A., Muilerman, H., Santos, T., *et al.* (2014). Risk assessment's insensitive toxicity testing may cause it to fail. *Environmental Research* **135**, 139–147.

37. EFSA. (2012). *EFSA's 17th Scientific Colloquium on Low Dose Response in Toxicology and Risk Assessment*. Summary Report EFSA Scientific Colloquium 17, 64pp. Parma, Italy: EFSA.

38. EFSA. (2013). Scientific opinion on the hazard assessment of endocrine disruptors: scientific criteria for identification of endocrine disruptors and appropriateness of existing test methods for assessing effects mediated by these substances on human health and the environment. *EFSA Journal* **11**(3132), 84.

39. SCCS. (2012). *Opinion on Use of the Threshold of Toxicological Concern (TTC) Approach for Human Safety Assessment of Chemical Substances With Focus on Cosmetics and Consumer Products. Joint Opinion of the Scientific Committee on Consumer Safety (SCCS), the Scientific Committee on Health and Environmental Risks (SCHER) and the Scientific Committee on Emerging and Newly Identified Health Risks (SCENIHR)*. SCCP/1171/08, 56pp. Luxembourg: European Commission.

40. Schrenk, D. (2016). Threshold of toxicological concern. *Toxicology Letters* **259**, S64–S65.

41. Bassan, A., Fioravanzo, E., Pavan, M., *et al.* (2011). Applicability of physicochemical data, QSARs and read-across in Threshold of Toxicological Concern assessment. *EFSA Supporting Publication* **8**(159), 745.

42. Boobis, A., Brown, P., Cronin, M.T.D., *et al.* (2017). Origin of the TTC values for compounds that are genotoxic and/or carcinogenic and an approach for their re-evaluation. *Critical Reviews in Toxicology*, 1–23.

43. Worth, A., Cronin, M., Enoch, S., *et al.* (2012). *Applicability of the Threshold of Toxicological Concern (TTC) Approach to Cosmetics – Preliminary Analysis*. JRC Report EUR 25162, 40pp.

44. Yang, C., Barlow, S.M., Muldoon Jacobs, K.L., *et al.* (2017). Thresholds of toxicological concern of cosmetics-related substances: New database, thresholds and enrichment of chemical space. *Food and Chemical Toxicology* **109**, 170–193.

45. Mostrag-Szlichtyng, A. (2017). *Development of Knowledge Within a Chemical-Toxicological Database to Formulate Novel Computational Approaches for Predicting Repeated Dose Toxicity of Cosmetics-Related Compounds* (Ph.D. thesis), 162pp. Liverpool, UK: Liverpool John Moores University.

46. Karmaus, A.L., Filer, D.L., Martin, M.T., *et al.* (2016). Evaluation of food-relevant chemicals in the ToxCast high-throughput screening program. *Food and Chemical Toxicology* **92**, 188–196.

47. Renwick, A. (2005). Structure-based thresholds of toxicological concern—guidance for application to substances present at low levels in the diet. *Toxicology and Applied Pharmacology* **207**, 585–591.

48. Munro, I.C., Renwick, A.G. & Danielewska-Nikiel, B. (2008). The threshold of toxicological concern (TTC) in risk assessment. *Toxicology Letters* **180**, 151–156.

49. Koster, S., Rennen, M., Leeman, W., *et al.* (2014). A novel safety assessment strategy for non-intentionally added substances (NIAS) in carton food contact materials. *Food Additives & Contaminants: Part A* **31**, 422–443.

50. Leeman, W.R., Krul, L. & Houben, G.F. (2014). Reevaluation of the Munro dataset to derive more specific TTC thresholds. *Regulatory Toxicology and Pharmacology* **69**, 273–278.

51. Pinalli, R., Croera, C., Theobald, A., *et al.* (2011). Threshold of toxicological concern approach for the risk assessment of substances used for the manufacture of plastic food contact materials. *Trends in Food Science & Technology* **22**, 523–534.

52. Feigenbaum, A., Pinalli, R., Giannetto, M., *et al.* (2015). Reliability of the TTC approach: Learning from inclusion of pesticide active substances in the supporting database. *Food and Chemical Toxicology* **75**, 24–38.

53. Lapenna, S. & Worth, A. (2011). *Analysis of the Cramer Classification Scheme for Oral Systemic Toxicity - Implications for Its Implementation in Toxtree*. JRC Report EUR 24898, 39pp.

54. Tluczkiewicz, I., Buist, H.E., Martin, M.T., *et al.* (2011). Improvement of the Cramer classification for oral exposure using the database TTC RepDose—a strategy description. *Regulatory Toxicology and Pharmacology* **61**, 340−350.

55. van Ravenzwaay, B., Jiang, X., Luechtefeld, T., *et al.* (2017). The Threshold of Toxicological Concern for prenatal developmental toxicity in rats and rabbits. *Regulatory Toxicology and Pharmacology* **88**, 157−172.

56. Laufersweiler, M.C., Gadagbui, B., Baskerville-Abraham, I.M., *et al.* (2012). Correlation of chemical structure with reproductive and developmental toxicity as it relates to the use of the threshold of toxicological concern. *Regulatory Toxicology and Pharmacology* **62**, 160−182.

57. Gatnik, M.F. (2016). *Computational Methods in Support of Chemical Risk Assessment* (Ph.D. thesis), 184pp. Liverpool, UK: Liverpool John Moores University.

58. Enoch, S.J. & Cronin, M.T.D. (2012). Development of new structural alerts suitable for chemical category formation for assigning covalent and non-covalent mechanisms relevant to DNA binding. *Mutation Research: Genetic Toxicology and Environmental Mutagenesis* **743**, 10−19.

59. Benigni, R., Bossa, C., Jeliazkova, N., *et al.* (2008). *The Benigni/Bossa Rulebase for Mutagenicity and Carcinogenicity − a Module of Toxtree*. JRC Report EUR 23241, 75pp.

60. Benigni, R. & Bossa, C. (2011). Mechanisms of chemical carcinogenicity and mutagenicity: a review with implications for predictive toxicology. *Chemical Reviews* **111**, 2507−2536.

61. Schüürmann, G., Ebert, R.-U., Tluczkiewicz, I., *et al.* (2016). Inhalation threshold of toxicological concern (TTC) — Structural alerts discriminate high from low repeated-dose inhalation toxicity. *Environment International* **88**, 123−132.

62. Hewitt, M., Enoch, S.J., Madden, J.C., *et al.* (2013). Hepatotoxicity: A scheme for generating chemical categories for read-across, structural alerts and insights into mechanism(s) of action. *Critical Reviews in Toxicology* **43**, 537−558.

63. Nelms, M.D., Ates, G., Madden, J.C., *et al.* (2015). Proposal of an in silico profiler for categorisation of repeat dose toxicity data of hair dyes. *Archives of Toxicology* **89**, 733−741.

64. Przybylak, K.R., Alzahrani, A.R. & Cronin, M.T.D. (2014). How does the quality of phospholipidosis data influence the predictivity of structural alerts? *Journal of Chemical Information and Modeling* **54**, 2224−2232.

65. Benfenati, E., Como, F., Manzo, M., *et al.* (2017). Developing innovative in silico models with EFSA's OpenFoodTox database. *EFSA Supporting Publication* **14**(1206), 19.

66. Partosch, F., Mielke, H., Stahlmann, R., *et al.* (2015). Internal threshold of toxicological concern values: enabling route-to-route extrapolation. *Archives of Toxicology* **89**, 941−948.

67. Gallegos, A., Patlewicz, G. & Worth, A.P. (2005). *A Similarity Based Approach for Chemical Category Classification*. JRC Report EUR 21867, 42pp.

68. Patlewicz, G., Jeliazkova, N., Safford, R.J., *et al.* (2008). An evaluation of the implementation of the Cramer classification scheme in the Toxtree software. *SAR and QSAR in Environmental Research* **19**, 495−524.

69. Bhatia, S., Schultz, T., Roberts, D., *et al.* (2015). Comparison of Cramer classification between Toxtree, the OECD QSAR Toolbox and expert judgment. *Regulatory Toxicology and Pharmacology* **71**, 52−62.

70. Roberts, D.W., Aptula, A., Schultz, T.W., *et al.* (2015). A practical guidance for Cramer class determination. *Regulatory Toxicology and Pharmacology* **73**, 971−984.

71. Brown, R., Carter, J., Dewhurst, I., *et al.* (2009). *Applicability of Thresholds of Toxicological Concern in the Dietary Risk Assessment of Metabolites, Degradation and Reaction Products of Pesticides. Scientific Report Submitted to the EFSA*. CFP/EFSA/PPR/2008/01, 146pp. London, UK: Chemicals Regulation Directorate, Health & Safety Executive.

72. Worth, A., Fuart-Gatnik, M., Lapenna, S., *et al.* (2011). Applicability of QSAR analysis to the evaluation of the toxicological relevance of metabolites and degradates of pesticide active substances for dietary risk assessment. *EFSA Supporting Publication* **8**(169E), 311.

73. Schilter, B., Benigni, R., Boobis, A., *et al.* (2013). Establishing the level of safety concern for chemicals in food without the need for toxicity testing. *Regulatory Toxicology and Pharmacology* **68**, 275−296.

74. Blaauboer, B.J., Boobis, A.R., Bradford, B., *et al.* (2016). Considering new methodologies in strategies for safety assessment of foods and food ingredients. *Food and Chemical Toxicology* **91**, 19−35.

Chapter 3.5

A Replacement Perspective on Inhalation Toxicology

Robert D. Combes[1] and Michael Balls[2]

[1]Independent Consultant, Norwich, United Kingdom; [2]University of Nottingham, Nottingham, United Kingdom

SUMMARY

In vivo inhalation methods for respiratory toxicity and disease in laboratory animals are time-consuming, technically demanding and of doubtful relevance for predicting effects in humans. They can also cause great suffering to the animals used. Fortunately, there has been increasing interest in developing *in vitro* alternatives. They can greatly simplify exposure and dosimetry, while using human cell lines and primary cells representative of all the cell types of the conducting airways. Maintained on membranes, fed basally and exposed apically at the air–liquid interface, the cells retain their *in vivo*-like properties long enough for even chronic exposure and response studies to be undertaken. The predictive performance of several models is showing encouraging signs of improvement, especially when undertaken in conjunction with the latest airway particle deposition and gaseous exchange algorithms. Additional improvements in test substance delivery, automation and miniaturisation continue to be made. However, there needs to be more guidance and harmonisation applied to: (a) exposure modelling; (b) the need for exogenous metabolic activation; and (c) the use of positive and negative controls. With levels of inhalation testing and pulmonary diseases increasing, the need to expedite validation is now urgent. There are signs that the necessary dialogue and cooperation between the principal stakeholders is starting to occur, but regulatory authorities need to take the initiative to ensure that 'actions speak louder than words'.

1. INTRODUCTION

There are sound logistical, scientific and animal welfare-related reasons why inhalation research and testing on laboratory animals needs to be replaced by alternative approaches, without delay.

The *in vivo* techniques for exposure and dosimetry are time-consuming, technically demanding, and suffer from unavoidable and inherent inaccuracies, in addition to the overriding need in toxicity testing in general for interspecies extrapolation. This is further confounded when inhalation is involved by pronounced interspecies differences in facial anatomy and other major respiratory anatomical and physiological parameters, including the breathing process itself and the extent of inhalation. In addition, where long periods of restraint are required, stress could well become a limiting factor, despite the practice of animal training prior to dosing. Animal welfare concerns also include the requirement, in some studies (e.g. on drug dependence), for the use of companion animals and non-human primates (NHPs), as well as some transgenic rodent strains.

It is not possible to avoid inhaling many kinds of substances in the air we breathe, and there is increasing concern about air pollution, especially in large cities with heavy car traffic. Recent press reports suggest that German car-makers have been testing diesel exhaust emissions on NHPs in poorly designed experiments of little merit, apparently aimed at showing that such emissions are not a significant risk to human health (1, 2).

One of the earliest discussions about alternative methods in inhalation toxicology took place at the Royal Society in London on 1–3 November 1982, at a meeting held to discuss the report of the FRAME Toxicity Committee (3).

David Clark introduced the topic as one of particular importance, as we are likely to inhale 250 million litres of air as we pass from the cradle to the grave, Robert Brown reviewed the availability and use of alternatives, then the two of them made the following four recommendations: (a) any inhalation toxicity study should begin with thinking in the human brain: 'Is this study really necessary?'; 'Has the work been done before?'; and 'Can possible toxic responses be predicted from the molecular structures and physical properties of the chemicals to be tested?'; (b) where good alternatives exist, they should be used; (c) if animal experiments are inevitable, the minimum number of animals should be used; and (d) more research should be done to validate promising *in vitro* tests. There then followed a discussion with Alastair Worden, founder of Huntingdon Research Centre, as rapporteur. These four recommendations could (still) be usefully applied to many other aspects of toxicology.

Also, there is increasing recognition of the value of using the respiratory route as an extremely efficient means of drug delivery, which has significant implications for drug discovery and toxicity testing. Similarly, the respiratory route is perceived as a means of delivering nicotine without the risks involved in conventional cigarette smoking, through, for example, the use of electronic cigarettes (ECs). Another important development is that the increasing use of carbon nanotubes (CNTs), which have many novel and useful properties, will lead to increased human exposure, not least by inhalation (4). This will require new approaches to toxicity testing, especially as CNTs appear to be potentially more toxic than other nanoparticles or larger fibres.

Fortunately, there has been considerable interest of late in the development of *in vitro* alternatives that greatly simplify exposure and dosimetry, while using all the human cell types found in the conducting airways that maintain their *in vivo*-like properties for extended periods in tissue culture long enough for even chronic exposure and response studies to be undertaken.

This chapter explains the rationale for developing *in vitro* alternatives for inhalation studies, and it briefly discusses how the field has developed, with the increasing complexity of the enabling technologies and of the methods involved in exposing organotypic human cells in culture systems to inhalable test materials. A generalised framework is presented for selecting the main study components and variables to maximise relevance and to optimise data extrapolation, and some suggestions are offered for the future work needed to facilitate validation and regulatory acceptance. Clinical testing has not been covered, but the principles are the same as those for new drugs (see 5, 6).

For more information, especially regarding practical details, the reader is referred to several reviews, some of which focus on specialised areas (7–12).

2. INHALATION STUDIES

2.1 Fulfilling a Need

Humans, at work and in the home, are constantly exposed to many diverse inhalable substances and complex mixtures, many of which need to be subjected to toxicity testing and safety evaluation in the same sorts of ways as those required for non-inhalable substances, according to product category and anticipated exposure levels. At present, these tests are predominantly conducted in animals, and, in common with most such methods, involve welfare issues and important scientific limitations, irrespective of the route of exposure, but which are particularly challenging when it is by inhalation.

Gases, volatiles, aerosols, dusts, smoke and exhaust fumes enter the body primarily via the respiratory route. Therefore, experimental exposure has to be via one of several techniques for inhalation, as is true for studies on the aetiology of respiratory-linked conditions, such as asthma, chronic obstructive pulmonary disease (COPD) and cardiovascular disease (CVD; 13).

2.2 Potential Target Cells for Inhalation Toxicity

Candidate sites in the airways for targeting by inhaled materials are related to the structure and function of the surfaces of the conducting airways (see 14). These are principally lined by bronchial epithelial cells, with cilia and mucus-producing goblet cells. In bronchioli, specialised epithelial Clara cells are found, which secrete a protein which modulates the inflammatory response, and, with olfactory cells of the nasal epithelium, act as the main sites of cytochrome P-450 (CYP) phase-I and phase-II biotransformation (15, 16). All epithelial cells reside on a basement membrane. Over-production of mucus can occur, due to a single mutation in the gene encoding the cystic fibrosis transmembrane conductance regulator. This is a membrane protein and chloride channel in vertebrates that is responsible for maintaining ion balance across epithelia (17).

A further cell secretion is surfactant, which is produced mainly by alveolar epithelial AT-II cells. It reduces surface tension, thereby facilitating transfer across the moist epithelial alveolar membrane to the endothelial layer of blood capillaries (18).

With the many advantages offered by *in vitro* methods, it is somewhat surprising that there has been such little involvement on the part of regulatory bodies in this area. In a review on inhalation toxicity, published by Dorato and Wolff in 1990 (19), there is no mention of the words '*in vitro*' or 'tissue culture', implying that, at that time, there was little or no use of non-animal methods in this area of safety testing. By 1996, the year of a European Centre for the Validation of Alternative Methods (ECVAM) workshop report on alternatives for respiratory toxicology (20), only sufficient information was known for a set of very general recommendations to be formulated, which can, with hindsight, be seen to have presaged, if not directly guided, subsequent phases in the development of inhalation toxicology. Key recommendations from the workshop included the following: *Toxicological appraisal should commence with a systematic evaluation of existing data, assessment of the physicochemical characteristics of the test material and the description of any structure-activity relationships....Cell lines need to be properly characterised to establish their usefulness as models of selected functions of the particular target cell of interest.... The use of primary cell cultures is encouraged to mimic as closely as possible the* in vivo *situation.... In vitro test systems maintaining appropriate biotransformation activities are essential.... Assays for cell viability and cell functionality need to be identified, optimised and validated for each cell type.* The situation at the time was such that the report also stated that *the use of cells isolated from laboratory animals, such as alveolar macrophages, Type II cells and Clara cells, is unavoidable at present.*

A similar situation was reflected in a review on inhalation toxicology, published in 2000 by Pauluhn and Mohr (21), in which the authors refer to the need sometimes to use different species as alternatives rather than *non-animal* alternatives.

2.3 General Drivers for Inhalation Studies

Several additional factors have driven the development of inhalation toxicology, including: (a) an increasing knowledge of the physicochemical properties of inhalable materials that affect their absorption, distribution, deposition and systemic circulation; (b) developments in exposure and dosimetry; (c) technological advances in the ability to isolate maintain, propagate and experiment on an ever-increasing diversity of cell types (22), particularly those obtainable as primary cells from human tissue banks; (d) the advent of new testing requirements due to the development of innovative products that require inhalation exposure, such as nanoparticles and reduced harm of smoking and tobacco-related products, and the need for the respective industries to demonstrate increased safety; and (e) legislation and ethical pressure in certain countries to avoid using animals for testing tobacco products and new cosmetic ingredients (see Ref. 23).

2.4 Scientific Limitations of the *In vivo* Methods

Each of the five basic types of *in vivo* inhalation toxicology exposure methods, namely, whole body, head only, nose only, lung only and partial lung, has its own unique set of advantages and disadvantages (14, 19, 21, 24, 25). For example, nose-only experiments are difficult to interpret due to interspecific variations in the physiology and anatomy of the respiratory tract, and other species-specific differences in breathing. Also, it is more difficult to measure the actual concentration at the target site after dosing an animal than it is during *in vitro* exposures. Furthermore, during whole-body exposure, differing portions of the dose applied enter the body via routes other than inhalation. The use of smoking machines is a crude approximation of the ways in which humans smoke, in terms of puff volume, dilution of each puff with air, tidal volume, rate of puffing and extent of inhalation.

With regard to *Refinement*, stress can be important whenever restraint is required, as it affects the welfare of the animals and could compromise the data obtained during the experiment. This a controversial area, especially concerning the alleged benefits of animal training, more-precisely referred to as positive reinforcement learning to engender cooperative behaviour (26). Inhalation studies are also conducted in relation to respiratory and associated conditions, such as CVD, which involve several important endpoints, like atherosclerosis, heart failure, hypertrophy, ischaemia, obesity, hyperlipidaemia, type 2 diabetes and insulin resistance (27).

3. NON-ANIMAL APPROACHES TO INHALATION TOXICITY AND RESPIRATORY DISEASE

3.1 Early Studies

Several papers involving animal cell lines, as well as alveolar macrophages, as targets, started to appear in print from 2000, together with studies on nanomaterials and publications describing *in vitro* models of respiratory disease (28–30), following the 1996 ECVAM workshop report (20).

Some of the first studies involved testing for bacterial mutagenicity by using modified Ames tests. At first, liquid pre-incubation protocols were altered to allow either aspiration with the test material or passive exposure by simply adding the test material to the pre-incubation mix. However, for gases, Dillon *et al.* (31) exposed the cells in a system which allowed the test material, at a range of concentrations in air, to have access to the cells, while preventing microbial contamination, with the whole system contained in desiccators inside incubators.

Early *in vitro* studies of the toxicity of volatiles, gases or dusts were undertaken by using either permanent cell lines or, more-rarely, primary cells, grown as monocultures in suspension in liquid media, through which the test substance, at different concentrations in the normal atmosphere used for tissue culturing, was bubbled (32). Genotoxicity and cyto-toxicity were endpoints in early experiments with mammalian cells. Such cultures were usually prepared in-house at that time. Also, there was great interest in modelling diseases such as COPD (33–35).

In 1997, Bombick *et al.* (36) published results obtained with a novel method for exposing cells directly to cigarette smoke introduced into a closed chamber containing open culture flasks, each with an adherent cell monolayer. To maintain cell viability, the culture flask was then placed on a rocking platform, where the cultures were exposed alternately to culture medium and the smoke/gas phase.

In another variant, called Cellular Smoke Exposure Technology, mainstream smoke from a smoke generator was diluted with a humidified high-efficiency particulate accumulation (HEPA) and charcoal-filtered air, and distributed to a two-tier exposure chamber originally designed for the nose-only exposure of animals (37).

3.2 Period of Transition to the Present

Inhalation toxicology was greatly influenced by the increasing commercialisation of systems for exposure, containment and dosimetry and the parallel marketing of reconstructed epithelial cell layer models, developed to satisfy the increasing demand, particularly for the *in vitro* testing of cosmetics (38).

Undoubtedly, the most significant innovation in *in vitro* inhalation toxicity testing was the idea to grow and expose cells on semi-porous filters at the air–liquid interface (ALI). Such transwell cultures were first used in permeability studies with intestinal Caco2 cells (39). Such bi-phasic cultures are supplied with fresh nutrients from below and retain their *in vivo*-like barrier functions and apical–basal orientation (40). One of the first commercially available systems, which involved exposure at the ALI, was CULTEX (41, 42), which was developed by using HFBE21 bronchial epithelial cells and LK004 human lung fibroblasts.

In vitro human cell-based models are now available for all the key endpoints and target sites of the respiratory system covered by the *in vivo* tests, as well as various disease conditions, including asthma and COPD.

At present, respiratory sensitisation is proving difficult to model satisfactorily, although progress is being achieved. Interestingly, this is an endpoint for which computational modelling models were first proposed in some detail in 1996 (43). Despite past studies with epithelial cells, macrophages and dendritic cells, and the fact that respiratory sensitisation was an endpoint included in the ECVAM-coordinated Sens-It-iv work programme, Rovida *et al.* (44) concluded, in their overall summary of the project, that: *Currently, there are no validated or widely recognized methods (animal or non-animal) for the identification of chemical respiratory allergens.* This was attributed, in part, to doubts over the immunological mechanisms involved.... In vitro *and* in silico *approaches inspire hope, but a lot of work and research has to be invested before coming to a conclusion.* The use of alveolar macrophages, particularly as targets for nanomaterials, is still actively being pursued (45).

3.3 Pattern of Progress

Over this period, therefore, there were several ongoing important developments in inhalation testing being progressed in parallel, starting with submerged cultures, usually of bacteria with mutagenicity as the endpoint (the Ames test in *Salmonella* as the indicator organism) to the use of human cell-derived organotypic cultures, maintained on filter inserts at the ALI, with continual improvements being made, especially to culture longevity (32).

The range of functional tests increased to meet the demand for a greater variety of cell types to act as target tissue. These assays were selected to be able to be measured in any cell type and in any type of culture system, including *in situ* in organotypic culture (e.g. UDS - unscheduled DNA synthesis), the Comet assay and micronucleus induction (see 46, 47). These assays were first applied to mono-culture, then to co-culture systems followed by 3-D tissue constructs. They can also be used with the 'lung-on-a-chip' system (see 48), developed by employing micro-lithography and micro-machining to result in a miniaturised device for modelling the responses of entire organ systems and to facilitate screening (49). Modifications to existing models have contributed to their gradual improvement, with respect to increasing longevity and viability, together with enhanced stability and recalcitrance to dedifferentiation, properties that hitherto had been limiting factors.

As these advances were being made, progress with dosimetry and dosing continued, especially with respect to automation, robotisation and greater design flexibility (provided by the availability of autoclavable strong plasticware). These features become increasingly important as the duration of experiments becomes longer.

3.4 Modelling Deposition, Uptake and Passage Across the Alveolar Gas-Blood System

A further key stage in the history of inhalation toxicology took place as greater understanding was gained of the physico-chemical factors influencing the passage of inhaled materials through, and deposition within, the conducting airways, and the ability to predict these phenomena by using simulation algorithms followed. However, this is a complex area, which probably remains the least transparent aspect of inhalation toxicity testing. For a much more-detailed account, the reader should consult Kleinstreur *et al.* (50), as well as Fröhlich *et al.* (51) and Crapo (52), plus other literature cited later on the effects of airway geometry, air-particle transport and simulation of the extent and uniformity of particle depositions.

Data from airway deposition modelling (ADM) and modelling of the partitioning and transfer of the gaseous phase across the alveolar blood–gaseous barrier are used to identify: (a) the proportion of the applied dose that enters the pulmonary blood system; and (b) the main sites where flow and passage through the airways is interrupted, and where greater deposition occurs than elsewhere, possibly to result in local effects (53–55). Such regions are known as 'hot-spots', which are potentially at greater risk from exposure than elsewhere.

Many factors have to be taken into account by the algorithms involved, including airway geometry, airflow rate air-particle transport and simulation of the extent and uniformity of particle depositions. In addition, tidal volume, breathing pattern and frequency, as well as the extent of inhalation, all need to be considered.

In their detailed review on nanoparticle toxicity testing, Fröhlich and Salar-Behzadi (14) identified the following mechanisms of particle deposition: *Large particles are subjected to inertial impaction, preferentially in large airways, smaller particles deposit by gravitational sedimentation and, for still smaller particles in the alveoli, deposition is by diffusion. Electrostatic deposition is seen for charged particles and interception for fibre-shaped particles.*

To make matters yet more complicated, single-path and multi-path models exist. A relatively straightforward example of the former type is a model that divides the respiratory system into three compartments as follows: (a) naso-otopharyngo-laryngeal; (b) tracheal-bronchial; and (c) alveolar. Multi-path models can become over-complex, when attempting to take all possible physicochemical factors into account.

The uptake and internalisation of different nanoparticles has been studied by scanning electron microscopy and confocal microscopy, in cultures of human epithelial cell lines, and in an immortalised cell line derived from primary tissue, as well as by live cell imaging by using scanning ion conductance microscopy (56).

Predictions from gas flow and blood–gas barrier modelling should be similar to those obtained by using an *in vitro*, alveolar–capillary barrier to test the substances of interest (57). It might, however, be appropriate to undertake ADM in addition, especially when the density of particulate matter in the test material is low.

The surfactant layer also needs to be modelled, as it can be damaged by chemicals (58), including impregnated spray-on pesticides, an observation that forms the basis for an *in vitro* test for such products (59).

3.5 Special Effects

Some exposures could possibly affect the epithelia of the conducting airways by specific mechanisms. One example is oxidative damage mediated by free radicals in conjunction with ultra-thin particles (e.g. nanoparticles). Interaction between the free radicals and nanoparticles generates reactive oxygen species (ROS), which induce oxidative damage and induction of the inflammatory cascade, which, in turn, could be linked to atherosclerosis if it occurred in the pulmonary capillary wall (60). These processes occur in smokers, and possibly in vapers, probably in the latter case due to the shedding of metal atoms of the heating element. This could account for the observation that EC vapour enhanced pneumococcal adherence to airway epithelial cells (61). The vapour increased both platelet-activating factor receptor (PAFR)-dependent pneumococcal adhesion to airway epithelial cells *in vitro*, and also pneumococcal colonisation in the mouse nasopharynx, as well as in the nasal epithelia in a small number of human volunteers (in comparison with un-exposed controls, or in the exposed group before treatment, used as internal controls). These effects were attributed to free radicals in the vapour, inducing oxidative stress in airway cells and increasing PAFR expression, with PAFR co-opted by pneumococci to adhere to host cells.

A further effect that can be induced by inhaling certain substances is squamous metaplasia (SM). This has been studied in organotypic models of the human tracheo–bronchial tract (TBT; 62). In common with other internal epithelial cell linings, the epithelium of the TBT is not normally terminally differentiated by keratinisation and cornification. However, these processes can be induced when SM occurs. Early markers of SM are the enzyme transglutaminase I (TGI) and involucrin. TGI is involved in cross-linking various proteins, including involucrin, with further keratinisation in cornified envelopes that arise with the induction of terminal differentiation.

The activity of TGI can be measured by the level of fluorescence incorporated into cornified envelopes by incubating epithelial preparations with fluorescein cadaverine, which acts as a substrate for the enzyme, in place of endogenous substrates. This forms the basis for an assay for inducers of SM, which itself is a condition that can ultimately result in squamous cell carcinoma.

4. MODELLING LONG-TERM EFFECTS

4.1 Sub-Chronic Toxicity

The use of an alternative for sub-chronic toxicity testing was described in a study (63), which entailed mice being exposed to nicotine-containing E-liquids, as vaporised in electronic cigarettes, for 1 h daily over 4 months. The exposures induced effects associated with the onset of COPD, including cytokine expression, airway hyper-reactivity and lung tissue destruction. The same results were obtained when normal human bronchial epithelial airway cells were cultured at the ALI and exposed to EC vapours or nicotine solutions by using a VITROCELL smoke exposure robot, a device described by Thorne *et al.* (64). This particular study is an illustration of parallel *in vivo–in vitro* testing.

4.2 Chronic Toxicity

In vitro modelling of longer-term chronic inhalation toxicity presents formidable technical challenges, especially with regard to the need for cultures to remain viable for extended periods. Epithelix has developed an *in vitro* cell model of the human airway epithelium (MucilAir; 65, 66), which can remain morphologically and functionally differentiated for over a year, exhibiting no abnormalities with respect to cilial activity, mucus production, endogenous levels of barrier function and CYP metabolising capacity. It is to be hoped that long-term data obtained by using MucilAir will be published in the near future, to enable the performance of the system to be evaluated.

5. SPECIAL CONSIDERATIONS

5.1 Biotransformation

If it is known, or strongly suspected, that the test material being investigated requires metabolic activation, then, whatever cell source and culture system is used, biotransforming capability should be fully characterised by using standard biochemical assays for mixed-function oxidase activity. If this is low, the addition of an exogenous source of metabolism should be considered (e.g. a postmitochondrial S9 fraction). If testing is for the rapid pre-screening of many candidates, when a low incidence of false positives can be tolerated, then the default source of the S9 fraction should be aroclor-induced rat liver. However, the enzymes induced in rats do not all have the same specific activities or substrate specificities as their counterparts which operate in humans, so, if the need is for a mechanistic study, consideration should be given to the possibility of using a human S9 fraction from the target tissue.

Precision-cut tissue slices have been used extensively for biotransformation studies, including slices derived from the lung (18), but their use in toxicology and disease studies is less well-documented. However, this might be about to change, with the appearance of a report that an *ex vivo* model of murine precision-cut lung tissue slices can be used to study *Mycobacterium tuberculosis* infections (67).

5.2 Controls

Controls are required to demonstrate that any resulting data are not false, and to comply with Good Laboratory Practice and Good Cell Culture Practice requirements. Ideally, negative controls should be HEPA-filtered air for smoke and dusts or charcoal-filtered air for non-particulates. The choice of control and diluent for testing nanoparticles should be another nanoparticle, which shares similar physicochemical properties to those of the test material, but which is inactive in the system and for the endpoint being investigated.

Positive controls should be selected according to the same criteria, except that they should be clearly positive in the system. Where the activity of the test sample is dependent on metabolic activation, two positive controls should be used. The first positive control consists of an S9 fraction, with the indirect-acting positive control chemical added to the reaction mix. The second positive control comprises the same reaction components, but without the indirect-acting positive control chemical. This must give a negative result to show that a positive with the test sample in the presence of the S9 fraction was not due to some spurious interaction of the enzyme mix with a component of the system, producing toxicity independently of the test material. The cytotoxicity of S9 fractions alone to certain cell lines is well-documented, and can itself be problematic.

All controls should be exposed and used in the same way as the test samples, and they should not interact with diluents, gases, vapours or aerosols.

6. VALIDATION

6.1 Need

In most cases, the use for regulatory purposes of the methods and techniques outlined in this chapter will require further characterisation, optimisation and standardisation, followed by their independent validation according to internationally agreed criteria to establish their relevance and reliability for their particular purposes (68). It might be possible to fast-track validation when the cell function assays, and the indicator cell component of the test method on which they are performed, have previously been validated for a protocol involving a different route of exposure.

The need for such further work and formal validation is now urgent, especially with newly introduced legislation in the USA, which requires the efficacy and safety testing of harm-reduction tobacco and tobacco-related products (23).

6.2 Assessing Predictive Performance

Surprisingly, one of the first attempts to assess the predictivity of in vitro inhalation toxicity methods (i.e. their relevance) was not published until 2002 (69). It was noted that the rankings from in vitro testing for pulmonary toxicity of diesel engine particulate extracts were poorly correlated with the order of toxicity obtained in in vivo experiments. Essentially similar disappointing results were obtained in another experiment concerning the relative toxicities of five different particulate preparations, ranging from 90 to 500 nm in size, when in vitro and in vivo data were compared (70). Because of ethical constraints on exposing human volunteers to the test samples, the above-mentioned in vivo experiments were undertaken in rats by using intra-tracheal instillation, and, for direct comparison, rat lung cell cultures in vitro were used. However, the in vitro–in vivo correlation might have been better had human volunteers and the appropriate human cells been used.

A low flow system, for generating and depositing airborne nanoparticles directly onto lung epithelial cells in transwells at the ALI, was shown by Kim et al. (71) to provide uniform and controlled dosing of particles of a reference nanoparticle with a count median diameter of 60 with 70.3% efficiency and without any cytotoxicity. By contrast, exposure to copper nanoparticles decreased cell viability to 73% ($P < .01$) and significantly ($P < .05$) elevated levels of lactate dehydrogenase, intracellular ROS and interleukin-8, that reflected findings from sub-acute in vivo inhalation studies in mice.

6.3 Involvement of Regulatory Agencies and Consortia

Interest in validating in vitro assays for inhalation toxicity has been gathering momentum over the last 5 years with: (a) the increasing involvement of regulatory agencies; and (b) the formation of several collaborative exercises between major stakeholders. As the US Food and Drug Administration has been mandated to regulate the sale of electronic cigarettes (ECs) in the USA, it is somewhat reassuring that the agency's National Center for Toxicological Research has recently initiated projects on method development for inhalation testing (23).

Another of the collaborative initiatives referred to earlier started in 2014, and involves the US Environmental Protection Agency (EPA), the US National Toxicology Program Interagency Center for the Evaluation of Alternative Toxicological Methods, industry and animal welfare organisations, with coordination provided by People for the Ethical Treatment of Animals (72). The first priority is sharing information on evaluating and optimising *in vitro* inhalation methods for acute toxicity. This is a biological endpoint, the *in vivo* determination of which has been extensively criticised, and for which basal cell cytotoxicity determination in cultured cells is gaining widespread credibility as an acceptable alternative to methods based on animal lethality as an endpoint.

At the first of a series of workshops commencing in March 2016, the following conclusions were agreed (73): (a) *a variety of available alternative test methods can reliably identify potential cytotoxicants, but none can single-handedly assess the multiple mechanisms of acute systemic toxicity following inhalation exposure*; (b) *applying multiple path particle dosimetry may be helpful for estimating inhalation toxicity*; (c) *a number of promising* in vitro *systems exist;* and (d) *integrated approaches to testing and assessment will be needed.* Working parties have been established to further explore each of these conclusions.

Another collaborative initiative involving the EPA is called the Next Generation Risk Assessment project (74). Ozone was chosen as the reference chemical in view of the extensive database available in the public domain, much of it involving humans. Radio-labelled ozone was used for the *in vitro* and *in vivo* study exposures so that the dose of ozone at the target sites in both cases could be adjusted to be equal. Volunteers were exposed to 0.3 ppm ozone, or clean air, on two separate occasions, followed by the taking of bronchial epithelium biopsies for cell culture. Also, epithelia from control volunteers were cultured and exposed to varying concentrations of ozone *in vitro* at the ALI. Preliminary results indicate that the inflammation seen following *in vitro* exposure was predictive of inflammation seen following human exposure to ozone. This very encouraging result is part of a larger collaborative project.

An additional collaborative initiative is focusing on COPD, and in December 2014, the Institute for *In Vitro* Sciences organised a workshop on *Assessment of In Vitro COPD Models for Tobacco Regulatory Science* (75). Four topics were discussed as follows: (a) inflammation and oxidative stress; (b) ciliary dysfunction and ion transport; (c) goblet cell hyperplasia and mucus production; and (d) parenchymal/bronchial tissue destruction and remodelling.

6.4 Data Interpretation

When interpreting data from inhalation studies, it should be remembered that the respiratory system, in common with other entry portals, acts as a target site for initial toxicity and also as a place where the inhaled substance is a potential substrate for extrahepatic biotransformation and distribution. Such metabolism can differ substantially from that occurring in the liver (depending on the test substance involved) due to the presence of different CYP isozymes and other biotransformation enzymes involved in both phase I and phase II reactions. Metabolism can alter the structure and physico-chemical properties of the parent chemical in such a way as to affect its subsequent biokinetics and distribution *in vivo*, as well as to modulate the outcome of subsequent hepatic biotransformation after the test chemical has reached the liver. This is because, in addition to non-metabolised parent compounds, the liver enzymes also receive, as substrates, metabolites derived from extrahepatic sources.

Furthermore, because the specific activities of extrahepatic biotransformation enzymes are generally considerably lower than those for the same substrates and corresponding enzymes in the liver (16), exposure to substances by routes other than orally delays the time between entry into the body and the first-pass effect (76). The latter effect arises as lower concentrations of substances re-enter systemic circulation, following metabolic clearance from the liver *en route* to the kidneys for excretion.

The first-pass effect mainly occurs with oral dosing, in which, following gut absorption, rapid transport to the liver occurs, via the hepatic portal vein. Breathing in a substance, on the other hand, leads to its efficient absorption into the pulmonary blood system, thence to the heart, and then, via the main aorta, to various tissues and organs, one of which is the liver, before the first-pass effect can occur.

All the above-mentioned processes have important consequences for toxicity, the nature of which can vary with the test sample as follows: (a) delaying the first-pass effect would be expected to increase the target-organ toxicity of the substance due to the longer time period during which higher internal doses would persist before hepatic clearance could occur (assuming that the parent chemical or a lung metabolite of it was toxic); and (b) exposed cells in the upper airways, including the buccal cavity, are themselves targets for toxicity and potential sites of metabolism, following the intake of a test substance.

The above-mentioned processes and their consequences are not always considered when comparing data obtained from tests in which different routes of exposure are involved.

7. DISCUSSION AND CONCLUSIONS

Potentially useful new tissue culture models of human airways are being described with increasing frequency. The relevance to human safety of inhalation data is increased by: (a) avoiding the problem of inter-species extrapolation through the use of human cells and assays based on human mechanistic data; (b) the ability to use all of the major target cells of the respiratory system in tissue culture; (c) conducting exposures at the ALI; and (d) facilitating *in vitro* to *in vivo* extrapolation by simplifying the kinetics and access of molecules of the test sample to the target site during exposure, such that the concentration applied and that actually received are closely related.

The most useful *in vitro* test system, in terms of predicting toxicity of human relevance, might not require all of the above-mentioned features. In other words, this could be an example of Russell and Burch's high fidelity fallacy (77). For example, the need for 3-D organotypic cultures could be less important than the target tissue site and the donor species, and a single layer of one cell type instead, exposed at the ALI, might yield equally useful, or even more-relevant, data. Such a situation would be expected to depend on the test material, and there should be information in the public domain which could be used to further investigate these possibilities, although that is beyond the scope of this chapter.

Nonetheless, inhalation toxicity testing provides substantial challenges for the development and validation of non-animal alternatives, as it requires specialised apparatus for exposure and dosimetry, as well as being subject to the fidelity of the test system selected to represent a wide range of different human exposure scenarios. Nevertheless, the available animal models are constrained by serious, and unchangeable, logistical, welfare and scientific limitations, a major portion of which are unique to this discipline of toxicity.

With the careful selection of target cells, partly depending on the *in vivo* data being used for benchmarking, used in conjunction with data from increasingly sophisticated particle deposition modelling, the predictive performance of several models is showing encouraging signs of improvement. However, more guidance and harmonisation need to be applied to the complex area of particle deposition and gaseous exchange modelling.

The choice of positive controls, especially when metabolic activation is required, is another area where more guidance is needed. This is likely to result from the fact that positive controls are rarely deemed necessary for *in vivo* inhalation testing, and they do not feature in the respective test guidelines. However, their judicious use would seem to represent the bare minimum required to be confident that lack of toxicity is not a false negative due to: (a) the way the test was performed; (b) lack of metabolic activation; or (c) an inherent insensitivity of the test. It should be noted that such controls are used routinely in other applications of *in vitro* toxicity testing.

With levels of inhalation testing rising, as well as the increasing incidence of pulmonary diseases, the need for expediting the validation of the evolving test methods has become urgent. There are signs that the necessary dialogue and cooperation between the principal stakeholders is starting to occur, but 'actions speak louder than words'.

An integrated testing strategy for inhalation toxicology testing has previously been proposed by Combes and Balls (78), and the principles involved in developing such strategies have been discussed by various authors, including Balls *et al.* (79) and Worth and Blaauboer (80). As discussed in the present chapter, such a scheme for inhalation toxicology should make maximum use of physicochemical properties and deposition modelling, as well cultures of the relevant human target cells and differentiated tissue models of the conducting airways, exposed at the ALI.

Because of our concerns about the safety assessment of innovative tobacco-related products (23) and about the unknown, but potentially serious, risks associated with vaping (81, 82), we were particularly interested to see the framework for the *in vitro* systems toxicology assessment of e-liquids discussed in detail by Isakander *et al.* (83).

While more work is required before the formal validation of both the component tests, and of the integrated strategies for their application, can take place, first steps for screening purposes could be taken, which should involve the use of weight-of-evidence (WoE) options at key steps, with a view to detecting and discarding candidate molecules with contraindications.

The focus should now be on coordinating the necessary future programme of fundamental and applied research to encourage the development of new methods, to improve hazard prediction and risk assessment, with the aim of improving public safety. However, for this to be realised, the regulatory agencies will need to recognise the limitations of the data that they have hitherto helped to generate, and have the conviction to effect the necessary changes, irrespective of objections based merely on tradition, inertia, and intransigence, as well as political and commercial interests, and biases.

REFERENCES

1. Charter, D. (2018). VW admits guilt over 'repulsive' tests on monkeys. *The Times*, 3, 31.01.2018.
2. Charter, D. (2018). Newer diesels caused test monkeys most suffering. *The Times*, 22, 01.02.2018.
3. Clark, D.G., Brown, R.C., Poole, A., *et al.* (1983). Inhalation toxicology. In M. Balls, R.J. Riddell, & A.N. Worden (Eds.), *Animals and Alternatives in Toxicity Testing*, pp. 299–312. London, UK and New York, NY, USA: Academic Press.

4. Donaldson, K., Aitken, R., Tran, L., *et al.* (2006). Carbon nanotubes: A review of their properties in relation to pulmonary toxicology and workplace safety. *Toxicological Sciences* **92**, 5–22.

5. Kenna, J.G. & Ram, R. (2018). *Safety Assessment of Pharmaceuticals* (This volume).

6. Burt, T. & Combes, R.D. (2018). *The Use of Non-invasive Imaging and Microdosing in Volunteers to Improve Drug Discovery and Safety Assessment* (This volume).

7. Costa, D.L. (2008). Alternative test methods in inhalation toxicology: Challenges and opportunities. *Experimental and Toxicologic Pathololology* **60**, 105–109.

8. Bakand, S. (2016). Cell culture techniques essential for toxicity testing of inhaled materials and nanomaterials in vitro. *Journal of Tissue Science and Engineering* **7**, 1000181-1–;1000181–1000185.

9. BéruBé, K., Aufderheide, M., Breheny, D., *et al.* (2009). *In vitro* models of inhalation toxicity and disease. The report of a FRAME workshop. *ATLA* **37**, 89–141.

10. Prytherch, Z. & BéruBé, K.A. (2015). Modelling the human respiratory system: Approaches for *in vitro* safety testing and drug discovery: Human-derived lung models; the future of toxicology safety assessment. *RSC Drug Discovery Series* **2015**(41), 66–87.

11. Manupello, J.R. & Sullivan, K.M. (2015). Toxicity assessment of tobacco products in vitro. *ATLA* **43**, 39–67.

12. Thorne, D. & Adamson, J. (2013). A review of *in vitro* cigarette smoke exposure systems. *Experimental and Toxicologic Pathology* **65**, 1183–1193.

13. Anon. (2018). *Respiratory Diseases in the World: Realities of Today — Opportunities for Tomorrow. Forum of International Respiratory Societies*, 35pp. Sheffield, UK: European Respiratory Society

14. Fröhlich, E. & Salar-Behzadi, S. (2014). Toxicological assessment of inhaled nanoparticles: role of *in vivo, ex vivo, in vitro*, and *in silico* studies. *International Journal of Molecular Sciences* **15**, 4795–4822.

15. Ling, G., Gu, J., Genter, M.B., *et al.* (2004). Regulation of cytochrome P450 gene expression in the olfactory mucosa. *Chemico-Biological Interactions* **147**, 247–258.

16. Coecke, S., Ahr, H., Blaauboer, B.J., *et al.* (2006). Metabolism: a bottleneck in *in vitro* toxicological test development. The report and recommendations of ECVAM Workshop 54. *ATLA* **34**, 49–84.

17. Fang, X., Song, Y. & Hirsch, J. (2006). Contribution of CFTR to apical–basolateral fluid transport in cultured human alveolar epithelial type II cells. *American Journal of Physiology - Lung Cellular and Molecular Physiology* **290**, 242–249.

18. Fisher, A.B. & Chander, A. (1985). Intracellular processing of surfactant lipids in the lung. *Annual Review of Physiology* **47**, 789–802.

19. Dorato, M.A. & Wolff, R.K. (1991). Inhalation exposure technology, dosimetry, and regulatory issues. *Toxicologic Pathology* **19**, 373–383.

20. Lambré, C.R., Aufderheide, M., Bolton, R.E., *et al.* (1996). *In vitro* tests for respiratory toxicity. The report and recommendations of ECVAM Workshop 18. *ATLA* **24**, 671–681.

21. Pauluhn, J. & Mohr, U. (2000). Inhalation studies in laboratory animals — current concepts and alternatives. *Toxicologic Pathology* **28**, 734–753.

22. Heinonen, T. & Verfaillie, C. (2018). *The Development and Application of Key Technologies and Tools* (This volume).

23. Combes, R.D. & Balls, M. (2015). A critical assessment of the scientific basis, and implementation, of regulations for the safety assessment and marketing of innovative tobacco-related products. *ATLA* **43**, 251–290.

24. Morrow, P.E. & Mermelstein, R. (1988). Chronic inhalation toxicity studies: Protocols and pitfalls. In U. Mohr, D. Dungworth, G. Kimmerle, J. Lewkowski, R. McClellan, & W. Stober (Eds.), *ILSI Monograph: Inhalation Toxicology*, pp. 103–117. New York, NY, USA: Springer-Verlag, Inc.

25. Coggins, C.R. (2007). An updated review of inhalation studies with cigarette smoke in laboratory animals. *International Journal of Toxicology* **26**, 331–338.

26. Hubrecht, R. (2014). *The Welfare of Animals Used in Research: Practice and Ethics*, 271pp. Hoboken, NJ, USA: Wiley Blackwell

27. Edwards, S. & Koob, G.F. (2012). Experimental psychiatric illness and drug abuse models: From human to animal, an overview. *Methods in Molecular Biology* **829**, 31–48.

28. Forbes, B. (2000). Human airway epithelial cell lines for *in vitro* drug transport and metabolism studies. *Pharmacutical Science & Technology Today* **3**, 18–27.

29. Forbes, B., Shah, A., Martin, G.P., *et al.* (2003). The human bronchial epithelial cell line 16HBE14o– as a model system of the airways for studying drug transport. *International Journal of Pharmaceutics* **257**, 161–167.

30. Paur, H.-R., Mülhopt, S., Weiss, C., *et al.* (2008). *In vitro* exposure systems and bioassays for the assessment of toxicity of nanoparticles to the human lung. *Journal für Verbraucherschutz und Lebensmittelsicherheit* **3**, 319–329.

31. Dillon, D., Combes, R., McConville, M., *et al.* (1992). Ozone is mutagenic in Salmonella. *Environmental and Molecular Mutagenesis* **19**, 331–337.

32. Hayes, A., Bakand, S. & Winder, C. (2007). Novel in-vitro exposure techniques for toxicity testing and biomonitoring of airborne contaminants. In U. Marx, & V. Sandig (Eds.), *Drug Testing In Vitro: Breakthroughs and Trends in Cell Culture Technology*, pp. 103–124. Weinheim, Germany: Wiley OnLine Library.

33. Adamson, J., Haswell, L.E., Phillips, G., *et al.* (2011). *In vitro* models of chronic obstructive pulmonary disease (COPD). In I.M. Ãn-Loeches (Ed.), *Bronchitis*, pp. 41–66. Rijeka, Croatia: InTech.

34. Fox, J.C. & Fitzgerald, M.F. (2004). Models of chronic obstructive pulmonary disease: a review of current status. *Drug Discovery Today: Disease Models* **1**, 319–328.

35. Pelagic, R. & Pahl, A. (2004). Smoke induced changes in epithelial cell gene expression: development of an in vitro model for COPD. *ALTEX* **21**, 3–7.

36. Bombick, D.W., Reed Bombick, B., Ayres, P.H., *et al.* (1997). Evaluation of the genotoxic and cytotoxic potential of mainstream whole smoke and smoke condensate from a cigarette containing a novel carbon filter. *Fundamental and Applied Toxicology* **39**, 11—17.

37. Bombick, D.W., Ayres, P.H. & Doolittle, D.J. (1997). Cytotoxicity assessment of whole smoke and vapour phase of mainstream and sidestream cigarette smoke from three Kentucky reference cigarettes. *Toxicology Methods* **7**, 177—190.

38. Combes, R.D. (2013). Progress in the development, validation and regulatory acceptance of in vitro methods for toxicity testing. In J. Reedijk (Ed.), *Reference Module in Chemistry, Molecular Sciences and Chemical Engineering*, pp. 1—25. Waltham, MA, USA: Elsevier.

39. Hidalgo, I.J., Raub, T.J. & Borchardt, R.T. (1989). Characterization of the human colon carcinoma cell line (Caco-2) as a model system for intestinal epithelial permeability. *Gastroenterology* **96**, 736—749.

40. Knebel, J.W., Ritter, D. & Aufderheide, M. (1998). Development of an *in vitro* system for studying effects of native and photochemically transformed gaseous compounds using an air/liquid culture technique. *Toxicology Letters* **96—97**, 1—11.

41. Aufderheide, M. (2001). In vitro exposure of isolated cells to native gaseous compounds-development and validation of an optimized system for human lung cells. *Experimental and Toxicologic Pathology* **53**, 373—386.

42. Aufderheide, M. & Mohr, U. (2000). CULTEX - An alternative technique for cultivation and exposure of cells of the respiratory tract to the airborne pollutants at the air/liquid interface. *Experimental and Toxicologic Pathology* **52**, 265—270.

43. Karol, M.H., Graham, C., Gealy, R., *et al.* (1996). Structure-activity relationships and computer-assisted analysis of respiratory sensitization potential. *Toxicology Letters* **86**, 187—191.

44. Rovida, C., Martin, S.F., Vivier, M., *et al.* (2013). Advanced tests for skin and respiratory sensitization assessment. *ALTEX* **30**, 231—252.

45. Wiemann, M., Vennemann, A., Sauer, U.G., *et al.* (2016). An *in vitro* alveolar macrophage assay for predicting the short-term inhalation toxicity of nanomaterials. *Journal of Nanobiotechnology* **14**, 16.

46. Phillips, J., Kluss, B., Richter, A., *et al.* (2005). Exposure of bronchial epithelial cells to whole cigarette smoke: assessment of cellular responses. *ATLA* **33**, 239—248.

47. Sassen, A.W., Richter, E., Marzell, P., *et al.* (2005). Genotoxicity of nicotine in mini-organ cultures of human upper aerodigestive tract epithelia. *Toxicological Sciences* **88**, 134—141.

48. Benam, K.H., Novak, R., Nawroth, J., *et al.* (2016). Matched-comparative modelling of normal and diseased human airway responses using a micro-engineered breathing lung chip. *Cell Systems* **3**, 456—466.

49. Dehne, E.M., Hickman, J. & Shuler, M. (2018). *Biologically-Inspired Microphysiological Systems* (This volume).

50. Kleinstreur, C., Zhang, Z. & Li, Z. (2008). Modeling airflow and particle transport/deposition in pulmonary airways. *Regulatory Physiology & Neurobiology* **163**, 128—138.

51. Fröhlich, E., Mercuri, A., Wu, S., *et al.* (2016). Measurements of deposition, lung surface area and lung fluid for simulation of inhaled compounds. *Frontiers in Pharmacology* **7**, 181.

52. Crapo, J.D. (1989). *Extrapolation of Dosimetric Relationships for Inhaled Particles and Gases*, 377pp. New York, NY, USA: Academic Press

53. Aufderheide, M. (2005). Direct exposure methods for testing native atmospheres. *Experimental Toxicology and Pathology* **57**, 213—226.

54. Olsson, B., Borgström, L., Lundbäck, H., *et al.* (2013). Validation of a general *in vitro* approach for prediction of total lung deposition in healthy adults for pharmaceutical inhalation products. *Journal of Aerosol Medicine and Pulmonary Drug Delivery* **26**, 355—369.

55. Isaacs, K.K., Rosati, J.A. & Martonen, T.B. (2012). Modelling deposition of inhaled particles. In L.S. Ruzer, & N.H. Harley (Eds.), *Handbook: Measurement, Dosimetry, and Health Effects* (2nd edn., pp. 83—127). Boca Raton, FL, USA: CRC Press.

56. Kemp, S.J., Thorley, A.J., Gorelik, J., *et al.* (2008). Immortalization of human alveolar epithelial cells to investigate nanoparticle uptake. *American Journal of Respiratory Cell & Molecular Biology* **39**, 591—597.

57. Hermanns, M.I., Unger, R.E., Kehe, K., *et al.* (2004). Lung epithelial cell lines in coculture with human pulmonary microvascular endothelial cells: development of an alveolo-capillary barrier in vitro. *Laboratory Investigation* **84**, 736—752.

58. Müller, B., Seifart, K. & Barth, F. (1998). Effect of air pollutants on the pulmonary surfactant system. *European Journal of Clinical Investigation* **28**, 762—777.

59. Sørli, J.B., Hansen, J.S., Nørgaard, A.W., *et al.* (2015). An *in vitro* method for predicting inhalation toxicity of impregnation spray products. *ALTEX* **32**, 101—111.

60. Valavanidis, A., Vlachogianni, T. & Fiotakis, K. (2009). Tobacco smoke: involvement of reactive oxygen species and stable free radicals in mechanisms of oxidative damage, carcinogenesis and synergistic effects with other respirable particles. *International Journal of Environmental Research and Public Health* **6**, 445—462.

61. Miyashita, L., Suri, R., Dearing, E., *et al.* (2018). E-cigarette vapour enhances pneumococcal adherence to airway epithelial cells. *European Respiratory Journal* **51**, 1701592.

62. Gray, A.C., McLeod, J.D. & Clothier, R.H. (2007). A review of *in vitro* modelling approaches to the identification and modulation of squamous metaplasia in the human tracheobronchial epithelium. *ATLA* **35**, 493—504.

63. Garcia-Arcos, I., Geraghty, P., Baumlin, N., *et al.* (2016). Chronic electronic cigarette exposure in mice induces features of COPD in a nicotine-dependent manner. *Thorax* **71**, 1119—1129.

64. Thorne, D., Kilford, J., Payne, R., *et al.* (2013). Characterisation of a Vitrocell® VC 10 in vitrosmoke exposure system using dose tools and biological analysis. *Chemistry Central Journal* **7**, 146.

65. Constant, S., Wiszniewski, L. & Huang, S. (2014). The use of in vitro 3D cell models of human airway epithelia (MucilAir™) in inhalation toxicology. In J. Haycock, A. Ahluwalia, & J.M. Wilkinson (Eds.), *Cellular In Vitro Testing: Methods and Protocols*, pp. 15—34. Boca Raton, FL, USA: CRC Press.

66. Huang, S. & Caulfuty, M. (2009). *A Novel In-vitro Cell Model of the Human Airway Epithelium. 3R Info Bulletin 41*, 2pp. Münsingen, Switzerland: 3R Research Foundation Switzerland

67. Carranza-Rosales, P., Carranza-Torres, I.E., Guzmán-Delgado, N., *et al.* (2017). Modeling tuberculosis pathogenesis through *ex vivo* lung tissue infection. *Tuberculosis* **107**, 126–132.

68. Balls, M., Worth, A. & Combes, R.D. (2018). *Validation* (This volume).

69. Seagrave, J.C., Mauderly, J.L. & Seilkop, S.K. (2003). *In vitro* relative toxicity screening of combined particulate and semivolatile organic fractions of gasoline and diesel engine emissions. *Journal of Toxicology & Environmental Health* **66**, 1113–1132.

70. Sayes, C.M., Reed, K.L. & Warheit, D.B. (2007). Assessing toxicity of fine and nanoparticles: comparing in vitro measurements to in vivo pulmonary toxicity profiles. *Toxicological Sciences* **97**, 163–180.

71. Kim, J.S., Peters, T.M. & O'Shaughnessy, P. (2013). Validation of an *in vitro* exposure system for toxicity assessment of air-delivered nanomaterials. *Toxicology in Vitro* **27**, 164–173.

72. Sprankle, C. (2016). NICEATM presents webinar series on inhalation toxicity. Newsletter, April 2016, 1p. Research Triangle Park, NC, USA: National Toxicology Program, NIEHS *UPDATE*. Available at: https://ntp.niehs.nih.gov/update/2016/4/iccvaminhaltox/index.html.

73. Allen, D., Wilson, D., Hotchkiss, J., *et al.* (2017). *Integrating Alternative Approaches to Replace Animals in Inhalation Toxicity Testing*. Poster, 1p. NICEATM News. Research. Triangle Park, NC, USA: NIEHS. Available at: https://ntp.niehs.nih.gov/iccvam/meetings/10wc/allen-inhtox-wc10-fd.pdf.

74. Cote, I., Andersen, M.E., Ankley, G.T., *et al.* (2016). The next generation of risk assessment multi-year study—highlights of findings, applications to risk assessment, and future directions. *Environmental Health Perspectives* **124**, 1671–1682.

75. Behrsing, H., Raabe, H., Manuppello, J., *et al.* (2016). Assessment of *in vitro* COPD models for tobacco regulatory science: Workshop proceedings, conclusions and paths forward for *in vitro* model use. *ATLA* **44**, 129–166.

76. Benet, L.Z. (1978). Effect of route of administration and distribution on drug action. *Journal of Pharmacokinetics and Biopharmaceutics* **6**, 559–585.

77. Russell, W.M.S. & Burch, R.L. (1959). *The Principles of Humane Experimental Technique*, 238pp. London, UK: Methuen

78. Combes, R.D. & Balls, M. (2011). Integrated testing strategies for toxicity employing new and existing technologies. *ATLA* **39**, 213–225.

79. Balls, M., Combes, R.D. & Bhogal, N. (2011). The use of integrated and intelligent testing strategies in the prediction of toxic hazard and in risk assessment. In M. Balls, R.D. Combes, & N. Bhogal (Eds.), *New Technologies for Toxicity Testing*, pp. 221–253. Georgetown, TX, USA: Landes Bioscience.

80. Worth, A. & Blaauboer, B. (2018). *Integrated Approaches to Testing and Assessment* (This volume).

81. Combes, R.D. & Balls, M. (2015). On the safety of e-cigarettes: "I can resist anything except temptation". *ATLA* **43**, 417–425.

82. Combes, R.D. & Balls, M. (2016). *Draft Response Regarding Comments Made by Clive Bates about one of our Publications on the Safety of Electronic Cigarettes and Vaping*. ResearchGate working paper, 6pp. Available at: https://www.researchgate.net/publication/307958871.

83. Iskandar, A.R., Gonzalez-Suarez, I., Majeed, S., *et al.* (2016). A framework for *in vitro* systems toxicology assessment of e-liquids. *Toxicology Mechanisms and Methods* **26**, 389–413.

Chapter 3.6

Alternative Approaches for Carcinogenicity and Reproductive Toxicity

Raffaella Corvi[1], Horst Spielmann[2] and Thomas Hartung[3,4]

[1]Joint Research Centre, European Commission, Ispra (VA), Italy; [2]Freie Universität Berlin, Berlin, Germany; [3]Johns Hopkins Bloomberg School of Public Health, Baltimore, MD, United States; [4]University of Konstanz, Konstanz, Germany

SUMMARY

The regulatory assessment of the complex endpoints, carcinogenicity and reproductive and developmental toxicity, still heavily relies on animal testing. This chapter reviews the alternative approaches that have been developed in these areas in the last decades to waive testing and reduce the number of animals used and summarises the lessons learned. The alternative approaches range from the individual test methods, such as the cell transformation assay for carcinogenicity and the embryotoxicity tests for reproductive toxicity, to reduction approaches, such as the International Conference on Harmonisation strategy for pharmaceuticals and the extended-one-generation assay. Currently, these areas are being revitalised due to the broad recognition of the shortcomings of current *in vivo* testing requirements and the current regulatory environment (e.g. the European Registration, Evaluation, Authorisation and Restriction of Chemicals and Cosmetics Regulations). More-recent developments aimed at a more human-relevant chemical assessment, which rely on the integration of different sources of information, are also described.

1. INTRODUCTION

The assessments of carcinogenicity and reproductive toxicity represent essential components of the safety assessment of all types of substances being among the endpoints of highest concern. Their assessment still relies mainly on animal tests.

Substances are defined as carcinogenic if, after inhalation, ingestion, dermal application or injection, they induce (malignant) tumours, increase their incidence or malignancy or shorten the time of tumour occurrence. It is generally accepted that carcinogenesis is a multi-hit/multi-step process from the transition of normal cells into cancer cells via a sequence of stages and complex biological interactions, strongly influenced by factors such as genetics, age, diet, environment and hormonal balance (1). Although attributing a number of the observed cancer rates to individual specific causes remains a challenge, the fraction of all cancers currently due to exposure to carcinogenic pollutants is estimated to range from less than 1% to as high as 5%–10% (2).

Reproductive toxicity is defined as *effects such as reduced fertility, effects on gonads and disturbance of spermatogenesis; this also covers developmental toxicity*, which itself is defined as *effects to, e.g. growth and developmental retardation, malformations and functional deficits in the offspring* (3). Often referred to in combination as DART (developmental and reproductive toxicity), the assessment of these endpoints aims to identify possible hazards to the reproductive cycle, with an emphasis on embryotoxicity. Only 2%–5% of birth defects can be associated with chemical and physical stress (4). This includes mainly the abuse of alcohol and other drugs. For the assessment of the prevalence of effects on mammalian fertility, the available database is even more limited.

2. GOLD STANDARDS AND THEIR DRAWBACKS

For nearly half a century, the 2-year rodent cancer bioassay has been widely regarded as the 'gold standard' for determining the carcinogenic potential of a chemical, and OECD Test Guidelines (TGs) have been in place since 1981 (5). However, its adequacy to predict cancer risk in humans is the subject of considerable debate (6, 7), with notable challenges and uncertainty associated with extrapolating from rodents to humans, with quantitative risk estimation and limited accuracy (8—10). Moreover, the rodent bioassay, as originally designed, does not take into account windows of susceptibility over the life-time, and so may not have adequate sensitivity to detect agents, such as endocrine-active chemicals, that alter susceptibility to tumours (11). Furthermore, these studies are extremely time-consuming and resource-consuming, and the high animal welfare burden has raised ethical concerns.

From a regulatory perspective, the gradual recognition of non-genotoxic mechanisms of carcinogenesis (not involving direct alterations in DNA) has complicated the established relationship between genotoxicity and carcinogenicity, and has also challenged the conventional interpretation of rodent carcinogenicity results in terms of their relevance to human cancer (12). Because of the default assumption in regulatory decision-making regarding the presumed linearity of the dose—response curve for genotoxic carcinogens, the classification of carcinogens as genotoxic or non-genotoxic became an essential, but highly controversial, component of cancer risk assessment.

The area of carcinogenicity has been very quiet for decades, but in recent years it has been revitalised due to broad recognition of the shortcomings of the current regulatory *in vivo* testing requirements and the awareness of information gaps in pieces of legislation, which limit or ban the use of animals (e.g. the European Registration, Evaluation, Authorisation and Restriction of Chemicals (REACH) and Cosmetics Regulations).

Similarly, DART was not in the foreground of safety assessments for many years after the shock of the thalidomide disaster (13) had died down. More recently, the European REACH legislation, which is extremely demanding in this field (14), has stirred discussion again, notably because tests like the two-generation study are among the most costly tests and require up to 3200 animals per substance (in a traditional two-generation study). In the drug development area, the discussion has focused mainly around a possible replacement of the second species by human mechanistic assays and the value of using non-human primates for biologicals. Another driving force is the European ban on testing for cosmetics ingredients (15). A series of activities by the European Centre for the Validation of Alternative Method (ECVAM) and Center for Alternatives to Animal Testing (CAAT), including several workshops, have tackled this challenge. The Integrated Project RePoTect (16) was one of its offsprings, pioneering several alternative approaches, followed by projects like ChemScreen and, most recently, the flagship program EU-ToxRisk (17).

Developmental processes are especially difficult to assess (18), as the timing of processes creates windows of vulnerability, the process is especially sensitive to genetic errors and environmental disruptions, simple lesions can lead to complex phenotypes (and *vice versa*) and maternal effects can have an impact at all stages.

The treatment of one or more generations of rats or rabbits with a test chemical is the most common approach for identifying DART, enshrined in seven OECD TGs. For specifically evaluating developmental toxicity, TGs were designed to detect malformations in the developing offspring, together with parameters such as growth alterations and prenatal mortality (19), but developmental toxicity tests are considered mainly as screening tests, especially for REACH (20). The shorter and less complex 'screening' tests, which combine reproductive, developmental and (optionally) repeat-dose toxicity endpoints into a single study design, are variants.

The fundamental relevance of the current testing paradigm has only recently been addressed in a more comprehensive way (21, 22). There is considerable concern about inter-species differences (of about 60% concordance), reproducibility (in part due to a lack of standardisation of protocols but also high background levels of developmental variants) and the value of the second generation in testing versus the costs, duration and animal use. An analysis for 254 chemicals suggests that 99.8% of chemicals show no-effect-levels for DART within a tenfold range of maternal toxicity, and thus might be simply covered by an assessment factor of 10 (23).

An analysis by Bremer and Hartung of 74 industrial chemicals (24), which had been tested in developmental toxicity screening tests and reported in the EU New Chemicals Database, showed that 34 chemicals have demonstrated effects on the offspring, but only two chemicals have been actually classified as developmentally toxic according to the standards applied by the national competent authorities. This demonstrates the lack of confidence in the specificity of this 'definitive' test. The same analysis showed that 55% of these chemical effects to the offspring could not be detected within multi-generation studies.

Overall, further discussion is needed as to the relevance of the current carcinogenicity and DART assessments. As the societal need to ensure the respective safety of drugs, chemicals and consumer products is recognised, this might make it difficult to abandon current testing but should lower the barrier for implementing alternative approaches.

3. ACTIVITIES AND ACHIEVEMENTS — CARCINOGENICITY

3.1 Genotoxicity Assays

In the late 1960s, highly predictive short-term genotoxicity assays were initially developed to screen for carcinogens. This led to a variety of well-established *in vitro* assays, and since the 1980s, to their respective OECD TGs that have been used successfully to predict genotoxicity, label chemical substances and inform the cancer risk assessment process. However, these tests are not at present considered to fully replace the animal tests currently used to evaluate the safety of substances (1). In the last decade, considerable activities have been carried out worldwide, with the aim of optimising strategies for genotoxicity testing, both with respect to the basic *in vitro* testing battery and to *in vivo* follow-up tests. This reflects the fact that the science has progressed substantially, and significant experience in 40 years of regulatory toxicology testing in this area has been acquired. The main gap identified was the need to ensure that *in vitro* tests do not generate a high number of false positive results, which trigger unnecessary *in vivo* follow-up studies, hence generating undesirable implications for animal welfare (25). The recommendations from a workshop organised by ECVAM (26) and from an EURL ECVAM strategy paper (27) on how to reduce genotoxicity testing in animals have contributed to several international initiatives aimed at improving the existing *in vitro* genotoxicity tests and strategies, and at identifying and evaluating new test systems with appropriate sensitivity and improved specificity. This acquired new knowledge led to the revision of the OECD TGs for genotoxicity. The *in vitro* micronucleus test, which was the first test to be evaluated by ECVAM through a retrospective type of validation (28), plays a prominent role in the genotoxicity strategy, as it has been proposed as the assay to be used in a two-test battery together with the Ames test (29, 30). Novel *in vitro* methods are being developed and validated, with the aim of full replacement and providing better understanding of modes of action, as in the case of genotoxicity assays in 3-D human reconstructed skin models, toxicogenomics-based tests and biomarker assays (30).

3.2 Transgenic Assays

Transgenic mouse model tests are possible alternatives to the classical 2-year cancer bioassay (31). The rationale for using transgenic mice in regulatory carcinogenicity testing is that transgenic mouse models may be more sensitive predictors of carcinogenic risk to humans. Indeed, these models have a reduced tumour latency period (6—9 months) to chemically induced tumours and may result in a significant reduction in the use of experimental animals (20—25 animals/sex/treatment group; (32)). A study coordinated by International Life Sciences Institute (ILSI)/Health and Environmental Sciences Institute (HESI) (33, 34) led to the initial acceptance by pharmaceutical regulatory agencies of three primary models, $p53^{+/-}$, Tg.AC and rasH2 to be used *in lieu* of a second species full carcinogenicity bioassay (35).

3.3 Cell Transformation Assays

In vitro cell transformation assays (CTAs) for the detection of potential carcinogens have been in use for about 40 years. Transformation involves several events in the cascade potentially leading to carcinogenesis and is defined as the induction of phenotypic alterations in cultured cells that are characteristic of tumorigenic cells (36, 37). Despite the long experience in the use of CTAs, the intense and lengthy activities at the OECD from 1997 to 2016 and the conduct of ECVAM and JaCVAM validation studies (38, 39), the assays were adopted as OECD Guidance Documents (40, 41), but they have so far failed to be adopted as TGs in their own right. Among the obstacles to development of an OECD TG for the SHE CTA was the lack of a coordinated full validation, but instead the combination of a Detailed Review Paper (DRP) and a prospective limited validation study, which triggered the need for additional analyses by the OECD expert group (42, 43). This also demonstrates that a DRP is not always equivalent to a retrospective validation. Moreover, no Integrated Approaches to Testing and Assessments (IATA) or alternative testing strategies were available for carcinogenicity, and because there was common agreement that the assay should not be used as a stand-alone, difficulties were encountered in defining how to apply it for regulatory decision-making. This can be seen as a dilemma: 'Which comes first: the chicken or the egg? ….the test method or the testing strategy (or IATA)?'. This created a precedent at the OECD, questioning whether in the future only new methods associated with a well-defined testing strategy or IATA should be accepted. Also, a better characterisation of the performance of the CTAs to detect non-genotoxic carcinogens was considered important because the data collected in the DRP were biased toward genotoxic carcinogens, which reflects the data available in the public domain. Another recurring concern was that the mechanistic bases of cell transformation are not yet completely elucidated. Consequently, the link to tumorigenesis is not fully understood, which hampers interpretation of the findings from the CTA.

During the course of the CTA activities at the OECD, the regulatory framework in Europe changed considerably with the ban on animal testing for cosmetics and the REACH evaluation of industrial chemicals. This has put a huge burden on industry that is limited in the use of *in vivo* tests to confirm results from *in vitro* tests, and on regulators that have to assess carcinogenicity potential with no *in vivo* data, leading to a more cautious uptake of *in vitro* tests to support the assessment of such a critical endpoint.

Finally, a clear position early on in the OECD process by the WNT (Working Group of National Coordinators) with two opposing countries (i.e. UK and The Netherlands) would have been desirable, as some of the concerns were raised only in very late phases of the process, despite an initial consensus by all countries to proceed with the drafting of the SHE CTA TG. Many of these considerations apply also to the CTA based on Bhas 42 cells.

3.4 Integrated Approaches to Testing and Assessment for Non-Genotoxic Carcinogens

Non-genotoxic carcinogens contribute to an increased cancer risk by a variety of mechanisms that are not yet directly assessed by international regulatory approaches. In April 2014, the OECD WNT recognised that the CTA alone was insufficient to address non-genotoxic carcinogenicity and that a more comprehensive battery of tests addressing different non-genotoxic mechanisms of carcinogenicity would be needed in the future. This discussion led to the identification for the need for an IATA to properly address the issue of non-genotoxic carcinogenicity and where the CTA, together with other relevant assays, could fit. Under the auspices of the OECD, an expert working group was set up to examine the current international regulatory requirements and their limitations in respect to non-genotoxic carcinogenicity, and how an IATA could be developed to assist regulators in their assessment of non-genotoxic carcinogenicity (44). Moreover, the working group was tasked to review, describe and assess relevant *in vitro* assays with the aim of tentatively organising them into levels of testing, following the Adverse Outcome Pathway (AOP) format, such as that possible structures of the future IATA can be created. Different *in vitro* methods are in fact already available as research tools to study a number of potential non-genotoxic mechanisms, such as oxidative stress, or inhibition of gap junction intercellular communication (22, 44). However, these methods cannot currently be used to reliably predict carcinogenic potential; rather, they are useful to improve understanding the mechanistic basis of effects elicited by a compound within a weight-of-evidence assessment strategy (i.e. an IATA).

3.5 Toxicogenomics-Based Test Methods for Carcinogenicity

Toxicogenomics for the study of carcinogenicity has been applied to several *in vitro* and short-term *in vivo* test systems (45–47). For example, the EU-Framework Project, carcinoGENOMICS, which aimed at developing toxicogenomics-*in vitro* tests to detect potential genotoxicants and carcinogens in liver, lung and kidney cells, also assessed the preliminary reproducibility of the assay by using different bioinformatics approaches (48, 49).

Potential applications of toxicogenomics-based assays are clarification of Mode of Action (MoA), hazard classification, derivation of points of departure and prioritisation (10, 12). Among these, the targeted use of transcriptomics tests for MoA determination seems to be the preferred application. However, there is still limited implementation of transcriptomics in regulatory decision-making, as discussed in a recent workshop to feature multi-sector and international perspectives on current and potential applications of genomics in cancer risk assessment, organised by the HESI, Health Canada and McGill University in Montreal, in May 2017. Even though companies make use of transcriptomics-based tests for guiding internal decisions, the uncertainty on how these data would be interpreted by regulators is among the main roadblocks identified for submission of data. In addition, lack of validation and regulatory guidance were considered as roadblocks (50).

3.6 Alternative Approaches to Rodent Long-Term Carcinogenicity Studies for Pharmaceuticals

Because of the deficiencies of animal carcinogenicity studies and based on several extensive data reviews, some proposals have been made by representatives of the pharmaceutical industry for refining the criteria for when carcinogenicity testing may or may not be warranted for pharmaceuticals. In August 2013, an International Conference on Harmonisation (ICH) Regulatory Notice Document has been posted by the Drug Regulatory Authorities (DRAs), announcing the evaluation of an alternative approach to the 2-year rat carcinogenicity test (51). This approach is based on the hypothesis that knowledge of pharmacological targets and pathways, together with toxicological and other data, can provide sufficient information to anticipate the outcome of a 2-year rat carcinogenicity study and its potential value in predicting the risk of human carcinogenicity of a given pharmaceutical. The rationale behind this proposal was supported by a retrospective evaluation of several datasets from Industry and DRAs, which suggests that up to 40%—50% rat cancer studies could be avoided (51—53).

A prospective evaluation study to confirm the above hypothesis is ongoing, where the industry sponsors are encouraged to submit to the DRAs a Carcinogenicity Assessment Document (CAD) to address the carcinogenic potential of an investigational pharmaceutical, and to predict the outcome and value of the planned 2-year rat carcinogenicity study prior to knowing the outcome of the carcinogenicity testing (51). Predictions in the submitted CADs will then be checked against the actual outcome of the 2-year rat studies as they are completed, and the results of this study are expected in 2019.

Currently, a project under the umbrella of the European Partnership for Alternative Approaches to Animal Testing is ongoing to evaluate whether this approach is applicable to the carcinogenicity assessment of pesticides.

4. ACTIVITIES AND ACHIEVEMENTS — REPRODUCTIVE AND DEVELOPMENTAL TOXICITY

The status of alternative methods for DART has been summarised by Adler *et al.* (1), endorsed by Hartung *et al.* (54) and in the context of developing roadmaps for the way forward (22, 55, 56). Some key developments are summarised here.

4.1 Extended One-Generation Reproductive Toxicity Study

Increasing doubt as to the usefulness of the second generation for testing of substances led to retrospective analyses by Janer *et al.* (57), who concluded that this made no relevant contribution to regulatory decision-making. The US EPA obtained similar data (23) supporting the development of an extended one-generation reproductive toxicity study (EORGTS; OECD TG 443; (58)), originally proposed by the ILSI-HESI Agricultural Chemicals Safety Assessment initiative (59), including a modular approach to the EOGRTS (60). The history of the EOGRTS assay was summarised by Moore *et al.* (61). This shows that (elements of) study protocols can indeed be useless and warrant critical assessment. This reduction alternative brings the number of animals down from 3200 to about 1400 per substance tested. Ongoing discussions concern the triggered new modules for neurodevelopmental and developmental immunotoxicity, which undo a lot of the reduction in terms of work and animal use.

4.2 Zebrafish Egg Assays

The most complete reflection of embryonic development apparently can be achieved with zebrafish embryos (62—65) by, for example, using dynamic cell imaging or frog eggs (the FETAX assay, (66)), with the latter having been evaluated quite critically by ICCVAM.

Currently, the Evidence-based Toxicology Collaboration is conducting a systematic review of available protocols and data. This retrospective analysis is also exploring whether such systematic reviews (67, 68) can substitute for traditional validation approaches (69).

4.3 Embryotoxicity Tests

Since 1970, reproductive toxicologists have developed *in vitro* assays covering the essential steps of the mammalian reproductive cycle (56), including the embryonic stem cell test (EST), the first toxicity test employing embryonic stem cells (ESCs, (70—72)).

By 2002, three well-established tests had already been validated, i.e. the mouse EST (mEST), the whole rat embryo test and the limb bud assay (73—75). The EST proved more predictive and reproducible than the other two assays. This validation process represented a radical departure from other ongoing validation studies at that time, as these covered only a small part of the reproductive cycle and only a small though critical part of the embryonic development. For this reason, none of the tests have received regulatory acceptance up to now. In 2003, as a first step following validation, a workshop was needed to define the use of such assays (76). The validation study was criticised because the validity statements had raised a lot of expectations which failed to understand that such partial replacements could only be used in a testing strategy (77, 78), as later attempted within ReProTect and other projects cited earlier. This prompted a restructuring of the validation process with earlier involvement of regulators and their needs (79), as well as the need to apply IATAs (80, 81). However, the embryotoxicity tests can also be seen as forerunners of such building blocks in testing strategies.

Other critical views concerned the low number of substances evaluated in the validation study due to the costs of these assays and the somewhat arbitrary distinction between weak and strong embryotoxicants, where a weak one was defined as being reported reprotoxic in one species, and a strong one in two or more species Among the embryotoxicity tests, the EST has attracted most interest, partly because it represents the only one of the three methods which is truly animal-free. Originally based on the counting of beating mouse heart cells formed, this test has been adapted to other endpoints and to human cells (82). It is also used in the pharmaceutical industry, with revised prediction models. A dedicated workshop on the EST (83) pointed out that its prediction model is driven by the cytotoxicity of the test compounds.

Meanwhile, regulatory agencies in Japan and the USA are considering the use of derivatives of the EST for regulatory purposes. For example, in Japan the Hand1-Luc EST, employing engineered mouse ES cells (84), has been validated, and Japan has submitted a peer review report to the OECD as a 'non-animal test for evaluating the developmental toxicity of chemicals' (85). The US FDA is concluding from in-house studies that transcriptional profiles are a sensitive indicator of early mouse ESC differentiation and that transcriptomics may improve the predictivity of the mEST by suggesting possible MoAs for tested chemicals (86).

Importantly, a variant of the EST using either human embryonic stem cells or human induced pluripotent stem cells and metabolite measurements, which were identified by metabolomics, was introduced by Stemina Biomarker Discovery. This assay was evaluated with very promising results for more than 100 substances and is undergoing validation by ICCVAM.

There is ongoing discussion with the FDA as to whether such assays might replace the second species in DART evaluations. Significantly, the FDA has recently launched a 'predictive toxicity roadmap' (87), and is proposing that once a new model or assay is considered qualified by FDA for a specific context of use, industry and other stakeholders can use it for the qualified purpose during product development, and FDA reviewers can be confident in applying it without needing to re-review the underlying supporting data. Thus, a new assay may "qualify" to be used within an IATA and not need to undergo a 'formal validation' exercise. The current revision of ICH *S5 Guideline on Detection of Toxicity to Reproduction for Human Pharmaceuticals* foresees *in vitro* tests for the registration of pharmaceuticals.

4.4 Endocrine Disruptor Screening Assays

Endocrine disruption is one key element of DART but may also constitute a pathway of carcinogenesis. These important assay developments in the context of chemical endocrine disruptor screening are discussed elsewhere and go beyond the scope of this short overview. However, they would form critical building blocks in an integrated test strategy for DART, as suggested first by Bremer *et al.* (88) and attempted in ReProTect for DART, and for carcinogenicity (89).

4.5 Computational Methods and the Threshold of Toxicological Concern

Developments of Quantitative Structure-Activity Relationship Models (see also Chapter 5.3) for reproductive toxicity are relatively meagre due to both the complexity of the endpoint and the limited data which are publicly available (90). The more-recent availability of larger toxicity data-sets might change this (91).

An alternative approach has been made by improving the Threshold of Toxicological Concern (TTC) for DART (92) by expanding earlier attempts by BASF (93–96), which avoid testing by defining doses that are very unlikely to produce a hazard across large numbers of chemicals (97). This work resulted in remarkably high TTCs (compared with other endpoints) of 100 µg/kg bw/day for rats, and 95 µg/kg bw/day for rabbits, for reproductive toxicity. If found acceptable, this approach could contribute to considerable test waiving.

5. CONCLUDING REMARKS

Because carcinogenicity and reproductive toxicity are two complex endpoints, the uptake of alternative *in vitro* test methods is still very limited. Rather, some approaches are being investigated or are already in place for waiving testing and reducing the number of animals, such as the ICH strategy for pharmaceuticals and the extended one-generation assay.

Promise for both hazards comes from the starting development of IATAs: by mapping the reproductive cycle and its disturbance or the array of pathways of carcinogenesis with a number of assays, the hope is to design a more human-relevant test strategy. These and other approaches form part of the emerging roadmap for replacement (22, 54, 98) and will contribute to the momentum for implementing alternative approaches, which is also helped by the increasing recognition of the shortcomings of current testing (99).

Given the importance of these hazards and the backlog of testing for most substances in daily use, more efforts in the development of tests, design of testing strategies and their validation are needed, as recently proposed by the US FDA.

REFERENCES

1. Adler, S., Basketter, D., Creton, S., *et al.* (2011). Alternative (non-animal) methods for cosmetics testing: current status and future prospects. *Archives of Toxicology* **85**, 367—485.
2. Anon. (2017). *Study on the Cumulative Health and Environmental Benefits of Chemical Legislations*, 529pp. London, UK: Amec Foster Wheeler Environment & Infrastructure UK Limited. Final report for the European Commission. KH-01-17-912-EN-N.
3. ECHA. (2011). *ECHA Guidance on Information Requirements and Chemical Safety Assessment. Part B: Hazard Assessment*, 68pp. Helsinki, Finland: ECHA.
4. Mattison, D.R. (2010). Environmental exposures and development. *Current Opinions in Pediatrics* **22**, 208—218.
5. Madia, F., Worth, A. & Corvi, R. (2016). Analysis of carcinogenicity testing for regulatory purposes in the European Union, 92pp. JRC Report EUR **27765**.
6. Gottmann, E., Kramer, S., Pfahringer, B., *et al.* (2001). Data quality in predictive toxicology: Reproducibility of rodent carcinogenicity experiments. *Environmental Health Perspectives* **109**, 509—514.
7. Alden, C.L., Lynn, A., Bourdeau, A., *et al.* (2011). A critical review of the effectiveness of rodent pharmaceutical carcinogenesis testing in predicting human risk. *Veterinary Pathology* **48**, 772—784.
8. Knight, A., Bailey, J. & Balcombe, J. (2006). Animal carcinogenicity studies: 1. Poor human predictivity. *ATLA* **34**, 19—27.
9. Paparella, M., Colacci, A. & Jacobs, M.N. (2016). Uncertainties of testing methods: What do we (want to) know about carcinogenicity? *ALTEX* **34**, 235—252.
10. Paules, R.S., Aubrecht, J., Corvi, R., *et al.* (2011). Moving forward in human cancer risk assessment. *Environmental Health Perspectives* **119**, 739—743.
11. Birnbaum, L.S. & Fenton, S. (2003). Cancer and developmental exposure to endocrine disruptors. *Environmental Health Perspectives* **111**, 389—394.
12. Waters, M.D. (2016). Introduction to predictive carcinogenicity. In M.D. Waters, & R.S. Thomas (Eds.), *Issues in Toxicology No. 28 Toxicogenomics in Predictive Carcinogenicity*, pp. 1—38. Cambridge, UK: Royal Society of Chemistry.
13. Kim, J.H. & Scialli, A.R. (2011). Thalidomide: the tragedy of birth defects and the effective treatment of disease. *Toxicological Sciences* **122**, 1—6.
14. Hartung, T. & Rovida, C. (2009). Chemical regulators have overreached. *Nature, London* **460**, 1080—1081.
15. Hartung, T. (2008). Toward a new toxicology — evolution or revolution? *ATLA* **36**, 635—639.
16. Hareng, L., Pellizzer, C., Bremer, S., *et al.* (2005). The Integrated Project ReProTect: a novel approach in reproductive toxicity hazard assessment. *Reproductive Toxicology* **20**, 441—452.
17. Daneshian, M., Kamp, H., Hengstler, J., *et al.* (2016). Highlight report: Launch of a large integrated European in vitro toxicology project: EU-ToxRisk. *Archives of Toxicology* **90**, 1021—1024.
18. Knudsen, T.B., Kavlock, R.J., Daston, G.P., *et al.* (2011). Developmental toxicity testing for safety assessment: new approaches and technologies. *Birth Defects Research B: Developmental Reproductive Toxicology* **92**, 413—420.
19. Collins, T.F. (2006). History and evolution of reproductive and developmental toxicology guidelines. *Current Pharmaceutical Design* **12**, 1449—1465.
20. Rovida, C., Longo, F. & Rabbit, R.R. (2011). How are reproductive toxicity and developmental toxicity addressed in REACH dossiers? *ALTEX* **28**, 273—294.
21. Carney, E.W., Ellis, A.L., Tyl, R.W., *et al.* (2011). Critical evaluation of current developmental toxicity testing strategies: a case of babies and their bathwater. *Birth Defects Research B: Developmental Reproductive Toxicology* **92**, 395—403.
22. Basketter, D.A., Clewell, H., Kimber, I., *et al.* (2012). A roadmap for the development of alternative (non-animal) methods for systemic toxicity testing. *ALTEX* **29**, 3—89.
23. Martin, M.T., Judson, R.S., Reif, D.M., *et al.* (2009). Profiling chemicals based on chronic toxicity results from the U.S. EPA ToxRef Database. *Environmental Health Perspectives* **117**, 392—399.
24. Bremer, S. & Hartung, T. (2004). The use of embryonic stem cells for regulatory developmental toxicity testing in vitro — the current status of test development. *Current Pharmaceutical Design* **10**, 2733—2747.
25. Kirkland, D., Aardema, M., Henderson, L., *et al.* (2005). Evaluation of the ability of a battery of three *in vitro* genotoxicity tests to discriminate rodent carcinogens and non-carcinogens I. Sensitivity, specificity and relative predictivity. *Mutation Research* **584**, 1—256.
26. Kirkland, D., Pfuhler, S., Tweats, D., *et al.* (2007). How to reduce false positive results when undertaking *in vitro* genotoxicity testing and thus avoid unnecessary follow up animal tests: Report of an ECVAM Workshop. *Mutation Research* **628**, 31—55.
27. EURL ECVAM. (2013). EURL ECVAM strategy to avoid and reduce animal use in genotoxicity testing, 48pp. JRC Report EUR **26375**.
28. Corvi, R., Albertini, S., Hartung, T., *et al.* (2008). ECVAM retrospective validation of in vitro micronucleus test (MNT). *Mutagenesis* **23**, 271—283.
29. Kirkland, D., Reeve, L., Gatehouse, D., *et al.* (2011). A core *in vitro* genotoxicity battery comprising the Ames test plus the *in vitro* micronucleus test is sufficient to detect rodent carcinogens and *in vivo* genotoxins. *Mutation Research* **721**, 27—73.
30. Corvi, R. & Madia, F. (2017). In vitro genotoxicity testing: can the performance be enhanced? *Food and Chemical Toxicology* **106**, 600—608.
31. Tennant, R.W., Stasiewicz, S., Mennear, J., *et al.* (1999). Genetically altered mouse models for identifying carcinogens. *IARC Scientific Publications* **146**, 123—150.
32. Marx, J. (2003). Building better mouse models for studying cancer. *Science, New York* **299**, 1972—1975.
33. ILSI HESI ACT. (2001). ILSI HESI Alternatives to carcinogenicity testing project. *Toxicologic Pathology* **29**(Suppl), 1—351.
34. MacDonald, J., French, J.E., Gerson, R.J., *et al.* (2004). The utility of genetically modified mouse assays for identifying human carcinogens: A basic understanding and path forward. *Toxicological Sciences* **77**, 188—194.

35. ICH.. (2009). S1B Guideline on Carcinogenicity Testing of Pharmaceuticals. *EMA Document CPMP/ICH/299/95*, 8pp. London, UK: European Medicines Agency.

36. LeBoeuf, R.A., Kerckaert, K.A., Aardema, M.J., *et al.* (1999). Use of Syrian hamster embryo and BALB/c 3T3 cell transformation for assessing the carcinogenic potential of chemicals. *IARC Scientific Publications* **146**, 409–425.

37. Combes, R., Balls, M., Curren, R., *et al.* (1999). Cell transformation assay as predictors of human carcinogenicity. *ATLA* **27**, 745–767.

38. EURL ECVAM. (2012). *EURL ECVAM Recommendation on Three Cell Transformation Assays Using Syrian Hamster Embryo Cells (SHE) and the BALB/c 3T3 Mouse Fibroblast Cell Line for In Vitro Carcinogenicity Testing*, 43pp. Ispra, Italy: EC Joint Research Centre.

39. EURL ECVAM. (2013). EURL ECVAM Recommendation on cell transformation assay based on the Bhas 42 cell line, 36pp. JRC Report EUR **26374**, 36.

40. OECD. (2015). *Guidance Document on the In Vitro Syrian Hamster Embryo (SHE) Cell Transformation Assay*. Series on Testing and Assessment No. 214, 24pp. Paris, France: OECD.

41. OECD. (2016). *Guidance Document on the In vitro Bhas 42 Cell Transformation Assay*. Series on Testing and Assessment No. 231, 35pp. Paris, France: OECD.

42. OECD. (2007). *Detailed Review Paper on Cell Transformation Assays for Detection of Chemical Carcinogens*. Series on Testing and Assessment No. 31, 164pp. Paris, France: OECD.

43. Corvi, R., Aardema, M.J., Gribaldo, L., *et al.* (2012). ECVAM prevalidation study on in vitro cell transformation assays: general outline and conclusions of the study. *Mutation Research* **744**, 12–19.

44. Jacobs, M.N., Colacci, A., Louekari, K., *et al.* (2016). International regulatory needs for development of an IATA for non-genotoxic carcinogenic chemical substances. *ALTEX* **33**, 359–392.

45. Vaccari, M., Mascolo, M.G., Rotondo, F., *et al.* (2015). Identification of pathway-based toxicity in the BALB/c 3T3 cell model. *Toxicology in Vitro* **29**, 1240–1253.

46. Schaap, M.M., Wackers, P.F., Zwart, E.P., *et al.* (2015). A novel toxicogenomics-based approach to categorize (non-)genotoxic carcinogens. *Archives of Toxicology* **89**, 2413–2427.

47. Worth, A., Barroso, J.F., Bremer, S., *et al.* (2014). Alternative methods for regulatory Toxicology — A State-of-the-art Review, 470pp. JRC Report EUR **26797**.

48. Doktorova, T.Y., Yildirimman, R., Celeen, L., *et al.* (2014). Testing chemical carcinogenicity by using a transcriptomics HepaRG-based model? *EXCLI Journal* **13**, 623–637.

49. Herwig, R., Gmuender, H., Corvi, R., *et al.* (2016). Inter-laboratory study of human *in vitro* toxicogenomics-based tests as alternative methods for evaluating chemical carcinogenicity: a bioinformatics perspective. *Archives of Toxicology* **90**, 2215–2229.

50. Corvi, R., Vilardell, M., Aubrecht, J., *et al.* (2016). Validation of transcriptomics-based *in vitro* methods. In C. Eskes, & M. Whelan (Eds.), *Advances in Experimental Medicine and Biology:* **856**. *Validation of Alternative Methods for Toxicity Testing*, pp. 243–257. Basel, Switzerland: Springer Verlag.

51. ICH.. (2016). *The ICHS1 Regulatory Testing Paradigm of Carcinogenicity in Rats - Status Report*, 5pp. Geneva, Switzerland: ICH. Safety Guidelines, 2 March 2016.

52. Sistare, F.D., Morton, D., Alden, C., *et al.* (2011). An analysis of pharmaceutical experience with decades of rat carcinogenicity testing: support for a proposal to modify current regulatory guidelines. *Toxicological Pathology* **9**, 716–744.

53. van der Laan, J.W., Kasper, P., Silva Lima, B., *et al.* (2016). Critical analysis of carcinogenicity study outcomes. Relationship with pharmacological properties. *Critical Reviews in Toxicology* **26**, 1–28.

54. Hartung, T., Blaauboer, G.J., Bosgra, S., *et al.* (2011). An expert consortium review of the EC-commissioned report "Alternative (Non-Animal) Methods for Cosmetics Testing: Current Status and Future Prospects — 2010". *ALTEX* **28**, 183–209.

55. Spielmann, H. (2009). The way forward in reproductive/developmental toxicity testing. *ATLA* **37**, 641–656.

56. Leist, M., Hasiwa, N., Rovida, C., *et al.* (2014). Consensus report on the future of animal-free systemic toxicity testing. *ALTEX* **31**, 341–356.

57. Janer, G., Hakkert, B.C., Slob, W., *et al.* (2007). A retrospective analysis of the two-generation study: What is the added value of the second generation? *Reproductive Toxicology* **24**, 97–102.

58. OECD. (2012). *OECD TG No. 443: Extended One-Generation Reproductive Toxicity Study*, 25pp. Paris, France: OECD.

59. Doe, J.E., Boobis, A.R. & Blacker, A. (2006). A tiered approach to systemic toxicity testing for agricultural chemical safety assessment. *Critical Reviews in Toxicology* **36**, 37–68.

60. Vogel, R., Seidle, T. & Spielmann, H. (2010). A modular one-generation reproduction study as a flexible testing system for regulatory safety assessment. *Reproductive Toxicology* **29**, 242–245.

61. Moore, N., Bremer, S., Carmichael, N., *et al.* (2009). A modular approach to the extended one-generation reproduction toxicity study: Outcome of an ECETOC task force and International ECETOC/ECVAM workshop. *ATLA* **37**, 219–225.

62. Selderslaghs, I.W.T., Blust, R. & Witters, H.E. (2012). Feasibility study of the zebrafish assay as an alternative method to screen for developmental toxicity and embryotoxicity using a training set of 27 compounds. *Reproductive Toxicology* **33**, 142–154.

63. Sukardi, H., Chng, H.T., Chan, E.C., *et al.* (2011). Zebrafish for drug toxicity screening: bridging the in vitro cell-based models and in vivo mammalian models. *Expert Opinion on Drug Metabolism and Toxicology* **7**, 579–589.

64. Weigt, S., Huebler, N., Braunbeck, T., *et al.* (2010). Zebrafish teratogenicity test with metabolic activation (mDarT): effects of phase I activation of acetaminophen on zebrafish Danio rerio embryos. *Toxicology* **275**, 36–49.

65. Yang, Q., Hu, J., Ye, D., *et al.* (2010). Identification and expression analysis of two zebrafish E2F5 genes during oogenesis and development. *Molecular Biology Reports* **37**, 1773–1780.

66. Hoke, R.A. & Ankley, G.T. (2005). Application of frog embryo teratogenesis assay-Xenopus to ecological risk assessment. *Environmental Toxicology & Chemistry* **24**, 2677−2690.
67. Stephens, M.L., Betts, K., Beck, N.B., *et al.* (2016). .The emergence of systematic review in toxicology. *Toxicological Science* **152**, 10−16.
68. Hoffmann, S., de Vries, R.B.M., Stephens, M.L., *et al.* (2017). A primer on systematic reviews in toxicology. *Archives of Toxicology* **91**, 2551−2575.
69. Hartung, T. (2010). Evidence based-toxicology − the toolbox of validation for the 21st century? *ALTEX* **27**, 241−251.
70. Laschinski, G., Spielmann, H. & Vogel, R. (1990). *In vitro* Testsystem in der Reproduktionstoxikologie: Zytotoxizitätstest an embryonalen Stammzellen der Maus. *Fertilität* **6**, 214−219.
71. Laschinski, G., Vogel, R. & Spielmann, H. (1991). Cytotoxicity test using blastocyst-derived euploid embryonal stem cells: a new approach to in vitro teratogenesis screening. *Reproductive Toxicology* **5**, 57−64.
72. Heuer, J., Bremer, S., Pohl, I., *et al.* (1993). Development of an in vitro embryotoxicity test using embryonic stem cell cultures. *Toxicology in Vitro* **7**, 551−556.
73. Genschow, E., Spielmann, H., Scholz, G., *et al.* (2004). Validation of the embryonic stem cell test in the international ECVAM validation study on three in vitro embryotoxicity tests. *ATLA* **32**, 209−244.
74. Piersma, A.H., Genschow, E., Verhoef, A., *et al.* (2004). Validation of the postimplantation rat whole-embryo culture test in the international ECVAM validation study on three in vitro embryotoxicity tests. *ATLA* **32**, 275−307.
75. Spielmann, H., Genschow, E., Brown, N.A., *et al.* (2004). Validation of the rat limb bud micromass test in the international ECVAM validation study on three in vitro embryotoxicity tests. *ATLA* **32**, 245−274.
76. Spielmann, H., Seiler, A., Bremer, S., *et al.* (2006). The practical application of three validated in vitro embryotoxicity tests. The report and recommendations of an ECVAM/ZEBET workshop (ECVAM workshop 57). *ATLA* **34**, 527−538.
77. Hartung, T., Luechtefeld, T., Maertens, A., *et al.* (2013). Integrated testing strategies for safety assessments. *ALTEX* **30**, 3−18.
78. Rovida, C., Alépée, N., Api, A.M., *et al.* (2015). Integrated testing strategies (ITS) for safety assessment. *ALTEX* **32**, 171−181.
79. Bottini, A.A., Amcoff, P. & Hartung, T. (2007). Food for thought... on globalisation of alternative methods. *ALTEX* **24**, 255−269.
80. OECD. (2016). *Guidance Document on the Reporting of Defined Approaches to be used within Integrated Approaches to Testing and Assessment.* Series on Testing and Assessment No. 255, 23pp. Paris, France: OECD.
81. Tollefsen, K.E., Scholz, S., Cronin, M.T., *et al.* (2014). Applying adverse outcome pathways (AOPs) to support integrated approaches to testing and assessment (IATA). *Regulatory Toxicology and Pharmacology* **70**, 629−640.
82. Leist, M., Bremer, S., Brundin, P., *et al.* (2008). The biological and ethical basis of the use of human embryonic stem cells for in vitro test systems or cell therapy. *ALTEX* **25**, 163−190.
83. Marx-Stoelting, P., Adriaens, E., Ahr, H.J., *et al.* (2009). A review of the implementation of the embryonic stem cell test (EST). The report and recommendations of an ECVAM/ReProTect Workshop. *ATLA* **37**, 313−328.
84. Le Coz, F., Suzuki, N., Nagahori, H., *et al.* (2015). Hand1-Luc embryonic stem cell test (Hand1-Luc EST): a novel rapid and highly reproducible in vitro test for embryotoxicity by measuring cytotoxicity and differentiation toxicity using engineered mouse ES cells. *Journal of Toxicological Sciences* **40**, 251−261.
85. Hall, W. (2017). *OECD Test Guidelines Programme Update*, 8pp. ICCVAM Public Forum, 23 May 2017.
86. Chen, X., Han, T., Fisher, J.E., *et al.* (2017). Transcriptomics analysis of early embryonic stem cell differentiation under osteoblast culture conditions: Applications for detection of developmental toxicity. *Reproductive Toxicology* **69**, 75−83.
87. FDA. (2017). *FDA's Predictive Toxicology Roadmap*, 16pp. Silver Spring, MD, USA: US FDA.
88. Bremer, S., Pellizzer, C., Hoffmann, S., *et al.* (2007). The development of new concepts for assessing reproductive toxicity applicable to large scale toxicological programs. *Current Pharmaceutical Design* **13**, 3047−3058.
89. Schwarzman, M.R., Ackerman, J.R., Dairkee, S.H., *et al.* (2015). Screening for chemical contributions to breast cancer risk: A case study for chemical safety evaluation. *Environmental Health Perspectives* **123**, 1255−1264.
90. Hartung, T. & Hoffmann, S. (2009). Food for thought on... in silico methods in toxicology. *ALTEX* **26**, 155−166.
91. Hartung, T. (2016). Making big sense from big data in toxicology by read-across. *ALTEX* **33**, 83−93.
92. van Ravenzwaay, B., Jiang, X., Luechtefeld, T., *et al.* (2017). The threshold of toxicological concern for prenatal developmental toxicity in rats and rabbits. *Regulatory Toxicology and Pharmacology* **88**, 157−172.
93. Bernauer, U., Heinemeyer, G., Heinrich-Hirsch, B., *et al.* (2008). Exposure-triggered reproductive toxicity testing under the REACH legislation: A proposal to define significant/relevant exposure. *Toxicology Letters* **176**, 68−76.
94. van Ravenzwaay, B., Dammann, M., Buesen, R., *et al.* (2011). The threshold of toxicological concern for prenatal developmental toxicity. *Regulatory Toxicology and Pharmacology* **59**, 81−90.
95. van Ravenzwaay, B., Dammann, M., Buesen, R., *et al.* (2012). The threshold of toxicological concern for prenatal developmental toxicity in rabbits and a comparison to TTC values in rats. *Regulatory Toxicology and Pharmacology* **64**, 1−8.
96. Laufersweiler, M.C., Gadagbui, B., Baskerville-Abraham, I.M., *et al.* (2012). Correlation of chemical structure with reproductive and developmental toxicity as it relates to the use of the threshold of toxicological concern. *Regulatory Toxicology and Pharmacology* **62**, 160−182.
97. Hartung, T. (2017). Thresholds of Toxicological Concern − setting a threshold for testing where there is little concern. *ALTEX* **34**, 331−351.
98. Corvi, R., Madia, F., Guyton, K.Z., *et al.* (2017). Moving forward in carcinogenicity assessment: Report of an EURL ECVAM-ESTIV workshop. *Toxicology in Vitro* **45**, 278−286.
99. Smirnova, L., Kleinstreuer, N., Corvi, R., *et al.* (2018). 3S - Systematic, systemic, and systems biology and toxicology. *ALTEX* **35**, 139−162.

Chapter 3.7

Biologicals, Including Vaccines

Thea Sesardic and Philip Minor

National Institute for Biological Standards and Control (NIBSC), Potters Bar, Hertfordshire, United Kingdom

SUMMARY

This chapter provides a historical and up-to-date insight into Three Rs initiatives related to the safety and potency testing of certain biological products, including vaccines, which cannot be fully characterised by chemical or physical methods because of their complex modes of action or manufacturing processes. As a consequence, bioassays in animals were the method of choice in the regulatory procedures laid down to assess product quality. Biological products, which rely on the most severe endpoints, such as the LD50 test (e.g. the safety tests for pertussis and tetanus vaccines and potency tests for therapeutic botulinum toxin) and direct challenge potency tests (e.g. for inactivated vaccines against diphtheria, tetanus and rabies), use the largest number of animals and animals of the highest orders (e.g. monkeys for safety tests on live viral vaccines), were in the frontline of replacement. This chapter considers the progress made toward the elimination of the use of animals for these and other general safety methods involved in the quality control of biologicals.

1. INTRODUCTION

Biologicals, including many vaccines, are medicines that are often complex in their properties, modes of action and manufacturing processes, to an extent that it is impossible to measure the 'active component' in the product through the use of chemical or physical methods. Consequently, many of the tests designed to assure safety and potency measure a biological property of the product. Originally, many of these tests could only be performed in animals because *in vitro* methods were often not suitable to provide assurance of a measure of the clinically relevant biological property of the product.

Animals play a critical role in the development of biological products, and are used at various stages of product development, from early development and pre-clinical studies to clinical studies and sometimes post-licensure as part of the batch release process. In this chapter, we focus on batch release testing, in which animals can be used at different stages, including: (a) testing the seed lots used for the production of live viral vaccines (historically all live viral vaccines had to be tested by intracranial inoculation of monkeys, whatever their pathogenesis); (b) testing on product intermediates, as part of in-process control; and (c) testing of the final product prior to batch release. All batches of vaccines, and in particular, paediatric vaccines, are also evaluated and certified by an independent regulatory authority (Official Control Medicines Laboratory) for Official Control Authority Batch Release, co-ordinated by the European Directorate for the Quality of Medicines and Healthcare (EDQM) that is responsible for quality standards for safe medicines and their use in Europe.

The purpose of the batch release test is to demonstrate that a given lot of a product is safe and effective. For some viral vaccines (e.g. flu vaccines) and well-defined vaccines (e.g. meningococcal polysaccharide conjugate vaccines), a potency test can be performed entirely *in vitro* via antigen quantification assays or tests to assure the presence of the conjugated molecule. For more-complex vaccines, testing may involve the immunisation of animals. After a given period, the immunised animals are challenged, or infected with the virulent agent, to measure protection against the disease. These assays are often multi-dilution assays, may use large numbers of animals and may involve severe pain and distress when the animals that are not sufficiently protected (i.e. those which receive a vaccine dilution) develop the disease. The methods of choice of assays for batch release are stipulated in European Pharmacopoeia (Ph. Eur.) monographs and are legally binding in European Member States.

Initiatives have been in motion for several decades, in recognition that, from an ethical standpoint, animal welfare needs to be considered, and the impact on animal use resulting from vaccine safety and potency testing should be assessed (1–5). Therefore, the focus was on test methods that are most severe, conducted with a high frequency of testing and involving higher order animal species (6). In the UK, some small reduction in total experimental procedure was noted between 2007 and 2016, but 532,000 procedures for regulatory procedures were recorded, which represented 26% of the total number of procedures undertaken for experimental purposes (2.02 million) in 2016. Of these, more that 50% were used for quality control and routine product evaluation.

In this chapter, in several sub-sections, we provide a historical and up-to-date insight on safety and potency procedures for certain biological products, where alternative methods have been extensively studied, validated and, in some cases, introduced as new regulatory standards.

2. ENDOTOXIN AND PYROGENICITY

One of the safety tests that all medicinal products must undergo is the detection and measurement of materials that can cause fever — so-called pyrogens. These agents, derived from bacteria, viruses and fungi, can occur in medicines and vaccines, either as contaminants or as an integral part of the formulation.

The rabbit pyrogen test (RPT) was developed in the 1900s as a test to be prescribed by the pharmacopoeias for monitoring pyrogenicity, as the sensitivity of rabbits to pyrogens is similar to that of humans. The test was originally designed for large-volume parenteral preparations with low pyrogen contents, administered intravenously and is considered less appropriate for products administered intramuscularly or for vaccines that are inherently pyrogenic (7).

The bacterial endotoxins test (BET) was developed (8) and included in the US Pharmacopoeia from 1942 for the detection of endotoxins from gram-negative bacteria (9). Although it was able to replace the RPT for recombinant vaccine components produced in bacterial cells, it could not replace the rabbit test completely because it failed to detect non-endotoxin pyrogens and is sensitive to matrix interference. Alternatives for the BET and RPT for pyrogen testing have been under development since the late 1980s (10–12).

A more-appropriate test for the replacement of the RPT is the monocyte activation test (MAT), which is based on the interaction of pyrogenic substances with human peripheral blood mononuclear cells and measurement of the cytokine response. The MAT has the advantage that it does not require the use of animals, is fully quantitative, is less sensitive to test interference caused by the product and, most importantly, is physiologically relevant to the human fever response (13–15). Since 2010, the MAT has been listed in the Ph. Eur. chapter on Biological Assays but not in vaccine monographs (e.g. hepatitis B, meningococcal polysaccharide, pneumococcal polysaccharide, rabies, tick-borne encephalitis vaccines), where the use of the MAT requires validation in comparison with the RPT for the given product.

In 2014, scientists at the UK National Institute for Biological Standards and Control (NIBSC) validated the use of the MAT as a replacement for the RPT for paediatric meningococcal B vaccine, which was included as part of the UK infant vaccination programme in October 2015. This vaccine contains outer membrane vesicles (OMVs) of *Neisseria menin-gitides* and so potentially contains all the membrane components, including endotoxin and non-endotoxin pyrogens, which generate a pyrogenic response in rabbits when delivered intravenously (7). An international collaborative study to evaluate the robustness and set specification of the MAT for testing OMV-based vaccines has concluded, which should lead to the replacement of RPT as part of the batch release evaluation of these types of vaccines. It has recently been proposed that cell-line systems exclusively expressing single pattern recognition receptors (PRRs), such as Toll-like receptors, could be used instead of primary cells to recognise and identify specific pyrogenic components or contaminants in therapeutic biological products.

3. ABNORMAL TOXICITY

The abnormal toxicity test (ATT), also known as the General Safety Test or innocuity test, is carried out in mice and/or guinea-pigs to detect non-specific contaminates causing adverse effects. The test was originally established around the 1900s, and the rationale at the time was to either titrate the level of the preservative phenol in antiserum preparations or to detect contamination with tetanus spores or toxins. With the introduction of Good Manufacturing Practice and stringent quality control for starting materials, as well as the existence of specific toxicity tests, the relevance and scientific rationale for continuing with the ATT was questioned, as it was considered that the test was not suitable for its intended purpose

(6, 16–18). Retrospective analysis of the ATT carried out in the 1990s (19) led to deletion of the ATT from numerous product monographs and introduced test exemptions. For example, testing on the final lot may be omitted as part of routine lot release, once the consistency of production has been demonstrated (1, 20).

Although the ATT has been deleted from the Ph. Eur. as a general safety test, it is still required in monographs for certain human vaccines and immunosera and as a test to be performed during product development. Further initiatives by experts (21, 22) considered the justification for completely eliminating the ATT from pharmacopoeias and other regulatory requirements, both as a final product test and from production and development. This step has recently been taken by the US FDA (23). At a meeting in September 2016, the Ph. Eur. Group of Experts 15 agreed with the proposal to completely remove reference to the ATT. The revised monographs were adopted by the European Pharmacopoeia Commission, during its 159th plenary session, in November 2017 (EDQM press release of 8 December 2017; https://www.edqm.eu/en/alternatives-animal-testing).

4. SPECIFIC TOXICITY

4.1 Neurovirulence Testing of Live Viral Vaccines

4.1.1 Oral Polio Vaccine

Live polio vaccines were developed by passage of wild polioviruses under suboptimal conditions (24–28) and then testing them for virulence in large numbers of Old World primates, and occasionally chimpanzees (26). The strains acquired attenuating mutations that could, in principle, be lost when the strains were grown, thus producing dangerous viruses (29, 30). Such revertant viruses are also a factor in the endgame of polio eradication (31–33). A vaccine safety test was therefore required and was based on the methods used by Sabin (24, 25, 28). The process was not standardised. Species of Old World monkeys differ in their susceptibility (3), and very large numbers of animals were used, many of which provided little or no information. For example, the intrathalamic route rarely resulted in any histological or clinical signs with the vaccines, in contrast to the wild-type strains, and the effect of dose was minimal.

In the early 1980s, the test was rationalised under the auspices of the World Health Organisation (WHO). The test that emerged (34) used a single dose (as the dose–response curve was very flat), used intraspinal inoculation (as this was the most sensitive route), did not score clinical signs (which were rare) and analysed the response by histological analysis of specified sections of the Central Nervous System. A homologous reference was tested at the same time, to control for the many variables, including inoculation and histological scoring. The reference permitted the establishment of statistical limits and clear and consistent criteria for passing or failing a batch. Consequently, all the animals provided useful information, far fewer animals were used, and more-meaningful results were obtained. However, the number of animals was still very significant. Polio occurs in three different serotypes, which do not protect from each other, so the vaccine must contain a vaccine strain of each type. About 40 monkeys were required for testing a type 3 vaccine, and about 20 monkeys for each of types 1 and 2.

Molecular biological studies were undertaken to change this situation (31, 35). The receptor site used by poliovirus to enter human and primate cells was identified (36, 37). The gene was cloned, and transgenic mice susceptible to infection by polio were developed (38). Extensive studies on the molecular basis of the attenuation and reversion of the Sabin vaccine strains had been carried out (35), and it was shown that mice and monkeys responded in the same way to strains carrying attenuating or reverting mutations (39, 40). Finally, the model was validated extensively with genuine vaccine lots (41, 42). The process involves inoculation of two dilutions of virus into the spine, followed by monitoring for clinical signs and comparison to an established reference strain (34). Although the process uses mice rather than monkeys, and is therefore considered to be ethically more acceptable, it uses large numbers of mice to achieve statistical significance – 128 mice are used for each test of one vaccine and one reference. The test was introduced into regulatory documents in the 1990s.

The mutations involved in the attenuated phenotype were identified, and a method was devised to measure the reversion at a particular position (43). This does not work for mutations where reversion can be by a second site mutation (35). However, for the type 3 strain, it was found that the reversion at a particular base in a non-coding region correlated very precisely with animal neurovirulence (43). The test, termed MAPREC (Mutant Analysis by PCR and Enzyme Cleavage), is elaborate (34), but it provides a precise measure of reversion and consistency of production. The relationship of reversion at the equivalent positions of the type 1 and 2 strains to a virulent phenotype is less clear, but the method is very valuable for assessing consistency.

Next Generation Sequencing could, in principle, be used to assess consistency across the entire genome. If a vaccine is consistently produced, the clinical findings from one batch can be applied to another.

4.1.2 Mumps and Live Vaccines

Other live vaccines were developed with less-perfect animal models than for polio. Mumps is a neurotropic infection in humans, and one of the tests for the attenuation of vaccine seed virus involved the intrathalamic inoculation of non-human primates (44–46). No control was used, and the pass/fail criteria were not defined. Different strains of mumps virus gave different results in monkeys. However, the test was poor at distinguishing between closely related mumps strains with different virulence for humans, as, for example, with vaccines and isolates from vaccine-associated diseases such as aseptic meningitis (45). A test involving neonatal rats gave similar results (46), in that mumps strains could be distinguished, but the meningitis isolate could not be distinguished from parental vaccine. Neither test seemed to predict the virulence of the virus for humans reliably. The primate test remains in the compendium as a way of characterising the virus.

4.2 Inactivated Toxoid Vaccines

DTP vaccines include chemically inactivated diphtheria, tetanus and pertussis toxins, which require a specific toxicity test to confirm absence of toxin and irreversibility. Animals are still required for the safety testing of tetanus toxoid as an in-process test and for pertussis vaccine as part of batch release on final product by the histamine sensitisation test (HIST; (47)).

The Paul Ehrlich Institute (Germany) developed an *in vitro* biochemical method, the so-called BINACLE (binding and cleavage) assay, which mimics two functional properties of intact tetanus toxin molecules: (a) binding via the heavy chain to toxin receptor; and (b) the proteolytic activity of the light chain, namely, the cleavage of synaptobrevin-2 (48, 49). After successful transfer to several laboratories and promising results with regard to reproducibility (50), validation of the BINACLE assay within the Biological Standardisation Programme (BSP) concluded that the method suffers from matrix-effects and is not applicable to all products. Scientists at the NIBSC are working on cell-based assays (CBAs) for tetanus toxin, by using neurons derived from mouse embryonic stem cells and transfected cell lines, as reported at the IABS Conference '3 Rs and Consistency Testing in Vaccine Lot Release Testing', held at Egmond aan Zee, The Netherlands, September 2015.

The HIST was developed in the 1950s (51, 52), as a pharmacopoeia test for monitoring the safety of pertussis vaccines. Over the last 15 years, a number of possible alternatives to the HIST have been extensively studied, which are broadly divided into: (a) assays that measure receptor binding (53, 54); (b) assays that measure the enzymatic activity of the toxin (55, 56) or a combination of the two assay systems (57, 58); and (c) CBAs that measure the whole pertussis toxin function (59–61). An assay that measure biomarkers, i.e. effects on the transcription profile of human cells after exposure to pertussis toxin (62, 63), is at an early stage of development.

Several expert review meetings and workshops dedicated to alternatives to the HIST have been convened over the past few years (60, 61, 64, 65). There was a consensus that it is unlikely that the HIST could be replaced by a single *in vitro* method due to differences in the vaccines manufactured (e.g. pertussis toxin detoxification, formulations, adjuvants). Biochemical assays were considered useful for monitoring pertussis toxin activity, but, because they only capture a single function of the pertussis toxin, preference was given to the further development of CBAs capturing the full function of pertussis toxin.

At a workshop held in London in March 2015, the findings of an International Collaborative study conducted by the EDQM were reviewed, and it was concluded that the modified CHO cell clustering assay (using a porous cell culture insert to prevent contact of the cells with the adjuvant), which, unlike the CHO cell assay, can be applied to final product testing, is sufficiently developed to be considered suitable for further regulatory consideration, subject to product validation (66). The Group of Experts 15 are currently in the process of revising the Ph. Eur. monograph to include the modified CHO cell clustering assay and have initiated discussions to consider the removal of requirements to perform testing on the final product.

5. POTENCY/EFFICACY

5.1 Botulinum Toxins for Therapy

Although highly toxic, and the causative agents of potentially deadly botulism, botulinum toxins (BoNT/s) in minute doses have been used for over 20 years in many medical interventions to treat muscle hyperactivity, such as dystonia and spastic conditions, exocrine gland hyperactivity, such as hyperhidrosis, and pain disorders (67). A number of licensed products are manufactured globally, and testing for potency to determine toxin activity per vial, monitor lot-to-lot variability and set shelf life stability, was dependent on an *in vivo* mouse lethal dose 50 (LD50) assay when the products were first licensed (68, 69), as this was the only model with sufficient sensitivity to detect very small doses of toxin.

Methods to replace the LD50 potency test have been sought for many years and have focused on the measurement of local flaccid paralysis in mice (70), the measurement of the digit abduction score in rats (71) or a mouse tissue *ex vivo* model to measure the activity of the phrenic nerve (72), as refinement alternatives. Methods for the replacement of animals have initially focused on immunodetection (73), which were later improved to measure enzyme activity by detecting cleavage of an intracellular substrate, SNAP25, by the toxin L-chain (74, 75) and further improved to include receptor binding and enzyme activity as a dual functional assay (76, 77).

Reviews of the existing methodologies by the group of experts in 2008 (78) and 2010 (79) concluded that only CBAs, which are capable of reflecting all the major steps of botulinum toxin action *in vivo*, can be considered as new gold standard methods to replace the use of animals. However, biochemical enzyme activity assays can be applied as a consistency test for monitoring the concentration of toxin in pharmaceutical preparations.

In the past decade, much effort has focused on the development of CBAs for BoNT/s that could provide a sensitivity equivalent to the mouse bioassay. These have initially focused on the detection by Western Blotting of cleaved substrate from primary rodent neuronal cells (80), and later from neurons derived from human stem cells (81), by incorporating ELISA detection (82). Several manufacturers have now validated product-specific CBAs and have implemented them in routine potency testing for their products (83–85).

5.2 Inactivated Viral Vaccines

5.2.1 Rabies

Rabies is almost invariably fatal after symptoms develop but can be prevented by immunisation with a vaccine of the right potency; therefore, potency assays are vitally important.

The NIH test involves immunising mice with either the test vaccine or the reference and then challenging them with a virulent virus (86, 87). The original endpoint of the test was death of the animals from rabies, which was modified to use clinical signs and humane endpoints, but the test is hard to reconcile with animal welfare, and the results are also variable.

Antigen assays include Single Radial Diffusion (SRD; (87, 88)) and an ELISA (89), and, for a given product, these may well be perfectly acceptable substitutes for the *in vivo* protection assays. However, the immunogenicity of the different rabies strains per unit of antigen varies (87): the Pitman Moore strain differs from the ERA or LEP strains in terms of the amount of antigen required to protect in the NIH test, which is still essential for a new vaccine in the absence of a clinical trial.

5.2.2 Inactivated Polio Vaccine

Similarly, potency assays for inactivated polio vaccine (IPV) originally involved immunising animals and measuring the response. At that time, the vaccines were impure and of low potency, but as high-potency IPV was developed in the 1980s (90, 91), the tests were improved and the *in vivo* tests now involve rats (92). A single assay is able to measure the potency of all the three components (types 1, 2 and 3).

D antigen is expressed on the intact virus particle, stimulates neutralising antibodies and provides an alternative to the animal model. The usual format is a variation on an ELISA, with an antibody to capture the antigens followed by detector antibodies. The assay has many variables (34), including the extent to which the detector antibody reacts with polio after it has been treated with formalin (93).

The usual strains in IPV are Mahoney (type 1), MEF (type 2) and Saukette (type 3), which were selected more than 60 years ago as common laboratory strains. There is increasing interest in using other strains, which may be safer in production. However, as for rabies, the different strains have different immunogenicities per antigen unit (94). For instance, the type 2 Sabin (live vaccine) strain is about 10-fold less immunogenic than the MEF strain, and the type 1 Sabin strain is rather more immunogenic than the Sabin 1 strain. Thus, the antigen assay must be calibrated against some form of *in vivo* immunogenicity assay, such as in rats or, ultimately, in a clinical trial.

5.3 Inactivated Toxoid Vaccines

Inactivated bacterial toxoid vaccines include paediatric vaccines that protect against diphtheria, tetanus and pertussis diseases. In contrast to polysaccharide vaccines, these vaccines are more difficult to characterise by physicochemical methods, and these alone cannot provide assurance that each toxoid lot can induce a protective immune response. Originally, each batch of vaccine was tested by immunising mice or guinea-pigs with graded doses of vaccine, and the animals were then challenged with a dose of toxin which could cause toxicity. Although the test worked very well, there was considerable inter-assay variability, which meant that large numbers of animals were needed to obtain reliable data. Furthermore, a proportion of unprotected animals would show symptoms associated with the effects of active toxin, hence such tests are considered as high priority tests for replacement (2, 5, 6, 95).

Since the late 1990s, scientists from several laboratories and the NIBSC worked closely with the EDQM to introduce refined potency tests for these vaccines, involving a switch from separate challenge test methods for each component, using guinea-pigs and mice, to a single serological test for all components, using guinea-pigs only (96−100). The procedure is considered an important refinement because animals do not suffer from direct challenge with active toxins, and instead, serum from individual animals is titrated *in vitro*. Furthermore, the precision and variability are superior to that obtained with the challenge methods, and the number of invalid assays is reduced. An additional reduction of animal use could be achieved by applying a single-dilution approach (100). The serological assays were introduced into Ph. Eur. monographs from 2007 but were not validated by many vaccine manufacturers on the grounds of a continuing need for animal testing.

The use of physicochemical and immunochemical antigen quantification techniques to characterise the diphtheria and tetanus antigen, and to apply them to vaccine quality control, has been discussed (101). Because most toxoid vaccines are adjuvanted and contain several vaccine components, only certain immunochemical approaches can be realistically applied to the final product, where antigen can be detected and quantified before or after desorption from the adjuvant (102−105). All these methods are dependent on the binding of monoclonal antibodies to some functional epitopes on the toxoid molecule but cannot realistically provide the same information as that generated by protection models in animals (106). Because of this limitation, the replacement strategies are now being focused on the so-called consistency approach, a topic of several workshops organised by EURL ECVAM (22, 107, 108) and the EPAA (22, 47).

The outcome of these efforts has led to funding from the Innovative Medicines Initiative for VAC2VAC, a 5-year project which commenced in April 2016. The consortium comprises 20 partners, including experts from the vaccine industry, academia and independent testing laboratories, who aim to develop tests and approaches that will permit the acceptance of the consistency approach by the regulatory agencies, thereby providing opportunities for the reduction of animal use in the batch testing of vaccines that currently relies on animals.

6. CONCLUSIONS

Advances in the development of new methods and their validation in recent decades have resulted in the acceptance and introduction of some alternative methods as new regulatory standards. The most significant contribution, expected to have a great impact from 2018, will be the acceptance of CBAs for the safety testing of pertussis vaccines and for the potency testing of therapeutic botulinum toxins. Removing the requirement for a General Safety Test across all biologicals will also have a global impact on animal use. Reducing animal testing is also evident when traditional vaccines (e.g. whole cell or chemically inactivated vaccines) are replaced with more-defined acellular or genetically attenuated products. Nevertheless, there remains a continuing need to explore new technologies and approaches for the improved characterisation of biological products and vaccines, which could reduce the reliance on animal testing.

REFERENCES

1. Castle, P. (1997). Replacement, reduction, refinement (3Rs): Animal welfare progress in European Pharmacopoeia monographs. *Pharmeuropa* **19**, 430−441.
2. Weisser, K. & Hechler, U. (1997). In K. Botrill (Ed.), *Animal Welfare Aspects in the Quality Control of Immunobiologicals: A Critical Evaluation of the Animal Tests in Pharmacopoeial Monographs*, pp. 137−152. Nottingham, UK: FRAME and PEI.
3. Brown, F., Hendriksen, C.F.M. & Sesardic, D. (Eds.). (1999), *Developments in Biological Standardization: Vol. 101. Alternatives to Animals in the Development and Control of Biological Products for Human and Veterinary Use*, 335pp. Basel, Switzerland: S. Karger AG.
4. Brown, F., Hendriksen, C.F.M., Sesardic, D., *et al.* (Eds.). (2002), *Developments in Biological Standardization: 111. Advancing Science and Elimination of the Use of Laboratory Animals for Development and Control of Vaccines and Hormones*, 340pp. Basel, Switzerland: S. Karger AG.
5. Stokes, W.S., Kulpa-Eddy, J. & McFarland, R. (2011). The International Workshop on Alternative Methods to Reduce, Refine and Replace the Use of Animals in Vaccine Potency and Safety Testing: Introduction and Summary. In *Procedia in Vaccinology* **5**, pp. 1−15. Bethesda, MD: NICEAM-ICCVAM. September 2010.
6. Hendriksen, C.F.M., Garthoff, B., Aggerbeck, H., *et al.* (1994). Alternatives to animal testing in the quality control of immunobiologicals: Current status and future prospects. *ATLA* **22**, 420−434.
7. Vipond, C., Findlay, L., Feavers, I., *et al.* (2015). Limitations of the rabbit pyrogen test for assessing meningococcal OMV based vaccines. *ATLA* **33**, 47−53.
8. Bang, F.B. (1956). A bacterial disease of Limulus polyphemus. *Bulletin of John Hopkins Hospital* **98**, 325−351.

9. Roberts, K.J. (1970). The pyrogen test. In K.L. Williams (Ed.), *Endotoxins — Pyrogens, LAL Testing and Depyrogenation*, pp. 261–271. Boca Raton, FL, USA: CRC Press.

10. Duff, G.W. & Atkins, E. (1982). The detection of endotoxin by *in vitro* production of endogenous pyrogen: comparison with limulus amebocyte lysate gelation. *Journal of Immunological Methods* **52**, 323–331.

11. Kirchner, H., Kleinicke, C. & Digel, W. (1982). A whole-blood technique for testing production of human interferon by leukocytes. *Journal of Immunological Methods* **48**, 213–219.

12. Pool, E.J., Johaar, G., James, S., *et al.* (1998). The detection of pyrogens in blood products using an ex vivo whole blood culture assay. *Journal of Immunoassay* **19**, 95–111.

13. Nakagawa, Y., Maeda, H. & Murai, T. (2002). Evaluation of the *in vitro* pyrogen test system based on proinflammatory cytokine release from human monocytes: comparison with a human whole blood culture test system and with the rabbit pyrogen test. *Clinical and Diagnostic Laboratory Immunology* **9**, 588.

14. Hartung, T., Aaberge, I., Berthold, S., *et al.* (2001). Novel pyrogen tests based on the human fever reaction. The report and recommendations of ECVAM Workshop 43. *ATLA* **29**, 99–123.

15. Hoffmann, S., Peterbauer, A., Schindler, S., *et al.* (2005). International validation of novel pyrogen tests based on human monocytoid cells. *Journal of Immunological Methods* **298**, 161–173.

16. Kraemer, B., Nagel, M., Duchow, K., *et al.* (1996). Is the abnormal toxicity test still relevant for the safety of vaccines, sera and immunoglobulins? *ATLA* **13**, 7–16.

17. Duchow, K. & Kramer, B. (1994). Abnormal toxicity — A relevant safety test under GLP- and GMP-conditions in the production of vaccines? *ATLA* **11**, 11–18.

18. Gupta, R.K. (1996). Is the test for abnormal toxicity, general safety or innocuity necessary for vaccines? *Vaccine* **14**, 1716.

19. Krämer, B., Nagel, M., Duchow, K., *et al.* (1996). Is the abnormal toxicity test still relevant for the safety of vaccines, sera and immunoglobulins? *ATLA* **13**, 7–16.

20. Schwanig, M., Nagel, M., Duchow, K., *et al.* (1997). Elimination of abnormal toxicity test for sera and certain vaccines in the European Pharmacopoeia. *Vaccine* **15**, 1047–1048.

21. Garbe, J.H.O., Ausborn, S., Beggs, C., *et al.* (2014). Historical data analyses and scientific knowledge suggest complete removal of the abnormal toxicity test as a quality control test. *Journal of Pharmaceutical Sciences* **103**, 3349–3355.

22. Schutte, K., Szczepanska, A., Halder, M., *et al.* (2017). Modern science for better quality control of medicinal products "Towards global harmonization of 3Rs in biologicals": The report of an EPAA workshop. *Biologicals* **48**, 55–65.

23. FDA. (2 July 2015). Implementation of revocation of general safety test regulations that are duplicative or requirements in biologics license applications. *Federal Register 37971*, (127), 80.

24. Sabin, A.B. (1957). Properties of attenuated polioviruses and their behaviour inhuman beings. In O.V. St Whitlock (Ed.), *Cellular Biology Nucleic Acids and Viruses*, pp. 113–127. New York, NY, USA: New York Academy of Sciences.

25. Sabin, A.B. (1956). Characteristics and genetic potentialities of experimentally produced and naturally occurring variants of poliomyelitis virus. *Annals of the New York Academy of Sciences* **61**, 924–938.

26. Sabin, A.B. (1956). Pathogenesis of poliomyelitis: reappraisal in the light of new data. *Science, New York* **123**, 1151–1157.

27. Sabin, A.B. & Boulger, L. (1973). History of Sabin attenuated poliovirus oral live virus vaccine strains. *Journal of Biological Standardization* **1**, 115–118.

28. Sabin, A.B., Hemessen, W.A. & Winsser, J. (1954). Studies on variants of poliomyelitis virus. I Experimental segregation and properties of avirulent variants of three immunologic types. *Journal of Experimental Medicine* **99**, 551–576.

29. Assad, F. & Cockburn, W.C. (1982). The relation between acute persisting spinal paralysis and poliomyelitis vaccine-result of a ten year enquiry. *Bulletin of the World Health Organization* **60**, 231–242.

30. Minor, P.D. (1980). Comparative biochemical studies of type 3 poliovirus. *Journal of Virology* **34**, 73–84.

31. Minor, P.D. (2012). The polio eradication programme and issues of the endgame. *Journal of General Virology* **93**, 457–474.

32. Kew, O., Morris-Glasgow, V., Landaverde, M., *et al.* (2000). Outbreak of poliomyelitis in Hispaniola associated with circulating type 1 vaccine-derived poliovirus. *Science, New York* **296**, 356–359.

33. Jorba, J., Campagnoli, R.De L. & Kew, O. (2008). Calibration of multiple poliovirus molecular clocks covering an extended evolutionary range. *Journal of Virology* **82**, 4429–4440.

34. WHO. (2017). *Poliomyelitis*, 1pp. Geneva, Switzerland: WHO.

35. Minor, P.D. (1992). The molecular biology of polio vaccines. *Journal of General Virology* **73**, 3065–3077.

36. Minor, P.D., Pipkin, P.A., Hockley, D., *et al.* (1984). Monoclonal antibodies which block cellular receptors of poliovirus. *Virus Research* **1**, 203–212.

37. Mendelsohn, C.L., Wimmer, E. & Racaniello, V.R. (1989). Cellular receptor for poliovirus: molecular cloning, nucleotide sequence, and expression of a new member of the immunoglobulin superfamily. *Cell* **56**, 855–865.

38. Koike, S., Taya, C., Kurata, T., *et al.* (1991). Transgenic mice susceptible to poliovirus. *Proceedings of National Academy of Science of the United States of America* **88**, 951–955.

39. Ren, R., Moss, E.G. & Racaniello, V.R. (1991). Identification of two determinants that attenuate vaccine related type 2 poliovirus. *Journal of Virology* **65**, 1377–1382.

40. Macadaam, A.J., Pollard, S.R., Ferguson, M., *et al.* (1993). Genetic basis of attenuation of the Sabin type 2 vaccine strain in primates. *Virology* **192**, 18−26.
41. Dragunsky, E., Gardner, D., Taffs, R., *et al.* (1993). Transgenic PVR Tg-1 Mice for testing of poliovirus type 3 neurovirulence: comparison with monkey test. *Biologicals* **21**, 233−237.
42. Wood, D.J., Marsden, S. & Nomoto, A. (1996). Transgenic mice: a new model for poliovirus vaccine testing. *Scandinavian Journal of Laboratory Animal Science* **23**, 263−267.
43. Chumakov, K.M., Powers, L.B., Newman, K.E., *et al.* (1991). Correlation between amount of virus with altered nucleotide sequence and the monkey test for acceptability of oral polio virus vaccine. *Proceedings of National Academy of Science of the United States of America* **88**, 199−203.
44. European Pharmacopoiea. (2013). *Mumps Vaccine (Live) Vaccinum Parotitidis Vivum 2004 07/2013/1356*. Strasbourg, France: European Pharmacopoiea.
45. Afzal, M.A., Marsden, S.A., Hull, R.M., *et al.* (1999). Evaluation of the neurovirulence test for mumps vaccines. *Biologicals* **27**, 43−49.
46. Rubin, S.A., Pletnikov, M., Taffs, R., *et al.* (2000). Evaluation of a neonatal rat model for prediction of mumps virus neurovirulence in humans. *Journal of Virology* **74**, 5382−5384.
47. Fabrizio, DeM., Hendriksen, C., Buchheit, K.-H., *et al.* (2015). The Vaccines Consistency Approach project: an EPAA initiative. *Pharmeuropa Bio & Scientific Notes* **2015**, 30−56.
48. Behrensdorf-Nicol, H., Bonifas, U., Hanschmann, K., *et al.* (2013). Binding and cleavage (BINACLE) assay for the functional *in vitro* detection of tetanus toxin: Applicability as alternative method for the safety testing of tetanus toxoids during vaccine production. *Vaccine* **31**, 6247−6253.
49. Behrensdorf-Nicol, H., Kegel, B., Bonifas, U., *et al.* (2008). Residual enzymatic activity of the tetanus toxin light chain present in tetanus toxoid batches used for vaccine production. *Vaccine* **26**, 3835−3841.
50. Behrensdorf-Nicol, H.A., Bonifas, U., Isbrucker, R., *et al.* (2014). Results of an international transferability study of the BINACLE (binding and cleavage) assay for *in vitro* detection of tetanus toxicity. *Biologicals* **42**, 199−204.
51. Maitland, H.B., John, R. & MacDonald, A.D. (1955). The histamine-sensitizing property of Haemophilus pertussis. *Journal of Hygiene* **53**, 196−211.
52. Parfentjev, I.A. & Goodline, M.A. (1948). Histamine shock in mice sensitized with Hemophilus pertussis vaccine. *Journal of Pharmacology and Experimental Therapeutics* **92**, 411−413.
53. Gomez, S.R., Xing, D.H.-L., Corbel, M.J., *et al.* (2006). Development of a carbohydrate binding assay for the B-oligomer of pertussis toxin and toxoid. *Analytical Biochemistry* **356**, 244−253.
54. Isbrucker, R., Bliu, A. & Prior, F. (2010). Modified binding assay for improved sensitivity and specificity in the detection of residual pertussis toxin in vaccine preparations. *Vaccine* **28**, 2687−2692.
55. Cyr, T., Menzies, A., Calver, J. & Whitehouse, L. (2001). A quantitative analysis for the ADP-ribosylation activity of pertussis toxin: an enzymatic-HPLC coupled assay applicable to formulated whole cell and acellular pertussis vaccine products. *Biologicals* **29**, 81−95.
56. Gomez, S.R., Yuen, C.T., Asokanathan, C., *et al.* (2007). ADP-ribosylation activity in pertussis vaccines and its relationship to the in vivo histamine-sensitisation test. *Vaccine* **25**, 3311−3318.
57. Yuen, C.-T., Horiuchi, Y., Asokanathan, C., *et al.* (2010). An *in vitro* assay system as a potential replacement for the histamine sensitisation test for acellular pertussis based combination vaccines. *Vaccine* **28**, 3714−3721.
58. Xing, D., Yuen, C.-T., Asokanathan, C., *et al.* (2012). Evaluation of an *in vitro* assay system as a potential alternative to current histamine sensitization test for acellular pertussis vaccines. *Biologicals* **40**, 456−465.
59. Hoonakker, M., Ruiterkamp, N. & Hendriksen, C. (2010). The cAMP assay: a functional *in vitro* alternative to the *in vivo* histamine sensitization test. *Vaccine* **28**, 1347−1352.
60. Bache, C., Hoonakker, M., Hendriksen, C., *et al.* (2012). Workshop on animal free detection of pertussis toxin in vaccines − alternatives to the histamine sensitisation test. *Biologicals* **40**, 309−311.
61. Isbrucker, R. (2012). Alternative safety testing strategies for acellular pertussis vaccines. In *Proceedings of the 8th World Congress on Alternatives and Animal Use in the Life Sciences, ALTEX Supplement*, pp. 77−80.
62. Vaessen, S., Verkoeijen, S., Vandebriel, R., *et al.* (2013). Identification of biomarkers to detect residual pertussis toxin using microarray analysis of dendritic cells. *Vaccine* **31**, 5223−5231.
63. Vaessen, S., Bruysters, M., Vandebriel, R., *et al.* (2014). Toward a mechanism-based *in vitro* safety test for pertussis toxin. *Human Vaccines & Immunotherapeutics* **10**, 1391−1395.
64. Isbrucker, R., Arciniega, J., McFarland, R., *et al.* (2014). Report on the international workshop on alternatives to the murine histamine sensitization test (HIST) for acellular pertussis vaccines: state of the science and the path forward. *Biologicals* **42**, 114−122.
65. Arciniega, J., Wagner, L., Prymula, R., *et al.* (2016). Report on an international workshop. Alternatives to HIST for acellular pertussis vaccines: progress and challenges in replacement. *Pharmeuropa Bio & Scientific Notes* **2015**, 82−96.
66. Wagner, L., Isbrucker, R., Locht, C., *et al.* (2016). In search of acceptable alternatives to the murine histamine sensitisation test (HIST): what is possible and practical? *Pharmeuropa Bio & Scientific Notes* **2016**, 151−170.
67. Dressler, D. (2012). Clinical applications of botulinum toxin. *Current Opinion in Microbiology* **15**, 325−336.
68. Sesardic, D. (2012). Bioassays for evaluation of medical products derived from bacterial toxins. *Current Opinion in Microbiology* **15**, 310−317.
69. Sesardic, D. & Gaines-Das, R.E. (2009). *Botulinum Toxin: Applying the 3Rs to Product Potency Testing*, 8pp. London, UK: N3CRs.
70. Sesardic, D., McLellan, K., Ekong, T.A.N., *et al.* (1996). Refinement and validation of an alternative bioassay for potency testing of therapeutic botulinum type A toxin. *Pharmacology & Toxicology* **78**, 283−288.

71. Broide, R.S., Rubino, J., Nicholson, G.S., *et al.* (2013). The rat digit abduction score (DAS) assay: a physiological model for assessing botulinum neurotoxin-induced skeletal muscle paralysis. *Toxicon* **71**, 18−24.

72. Rasetti-Escargueil, C., Jones, R.G.A., Liu, Y., *et al.* (2009). Measurement of botulinum types A, B and E neurotoxicity using the phrenic nerve-hemidaphragm: improved precision with in-bred mice. *Toxicon* **53**, 503−511.

73. Ekong, T.A.N., McLellan, K. & Sesardic, D. (1995). Immunological detection of Clostridium botulinum toxin type A in therapeutic preparations. *Journal of Immunological Methods* **180**, 181−191.

74. Ekong, T.A.N., Feavers, I. & Sesardic, D. (1997). Recombinant SNAP-25 is an effective substrate for Clostridium botulinum type A endopeptidase activity. *Microbiology* **143**, 3337−3347.

75. Jones, R.G.A., Ochiai, M., Liu, Y., *et al.* (2008). Development of improved SNAP25 endopeptidase immune-assays for botulinum type A and E toxins. *Journal of Immunological Methods* **329**, 92−101.

76. Liu, Y., Rigsby, P., Marks, J.D., *et al.* (2012). A functional dual-coated (FDC) microtiter plate method to replace the Botulinum toxin LD50 test. *Analytical Biochemistry* **425**, 28−35.

77. Rosen, O., Ozeri, E., Barnea, A., *et al.* (2016). Development of an innovative *in vitro* potency assay for anti-botulinum antitoxins. *Toxins* **8**, 276.

78. NIEHS. (2008). *Report on the ICCVAM-NICEATM/ECVAM Scientific Workshop on Alternatives Methods to Refine, Reduce or Replace the Mouse LD50 Assay for Botulinum Toxin Testing.* NIH Publication number 08-6416, 173pp. Research Triangle Park, NC, USA: NIEHS.

79. Adler, S., Bicker, G., Bigalke, H., *et al.* (2010). Current scientific and legal status of alternative methods to the LD50 test for botulinum neurotoxin potency testing. Report and Recommendation of the ZEBET Expert meeting. *ATLA* **38**, 315−330.

80. Pellett, S., Tepp, W., Toth, S.I., *et al.* (2010). Comparison of the primary rat spinal cord cell (RSC) assay and the mouse bioassay for Botulinum neurotoxin type A potency determination. *Journal of Pharmaceutical and Toxicological Methods* **61**, 304−310.

81. Whitemarsh, R.C.M., Strathman, M.J., Chase, L.G., *et al.* (2012). Novel application of human neurons derived from induced pluripotent stem cells for highly sensitive Botulinum neurodetection. *Toxicological Sciences* **126**, 426−435.

82. Pellett, S., Tepp, W.H., Johnson, E.A., *et al.* (2017). Assessment of ELISA as endpoint in neuronal cell-based assay for BoNT detection using hiPSC derived neurons. *Journal of Pharmaceutical and Toxicological Methods* **88**(Pt 1), 1−6.

83. Fernandez-Salas, E., Wang, J., Molina, Y., *et al.* (2012). Botulinum neurotoxin serotype A specific cell based potency assay to replace the mouse bioassay. *PLoS One* **7**, e49516.

84. Allergan Press Release. (2011). *Allergan Receives FDA Approval for First-of-Its-Kind, Fully In Vitro, Cell-based Assay for BOTOX® and BOTOX® Cosmetic (OnabotulinumtoxinA).* Dublin, Ireland: Allergan.

85. Merz Press Release. (2015). *Alternative Test Method for Botulinum Neurotoxin now Approved in Europe*, 2pp. Frankfurt am Main, Germany: Merk Pharma GmbH.

86. LII, Cornell. (2017). *9 CFR 113.209 Rabies Vaccine, Killed Virus*, 2pp. Ithanca, NY, USA: Legal Information Institute, Corbell Law School.

87. Lyng, J., Bentzon, M.W., Ferguson, M., *et al.* (1992). Rabies vaccine standardization: International collaborative study for the characterization of the fifth International Standard for rabies vaccine. *Biologicals* **20**, 310−313.

88. Ferguson, M. & Schild, G.C.A. (1982). Single radial diffusion technique for the assay of rabies glycoprotein antigen: Application for the potency tests of vaccines against rabies. *Journal of General Virology* **59**, 197−201.

89. Morgeaux, S., Poirier, B., Ragan, C.I., *et al.* (2017). Replacement of in vivo human rabies vaccine potency testing by in vitro glycoprotein quantification using ELISA − Results of an international collaborative study. *Vaccine* **35**, 966−971.

90. Van Wezel, A.L., van Herwaarden, J.A.M. & van de Heuvel-de-Rijk, E.W. (1979). Large scale concentration and purification of virus suspension from microcarrie culture for the preparation of inactivated virus vaccines. *Developments in Biological Standardization* **42**, 65−69.

91. Van Wezwl, A.L., van Steenis, G., Hannick, C.A., *et al.* (1978). New approach to the production of concentrated and purified inactivated polio and rabies tissue culture vaccines. *Developments in Biological Standardization* **41**, 159−168.

92. Van Steenis, G., van Wezel, A.L. & Sekhuis, V.M. (1981). Potency testing of killed polio vaccine in rats. *Developments in Biological Standardization* **47**, 119−128.

93. Ferguson, M., Wood, D.J. & Minor, P.D. (1993). Antigenic structure of poliovirus in inactivated vaccines. *Journal of General Virology* **74**, 685−690.

94. Dragunsky, E.M., Ivanov, A.P., Wells, V.R., *et al.* (2004). Evaluation of immunogenicity and protective properties of inactivated poliovirus vaccines: a new surrogate method for predicting vaccine efficacy. *Journal of Infectious Diseases* **190**, 1404−1412.

95. Stokes, W.S., Kulpa-Eddy, J. & McFarland, R. (2011). The international workshop on alternatives methods to reduce, refine and replace the use of animals in vaccine potency and safety testing: introduction and summary. *Procedia in Vaccinology* **5**, 1−15.

96. Winsnes, R. & Hendriksen, C. (2000). Collaborative study for the validation of serological methods for potency testing of tetanus toxoid vaccines for human use. *Pharmeuropa Bio* **2000**(1), 83−124.

97. Winsnes, R., Sesardic, D., Dass, A., *et al.* (2004). Collaborative study for the validation of serological methods for potency testing of diphtheria toxoid vaccines. Part 1. *Pharmeuropa Bio* **2003**(2), 35−68.

98. Winsnes, R., Sesardic, D., Dass, A., *et al.* (2006). Collaborative study for the validation of serological methods for potency testing of diphtheria toxoid vaccines. Part 2. *Pharmeuropa Bio* **2006**(1), 73−88.

99. Winsnes, R., Sesardic, D., Daas, A., *et al.* (2009). Collaborative study on a guinea pig serological model for the assay of acellular pertussis vaccines. *Pharmeuropa Bio* **2009**(1), 27−40.

100. Stickings, P., Rigsby, P., Coombes, L., *et al.* (2011). Animal refinement and reduction: alternative approaches for potency testing of diphtheria and tetanus vaccines. *Procedia in Vaccinology* **5**, 200−212.

101. Metz, B., Brunel, F., Chamberlin, C., *et al.* (2007). The potential of physicochemical and immunochemical assays to replace animal tests in the quality control of toxoid vaccines. The report and recommendations of ECVAM workshop 61. *ATLA* **35**, 323–331.

102. Coombes, L., Tierney, R., Rigsby, P., *et al.* (2012). *In vitro* antigen ELISA for quality control of tetanus vaccines. *Biologicals* **40**, 466–472.

103. Coombes, L., Stickings, P., Tierney, R., *et al.* (2009). Development and use of a novel *in vitro* assay for testing of diphtheria toxoid in combination vaccines. *Journal of Immunological Methods* **350**, 142–149.

104. Zhu, D., Huang, S., Gebregeorgis, E., *et al.* (2009). Development of a direct alhydrogel formulation immunoassay (DAFIA). *Journal of Immunological Methods* **344**, 73–78.

105. Westdijk, J., Metz, B., Spruit, N., *et al.* (2017). Antigenic fingerprinting of diphtheria toxoid adsorbed to aluminium phosphate. *Biologicals* **47**, 69–75.

106. Keller, J.E. (2011). Overview of currently approved serological methods with a focus on diphtheria and tetanus toxoid potency testing. *Procedia in Vaccinology* **5**, 192–199.

107. Hendriksen, C., Arciniega, J., Bruckner, L., *et al.* (2008). The consistency approach for the quality control of vaccines. *Biologicals* **36**, 73–77.

108. De Mattia, F., Chapsal, J., Descamps, J., *et al.* (2011). The consistency approach for quality control of vaccines — a strategy to improve quality control and implement 3Rs. *Biologicals* **39**, 59–65.

Chapter 3.8

The Use of Imaging, Biomonitoring and Microdosing in Human Volunteers to Improve Safety Assessments and Clinical Development

Tal Burt[1] and Robert D. Combes[2]

[1]Burt Consultancy, LLC, Durham, NC, United States; [2]Independent Consultant, Norwich, United Kingdom

SUMMARY

The scientific rationale for undertaking first-in-human volunteer studies at earlier than the usual stages of pharmaceutical development involving efficacy and safety assessment, within the stipulations of the Declaration of Helsinki, is discussed. The advantages and disadvantages of various clinical techniques, including diagnostic imaging, biomonitoring to estimate levels of endogenous exposure from levels of biomarkers in body fluids, and the administration of microdose levels (<100 μg/each administration) of drug candidates (phase 0 trials), coupled with ultra-sensitive analytical detection methods, are considered, with the use of examples. It is concluded that: (a) the above-mentioned techniques offer substantial scientific, financial and logistical benefits, while remaining largely non-invasive to volunteers; (b) recently developed procedures for real-time imaging, at the single cell level in humans require simplification; and (c) these advantages need to be more-widely publicised to increase the adoption of the methods into practice.

1. GENERAL INTRODUCTION

One reason given for using animals in many types of biomedical and toxicological research and testing is to avoid the possibility that human volunteers could be subjected to unacceptably high risks, when insufficient prior safety information is available. This is despite the fact that the target species is most often the human being, in which case, species extrapolation is by-passed, when using humans as surrogates for the effects arising in other humans (1, 2). However, approaches have been suggested, which, in some cases, might replace the use of animals with studies on humans at earlier than the usual stages of pharmaceutical development. Phase-0/microdosing studies, with their sub-therapeutic exposure and lack of therapeutic intent, are examples of such approaches.

Some of these strategies were discussed at a symposium in 1995, organised by a group of individuals in the UK called Volunteers in Research and Testing (VRT; 3). The methods included non-invasive brain scanning, particularly for monitoring and studying neurodegenerative diseases, and in the application of therapeutic treatments for them, and to characterise various mechanistic processes occurring in response to endogenous exposure to new drugs. The methods included real-time imaging of drug—receptor interactions and microdosing (4, 5). Yet a further approach to investigating endogenous levels, and potential adverse effects, of chemical exposures is to undertake non-invasive biomonitoring by analysis of body fluids for biomarkers specific for the chemicals involved, and the toxic endpoints of interest (6).

In the UK, in particular, the first administration to humans (phase I testing) of a candidate drug, to assess absorption, distribution, metabolism and excretion, has traditionally been possible at a reasonably early stage of pre-clinical testing,

The History of Alternative Test Methods in Toxicology. https://doi.org/10.1016/B978-0-12-813697-3.00026-3

with further, longer-term clinical studies being contingent on the results of subsequent animal testing, involving an increased number of toxicity endpoints. While the first few doses of a candidate pharmaceutical, administered during phase 1 of a clinical study, are escalating, the first, lowest dose is usually, but not necessarily, known, or assumed, to be safe.

Permission to proceed with any research and testing, involving human subjects, should not be granted, if the importance of the objective is disproportionate to the inherent risks to the subject. Moreover, even if the go-ahead were to be granted at this stage, each volunteer entering a study must be fully informed of the trial protocol, so that he or she would be able to make a balanced judgement about participation: and volunteers should also be informed of their right to withdraw from a study at any time. The volunteer's written informed consent should be obtained prior to the commencement of the study.

These issues, and those dealing with encouragement protection, are fully covered by the requirements for clinical research, as presented in the World Medical Association's Declaration of Helsinki, as adopted by the 18th World Medical Assembly in 1964, with subsequent amendments (7). In practice, studies must not carry more than minimal risk, they must not be more than minimally painful or unpleasant, they should not cause any permanent disfigurement, or hidden irreversible toxic effect (such as sensitisation), and they must not be degrading or offensive.

The rationale for the conference, organised by VRT in 1995, was to discuss the benefits and limitations of human studies, in relation to the possible subsequent effects on reducing the numbers of animals required in research and testing. To this should be added, the very important scientific benefit that studies in the target species, earlier than usually thought possible, should provide more-relevant information at critical stages in the development of new pharmaceuticals, when crucial decisions have to be made about selecting drug candidates, for further development. The proceedings of the VRT conference show that, even some 22 years ago, there was considerable scope for clinical studies in humans, of substances for which toxicological profiles in other test systems were incomplete.

2. CLINICAL IMAGING

The prediction that the application of clinical imaging techniques to patients is likely to be of increasing value, made in several reviews published in the 1990s, has certainly come to fruition. Such imaging is largely non-invasive, and electrode probes have been miniaturised and made to be more-sensitive, thereby further enabling studies to be performed in real-time. Such has been the pace of progress in this field over the last two decades that Matthews et al. (8) noted that *Clinical imaging offers a range of methods for the support of drug development that are able to address major questions related to target validation and molecule biodistribution, target interactions and pharmaco-dynamics.* Also, in 2011, Asbury (9) began a comprehensive review with the words, *Imaging technologies now provide unprecedented sensitivity to visualisation of brain structure and function from the level of individual molecules to the whole brain. Many imaging methods are noninvasive and allow dynamic processes to be monitored over time. Imaging is enabling researchers to identify neural networks involved in cognitive processes; understand disease pathways; recognise and diagnose diseases early, when they are most effectively treated; and determine how therapies work.*

Some examples of imaging and its applications in the pharmaceutical industry are summarised in Table 1, whereas a more-detailed discussion can be found in ref. (10). With some imaging techniques, it is possible to analyse effects, not only in real-time, but also in different layers through an organ or the whole, or part, of the body (e.g. Computer Tomography), but also to monitor recovery, and the effects of repeat-dose exposure. PET imaging, through the labelling of the test drug or the biomarkers associated with the drug effects, can enable real-time study of core features relevant to drug development decision-making: tissue distribution, receptor binding, and post-receptor modulation. These studies can apply to both therapeutic and toxicity targets simultaneously as a single administration of a radiotracer would allow PET imaging of the entire body. Magnetic resonance imaging (MRI) can also be used to visualise internal structures, and is especially useful in showing what is happening in brain tissues. Thus, by applying clinical imaging techniques, the nature and progression of events can be followed as they happen, at the molecular level, and within the human body. Imaging studies with volunteers can also reduce the duration and financial costs of clinical trials.

3. BIOMONITORING

3.1 Background

Biomonitoring is a way of assessing internal exposure to, and the possible systemic effects of, a substance to which an individual is exposed, thereby strengthening the link between exposure and effect (6). It is most commonly undertaken by analysing body fluids (including, most frequently, blood and urine, and occasionally, bile, semen, amniotic fluid and cerebrospinal fluid). Biomonitoring sometimes involves the analysis and processing of faecal stool samples, when there is a focus on the intestinal tract as a target (11, 12).

TABLE 1 Some Non-invasive Approaches for Undertaking Pharmaceutical Characterisation and Prospective (P) and Retrospective (R) Safety Testing by Using Healthy Volunteers and Patients Early in Product Development

Description (P/R)	Technology	Main Outcome
Drug imaging — low dose studies (P)	PET[a] visualisation of radiolabelled drug (*in vivo*)[b]	Can work with picomole amounts, as in microdosing
Drug imaging — early PK[c] studies (P)	PET visualisation of drug-target receptor binding	Prediction of optimal dose levels for subsequent clinical trials
Drug imaging — mechanistic studies[d] (P)	PET or MRI[e] quantification of receptor binding and receptor occupancy	Provides better measure of drug efficacy at doses below toxic threshold
Drug imaging — levels of drug in brain (P)	Imaging of brain levels of enkephalinase inhibitors in humans	Highly toxic in animals halting preclinical studies; but not so in humans due to lack of passage across BBB[f] (see Ref. (10))
Endogenous exposure studies via biomonitoring of body fluids (especially urine; R)	Biomarkers of exposure (e.g. NNAL[g] — principal metabolite of TSNA[h] lung carcinogen — NNK[i])	E.g. safety studies on vaping; occupational exposures (see Ref. 17. for example)
	Biomarkers of effect (e.g. DNA adducts; methylated bases; *Salmonella* mutagenicity/activity in other genetox assays)	Endogenous exposure to potential carcinogens — either via parent chemicals or their reactive metabolites; detection further enhanced by fractionation on resin column and deconjugation before assaying
Imaging biomarkers (P)	Target validation for new drug candidates; pharmacodynamic studies	See Ref. (8) for further discussion
Using cytokines as biomarkers for inflammation (P)	Cytokines control cell growth and differentiation and predict an inflammatory response in volunteers subjected to diesel exhaust and ozone	Validation of system to work with lung cells in culture (see Ref. 15)

[a]*PET, positron emission tomography.*
[b]*See section 5.2 of this chapter.*
[c]*PK: pharmacokinetics.*
[d]*e.g. agonist studies.*
[e]*MRI, magnetic resonance imaging.*
[f]*BBB, blood–brain barrier.*
[g]*NNAL, 4-(methylnitrosamino)-1-(3-pyridyl)-1-butanol.*
[h]*TSNAS, tobacco-specific nitrosamines.*
[i]*NNK, 4-(methylnitrosamino)-1-(3-pyridyl)-1-butanone.*

The evidence for a link between exposure and effect is normally the positive detection of a biomarker, the level of which can be quantified (13, 14). An example of a biomarker of exposure is 4-(methylnitrosamino)-1-(3-pyridyl)-1-butanone (NNAL), the urinary metabolite of the carcinogen, nicotine-derived nitrosamine ketone (NNK; Table 1); examples of biomarkers of effect are chemically modified bases, or the genotoxicity of urine extracts.

Biomarkers can also be disease-related and drug-related, and they can be further subdivided into various categories, such as biomarkers of susceptibility, of drug efficacy, of toxicity, and of patient response, or used as diagnostic biomarkers. The fact that imaging biomarkers have now been proposed as a new type of biomarker (8) links imaging with biomonitoring (Table 1), involving two ways of maximising the use of human studies.

The scope for such studies is potentially large, especially when the procedures used involve the simple collection of fluids, such as blood and urine. The results from such investigations can be related to levels of parent compound and its metabolites, in body fluids, to facilitate safety assessment (6). Detection resolution can be enhanced by fractionation on resin columns, by incubation with beta-glucuronidases to yield potentially reactive metabolic intermediates from their conjugates and by genotoxicity testing with and without an exogenous biotransformation system, with the appropriate cofactors. When the objective is to compare different populations of exposed subjects, it is recommended that levels of biomarkers be expressed relative to the concentration of creatinine in the same body fluid. This substance is a breakdown product that is produced continuously from creatine in muscles, and is an indicator of muscle mass, which also varies with age, gender and ethnicity.

3.2 Potential Opportunities and Problems

Biomonitoring studies involving healthy volunteers, who were inhaling diesel exhaust and ozone, have recently been reported to exhibit a series of changes in the expression of some 10 key cytokines, which control cell growth and differentiation and the inflammatory response (Table 1), as revealed by gene expression profiling (15). The same biomarkers have been analysed, after the *in vitro* exposure of lung cells in culture, and the results were sufficiently similar to those obtained in the biomonitoring exercise to suggest that meaningful data could be obtained by using such cells and biomarkers *in vitro*, at even earlier stages of drug development. Further characterisation of the biomarkers is taking place.

Substantial amounts of inter-individual variation and other confounding factors, such as additional exposures (e.g. unregulated dietary and liquid intake, as well as uncontrolled exposure to other drugs), and the time of day at which samples are collected, can all complicate the interpretation of biomonitoring data (16). Such problems can be minimised, particularly by using each volunteer as his/her own control, by adhering to strict sample collection times, and by exerting more control over dietary intake, where this is possible. It is also very important to subject negative control body fluid samples to the same processing steps as are used for all other treatment samples, involving all the post-collection stages of fractionation, concentration and enzymatic exposures to investigate the possibility of spurious formation of active chemicals from sample processing itself, rather than by endogenous exposure to substances in the environment (11).

Also, the relevance and specificity of the biomarker in question to the process being predicted need to be established by some sort of validation step before acceptance for use (12). This also establishes the biomarker as being able to act as an objectively defined measure of a particular biological effect, process or pathogenic state. Biomarkers should be specific, and/or readily detected, and quantifiable.

Finally, it should be noted that most biomonitoring studies are retrospective, although there are a few situations where prospective work can be undertaken, for various reasons. Modified-risk tobacco products and electronic cigarettes are a case in point, due to the already extensive recreational use of smoking and vaping by the general population, so any proposal for clinical studies is not a first-administration-to-humans situation (17).

4. MICRODOSING

4.1 Background

Microdosing, or phase-0 clinical trials, is a regulatory pathway to first-in-human (FIH) studies that employs sub-therapeutic pharmacological exposures, to study the effects of novel drugs in humans. Microdosing is based on two main principles: first, that human data are superior to animal and *in-vitro* data when modelling the effects of human disease and therapeutics, and, second, that data obtained with limited pharmacological exposure can be reliably extrapolated to the therapeutic dose range.

These approaches have several operational advantages, most notably, the implied safety, which in turn is translated into quicker and less-expensive human testing, and reduced testing in animals. While these approaches were originally used primarily to study pharmacokinetics (PK), the direction and interest in phase-0/microdosing has recently been broadened to include pharmacodynamics (PD), focusing on biomarkers of efficacy and toxicity, and information relevant to drug mode of action (MoA; 18).

The term '*in humano*' has recently been coined to describe such studies as pre-clinical trials in humans, in the vein of terms such as '*in vivo*', '*in vitro*' and '*in silico*' (18). Notwithstanding the lack of therapeutic intent, these approaches produce sufficient pharmacological exposure to quantify the PK and PD properties of test items, including concentrations in target organs and tissues, binding to receptors and post-receptor modulation (19). Such approaches can include non-invasive imaging, with the test compound labelled with radionuclides, for monitoring and studying drug effects in real-time, with the potential to replace some experiments on animals, including non-human primates (NHPs; 10, 20). Phase-0/microdosing studies have also been called 'exploratory clinical trials' and 'exploratory Investigational New Drug' (eIND) trials (21, 22).

4.2 Volunteer and Clinical Studies

The ethical use of humans, particularly for the efficacy and safety testing of pharmaceuticals (23), together with biomonitoring, has long been an important way of obtaining information of direct relevance to the development of therapeutics, and there have been many discussions as to how this could be expanded without compromising volunteer safety, especially in the wake of FIH studies with serious adverse outcomes (3, 24, 25; see later, under *Safer development*). Phase-0/microdosing offers the possibility of testing novel drugs in human volunteers in a safer manner than in traditional phase-1 studies, and hence with less prior animal testing (26). The exceedingly small amounts of a substance can still be detected by using ultra-sensitive analytical methods (5, 19, 27; and see later, under *Analytical methodologies*, 4, 19, 27—29; see also, 23).

4.3 Definitions of Phase-0/Microdosing Approaches

Phase-0/microdosing approaches are defined in the International Conference on Harmonisation, Guidance on Nonclinical Safety Studies for the Conduct of Human Clinical Trials and Marketing Authorisation for Pharmaceuticals M3 (ICH M3 guidelines; 22). The document contains five approaches under the category of 'exploratory clinical trials' (synonymous with phase-0/microdosing trials), but also emphasises that other, intermediate approaches on the continuums of dosage and duration of exposure are possible (Fig. 1).

The first approach involves a total dose (single or divided) of <100 μg, supported by a 14-day extended single-dose toxicity study in one species, usually a rodent, by the clinical route of administration. A second microdosing approach permits a total of <500 μg per subject, divided into five doses, each no more than 100 μg and separated by at least six half-lives. This approach should be supported by a 7-day repeated-dose toxicity study in one species, usually a rodent. Neither approach requires genotoxicity studies. The other approaches are described in Table 2.

4.4 Reception and Regulatory Position

4.4.1 A Mixed Reception

While phase-0/microdosing approaches have been welcomed by many, for both scientific and animal welfare reasons, they are not without some controversy, and in particular, with regard to concerns over the extrapolation of study data from sub-

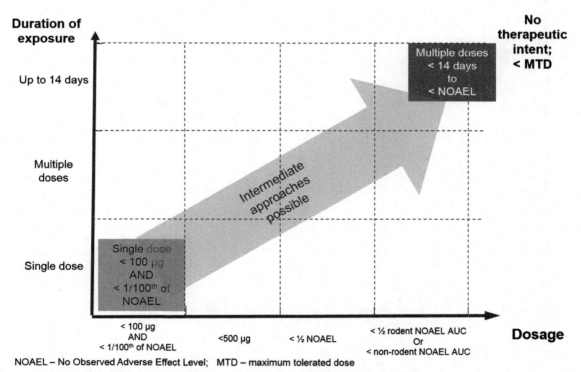

FIGURE 1 **Continuum of increasing dosages and duration of exposure in phase-0 approaches.** Higher dosages and duration of exposure involve greater pre-clinical requirements (animal and *in vitro* testing, genotoxicology), drug substance production costs, and increased duration of IND application preparation and hence reduced operational advantages versus traditional phase-1 approaches. At no point do phase-0/microdosing studies have therapeutic intent, even though there may be entry into the therapeutic-level range.

TABLE 2 Phase-0, Including Microdosing Approaches From ICH M3 Guidelines (ICH 2009). Intermediate Forms are Possible and the Optimal Approach Should be Arrived at Based on Discussions With Local Regulators

	Approach 1	Approach 2	Approach 3	Approach 4	Approach 5
	Microdosing				
Dose definition	≤1/100th NOAEL and ≤1/100th of pharmacologically active dose (scaled on mg/kg for IV and mg/m² for oral)	Same as approach 1	Starting at subtherapeutic dose and moving into the anticipated therapeutic range but < ½ NOAEL	Starting dose: <1/50 of NOAEL AUC; into the anticipated therapeutic range, but <10th pre-clinical AUC if no toxicity, or < NOAEL	Starting dose: <1/50 NOAEL; into the anticipated therapeutic range, but < non-rodent NOAEL AUC, or <½ rodent NOAEL AUC
Cumulative dose	100 µg	500 µg			
Limit per dose	100 µg	100 µg			
Maximal daily dose	100 µg	100 µg			
Number/duration of dosing	1 Could be divided into multiple doses with a total of 100 µg	5	1	Multiple <14 days	Multiple <14 days
Washout	No washout	Six or more half-lives between doses	No washout	No washout	No washout
Pharmacology	In vitro and receptor profiling PD model supporting human dose	Same as Approach 1	Same as Approach 1 + Core battery of safety pharmacology	Same as Approach 1 + Core battery of safety pharmacology	Same as Approach 1 + Core battery of safety pharmacology
General toxicity studies	14-day extended single dose toxicity	7-day repeated-dose toxicity	Extended single-dose toxicity; in rodent and non-rodent	14-day repeated-dose toxicity in rodent and non-rodent	14-day repeated-dose toxicity in rodent and non-rodent
GLP	Yes	Yes	Yes	Yes	Yes
Genotoxicity studies	Not recommended SAR included, if available	Same as Approach 1	Ames assay	Ames assay + chromosomal damage test	Ames assay + chromosomal damage test
Dosimetry estimates	For highly radioactive agents	Same as Approach 1	Same as Approach 1	Same as Approach 1	Same as Approach 1

AUC, area under the curve; GLP, good laboratory practice; NOAEL, no observed adverse effect level.
Adapted from Burt, T, John, C.S., Ruckle, J.L., et al. (2016). Phase-0/microdosing studies using PET, AMS, and LC-MS/MS: A range of study methodologies and conduct considerations. Accelerating development of novel pharmaceuticals through safe testing in humans - a practical guide. Expert Opinion on Drug Delivery. 4, 657–672.

therapeutic to therapeutic levels of exposure. In other words, doubt has been expressed as to whether a substance in tiny amounts behaves in the same way, pharmacologically, as it does in larger amounts (30, 31; and see later, under *Extrapolating phase-0/microdose study results*).

4.4.2 Regulatory Interest

The phase-0/microdosing framework was endorsed by regulatory authorities, including the European Agency for the Evaluation of Medicinal Products (4), the US Food and Drug Administration (FDA; 21) and Japanese (Ministry of Health, Labour and Welfare; 32) and was subsequently internationally harmonised and adopted by other authorities as well (22). This is compatible with the recommendations in the FDA's oft-quoted and much-welcomed 2004 report on innovation and stagnation in clinical development, which called for a greater emphasis on *in vitro*, computational and clinical tools, one of which was said to be microdosing (33, 34).

The FDA has been explicit in its encouragement of flexibility and efficiency in FIH studies and IND applications, stating the following in the introduction to the 2006 Exploratory eIND Guidelines, the first to define phase-0/microdosing approaches in the USA: *Existing regulations allow a great deal of flexibility in the amount of data that needs to be submitted with an IND application, depending on the goals of the proposed investigation, the specific human testing proposed, and the expected risks. The Agency believes that sponsors have not taken full advantage of that flexibility and often provide more supporting information in INDs than is required by regulations* (21).

5. A GENERALISED APPLICATION OF MICRODOSING

5.1 Study Procedures

A microdose is typically administered to 4−10 healthy male subjects, although female subjects and patients have also been used. The use of patients is attractive, as they are often excluded from FIH studies due to safety concerns. This is followed by the collection of plasma and sometimes, excreta, biopsy samples and positron emission tomography (PET) imaging (30; Table 3). Some applications, for example, trials for chemopreventives, might require modified protocols (35). The samples are analysed for target analytes, such as parent drug or metabolites, to ascertain the PK profile.

5.2 Analytical Methodologies

Sensitive analytical tools are required to detect the consequences of low drug exposures. Originally, ^{14}C-labelled drugs and accelerator mass spectrometry (AMS) were used, due to the extreme sensitivity of AMS (down to attogram 10^{-18} g/mL levels; 36−38). Recently, the increased use of PET and LC-MS/MS methodologies was driven by the development of PET-specific radionuclide labelling techniques and improvements in assay sensitivity, respectively (39).

PET-imaging permits the simultaneous study of the drug non-invasively in every organ/tissue in the body in real-time. LC-MS/MS has the advantage of non-radioactivity and wide availability in research centres, but is not as sensitive as AMS and PET. Combinations of these analytical approaches in the same study are both possible and encouraged, and could provide various complementary and synergistic advantages (40).

5.3 Extrapolating Phase-0/Microdose Study Results to Therapeutic-Range Exposures

A comprehensive analysis of the peer-reviewed literature on comparing human microdose with therapeutic dose PK was undertaken by Lappin *et al.* (30). A total of 35 compounds for which oral, intravenous, human and animal microdose and therapeutic dose data were available, were compared. Among those tested orally, 79% (N = 27), and among those tested intravenously, 100% (N = 12), showed scalable PK within a twofold range, the industry standard for valid extrapolation. Rowland analysed the available human data, and also found evidence to support the above-mentioned uses of microdosing (41). The relationship between the phase-0/microdosing data and the therapeutic-level exposures does not have to be linear to be scalable. If the relationship is known with sufficient detail and confidence, extrapolation can be performed (18).

TABLE 3 Comparison of Phase-0/Microdosing With Traditional Phase-1 Approaches

	Phase-0/Microdosing (eIND)	Traditional Phase-1 (IND)
Therapeutic intent	None	Possible
Study of systemic tolerability	None	Yes
Proof of mechanism	Possible (e.g. PET receptor binding and displacement)	Possible
Preclinical package	Limited, variable; depends on extent of exposure to the test article and experimental goals	Full requirements
• *In vitro* models	Full requirement	Full requirements
• Toxicology	Limited, variable	Full requirements
• Genotoxicology	None or limited	Full requirements
GMP	Flexible, depending on available preclinical information and route of administration (e.g. sterility ensured for IV route)	Full requirements
Regulatory review	30 days	30 days
Usual duration of programme	4–12 months	12–24 months
Cost of programme	$0.5–0.75M	$1.5–2.5M
Studies		
• Size (typical)	4–10 participants	6–30 participants
• Duration (per participant)	1–14 days[a]	6–60 days[a]
• Number of study sites	Single	Single/Multiple
• Maximal dose	<MTD	MTD
• Exposure	Limited (see Table 1)	Multiple doses allowed
• Population	Healthy volunteers or patients Vulnerable populations	Usually healthy volunteers (unless toxicity risk is high, e.g. in oncology trials)

MTD: maximum tolerated dose; *PET*: positron emission tomography.
[a]*On average, could be longer with longer half-life drugs.*
Adapted from Burt, T., John, C.S., Ruckle, J.L., et al., (2016). Phase-0/microdosing studies using PET, AMS, and LC-MS/MS: A range of study methodologies and conduct considerations. Accelerating development of novel pharmaceuticals through safe testing in humans - a practical guide. *Expert Opinion on Drug Delivery*, 4, 657–672.

6. DISCUSSION

6.1 Applications and Benefits of Phase-0/Microdosing Approaches

The original concept of microdosing — to provide PK data in humans as early as possible — has moved on to several other applications, including the study of drug–drug interactions, measuring drug concentrations at the site of action, metabolic profiling, receptor binding and post-receptor modulation effects (see also, 39). In addition, several new applications have been proposed, in which the technique is used in conjunction with other methodologies, such as intra-target drug delivery (an application called 'Intra-Target Microdosing') and physiologically-based modelling, to improve PK scalability and to permit the study of PD effects and drug MoA (42, 43).

Different drug development stakeholders have different motivations for using phase-0/microdosing approaches. In addition to the previously-mentioned pharmaceutical developers, academics and regulators, other stakeholders include patient advocacy and disease-dedicated non-profit groups, organisations that promote the Three Rs, and the public at large. For example, the Alzheimer's Drug Discovery Foundation, a venture philanthropy supporting drug discovery and development for Alzheimer's disease and related dementias, includes and encourages phase-0/microdosing approaches as part of its research funding strategies and portfolios (personal communication). Collaborations among the various stakeholders are encouraged, to maximise the application potential of these approaches, especially given the oft-fragmented translational environment, and dependence on multi-disciplinary expertise (30).

6.2 Operational Advantages

The reduced pharmacological exposures drive most of the operational advantages of phase-0/microdosing approaches. The implied safety to human research participants means that less-extensive pre-clinical testing is required by the regulators (e.g. animal, *in vitro* and genotoxicology studies), making possible, a quicker and less expensive entry into human testing. In addition, the production of the drug substance is facilitated by the reduced amount and preparation rigour (i.e. according to Good Manufacturing Practices (GMP; 19)).

Requirements increase proportionally along the spectrum of phase-0 studies, as dosages, duration of exposure and associated risks increase as well, with the single-dose microdose approach associated with the least requirements. The specific requirements for any developmental scenario should be discussed and agreed with the regulators well in advance, preferably at least 2.5 years prior to the initiation of the human studies (18).

6.3 Safer Development

Safer development has been welcomed, not only by regulators, but also by disease advocacy and non-profit research groups, especially when concerned with the development of treatments for vulnerable populations (e.g. paediatrics, women, the frail and the elderly, and, importantly, patients in general), who are often excluded from FIH studies due to safety considerations (44, 45). The potential of phase-0/microdosing to enhance the safety of FIH studies is emphasised by the consideration of their application in the following two historical FIH studies that ended in disaster:

1. *The TGN1412 study* (46). The dose of TGN1412, a T-cell activator monoclonal antibody that was given to volunteers, was 0.1 mg/kg, based on data from rats and cynomolgus monkeys. All six human subjects proceeded to multi-organ failure within 24 hours, but survived after 30 days in intensive care. Had a microdose (0.1 mg) been administered instead, the exposure would have been ~50−70 times lower, depending on the weight of the research subjects. This would almost certainly have resulted in a much more-benign clinical outcome, possibly even an asymptomatic one. Nevertheless, it would have provided an opportunity to study the drug in relative safety, and to conclude that the response in humans was different than that of animals, leading to a reduced full-dose exposure, or to termination of the development of the drug.
2. *The BIA 10−2474 study* (25). Notwithstanding a lack of toxicity in pre-clinical testing in four animal species (mouse, rat, dog and monkey; 25), five of six healthy human volunteers given the novel biologic, BIA 10−2474, in the FIH study experienced a rapidly progressive neurological syndrome, ending with one death. A recent report identified off-target proteins as likely targets of BIA 10−2474 neurotoxicity, by using Activity-Based Protein Profiling (ABPP; 47). These off-target proteins were not identified in any of the animal models, but a phase-0/microdosing study, involving the use of ABPP or similar methodologies, may have identified biomarkers suggesting a unique human response to BIA 10−2474 or may have concluded against progression for other reasons (e.g. PK/PD findings), all, again, conducted in relative safety.

6.4 Cheaper Development

In addition to substantial savings in the number and extent of pre-clinical studies, drug substance production as well as size and complexity of the human studies, an important consideration is savings to patent-lives of back-up compounds. Drug development companies often have multiple analogues of the same compound, and cannot test them all simultaneously in full-dose phase-1 programmes. Cassette microdose studies permit the study of multiple analogues contemporaneously, i.e. up to five compounds in the same individual, under the same IND application, whereas a phase 1-programme would require five separate studies and IND applications (48).

At this point in development (i.e. the pre-IND stage), drug compounds are usually already patented and companies risk losing market exclusivity by spending precious patent-life while they are put 'on hold' as back-up compounds. The sooner a drug in development can be identified as non-viable, the sooner a potentially successful back-up compound can be developed. This principle, sometimes termed 'kill-early-kill-cheap', not only results in savings in costs of the full phase-1 programme, but also much more substantially in savings due to patent-life preservation, calculated to be in the range of $300M per successful compound brought to market (19).

6.5 Quicker Development

Reduced regulatory and drug production requirements, simpler design and smaller size (see Table 3) mean that phase-0/microdosing studies can be initiated more quickly than traditional phase-1 studies, with the results available 8—12 months earlier (19, 49).

7. CONCLUDING REMARKS

Clearly, imaging, particularly that of the brains of volunteers, and biomonitoring of the presence of biomarkers of exposure and effect in the body fluids of individuals exposed, either as consumers or patients, to chemicals during, or following the development of new drug entities, both offer many opportunities for early studies in humans. This is due, in large part, to the fact that the majority of procedures involved are non-invasive or only minimally invasive.

Until comparatively recently, one key drawback has been the difficulty in developing imaging technology that reliably permits events, occurring at the single neuron level in the human brain to be followed as they happen. This was due to restrictions in spatial resolution. While this has been possible in animals, including NHPs, for some time, the methodologies recently devised are complex, although effective (50). Their simplification would enable imaging to provide even more advantages for drug testing in the future. Advances in related technologies have been reported (51), such that, for example, the progressive loss of retinal ganglion cells by apoptosis, leading to loss of vision, has been followed at the single neuronal level in real-time, by using fluorescently labelled annexin 5 (ANX776) with confocal laser scanning ophthalmoscopy. It is hoped that this technique will permit visualisation of therapeutic intervention to halt the disease before it becomes irreversible.

As for biomonitoring, there is the possibility of applying it prospectively by incorporating it into standard clinical testing schemes, and combining it with microdosing. However, many checks and balances need to be implemented to facilitate data interpretation, and this could well account for its rather limited use, thus far.

Microdosing has prompted considerable debate, with some commentators believing that it has little value in drug development, while others see great potential for benefit. The adoption of microdosing, as with any similar technique, will largely be driven by economics, with the value of the data assessed against the costs of obtaining them. The value of the data depends on the scalability of the results from sub-therapeutic to therapeutic levels, and this has been shown to be in the range of 80% for orally administered drugs, and virtually 100% for intravenously administered drugs, a considerable advantage over inter-species scalability (52). To assist this quest, algorithms, aimed at ruling out poor predictability, as well as modelling and simulation methodologies, have been developed (18, 31).

The application of phase-0/microdosing studies has expanded in recent years, and the sensitivity, efficiency and availability of the required analytical tools have improved, and this has increased the utility of these tools, alone and in combination.

Finally, it is recommended that regulatory bodies, industry, medical profession practitioners and academics, as well as advocacy and public non-profit organisations, should collaborate to facilitate the validation of phase-0/microdosing, thereby leading to its wider regulatory acceptance to enable the benefits of its many applications in new drug development to be gained (18).

REFERENCES

1. Olson, H., Betton, G., Robinson, D., *et al.* (2000). Concordance of the toxicity of pharmaceuticals in humans and in animals. *Regulatory Toxicology and Pharmacology* **32**, 56—67.
2. Mak, I.W., Evaniew, N. & Ghert, M. (2014). Lost in translation: Animal models and clinical trials in cancer treatment. *American Journal of Translational Research* **6**, 114—118.
3. Close, B., Combes, R., Hubbard, A., *et al.* (1997). *Volunteers in Research and Testing*, 194pp. Boca Raton, FL, USA: CRC Press
4. EMEA. (2004). *Position Paper on Non-clinical Safety Studies to Support Clinical Trials With a Single Microdose*, 4pp. London, UK: European Agency for the Evaluation of Medical Products
5. Combes, R.D., Berridge, T., Connelly, J., *et al.* (2003). Early microdose drug studies in human volunteers can minimise animal testing. *European Journal of Clinical Pharmacology* **19**, 1—11.
6. Combes, R.D. (1991). Use of clinical samples for biomonitoring of genotoxic exposure to pharmaceuticals. In W. Nimmo (Ed.), *Clinical Measurement in Drug Evaluation*, pp. 173—191. London, UK: Wolfe Medical Publications Limited.
7. Smith, P., Berger, B. & Heller, A. (2000). Concordance of the toxicity of World Medical Association, 2000. The Declaration - of Helsinki. Adopted pharmaceuticals in humans and animals. *Regulatory Toxicology and Pharmacology* **32**, 56—67.

8. Matthews, P.M., Rabiner, I. & Gunn, R. (2011). Non-invasive imaging in experimental medicine for drug development. *Current Opinion in Pharmacology* **11**, 501–507.

9. Asbury, C. (2011). *Brain Imaging Technologies and Their Applications in Neuroscience*, 45pp. New York, NY, USA: The Dana Foundation

10. Langley, G., Harding, G., Hawkins, P., *et al.* (2000). Volunteer studies replacing animal experiments in brain research - Report and recommendations of a Volunteers in Research and Testing workshop. *ATLA* **28**, 315–331.

11. Combes, R.D., Anderson, D., Brooks, T., *et al.* (1984). The detection of mutagens in urine, faeces and body fluids. In B.J. Dean (Ed.), *Guidelines for Mutagenicity Testing, Part II, Supplementary Tests, Mutagens in Body Fluids and Excreta, Nitrosation Products*, pp. 203–244. Swansea, UK: United Kingdom Environmental Mutagen Society.

12. Combes, R.D., Edwards, C.N. & Walters, J.M. (1981). An assessment of faecal mutagen analysis for predicting genotoxic exposure of rats to some orally administered carcinogens. In B.A. Bridges, & B. Butterworth (Eds.), *Indicators of Genotoxic Exposure in Man and Animals*, pp. 49–65. Cold Spring Harbor, New York, USA: Cold Spring Harbor Press. Banbury Report 13.

13. Dakubo, G.D. (2016). *Cancer Biomarkers in Body Fluids - Principles*, 509pp. Cham, ZG, Switzerland: Springer International Publishing

14. Gupta, R.C. (Ed.). (2014). *Biomarkers in Toxicology*. NY, USA: Academic Press, 1152pp. New York.

15. Stiegel, M.A., Pleil, J.D., Sobus, J.R., *et al.* (2017). Linking physiological parameters to perturbations in the human exposome: Environmental exposures modify blood pressure and lung function via inflammatory cytokine pathway. *Journal of Toxicology and Environmental Health A* **80**, 485–501.

16. Benford, D.J., Hanley, A.B., Bottrill, K., *et al.* (2000). Biomarkers as predictive tools in toxicity testing. The report and recommendations of ECVAM workshop 40. *ATLA* **28**, 119–131.

17. Combes, R.D. & Balls, M. (2015). A critical assessment of the scientific basis, and implementation, of regulations for the safety assessment and marketing of innovative tobacco-related products. *ATLA* **43**, 251–290.

18. Burt, T., Yoshida, K., Lappin, L., *et al.* (2016). Microdosing and other Phase-0 clinical trials: Facilitating translation in drug development. *Clinical and Translational Science* **9**, 74–88.

19. Burt, T., John, C.S., Ruckle, J.L., *et al.* (2016). Phase-0/microdosing studies using PET, AMS, and LC-MS/MS: A range of study methodologies and conduct considerations. Accelerating development of novel pharmaceuticals through safe testing in humans - a practical guide. *Expert Opinion on Drug Delivery* **4**, 657–672.

20. Bergstrom, M. (2017). The use of microdosing in the development of small organic and protein therapeutics. *Journal of Nuclear Medicine* **58**, 1188–1195.

21. FDA. (2006). *Guidance for Industry, Investigators, and Reviewers. Exploratory IND Studies*, 16pp. Rockville, MD, USA: US FDA

22. ICH. (2009). *Guidance on Nonclinical Safety Studies for the Conduct of Human Clinical Trials and Marketing Authorisation for Pharmaceuticals M3(R2)*, 22pp. London, UK: European Medicines Agency

23. Garner, R.C. (2014). Human microdosing/phase 0 studies to accelerate drug development. In R. Coleman (Ed.), *Human-based systems for Translational Research*, pp. 241–266. London, UK: Royal Society of Chemistry.

24. Kenter, M.J. & Cohen, A.F. (2006). Establishing risk of human experimentation with drugs: Lessons from TGN1412. *Lancet* **368**, 1387–1391.

25. Chaikin, P. (2017). The Bial 10-2474 Phase 1 Study - A drug development perspective and recommendations for future first-in-human trials. *The Journal of Clinical Pharmacology* **57**, 690–703.

26. Langley, G. & Farnaud, S. (2010). Opinion: Microdosing: Safer clinical trials and fewer animal tests. *Bioanalysis* **2**, 393–395.

27. Tewari, T. & Mukherjee, S. (2010). Microdosing: Concept, application and relevance. *Perspectives in Clinical Research* **1**, 61–63.

28. Rani, P.U. & Naidu, M.U.R. (2008). Phase 0-microdosing strategy in clinical trials. *Indian Journal of Pharmacology* **40**, 240–242.

29. Anon. (2013). *Microdosing Trials Point the Way to Smarter Drug Development*, 1p. London, UK: ScientistLive, Setform Limited

30. Lappin, G., Noveck, R. & Burt, T. (2013). Microdosing and drug development: Past, present and future. *Expert Opinion on Drug Metabolism and Toxicology* **9**, 817–834.

31. Bosgra, S., Vlaming, M.L. & Vaes, W.H. (2016). To apply microdosing or not? Recommendations to single out compounds with non-linear pharmacokinetics. *Clinical Pharmacokinetics* **55**, 1–15.

32. MHLW. (2008). *Microdose Clinical Studies: Pharmaceutical and Medical Safety Bureau, Ministry of Health Labour and Welfare. see: English Regulatory Information Task Force Japan Pharmaceutical Manufacturers Association: Pharmaceutical Administration and Regulations in Japan*, 211pp. Tokyo, Japan: Ministry of Health Labour and Welfare http://apps.who.int/medicinedocs/documents/s18577en/s18577en.pdf

33. FDA. (2004). *Innovation or Stagnation? Challenge and Opportunity on the Critical Path to New Medical Products*, 38pp. Rockville, MD, USA: US FDA

34. LoRusso, P.M. (2009). Phase 0 clinical trials: An answer to drug development stagnation? *Journal of Clinical Oncology* **27**, 2586–2588.

35. Kummar, S., Rubinstein, L., Kinders, R., *et al.* (2008). Phase 0 clinical trials: Conceptions and misconceptions. *Cancer Journal* **14**, 133–137.

36. Turteltaub, K.W. & Vogel, J.S. (2000). Bioanalytical applications of accelerator mass spectrometry for pharmaceutical research. *Current Pharmaceutical Design* **6**, 991–1007.

37. Young, G., Ellis, W., Ayrton, J., *et al.* (2001). Accelerator mass spectrometry (AMS): Recent experience of its use in a clinical study and the potential future of the technique. *Xenobiotica* **31**, 619–632.

38. Hellborg, R. & Skog, G. (2008). Accelerator mass spectrometry. *Mass Spectrometry Reviews* **27**, 398–427.

39. Lappin, G. (2015). The expanding utility of microdosing. *Clinical Pharmacology in Drug Development* **4**, 401–406.

40. Wagner, C., Simpson, M., Zeitlinger, M., *et al.* (2011). Combined accelerator mass spectrometry and positron emission tomography human microdose study with ^{14}C- and ^{11}C-labelled verapamil. *Clinical Pharmacokinetics* **50**, 111–120.

41. Rowland, M. (2012). Microdosing: A critical assessment of human data. *Journal of Pharmaceutical Sciences* **101**, 4067—4074.

42. Burt, T., Noveck, R.J., MacLeod, D.B., *et al.* (2017). Intra-target microdosing (ITM): A novel drug development approach aimed at enabling safer and earlier translation of biological insights into human testing. *Clinical and Translational Science* **10**, 337—350.

43. Nandal, S. & Burt, T. (Feb 19 2017). Integrating pharmacoproteomics into early-phase clinical development: State-of-the-art, challenges, and recommendations. *International Journal of Molecular Sciences* **18**(448), 24. https://doi.org/10.3390/ijms18020448.

44. Roth-Cline, M. & Nelson, R.M. (2015). Ethical considerations in conducting paediatric and neonatal research in clinical pharmacology. *Current Pharmaceutical Design* **21**, 5619—5635.

45. Turner, M.A., Mooij, M.G., Vaes, W., *et al.* (2015). Paediatric microdose and microtracer studies using (14)C in Europe. *Clinical Pharmacology & Therapeutics* **98**, 234—237.

46. Suntharalingam, G., Perry, M.R., Ward, S., *et al.* (2006). Cytokine storm in a phase 1 trial of the anti-CD28 monoclonal antibody TGN1412. *New England Journal of Medicine* **355**, 1018—1028.

47. van Esbroeck, A.C.M., Janssen, A.P.A., Cognetta, A.B., 3rd, *et al.* (2017). Activity-based protein profiling reveals off-target proteins of the FAAH inhibitor BIA 10-2474. *Science, New York* **356**, 1084—1087.

48. Maeda, K. & Sugiyama, Y. (2011). Novel strategies for microdose studies using non-radiolabelled compounds. *Advanced Drug Delivery Reviews* **63**, 532—538.

49. Wilding, I.R. & Bell, J.A. (2005). Improved early clinical development through human microdosing studies. *Drug Discovery Today* **10**, 890—894.

50. Cash, S.S. & Hochberg, L.R. (2015). The emergence of single neurons in clinical neurology. *Neuron* **86**, 79—91.

51. Cordeiro, M., Normando, E., Cardoso, M., *et al.* (2017). Real-time imaging of single neuronal cell apoptosis in patients with glaucoma. *Brain* **104**, 1757—1767.

52. Rowland, M. & Benet, L.Z. (2011). Lead PK. Commentary: PhRMA PISC — prediction of human pharmacokinetics. *Journal of Pharmaceutical Sciences* **100**, 4047—4049.

Section 4

Data Mining and Data Sharing

Chapter 4.1

Scientific Journals as Beacons on the Journey Toward Global Three Rs Awareness

Susan Trigwell[1], Franz P. Gruber[2,3], Sonja von Aulock[3] and Koichi Imai[4]

[1]Fund for the Replacement of Animals in Medical Experiments (FRAME), Nottingham, United Kingdom; [2]Doerenkamp-Zbinden Foundation and ALTEX Edition, Kuesnacht ZH, Switzerland; [3]ALTEX Editorial Office, ALTEX Edition, Kuesnacht, Switzerland; [4]Osaka Dental University, Osaka, Japan

SUMMARY

The editors of three current journals that specialise in publishing peer-reviewed articles, reporting on the development, validation and implementation of Three Rs alternatives, describe the evolution of each of their journals from its inception to its current form, and consider its contribution to the end-goal of increasing global awareness of the Three Rs concept. The journals are *Alternatives to Laboratory Animals*, *Alternatives to Animal Experimentation* and *Alternatives to Animal Testing and Experimentation*, published in the UK, Switzerland and Japan, respectively. These journals were established as a result of a common recognition of the importance of the Three Rs concept, and the need to promote awareness of its principles. Each journal has evolved, in its own manner, from modest beginnings into its present form. Other initiatives, which stand out as particular distinguishing strengths of the individual journals, in terms of working toward the desired end-goal, are also highlighted.

1. INTRODUCTION

The Three Rs (*Reduction, Refinement, Replacement*) concept was introduced by William Russell and Rex Burch in their ground-breaking book, *The Principles of Humane Experimental Technique* (1), in 1959. Since then, awareness of ways in which to implement the reduction, refinement and replacement of animal use in experiments has been increasing, with gathering momentum — first in the West (e.g. the UK, Europe and the USA), and later in other parts of the world. It is interesting to consider how this journey toward global awareness has been guided by the output of certain scientific journals that specialise, to a greater or lesser extent, in publishing peer-reviewed articles that report on the development, validation and implementation of the Three Rs.

Over the years, there have been a number of such journals in existence, some of which are now discontinued (see Table 1). The editors, of three of the seven current journals listed, have described the evolution of their journals from their inception to their current form, and have considered their contributions to the end-goal of increasing worldwide awareness of the Three Rs. To give a balanced view, one of the chosen journals is published in the UK, one in Switzerland, and one in Japan. They are featured here in chronological order of their inception, the first being established in 1973.

2. ALTERNATIVES TO LABORATORY ANIMALS

2.1 Beginnings

Alternatives to Laboratory Animals (ATLA) is a peer-reviewed journal that has been published for over 40 years by the Fund for the Replacement of Animals in Medical Experiments (FRAME), now based in Nottingham, UK. FRAME was

TABLE 1 Journals that Have Contributed to the Widespread Global Awareness of the Three Rs

Journal Title	Current Language	Start Year	Country of Publication
In Vitro	English	1965 (ended 1984)	USA
In Vitro. Monograph	English	1970 (ended 1984)	USA
Alternatives to Laboratory Animals (ATLA)	English	1973 (current)	England
Alternatives to Animal Experimentation (ALTEX)	English	1984 (current)	Switzerland
In Vitro Cellular and Developmental Biology	English	1985 (ended 1993)	USA
Toxicology in Vitro	English	1987 (current)	The Netherlands
In Vitro Toxicology	English	1987 (ended 1997)	USA
Alternatives to Animal Testing and Experimentation (AATEX)/AATEX–JaCVAM	English/Japanese	1990 (current)	Japan
In Vitro Cellular and Developmental Biology - Animal	English	1993 (current)	Germany
Methods in Cell Science	English	1995 (ended 2004)	The Netherlands
In Vitro and Molecular Toxicology	English	1998 (ended 2001)	USA
PLoS One	English	2006 (current)	USA
Applied In Vitro Toxicology	English	2015 (current)	USA

established in 1969 by Mrs Dorothy Hegarty. FRAME quite rightly recognised that 'the exchange of information, and its ready availability, are of paramount importance, if new techniques are to be adopted rapidly' (2). To help achieve this, the biannual *ATLA Abstracts* was launched in June 1973 (see Fig. 1). This way of informing scientists may seem rather naïve today, but at that time there were few abstracting services, and no personal computers or Internet. Scientists kept themselves informed by going to the library, and looking through hard copies of the scientific journals. In contrast, current *ATLA* articles are now listed in databases such as PubMed and EBSCOhost, as well as being available online at www.atla.org.uk.

Interestingly, in 1976, the expanded volume **4** included one of the first of many discussions, in *ATLA* and elsewhere, on *What is an 'alternative'?* (3). In 1981, *ATLA Abstracts* became *ATLA (Alternatives to Laboratory Animals)*. Editorials were introduced, and the original abstracts were replaced by *Selected Titles*. The journal was re-launched in 1983 as a quarterly journal. It would now consider submitted articles for peer-review and have an international Editorial Board. The *Trends...* series of journals had been established by Elsevier in 1976 to feature short reviews on a particular research area. The series began with *Trends in Biological Sciences*, and was subsequently expanded to cover a range of fields. The aim was for the new *ATLA* to cover *Trends in Alternatives Research*, on a par with these *Trends...* journals. In 1994, with the support of the European Centre for the Validation of Alternative Methods (ECVAM), the number of issues per volume rose from four to six.

2.2 Collaboration with ECVAM

ECVAM's support was conditional on the inclusion in *ATLA* of the reports of ECVAM Workshops, Task Forces and validation studies, which resulted in a partnership of great significance to both FRAME and ECVAM. These reports, dating from 1994, were notable contributions to the development, validation and acceptance of many alternative toxicity tests, and those on topics, such as target organ toxicity and validation, are still of great significance today. The first issue of volume **22** (1994) contained an outline of ECVAM's initial activities (4).

In addition to reporting on the work of ECVAM, the timely dissemination of the findings and recommendations from other significant workshops and meetings, in non-animal test methods, and procedures has been a key role of *ATLA*. For example, volume **18** (1990) included the reports of two important workshops, namely, the CAAT/ERGATT (Centre for Alternatives to Animal Testing/European Research Group for Alternatives to Animal Testing) Workshop on the Validation of Toxicity Test Procedures ((5); 'Amden 1'), and the International Workshop on Promotion of the Regulatory Acceptance of Validated Non-animal Toxicity Test Procedures ((6); 'the Vouliagmeni workshop'). The programmes and abstracts for

1970s	1980s	1990s	2000s	2010s
1973: *ATLA Abstracts* launched by FRAME, as an A4, single-column journal. The abstracts were written by abstracting staff, who were initially located at the British Library, Boston Spa, Wetherby, Yorkshire, UK. 1976: *ATLA Abstracts* expanded to include news and views, reviews, and opinions.	1981: *ATLA Abstracts* becomes *ATLA* *(Alternatives to Laboratory Animals)* (ISSN 0261-1929) and the A4 size reduced to 7 × 10 inches. 1981: Abstracts content replaced by *Selected Titles*, from issue **9**(2). This was the first issue published from FRAME's Nottingham office, following the move from London. 1983: With the support of the Maurice Laing Trust, *ATLA* is now published four times each year, has an international Editorial Board, and considers submitted articles. Now includes news and views, book reviews, and meeting reports. 1983: Format changed to being type-set and bound, rather than camera-ready and stapled (mainly in a single-column format).	1990: With a change to a two-column format, this was a single-issue volume to mark FRAME's 21st Anniversary. 1994: Increase from four to six issues per year, with the support of the newly-created European Centre for the Validation of Alternative Methods (ECVAM). 1995: FRAME's 25th Anniversary volume.	2002: Format change from 7 × 10 inches, back to the original A4 size. This was mainly to allow for large and complicated tables in pre-validation/validation study reports, and for easier photocopying and printing. 2006: The *Selected Titles* section is discontinued. 2007: *ATLA* articles are available on the FRAME website, www.frame.org.uk. 2009: FRAME's 40th Anniversary volume.	2010: *ATLA* was presented with the William and Eleanor Cave Award by the ARDF, for "extraordinary contributions to the advancement of Alternatives and the Three Rs in the United States and worldwide". 2012: The inclusion in *ATLA* of a special supplement, *Perspectives in Laboratory Animal Science (PiLAS)*, funded by The Phoebe Wortley Talbot Charitable Trust. 2014: A new website, www.*atla*.org.uk, is set up to provide access to *ATLA* articles.

FIGURE 1 *ATLA* development timeline.

the second and third World Congresses on Alternatives and Animal Use in the Life Sciences (Utrecht, The Netherlands, 1996; Bologna, Italy, 1999) also appeared in *ATLA*, and the proceedings of the fourth World Congress (New Orleans, USA, 2002) formed Supplement 1 of volume **32** (7).

ATLA has also regularly included meeting reports on the activities of other organisations, including the Scandinavian Society for Cell Toxicology, the European Society of Toxicology *In Vitro*, and the Safer Medicines Trust. FRAME itself has organised many of its own workshops and meetings, the conclusions of which have been published in *ATLA*. These include reports on the implications of the EU Registration, Evaluation, Authorisation and Restriction of Chemicals system (8), new approaches to chemical risk assessment (9), and *in vitro* models of inhalation toxicity and disease (10).

2.3 Reporting Large Interlaboratory Studies

In addition to the reporting of formal workshops and meetings, the publication in *ATLA* of peer-reviewed research papers on alternatives represents the day-to-day, hands-on work of the scientist at the bench. The findings of various large-scale laboratory projects have been particularly significant. One such early publication was the eight-part report of the *MEIC Evaluation of Acute Systemic Toxicity* (11−14). More recently, the findings from the EU *CADASTER project on* in silico *techniques for environmental hazard and risk assessment* (15), the EU *Environmental ChemOinformatics (ECO) project* (16), and the *SearchBREAST project* (17) have all featured in *ATLA*. From 2013, the Lush Prize Conference proceedings and awards, which recognise the active development, promotion and implementation of *replacement* alternatives, have appeared in an annual special issue.

Russell and Burch were the first proponents of the Three Rs concept (18), and thus could be viewed as the two people who, of their contemporaries, probably knew the Three Rs better than anyone. A number of articles on the subject were written by them for *ATLA*, both together and separately, with the Prefatory Note in volume **23** (19) being their first joint publication since *The Principles of Humane Experimental Technique* in 1959. One particularly memorable article was an ECVAM workshop report on *The Three Rs: The Way Forward* (20). This workshop was the first meeting that Russell and Burch had attended together since 1959. When Rex Burch died in 1996, William Russell was among those who commented in *ATLA* on his life and contributions; 10 years later, tributes were paid in *ATLA* to the late William Russell.

2.4 Promoting the Three Rs Further Afield

In recent years, *ATLA* has been dedicated to the promotion of the Three Rs in 'developing' countries, such as India and China (i.e. 'developing' in terms of their awareness and implementation of the Three Rs). To this end, the journal editors welcome submissions from authors, whose first language is not English, and aim to assist them, as much as possible, via copy editing. As part of FRAME's continuing mission, free hard copies of the journal are distributed world-wide to a range of 'developing' countries or, where convenient, researchers are provided with free online access via the *ATLA* website, www.atla.org.uk. In recognition of FRAME's founder, the annual Dorothy Hegarty Award is presented to the authors of the paper in that year's volume, which is deemed likely to have made the most significant contribution to the reduction, refinement and/or replacement of animal experimentation, based on nominations, and votes submitted by the members of the *ATLA* Editorial Board.

ATLA aims to consider the scientific basis of new techniques, and their validation and application. It also strives to cover the wider ethical and social aspects of the continuing dependence on the use of animal models. This means questioning and challenging current attitudes and procedures, and the fact that *ATLA* can achieve this is based on its high degree of openness, combined with a willingness to consider opinions from across the spectrum, on what are often controversial subjects.

3. ALTERNATIVES TO ANIMAL EXPERIMENTATION

3.1 Introduction

ALTEX — Alternatives to Animal Experimentation (www.altex.org) — is a peer-reviewed, open access journal informing readers about scientific advances in the research and development, as well as the promotion, of alternatives to animal experiments. A variety of formats provide information and viewpoint exchange for all stakeholders in the field, i.e. academics, regulators, industry scientists, animal welfare and Three Rs organisations, members of ethics committees, educators, and interested laypersons. Edited by the Swiss not-for-profit society, ALTEX Edition, and published by Springer Spektrum, *ALTEX* is the official journal of CAAT (Center for Alternatives to Animal Testing), via CAAT-Europe, the Doerenkamp chairs and t^4 (The Transatlantic Think-tank for Toxicology). All the content of *ALTEX* is available online without charge, whereas hard copies are available by subscription. New issues are announced to registered users of www.altex.org, and via the *Altweb Newsletter* (21).

3.2 Origins

The Fonds für Versuchstierfreie Forschung (FFVFF, Zurich, now Animalfree Research, Berne, Switzerland), first published *Alternativen zu Tierversuchen* (*Alternatives to Animal Experimentation*) in December 1984 (see Fig. 2). The biannual issues in German, later with English summaries, were compiled by Christoph Reinhard, in his role as editor, with enthusiastic support from the foundation's board members, Susi Goll and Irène Hagmann. The editorial of the first issue explains how public sentiment questioning the ethics of animal experiments had motivated many scientists to find practical solutions to replace or refine animal experiments, and reduce them to the indispensable minimum.

The increasing interest and recognition of ALTEX, which gained this acronym in 1991, led to the decision to further professionalise the journal. This was implemented by the second Editor-in-Chief, Franz Gruber. From 1994 onwards, *ALTEX* was published four times a year, in a new high-quality format. Articles were published in German or English, with summaries in both languages. Supplements containing contributions to conferences or seminars were published in co-operation with the respective organisers. Starting in 1995, the fourth yearly issue also carried an annual literature review, on the relationship between man and animals, compiled by Gottlieb Teutsch.

3.3 An International Open Access Journal

ALTEX has published numerous Abstract Books and Proceedings of the World Congresses on Animal Use and Alternatives (WC5 to WC10), and of the EUSAAT Congresses (since 2002), formerly as supplements, and, from 2012, in the journal *ALTEX Proceedings* (22), which also publishes abstracts or proceedings of other scientific meetings, in co-operation with their respective organisers. Since 1998, the FFVFF, and, since 2006, ALTEX Edition, have presented the annual *ALTEX* Award, either at the World Congress or at the EUSAAT Congress, for the best article published in *ALTEX* during the previous year (23).

1980s	1990s	2000s	2010s

1984: The FFVFF first publishes *Alternativen zu Tierversuchen*. Biannual issues are published in German, with English summaries.

1991: The journal acquires the acronym *ALTEX* and its first ISSN (1018-4562).

1994: *ALTEX* is published by Spektrum Akademischer Verlag (Heidelberg, Germany) four times per year in a new format, with articles in German or English and summaries in both languages (under ISSN 0946-7785).

1995: Start of the publication of an annual literature review on the human–animal relationship.

1998: Establishment of the annual *ALTEX* Award for best article.

2003: The Fondation E. Naef pour la recherche *in vitro* awards a Special Prize of CHF 5,000 to *ALTEX* for work in the field of alternative methods.

2004: *ALTEX* is now published by Elsevier (Amsterdam, The Netherlands).

2006: The Society *ALTEX* Edition is founded.

2007: *ALTEX* starts open access publication of content; start of the *Food for Thought...* series.

2007: *ALTEX* is again published by Spektrum Akademischer Verlag.

2008: Start of the publication of t^4 (workshop) reports; the North American Editorial Office is established.

2009: All articles are now in English (under ISSN 1868-596X); the literature review becomes a supplement; 25th Anniversary issue.

2011: The journal *TIERethik* is established (www.tierethik.net; published biannually in German, with English summaries; edited by Petra Mayr).

2012: The journal *ALTEX Proceedings* is established.

2012: *ALTEX* is now published by Springer Spektrum (Heidelberg, Germany).

2013: *ALTEX* is recognised as a gold open access journal by DOAJ.

2016: *ALTEX* receives LUSH Prize commendation in the Public Awareness category.

2018: The website is redesigned and moves to www.altex.org

FIGURE 2   *ALTEX* development timeline.

A major factor in the development of *ALTEX* into an international journal was the establishment in 2006, of the not-for-profit society, *ALTEX* Edition, based in Küsnacht, Switzerland (24), in 2006, for the purpose of broadening the journal's financial backing. The members of the society are national and international organisations promoting animal welfare and/or alternatives to animal experiments, or they are private individuals. The society owns and issues the three journals — *ALTEX*, *TIERethik* and *ALTEX Proceedings*.

The *ALTEX* website was set up in 2007, and since then, all the main articles of *ALTEX* have been published with open access upon print publication of each issue. In the same year, the *Food for Thought...* series — opinion articles mapping out the future of the Three Rs field — was initiated by Thomas Hartung (available as a collection of articles on the webpage; (25)). The t^4 reports and workshop reports, which started to appear in 2008, are unique strategic roadmaps, developed in constructive cooperation by experts in the field, invited by the transatlantic think tank for toxicology (t^4; see the dedicated webpage; (26)).

3.4 Mission to Promote the Three Rs

Since 2009, all the content of *ALTEX* has been published in English, and the name of the journal was changed that year to *ALTEX — Alternatives to Animal Experimentation*. Sonja von Aulock took over as Editor-in-Chief of *ALTEX* in 2011, and Joanne Zurlo became the journal's North American Editor in 2012, followed by Martin L. Stephens in 2018. The philosophical and ethical articles submitted to *ALTEX*, together with the literature review by Gottlieb Teutsch, were published as separate *ALTEX* supplements in 2009 and 2010. This led to the establishment of the German-language journal, *TIERethik*, in 2011. Since 2013, *ALTEX* has also published unedited open access Epub versions of main articles and short communications, immediately upon their acceptance. The full content of each issue is published with open access upon its completion. Since 2013, *ALTEX* has been recognised as a gold open access journal by the Directory of Open Access Journals (DOAJ).

The *ALTEX* staff are dedicated to professional, personal communication with authors, assisting in presenting data in high quality with regard to consistency, text flow, language editing, and figure quality. Scientific manuscripts submitted to *ALTEX* are evaluated on the basis of scientific merit and contributions to animal welfare, and the Three Rs principles. Although reduction and refinement articles are also welcomed, most of the articles, recently published in *ALTEX*, dealt with non-animal testing methods. Authors reporting on animal experiments must adhere to the ARRIVE guidelines on the reporting of *in vivo* experiments (27).

3.5 Recognition

The publication of highly cited articles, which especially include the Food for Thought ..., and t[4] workshop reports, as well as the switch to open access publication, led to a sharp rise in the Journal Citation Reports Impact Factor for *ALTEX* for 2010, from around 1 to 4.4. The high Impact Factor, which has remained around this level since then, and ranks highly in the journal category 'Medicine, Research and Experimental Science', has led to a considerable increase in the submission of high quality scientific manuscripts to *ALTEX*, perhaps in some cases also leading to scientists recognising the relevance of their work for the field of alternatives to animal experiments, and further raising the interest of scientists from outside the alternatives field in the work done, and opportunities offered by this field. This increased interest is helping to move research on alternatives to animal experiments from a niche into mainstream science.

4. ALTERNATIVES TO ANIMAL TESTING AND EXPERIMENTATION

4.1 Japanese Society for Alternatives to Animal Experiments' Role

AATEX (*Alternatives to Animal Testing and Experimentation*) is the official journal of the Japanese Society for Alternatives to Animal Experiments (JSAAE). The JSAAE is a scientific organisation, engaged in research, development, education, and surveillance activities, to promote and disseminate the Three Rs as international principles for animal experimentation. It was founded in Japan in 1984, as a study group to help disseminate the Three Rs principles nationwide via a newsletter, and it was established as a formal academic society in 1989. Currently, there are around 500 regular members of the JSAAE in Japan, and a meeting is held in Japan every year. International events held by the society have included the *sixth World Congress on Alternatives and Animal Use in the Life Sciences* (WC6; Tokyo, 2007), and the *Asian Congress on Alternatives and Animal Use in the Life Sciences* (Karatsu City, 2016).

The JSAAE is registered as a scientific research institute, collaborating with the Science Council of Japan. One of the requirements for such a registration is the publication of an academic periodical journal. As there was previously no scientific journal addressing the Three Rs principles in Japan, or indeed, in any other country outside the West, the foundation of an English journal belonging to the society was planned (see Fig. 3). In 1990, a new journal, named *AATEX*, was founded by Tsutomu Sugawara, President of the JSAAE, and Professor Emeritus of Kyoto University. The aims and scope of the journal are as follows: '*AATEX* is an international journal on new and novel developments, methods, techniques, validation, and use of alternatives to animal experimentation and testing. The journal's editorial policy is firmly rooted in the need for high-quality work in support of health and safety decisions, and emphasis will be placed on results that facilitate the use of alternatives to laboratory animals in biomedical research and toxicity testing'.

The JSAAE bears all the publishing costs of the journal. In the early days, *AATEX* was published four times a year, and several supplements were also published. In principle, all the articles were to be written in English. However, its editors

1980s	1990s	2000s	2010s
1985: In Japan, a small group of scientists was organised who were interested in alternatives to animal testing. This group published a newsletter. 1989: The Japanese Society for Alternatives to Animal Experiments (JSAAE) was established.	1990: *AATEX (Alternatives to Animal Testing and Experiments)* was launched as an English journal by the JSAAE. Journal size was 182 × 257mm. Proceedings of the 3rd JSAAE annual meeting were published (in English), with many original papers. The first Editor-in-Chief was Tsutomu Suguwara. 1998: Editor-in-Chief now Tadao Ohno (RIKEN, Tsukuba). Many papers on validation studies in the JSAAE were published. The journal cover design was changed. 1999: Editor-in-Chief now Hiroshi Ono (Hatano Research Institute, Food and Drug Safety Center, Kanagawa). The journal cover design was again changed.	2001: Editor-in-Chief now Isao Yoshimura (Tokyo University of Science). 2003: Editor-in-Chief now Tsutomu Miki Kurosawa (Osaka University). 2005: Editor-in-Chief now Koichi Imai (Osaka Dental University). The size of the journal changed to the international standard (7 × 10 inches). The design of the journal cover was also changed. 2006: Online ISSN was acquired and *AATEX* content published on J-STAGE.	2012: *AATEX–JaCVAM* (with a new ISSN) was launched to promote co-operation with JaCVAM. The *AATEX* cover design was used for this sister journal, but the colour scheme changed from yellow to light green. *AATEX–JaCVAM* publishes Japanese manuscripts, each with an English abstract. From 2012, four *AATEX* and *AATEX–JaCVAM* issues in total are published per year. 2013: Editor-in-Chief now Yuzi Yoshiyama (Kitasato University, Tokyo). 2015: Editor-in-Chief now Taku Matsushita (Sojo University, Kumamoto).

FIGURE 3 *AATEX* development timeline.

occasionally needed to adopt certain measures in order to address an insufficient number of submitted manuscripts. These measures included publishing (in English) the proceedings of the JSAAE annual meetings, and including articles in Japanese in some later volumes and supplements. After the publication of volume 6 (in 1999), the number of submitted manuscripts further decreased, and thus the publication frequency was reduced to three times a year. As for the two issues of volume 10, published in 2004, one contains both English and Japanese articles, whereas the other is a collection of Japanese abstracts. During that time, the society continued to face difficulty in maintaining the journal, due to the small number of submitted manuscripts.

4.2 A Second Beginning

Volume 11(1) was published in 2005, with Koichi Imai (Osaka Dental University) as a new Editor-in-Chief. This was a turning point for JSAAE, who were able to resume the publication of four issues per year, while discontinuing the inclusion of Japanese articles, and only accepting English manuscripts. The entire society was reinvigorated by the plan of Yasuo Ohno, of the National Institute of Health Sciences, to launch the Japanese Centre for the Validation of Alternative Methods (JaCVAM), as well as to prepare for WC6, to be held in Tokyo in 2007. Volume 11(1) contains a large number of manuscripts, including those from Michael Balls (FRAME, UK; (28)), Valerie Zuang and Thomas Hartung (ECVAM, Italy; (29)), and Alan Goldberg (CAAT, USA; (30)). In that same volume, 11(2) and 11(3) feature manuscripts from renowned international authors such as Horst Spielmann (ZEBET, Germany; (31)), Jon Richmond (Animals Scientific Procedures Division, UK; (32)), Coenraad Hendriksen (Netherlands Vaccine Institute; (33)), and Robert Coleman (Asterand UK Ltd; (34)). At the same time, Japanese researchers also began to actively submit their original manuscripts to the journal. Through these approaches, the society aimed to improve the quality of the journal, while continuing to deliver four issues annually, including one supplementary issue, containing the proceedings of the JSAAE annual meetings. In March 2012, the society obtained an online ISSN to publish *AATEX* in the Japanese digital journal system, J-STAGE (https://www.jstage.jst.go.jp/browse/aatex). Online publication started from Volume 11(1), meeting the requirement of its content being solely in English.

The number of manuscripts submitted to *AATEX* began to decrease around 2007, and the situation had become serious by 2010. As a general rule, non-IF journals are increasingly being forced to publish manuscripts rejected by international journals with an IF, those requiring acceptance by a certain date, or those from inexperienced researchers, making it difficult for these journals to maintain sufficient quality. Belonging to JSAAE, as a relatively minor publisher, *AATEX* lacked knowledge of the procedures needed to be considered for an IF rating, and of ways to maintain sufficient numbers of manuscripts and citations. The society is attempting to improve this situation by indexing the journal in PubMed, and consequently increasing the number of citations. Taku Matsushita (of Sojo University, Kumamoto), as the Editor-in-Chief, is currently co-ordinating an application to PubMed Central.

JaCVAM advises on the implementation of new alternatives to animal use in Japan, according to the Three Rs principles. Thus, in 2012, the JSAAE obtained another ISSN (2187-3690) and launched *AATEX*—*JaCVAM* to promote collaboration with this centre. The *AATEX* cover design was slightly modified in the colour scheme, for use as the cover for the sister journal. Since that time, the JSAAE has published an annual report of JaCVAM's activities in Japanese, in the form of *AATEX*—*JaCVAM*. In addition to this, two further issues of *AATEX* per year are published solely in English, and one supplementary issue is published (in English), featuring proceedings of academic meetings; thus, the society currently delivers four issues annually.

In countries outside the West, there are few academic societies, corresponding to the JSAAE, that focus on alternatives to animal testing. In the field of technological development, new drugs and biomaterials cannot be used for humans, unless their safety is accurately evaluated. Accordingly, those who aim to evaluate and help implement alternatives to animal experimentation are drawing global attention. The development and implementation of animal alternatives markedly contribute to the promotion of new industries. In this respect, it is expected that the *AATEX* journal will expand further in the future.

5. DISCUSSION

The three featured journals were each established as a result of a common recognition of the importance of the Three Rs, and the need to promote awareness of its principles. From modest beginnings, each journal has evolved in its own manner. At the heart of this evolution has been the desire to achieve the end-goal of increasing global awareness of the Three Rs. In addition to the timely publication of reports on workshops and validation studies, and scientific papers on the development of alternative methods, the publication of the proceedings of a vast number of conferences has also helped to get the information presented at such meetings into the wider arena for discussion, rather than remaining 'behind closed doors'.

Other initiatives stand out as particular distinguishing strengths of the individual journals in terms of working toward the desired end-goal. These include publishing early papers on the Three Rs, by Russell and Burch themselves; distributing hard copies to 'developing' countries, who are new to the Three Rs concept; establishing free open access of published content; encouraging scientists outside the field to publish in a high-IF 'alternatives' journal, and having initiative and strength under adversity in countries where knowledge of the Three Rs is not yet widespread.

Peer-reviewed scientific journals have always played an invaluable role in the dissemination of information relating to their specific field, not least in the illustrated case of Three Rs alternatives. In view of this, their existence should be safeguarded for the future by developing further evolutionary strategies to ensure their long-term survival.

REFERENCES

1. Russell, W.M.S. & Burch, R.L. (1959). *The Principles of Humane Experimental Techniques*, 238pp. London, UK: Methuen.
2. Anon. (1973). About FRAME. *ATLA Abstracts*, 1(1), i.
3. Anon. (1977). Editorial. What is an "alternative"? *ATLA Abstracts*, 5(2), ii.
4. Anon. (1994). ECVAM News and Views. *ATLA* **22**, 7−11.
5. Balls, M., Blaauboer, B., Brusick, D., *et al.* (1990). Report and recommendations of the CAAT/ERGATT Workshop on the validation of toxicity test procedures. *ATLA* **18**, 313−337.
6. Balls, M., Botham, P., Cordier, A., *et al.* (1990). Report and recommendations of an international workshop on the promotion of the regulatory acceptance of non-animal toxicity test procedures. *ATLA* **18**, 339−344.
7. Various authors. (2004). The Three Rs at the Beginning of the 21st Century. In, *ATLA: 32. Proceedings of the Fourth World Congress on Alternatives and Animal Use in the Life Sciences. 11−15 August 2002, New Orleans, Louisiana, USA.* Supplement 1A and 1B, 758pp.
8. Balls, M. & Combes, R. (ed.) (2006). The REACH system: scientific and animal welfare implications of EU legislation on chemicals testing. *ATLA* **34** (Suppl 1), 158pp.
9. Combes, R., Balls, M., Illing, P., *et al.* (2006). Possibilities for a new approach to chemicals risk assessment — The report of a FRAME Workshop. *ATLA* **34**, 621−649.
10. BéruBé, K., Aufderheide, M., Breheny, D., *et al.* (2009). *In vitro* models of inhalation toxicity and disease. The report of a FRAME Workshop. *ATLA* **37**, 89−141.
11. Walum, E., & Ekwall, B. (Eds.). (1996). MEIC Evaluation of Acute Systemic Toxicity. Part I: Methodology of 68 *in vitro* toxicity assays used to test the first 30 reference chemicals. Part II: *In vitro* results from 68 toxicity assays used to test the first 30 reference chemicals and a comparative cytotoxicity analysis. *ATLA* **24** (Suppl 1), 62.
12. Walum, E., & Ekwall, B. (Eds.). (1998). MEIC Evaluation of Acute Systemic Toxicity. Part III: *In vitro* results from 16 additional methods used to test the first 30 reference chemicals and a comparative cytotoxicity analysis. Part IV: *In vitro* results from 67 toxicity assays used to test reference chemicals 31e50 and a comparative cytotoxicity analysis. *ATLA* **26** (Suppl 1), 91.
13. Walum, E., & Ekwall, B. (Eds.). (1998). MEIC Evaluation of Acute Systemic Toxicity. Part V: Rodent and human toxicity data for the 50 reference chemicals. Part VI: The prediction of human toxicity by rodent LD50 values and results from 61 *in vitro* methods. *ATLA* **26** (Suppl 2), 89.
14. Walum, E., & Ekwall, B. (Eds.). (2000). MEIC Evaluation of Acute Systemic Toxicity. Part VII: Prediction of human toxicity by results from testing of the first 30 reference chemicals with 27 further *in vitro* assays. Part VIII: Multivariate partial least squares evaluation, including the selection of a battery of cell line tests with a good prediction of human acute lethal peak blood concentrations for 50 chemicals. *ATLA* **28** (Suppl 1), 75.
15. Peijnenburg, W.J.G.M. & Tetko, I.V. (2013). CADASTER Workshop proceedings. Preface. *ATLA* **41**, 13−17.
16. Tetko, I.V., Schramm, K.-W., Knepper, T., *et al.* (2014). Preface — Experimental and theoretical studies in the EU FP7 Marie Curie Initial Training Network Project, Environmental ChemOinformatics (ECO). *ATLA* **42**, 7−11.
17. Morrissey, B., Blyth, K., Carter, P., *et al.* (2015). SEARCHBreast Workshop proceedings: 3D modelling of breast cancer. *ATLA* **43**, 367−375.
18. Balls, M. (2009). The origins and early days of the Three Rs concept. *ATLA* **37**, 255−265.
19. Russell, W.M.S. & Burch, R.L. (1995). Prefatory Note. *ATLA* **23**, 11−13.
20. Balls, M., Goldberg, A.M., Fentem, J.H., *et al.* (1995). The Three Rs: The way forward. The report and recommendations of ECVAM Workshop 11. *ATLA* **23**, 838−866.
21. Anon. (2018). *CAATwalk Newsletter Homepage.* Baltimore, MD, USA: CAAT, Johns Hopkins University. http://altweb.jhsph.edu/newsletter/.
22. Anon. (2018). *ALTEX Proceedings.* Zurich, Switzerland: ALTEX Edition. https://www.altex.org/index.php/altex/index.
23. Anon. (2018). *ALTEX Award*, 2pp. Zurich, Switzerland: ALTEX Edition. https://www.altex.org/index.php/altex/ALTEX_Award.
24. Anon. (2018). *ALTEX Edition*, 2pp. Zurich, Switzerland: ALTEX Edition. https://www.altex.org/index.php/altex/article/view/94/149.
25. Anon. (2018). *Food for Thought... in ALTEX*, 2pp. Zurich, Switzerland: ALTEX Edition. https://www.altex.org/index.php/altex/FFT.
26. Anon. (2018). *Transatlantic Think Tank for Toxicology*, 2pp. Zurich, Switzerland: ALTEX Edition. https://www.altex.org/index.php/altex/t4.
27. Kilkenny, C., Browne, W.J., Cuthill, I.C., *et al.* (2013). *The ARRIVE Guidelines*, 2pp. London, UK: NC3Rs. https://nc3rs.org.uk/arrive-guidelines.
28. Balls, M. (2005). Alternatives to animal experiments: Serving in the middle ground. *AATEX* **11**, 4−14.
29. Zuang, V. & Hartung, H. (2005). Making validated alternatives available — The strategies and work of the European Centre for the Validation of Alternative Methods (ECVAM). *AATEX* **11**, 15−26.

30. Goldberg, A.M. (2005). TestSmart DNT — Creating a humane and efficient approach to developmental neurotoxicity testing. *AATEX* **11**, 27–30.
31. Spielmann, H. (2005). Progress in establishing in vitro alternatives to animal experiments — Ethical and scientific challenges. *AATEX* **11**, 89–100.
32. Richmond, J.D. (2006). A personal perspective. *AATEX* **11**, 150–154.
33. Hendriksen, C.F.M. (2006). Replacement, reduction and refinement in the production and quality control of immunobiologicals. *AATEX* **11**, 155–161.
34. Coleman, R.A. (2006). Regulation and practice of human tissue research in the UK. *AATEX* **11**, 162–169.

Chapter 4.2

Dissemination of Information on Alternative Methods: Databases and Systems

Annett J. Roi[1] and Roman Kolar[2]

[1]Joint Research Centre, European Commission, Ispra, Italy; [2]German Animal Welfare Federation - Animal Welfare Academy, Neubiberg, Germany

SUMMARY

In the 1980s, the demand for specific information on alternatives to animal experiments grew steadily. At the same time, the increasingly faster evolution of the Internet and technological advances have had a significant impact not only on the scientific research itself but also very importantly on the transformation of online databases and the changing attitude on how information is accessed by end-users. The steadily increasing number of information resources represents a powerful tool for research projects, but the satisfactory identification of the desired information has become a real challenge. The area of toxicology was one of the first that considered the use of alternative methods in its research projects and consequently pioneered the establishment of specialised resources that received a significant initial impulse with the establishment of the European Centre for the Validation of Alternative Methods. The historical development of selected specialised databases on advanced and alternative non-animal approaches is described in this chapter.

1. THE EUROPEAN DRIVE TO PROMOTE THE USE OF ALTERNATIVE METHODS

In the early 1990s, driven by both scientific needs and public concern on animal welfare, the European Commission was called upon to further accelerate the implementation of the European policy dedicated to the protection of animals used for scientific purposes (1, 2). The Commission responded by putting a system in place that would actively support the development and validation of alternative methods, as well as information dissemination and knowledge management.

This was the beginning of the European Centre for the Validation of Alternative Methods (ECVAM) established at the Commission's Joint Research Centre (JRC) in Ispra, Italy, in 1991. Among ECVAM's core tasks, particular emphasis was given to knowledge sharing and information dissemination to enhance the acceptance and use of alternative methods, in addition to its main duty regarding test development and validation activities (see also, Chapter 2.10). ECVAM later became the European Union (EU) Reference Laboratory for Alternatives to Animal Testing (EURL ECVAM) under EU *Directive 2010/63* (3), which reinforced and further extended its mandate to cover methods used in biomedical research, as well as in regulatory testing.

It was recognised at an early stage that ready access to reliable and comprehensive information on alternatives would be a prerequisite for their acceptance and practical application by any end-user. Consequently, from the outset it was a clearly defined duty of ECVAM to establish a computer-based service for the collection, analysis and review of relevant information, to then be prepared for re-dissemination, tailored for its use by scientific communities, regulatory entities and authorities, policy makers and/or the animal welfare movement. This pillar of ECVAM's activities was first realised by establishing its Scientific Information Service (SIS) in 1996 (4), which was relaunched as ECVAM's DataBase service on ALternative and advanced Methods to animal experimentation (DB-ALM; https://ecvam-dbalm.jrc.ec.europa.eu) in 2006.

The History of Alternative Test Methods in Toxicology. https://doi.org/10.1016/B978-0-12-813697-3.00028-7

2. THE START OF THE COLLABORATION AMONG INFORMATION PROVIDERS

2.1 Introduction

Technological advances over the past 4 decades have had a significant impact not only on the scientific research itself but also on the transformation of online databases and the change in attitudes on how information is accessed by end-users. Online resources have increasingly been offered via the World Wide Web, and end-users have increasingly been carrying out their own searches, without the help of the trained personnel of libraries or by information specialists. Technological progress in storage capabilities, the processing power of computers, and improvements in the software used for searching databases, have led to an unprecedented proliferation of resources (5–13). Although the multitude of information sources is undoubtedly of great value, and the information has never been brought so close to the end-user, the identification of the relevant information, and particularly on the Three Rs (*Replacement, Reduction* and *Refinement* of animal use for scientific purposes), has become a real challenge.

While the nature of problems has evolved over time, ready access to reliable information continues to be the core of the end-user's needs and has consequently been the driving force for ECVAM's activities in the area of information dissemination and knowledge management.

2.2 Getting Started

In 1996, an international ECVAM workshop was organised in collaboration with the German Animal Welfare Academy and the Dutch University of Utrecht, on the *Current Status and Future Developments of Databases on Alternative Methods*. It was the first official meeting involving experts from Europe and the USA, who had been involved in the creation and maintenance of databases that contribute to the aims of the Three Rs. The scope of the meeting was to: (a) review the current situation; (b) identify the types of information needed; (c) discuss possibilities for collaborations; and (d) agree on a strategy for improving the dissemination of information on alternatives (6). A first collection of about 20 databases was made available on the Internet immediately after the workshop.

In the early years, electronic forms of both large bibliographic databases containing references to publications, and factual databases containing real data and/or information on publications, were increasingly being developed in the various fields of biosciences (e.g. AGRICOLA, BIOSIS, CAB Abstracts EmBase, MEDLINE, the ECDIN Data Bank (European Chemicals Data and Information Network), the Toxnet Databases, RTECS (the Registry of Toxic Effects of Chemical Substances) or the US Toxicology Data Bank project). In 1998, the US National Library of Medicine (NLM) published ALTBIB (https://toxnet.nlm.nih.gov/altbib.html), a searchable bibliographic collection on alternatives to animal testing from 1980 to 2001, later offering access to additional sources and a search strategy for scanning publications on alternatives in PubMed, with particular attention to toxicology. Taken together, the databases and services have provided a wealth of information from various fields of study, with different levels of detail or focus, and most of them have undergone considerable innovation in the succeeding years. It was recognised that the use of public resources, together with in-house databases, represents a powerful and essential tool in a step-wise approach for any toxicology research project or regulatory toxicity application (6). However, the problem of retrieving relevant information has increasingly become an issue. The level of scientific output has grown constantly. In 1997, an estimated 3,000,000 articles were being published annually in the biosciences (6), and estimates for biomedicine showed an increase in publications of over 80% for Europe alone in a 10-year period (14). Whatever the exact numbers for the individual disciplines may be, the volume of information to be dealt with would be beyond the 'average' database user without specific skills in information retrieval or knowledge of relevant information sources. Pubmed alone allows for the simultaneous searching of about 20 million records with simple keywords (15). Therefore, it was evident that electronic sources, seen as a potential solution to this problem, were undergoing a similar proliferation, so it was becoming more and more difficult to locate the desired information, a problem further aggravated for an emerging area such as the Three Rs.

This situation, together with the increasing demands from various quarters for access to recent advances in methodologies, including methods undergoing validation, led to the first specialised value-added services, often developed on an *ad hoc* basis, to contribute to a better and tailored dissemination of information on alternatives to animal experimentation, as described in the ECVAM Workshop Report (6).

Some other specialised sources of information on alternative methods in toxicology are reported in this section, and ECVAM's activities are briefly described in Section 3.

2.2.1 The AnimAlt-Zebet Database on Alternatives to Animal Experiments

Located within the German Federal Institute for Risk Assessment (BfR), the former Centre for Documentation and Evaluation of Alternative Methods to Animal Experiments (ZEBET), now the German Centre for the Protection of Laboratory Animals (Bf3R), produced the publicly accessible AnimAlt-Zebet Database in response to the amendment to the German Animal Welfare Act of 1986. From 2000 to 2014, AnimAlt-ZEBET was hosted by the German Institute of Medical Documentation and Information (DIMDI). It is an English full-text database and provides 150 documents on reduction, refinement or replacement alternatives in all fields of biomedicine, together with 4300 bibliographic references (16, 17). The database provides expert-written documents that have been evaluated by ZEBET's staff according to the Three Rs principles and the current stage of development, validation and acceptance. The database was used to provide advice and information to scientists and animal welfare officers during the process of authorisation of animal experimentation (18). The database (http://www.bfr.bund.de/de/animalt_zebet___datenbank_fuer_alternativmethoden_zu_tierversuchen-59741.html) is available via the BfR website but has not been updated since 2013.

2.2.2 The 'Gelbe Liste', the Animal Welfare Academy Database on Alternatives to Animal Experiments

At the time when the German Animal Welfare Act came into force, there was almost no means for scientists, authorities or ethical committees to search for possible alternative approaches in scientific literature or to gain an overview to identify gaps and priorities for filling them. Therefore, the Animal Welfare Academy of the German Animal Welfare Federation (a German non-profit organisation), located at Neubiberg, established a computer-based literature database on alternatives in 1986 that ultimately provided about 20,000 searchable entries with relevance to research, testing and education, together with a thesaurus, the first specific one for alternative methods. Each database entry involved a critical evaluation with regard to the Three Rs (19, 20).

The database was widely used by authorities, universities and ethical committees. Free searches were performed on request by the Animal Welfare Academy, and details of the database were regularly presented at scientific conferences (20, 21). Annotated excerpts from the database were published as paperbacks, the so-called 'Gelbe Liste' (Yellow Lists), which were sent free-of-charge to all German universities, as well as to interested organisations and individuals, both inside and outside Germany.

At the end of the 1990s, international cooperation and combined efforts became a priority for the academy, which also contributed actively to the establishment of the ECVAM database. Consequently, its own project ceased, but considerable effort was invested in supporting international initiatives for the better dissemination of scientific information on alternatives to animal experiments.

2.2.3 INVITTOX, the Database on In Vitro Techniques in Toxicology

This service, which was established by the Fund for the Replacement of Animals in Medical Experiments (FRAME, Nottingham, UK), in collaboration with the European Research Group for Alternatives in Toxicity Testing, following a survey of potential users in 1986, provided protocols for methods of *in vitro* toxicity testing at a level of detail not normally found in the published literature. The protocols were written by *INVITTOX* staff in collaboration with the test developer, with the aim of minimising the inconvenience to the information provider, which was considered fundamental for keeping the database up to date. Up to 1996, about 5000 protocols were sent out at the request of these users, and a survey confirmed the success of the project (22, 23). *INVITTOX* was initially financially supported by Directorate General (DG) XI (today DG Environment) of the European Commission, and was transferred to ECVAM in 1996.

2.2.4 The Altweb Web Site on Alternatives to Animal Testing

Altweb (http://altweb.jhsph.edu), created in 1997 after the ECVAM workshop (6), serves as a gateway to alternatives news, information and resources on the Internet. Altweb's Research Resources for scientists and technicians cover specific topics across the entire range of the Three Rs and also provide access to the *ALTEX* journal. Altweb was established by the Center for Alternatives to Animal Testing at Johns Hopkins University, Baltimore, MD, USA, and is steered by an international advisory team (24). The website is designed for open access and is continuously updated.

2.3 Information Dissemination Grows out of Its Infancy

The ECVAM workshop gave a significant impulse to start discussions aimed at improving the information coverage on alternative methods at all stages of development and availability. The awareness that ready access to reliable information is an integral part of any research project was recognised as an argument that deserved attention. The theme then occupied a firm place in nearly all the World Congresses on alternatives to animal use in the life sciences, even though the 'information' topic has rarely received its own session and has never been the subject of a plenary lecture. The commitments made by organisations often lacked the continuity essential for the provision of evolved and updated databases (25). However, the operators continued to seek improvements to data retrieval, including the scientific vocabularies for indexing publications, as well as the possibility of inventorying, categorising and coordinating information sources (e.g. 4, 7, 9, 12, 13, 26–29).

The European Partnership on Alternative Approaches to Animal Testing (EPAA), launched in 2005 as a joint initiative of the European Commission and European industries, created a Platform dedicated to the Dissemination of Information on the Three Rs. The resulting EPAA Workshops on Dissemination Strategies in 2008 and 2009 pointed to the need for stakeholders to be able to access information with different levels of detail, presented as easy-to-read, pre-digested reviews, and more-detailed information, as well as the need for a 'marketplace' for sharing ideas and finding out what is in the research pipeline. Education in the Three Rs was also considered as a fundamental need for scientists. In this context, stakeholders appreciated the provision of thematic reviews via ECVAM's DB-ALM (30).

In due course, the development of knowledge-based search engines such as Go3R began (31). The AltTox website (http://alttox.org) was created in 2007, as a joint initiative of a non-governmental organisation and industry in the USA, with information on alternative methods. The website of the UK National Centre for the Three Rs (NC3Rs) also includes structured Three Rs resources (https://www.nc3rs.org.uk/3rs-resources).

The European Commission (Directorate General Environment) organised the *Expert Group Meeting on Dissemination of Information on Alternatives* in 2012 to discuss information availability and needs resulting from the introduction of *Directive 63/2010/EU*. (http://ec.europa.eu/environment/chemicals/lab_animals/3r/alternatives_information_en.htm). An overview of information resources is available from the website. Indeed, links to lists of resources from websites are common today, and several repositories for experimental protocols are available online in various forms. In its 2015 response to the EU Citizens' Initiative *Stop Vivisection* (32), the Commission committed to enhancing knowledge-sharing as means of accelerating progress in the Three Rs. Accordingly, EURL ECVAM conducted a survey on the use of resources and created an inventory (12). Norway's Three Rs Centre, NORECOPA, founded in 2007, established a web-based portal on various aspects of alternatives, including the database, 3R Guide, accessible on the Internet since 2016 (https://norecopa.no/3r-guide) and continues to maintain Norina, a database containing over 3500 audiovisuals.

Information dissemination and knowledge-sharing have become indispensable parts of all discussions on the Three Rs not only in Europe, but involving all continents as reflected in future World Conferences and international activities. The message to deliver was that improved information storage, exchange and use should be considered as a replacement method in its own right, as already noted by Balls (33) long ago, in 1994.

3. THE WAY FORWARD FOR ECVAM

To follow up the progress of ECVAM's SIS, established in 1996 (4), a special international advisory body was created in 2000 within ECVAM's Scientific Advisory Committee (ESAC), to provide feedback and discuss general strategic aspects. Representatives from ZEBET, FRAME, the University of Graz (Austria) and the University of Utrecht (The Netherlands) were involved.

The following activities were undertaken in response to the recommendations of the ECVAM workshop (6) and subsequent international input:

1. The launch of ECVAM's SIS on the Internet in 2001, together with a survey, including: (a) standard operating procedures of non-animal approaches at all stages of development, including from ECVAM's validation studies; and (b) a factual proposal on how the information on validation studies/projects could best be made available for public access. The idea of 'pre-digested, ready-to-use' information was put into practice, complementing the collection of protocols with contextual information based on a bibliographic review including the development status and applications of the methods. A new sector, *Method-Summaries*, was created to address scientists as well as authorities and regulatory communities.

   The response to ECVAM's SIS was immediate and very positive, leading to a steadily increasing user community. The Commissioner for Research at the time, Philippe Busquin, included it as a highlight in his newly launched Newsletter, *JRC in Action*.

2. In 2000, as a result of ECVAM's Task Force activities on Alternatives Databases, a joint feasibility study was undertaken with the Head of the Thesaurus section of the US National Library of Medicine (NLM) to investigate possible improvements of the scientific vocabulary in use by database providers in biomedical sciences with regard to alternative methods to enhance the retrieval of the indexed papers. It involved the analysis, selection and comparison of the terminology used in published documents/articles against respective thesauruses in a semi-automatic manner. The result was made available via the DB-ALM website for comments and open access (https://ecvam-dbalm.jrc.ec.europa.eu/thesaurus).

   A major milestone for improving access to alternative methods through literature databases resulted from the US NLM expert group meeting on alternatives terminologies triggered by ECVAM, in which ECVAM participated, together with a representative from ZEBET, to provide the expertise on alternative methods in biomedical sciences. It led to the following actions by the US NLM: (a) nine scientific journals covering animal alternatives were included in MEDLINE, Toxline and related sources; (b) the alternatives index term was changed to better identify papers on all Three Rs, from *Animal testing alternatives* to *Animal use alternatives*; and (c) search filters covering the Three Rs were developed.

   The importance of these developments should not be underestimated, as the MeSH (Medical Subject Headings) thesaurus was, and is, one of the most extensive thesauruses for indexing major literature databases in the biomedical sciences, with an impact on other databases and their indexing policies.

3. The first ECVAM website was launched in 2002, covering all the activities of ECVAM, together with a dedicated sector on all the methods included in ECVAM validation studies, including the ESAC statements on their validation status and readiness for regulatory acceptance, complemented with full method descriptions for ready implementation in laboratories.

4. Based on the success achieved with ECVAM's SIS, a more extensive database, DB-ALM, was formally launched in 2006 by the JRC, on the occasion of the 15th Anniversary of ECVAM. The database services include a comprehensive computerised information service on non-animal methods, covering *in vitro* and *in silico* methods, along with a special database on Quantitative Structure-Activity Relationship (QSAR) models, a tracking system on methods proposed for validation, and a search guide, all briefly described in the following section.

3.1 EURL ECVAM Databases on Alternative Methods Today

3.1.1 The DB-ALM: The DataBase Service on ALternative Methods to Animal Experimentation

The DB-ALM (https://ecvam-dbalm.jrc.ec.europa.eu) is a public, factual database service that provides ready-to-use information on animal alternatives in use in the life sciences. The content is presented as expert-written reviewed data sheets in the form of summary records and/or more-detailed information. Information on underlying scientific principles, development, applications and acceptance status is provided as method summaries or detailed protocols that facilitate method transfer to another laboratory without the need for additional information (Fig. 1). Contact information for the method user/developer is always provided, together with descriptions of research or validation projects, compounds tested and individual investigations.

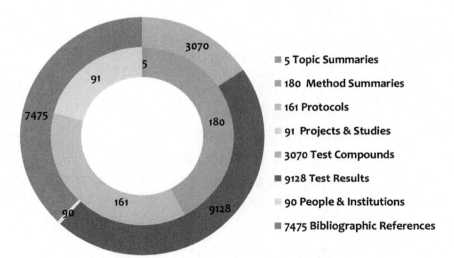

FIGURE 1 DB-ALM information content (Dec.2017).

The initial focus was on *in vitro* methods for toxicological evaluations of chemicals and formulations, but the database also includes biological substances, medical devices and other approaches to reduce animal use. An extension to models used in biomedical research is currently ongoing. Moreover, since 2015 the DB-ALM has provided a harmonised framework for comprehensively describing *in vitro* methods compliant with OECD Guidance Document 211 (34). An entirely revised version was launched in 2016, together with an online questionnaire (35). The database's subscribers are regularly updated with the latest news.

The collected information originates from national and international research projects, validation studies, individual submissions from scientists and thematic bibliographic reviews. All the documents are compiled by experts in the field and are reviewed by JRC staff before inclusion in the database.

3.1.2 The QSAR Model Database

The QSAR Model Database (http://qsardb.jrc.ec.europa.eu) is a freely accessible web application that enables users to submit, publish and search for peer-reviewed summary descriptions of QSAR models. It was initially established to support the use of QSARs under the REACH regulation. An internationally accepted reporting standard (the QSAR Model Reporting Format; QMRF) is used to ensure the provision of comprehensive and consistent information. Developers and users of QSAR models can submit a QMRF, which is reviewed for adequacy and completeness by EURL ECVAM before publishing it through the database. The descriptions are provided as robust summaries, including results of any validation studies. However, publication of the model does not imply acceptance or endorsement by the JRC or the European Commission, and responsibility for the use of the models lies with the end-users.

The online information content (Fig. 2) covers more than 140 QSAR model descriptions, grouped according to OECD-defined (regulatory) endpoints. A progress report summarising the activities of the QSAR model database during 2014–16 is available on request (JRC102362).

3.1.3 The Tracking System for Alternative Methods Toward Regulatory Acceptance

The revised Tracking System for Alternative methods toward Regulatory acceptance (TSAR; https://tsar.jrc.ec.europa.eu) was published by the JRC on the occasion of the Commission's scientific conference on *Non-animal Approaches-The Way Forward*, held in Brussels in December 2016. TSAR provides full transparency on the progress a test method makes from first being proposed for validation through to its eventual acceptance for the regulatory safety and efficacy testing of chemicals or biological agents. It includes all available records associated with different steps of the validation and acceptance process, and short summary descriptions of individual methods being integrated with the DB-ALM. TSAR disseminates information on test methods not only under consideration in Europe but also by all member and observer organisations of the International Collaboration on Alternative Testing Methods (ICATM), representing the EU, Canada, USA, Republic of Korea, Japan, Brazil and China. This first release of the revised TSAR includes the majority of methods submitted to ECVAM since 2008. The remaining methods will progressively be made available, together with those from ICATM partners.

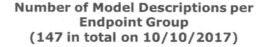

Number of Model Descriptions per Endpoint Group (147 in total on 10/10/2017)

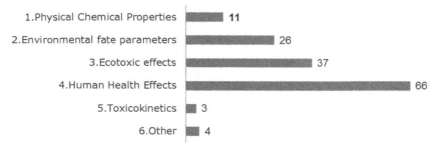

FIGURE 2   QSAR model database information content.

3.1.4 The Use and Outreach of ECVAM's Databases

ECVAM's databases provide a reference point for regulatory application and research studies, and are cited in scientific papers, books, OECD test guidelines and guidance documents, and on websites in various geographical areas. Taking as an example the DB-ALM, a steadily increasing interest in the services has been observed. Even though DB-ALM provides access to some information without the need to register, the service has a large number of registrants, totalling over 5000 from 82 countries (Fig. 3). Furthermore, its use is continuously growing, with more than 53,000 accesses from 7532 unique visitors during July 2016 to June 2017, corresponding to an increase of about 30% compared with the previous year. Over 3800 documents were downloaded during the same period, showing a similar increase of over 30% compared with the year before, the highest during 11 years of public online access.

3.2 The EURL ECVAM Search Guide

The *EURL ECVAM Search Guide* (SG; (36)) was specifically developed to inform and support untrained database users in finding high-quality information on relevant alternative methods and strategies from the large amount of available information resources. It provides advice on a structured and systematic data retrieval approach in the biomedical sciences, together with supporting information, offered in a way that allows users to select according to their needs (e.g. an inventory of selected information sources and their descriptions, suggested search terms or basic search principles). The essentials are summarised in the *Seven Golden Steps to Successful Searching*.

The SG (first published in 2012, with a revised edition in 2013) reached fourth place in the top 10 most downloaded publications of the EU Bookshop, only 2 months after its first publication. It has become a valuable resource for higher education in the life sciences and during scientific project preparation or evaluation that might involve animal use. It has also entered the Asian market, where it has been translated and re-published as a handbook and E-book in Korean. A Brazilian version was published in 2017, within the framework of ICATM.

4. CONCLUSIONS

The field of toxicology, including mechanistic evaluations, was one of the first that considered the use of alternative methods in its research projects and, consequently, pioneered the establishment of specialised resources. The increasing amount and diversity of information on the Internet changed the attitudes of end-users on how to access such information. Information providers have made efforts to group resources, providing a single search interface, and have started to develop semantic search engines. In addition, publishers have increasingly provided open-access resources together with experimental protocols, along with specialised websites and discussion forums. In spite of these developments, it remains a major challenge for the average database user to find relevant and adequate information, particularly in relation to the Three Rs. The ability to access such information sources is key when preparing or reviewing scientific projects ("I can only use what I know!"). Consequently, specialised subject-specific information resources on alternatives providing the context to the Three Rs for research projects, together with updates on methodological developments, are obvious first choices when starting scientific projects that might entail animal use. However, it must also be said that the reliance on such services is

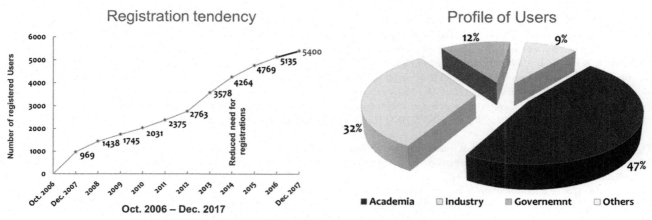

FIGURE 3 DB-ALM usage statistics.

very much dependent on their updating policy. Value-added and specialised services represent labour-intensive activities that require specific professional skills to ensure the quality of the information provided, as well as user-friendly means of dissemination. This is only achievable with a sincere long-term commitment by the providers.

REFERENCES

1. EEC. (1986). Council Directive 86/609/EEC on the approximation of the laws, regulation and administrative provisions of the Member States regarding the protection of animals used for experimental and other scientific purposes. *Official Journal of the European Union* **L358**, 1—28.
2. EC. (1991). *Communication from the Commission to the Council and the European Parliament on the establishment of a European Centre for the Validation of Alternative Methods.* Brussels, Belgium: European Commission. SEC (91) 1794, 29 June 1991.
3. EU. (2010). Directive 2010/63/EU of the European Parliament and of the Council of 22 September 2010 on the protection of animals used for scientific purposes. *Official Journal of the European Union* **L276**, 33—79.
4. Janusch-Roi, A. & Balls, M. (1999). The ECVAM Scientific Information Service (SIS). Symposium "ZEBET's 10 Year Anniversary" 21/22 June 1999, Bundesinstitut für gesundheitlichen Verbraucheschutz und Veterinärmedizin (BgVV), Zentralstelle zur Erfassung und Bewertung von Ersatz- und Ergänzungs. *ALTEX* **16**, 114—116.
5. Bawden, D. (1990). Information systems and databases as alternatives. *ATLA* **18**, 83—89.
6. Janusch, A., Kamp, M.D.O., Van Der, Bottrill, K., *et al.* (1997). Current status and future developments of databases on alternative methods. *ATLA* **25**, 411—422.
7. Mohapatra, A. & Wexler, P. (2009). Web-based databases. In P.J.B. Hakkinen, A. Mohapatra, & S.G.G. Gilbert (Eds.), *Information Resources in Toxicology* (4th ed., pp. 619—630). Cambridge, MA, USA: Elsevier Inc.
8. Bawden, D. & Robinson, L. (2016). Information and the gaining of understanding. *Journal of Information Science* **42**, 294—299.
9. Janusch-Roi, A., Libowitz, L., Grune, B., *et al.* (2000). Alternative methods databases-specialised information sources on alternatives to support scientists and authorities responsible for granting project licences. In M. Balls, A.-M. van Zeller, & M.E. Halder (Eds.), *Proceedings of the 3rd World Congress on Alternatives and Animal Use in the Life Sciences. Progress in Reduction, Refinement and Replacement of Animal Experimentation*, pp. 1731—1736. Amsterdam: Elsevier Science.
10. Hakkinen, P.J. & Green, D.K. (2002). Alternatives to animal testing: Information resources via the internet and world wide web. *Toxicology* **173**, 3—11.
11. Grune, B., Dörendahl, A., Köhler-Hahn, D., *et al.* (2004). New sources for alternative methods on the Internet: the objectives of databases and web sites. *ATLA* **32**(Suppl. 1), 573—582.
12. Holley, T., Bowe, G., Campia, I., *et al.* (2016). *Accelerating Progress in the Replacement, Reduction and Refinement of Animal Testing Through Better Knowledge Sharing.* JRC report EUR 28234, 64pp.
13. Smith, A.J. & Allen, T. (2005). The use of databases, information centres and guidelines when planning research that may involve animals. *Animal Welfare* **14**, 347—359.
14. Rahman, M. & Fukui, T. (2003). Biomedical publication — Global profile and trend. *Public Health* **117**, 274—280.
15. Butzke, D., Doerendahl, A., Skolik, S., *et al.* (2010). The threefold strategy of ZEBET at the BfR to improve dissemination of information on alternative methods to animal experiments (Aalborg University Press). In *Proceedings of the 10th International Conference on Current Research Information Systems, CRIS 2010, Connecting Science with Society, The Role of Research Information in a Knowledge-Based Society*, pp. 21—26.
16. Grune-Wolff, B., Doerendahl, A., Skolik, S., *et al.* (1995). Welche Unterstuetzung koennen ZEBET und DIMDI Wissenschaftlern bei der Suche nach Alternativmethoden zu Tierversuchen geben. In H. Schoeffl, H. Spielmann, & H.A. Tritthart (Eds.), *Ersatz und Ergaenzungsmethoden zu Tierversuchen*, pp. 282—288. Vienna: Springer Verlag.
17. Grune-Wolff, B., Doerndahl, A., Skolik, S., *et al.* (1996). ZEBET databank and information service on alternative methods to animal experiments. *ATLA* **24** (special issue, 124).
18. Butzke, D., Doerendahl, A., Skolik, S., *et al.* (2010). The AnimALT-ZEBET database: A unique resource for comprehensive and value-added information on 3R alternatives. *ALTEX* **27**, 133—135.
19. Rusche, B. & Sauer, U.G. (1994). Reviewed literature databank for alternatives to animal experiments — "Gelbe Liste". In C.A. Reinhardt (Ed.), *Alternatives to Animal Testing. New Ways in the Biomedical Sciences, Trends and Progress*, pp. 8—88. Weinheim: VCH.
20. Kolar, R. & Rusche, B. (1996). The database of the Deutscher Tierschutzbund e.V. for alternatives to animal experiments. In , *ATLA: Vol. 24. Second world congress on alternatives and animal use in the life sciences* (special issue, 336).
21. Kolar, R., Rusche, B., Ruhdel, I.W., *et al.* (1999). The work of the Deutscher Tierschutzbund e.V. (German animal welfare association) toward the Three Rs. *In Third World Congress on Alternatives and Animal Use in the Life Sciences. ATLA* **27** (special issue, 400).
22. Warren, M., Atkinson, K. & Steer, S. (1990). INVITTOX: The ERGATT/FRAME data bank of *in vitro* techniques in toxicology. *Toxicology in Vitro* **4**, 707—710.
23. Ungar, K. (1992). The INVITTOX data bank of in-vitro techniques in toxicology. *Human & Experimental Toxicology* **11**, 151—154.
24. Libowitz, L.A. (2004). Proposal for international recognition, support and coorperation with the internet clearinghouse on the Three Rs (Altweb). *ATLA* **32**, 583—584.
25. Bottrill, K. (2002). Information: needs for the future. *ATLA* **30**(Suppl. 2), 145—149.
26. Langley, G., Broadhead, C., Bottrill, K., *et al.* (1999). Accessing information on the reduction, refinement and replacement of animal experiments: Report and recommendations of a focus on alternatives workshop. *ATLA* **27**, 239—245.

27. Grune, B., Fallon, M., Howard, C., *et al.* (2004). Report and recommendations of the international workshop "Retrieval approaches for information on alternative methods to animal experiments." *ALTEX* **21**, 115–127.

28. Nesdill, D. & Adams, K.M. (2011). Literature search strategies to comply with institutional animal care and use committee review requirements. *Journal of Veterinary Medical Education* **3**, 150–156.

29. Choe, B.I. & Lee, G.H. (2013). Searching and review on the Three Rs information in Korea: Time for quality assessment and continued education. *BMB Reports* **46**, 335–337.

30. EPAA. (2012). *EPAA Activity Report on the Dissemination Platform: In EPAA Annual Report 2012*, 10pp.

31. Sauer, U.G., Kneuer, C., Tentschert, J., *et al.* (2011). A knowledge-based search engine to navigate the information thicket of nanotoxicology. *Regulatory Toxicology and Pharmacology* **59**, 47–52.

32. EC. (2015). *Communication from the Commission on the European Citizens' Initiative "Stop Vivisection"*, 14pp. Brussels, Belgium: European Commission. C (2015) 3773 final.

33. Balls, M. (1994). Replacement of animal procedures: alternatives in research, education and testing. *Laboratory Animals* **28**, 193–211.

34. OECD. (2014). Guidance document for describing non-guideline in vitro test methods. In *Series on Testing and Assessment No. 211*, 17pp. Paris, France: OECD.

35. EURL ECVAM. (2016). *DB-ALM Status Report 2014–2016*. JRC report EUR 28062, 70pp.

36. EURL ECVAM. (2013). *EURL ECVAM Search Guide*. JRC report EUR 24391, 179pp.

Key Technologies and Tools

Chapter 5.1

The Development and Application of Key Technologies and Tools

Tuula Heinonen[1] and Catherine Verfaillie[2]

[1]University of Tampere, Tampere, Finland; [2]Stem Cell Institute, Leuven, Belgium

SUMMARY

An interest in understanding the cellular and molecular mechanisms behind biological processes, and diseases, and the toxicity of chemicals, and the need to develop effective pharmaceuticals, have been the key drivers for the development of cellular models and related technologies. Public concern about laboratory animal welfare and the recognition that animals and humans have substantial physiological differences have also encouraged and promoted the shift from animal-based tests toward human-based cell, organ and tissue models. In Europe, the European Commission has been one of the key players.

The standardised production of human stem cells and induced human pluripotent cell-based differentiated cells with human *in vivo*-like properties has, and will be, a key factor, in addition to other key technologies, e.g. in relation to biomaterials and culture media, in developing adequate models. A very important milestone and promoter for cellular models was the mapping of all the genes of the human genome, which, via the development of omics technologies, helped to increase understanding of the biological processes behind normal functions, adverse effects and diseases. This has also laid the basis for systems toxicology-based risk assessment.

1. THE NEED FOR HUMAN-RELEVANT TESTS

Awareness of toxicity of chemicals, their mixtures and even natural extracts, has been the key driver for development of safety tests. Another key driver has been the need for pharmaceuticals. Development of cellular models and methods to be used in toxicity tests and as general research models, has been influenced by factors such as the costs of testing and the legislation that requires it, recognition that animals and humans have substantial biophysiological differences, and public concern about animal welfare. A big step forward for non-animal approaches has been the possibility to use human cells and tissues instead of animal cells and tissues. Major efforts are therefore afoot to establish cell culture models and related technologies that can accurately predict the responses of human organs to chemical exposure.

2. THE DEVELOPMENT OF *IN VITRO* METHODS WITH THEIR KEY COMPONENTS AND ANALYTICS

2.1 The Development of *In Vitro* Methods in Response to Societal Needs

Table 1 presents some of the milestones for the key biological and technological developments, partly in response to the increasing awareness of toxic effects of natural products and their extracts.

Paracelcus (1493–1541; 1) is widely regarded as the 'father of toxicology'. In the late 18th century, scientists managed to culture isolated organs and fragments of tissue, which gave rise to the name 'tissue culture'. The prerequisite for this was the adequate physiological medium developed by Ringer (2) in the 1880s, while true cell culture was started by Roux (3),

The History of Alternative Test Methods in Toxicology. https://doi.org/10.1016/B978-0-12-813697-3.00029-9

TABLE 1 Key Milestones in the Development of Cellular Methods

Year	Technological Milestone
1860s	Organ perfusion techniques – perfusion of the isolated heart
1882–85	Chick embryo cells maintained in saline culture medium
1903	Division of salamander cells seen *in vitro*
1906	Culture of frog nerve cells by the hanging-drop method
1910	Long-term culture of chick embryo cells in plasma clots
1911	Development of an artificial culture medium
1912–13	*Vaccinia* virus grown in guinea-pig corneal tissue fragments
	Development of D-flask made of Pyrex glass
1916	Cell dissociation by trypsinisation
1923	Development of Carrel flasks improves microscopic evaluation of cultures
1927	*In vitro* production of *Vaccinia* virus vaccine
1933	Development of the roller-tube culture method
1940s	Introduction of use of antibiotics to prevent contamination of cultures
1948	Clones formed from single mouse fibroblasts
	Development of a chemically-defined culture medium, CMRL 1066
1951	The first human immortal cell line, HeLa, developed from an adenocarcinoma
1954	Discovery of contact inhibition of cell movement
1955	Improvements if chemically-defined media
1956	Collagen coating of glass surfaces to improve cell adhesion and growth
	Development of protein-free defined culture media
1959	Formulation of Eagle's Minimum Essential Medium
1960s	Commercial development of disposable plastic culture flasks and plates
1961	Recognition of finite lifespan of normal human cells
	Development of techniques for somatic cell hybridisation by cell fusion
1963	Sendai virus induction of cell fusion
1964	Development of HAT medium for cell selection
1970	Development of a hormone-responsive cell line, MCF-7
1975	Monoclonal antibody production *in vitro*
1978	Use of recombinant DNA techniques to produce human insulin
1996	*Ex vivo* growth of a new organ, the urethra
2001	Start of the human genome project

who managed to maintain embryonic chick cells in culture for a few days. In 1903, Jolly found that salamander leucocytes could survive for a longer time in culture and showed mitotic cell division. One key milestone for cell culture was the discovery in 1916 that cells could be dissociated by using a proteolytic enzyme, trypsin (3). The pioneering work of Carrel (4) resulted in a specific cell culture flask (the D-flask, and later, the T-flask), which provided aseptic culture conditions and the monitoring of cell growth by a microscopy. Cell cultures then started to be used as production platforms — vaccine production started as early as 1927 (5). One of the most significant uses of cells as biological production platform is the production of monoclonal antibodies and recombinant gene products, which began in 1975 (6). From the 1930s to the 1950s, the discovery of antibiotics, the development of plastic culture vessels, and the formulation of new media, such as Eagle's medium (7), permitted longer-time cultures.

Until 1951, the cell cultures had involved isolated primary cells, but then the isolation of the HeLa cell line from the cervical adenomacarcinoma of Henrietta Lacks was achieved (8). In the 1960s, research on cellular mechanisms and cell growth progressed, and the discovery of how to fuse cells was a crucial step.

The interest in cell cultures was primarily due to use as test systems or cellular production platforms, but it was in 1959 that Russell and Burch emphasised their use in research and testing as a more ethical approach than animal experiments. Their proposals for reducing, refining and replacing animal use were the basis of a paradigm shift from animal experiments to non-animal approaches (9). This was taken up by European animal welfare organisations, which, together with public pressure and convincing scientific evidence, have encouraged legislators to favour such alternative approaches. *Directive 86/609/EEC* on the protection of animals used for experimental and other scientific purposes was the first legislation to specifically promote the Three Rs. The European Centre for the Validation of Alternative Methods (ECVAM), with Michael Balls as its first Head, was established by a communication of the European Commission to the European Parliament and the Council in 1992, which referred to Article 7.2 and Article 23 of the Directive. An updated directive, *Directive 2010/63/EU*, came into force in 2010. A second key step was when the EU cosmetics legislation banned the sale of cosmetic products and ingredients which had been tested in animals. Then the REACH legislation on chemicals had a strong promotional effect on the use of non-animal approaches in regulatory toxicity testing. In the USA, the National Academy of Sciences published a report on *Toxicity Testing in the 21st Century: A Vision and a Strategy* (10), and the Adverse Outcome Pathway concept was published by the OECD (11). A Stop Vivisection initiative on behalf of EU citizens in 2015 further encouraged politicians to take up a more-positive stance on animal tests and non-animal approaches (12).

The MEIC project, begun in 1989 and led by Björn Ekwall, was among the first large attempts to find a way of replacing animal testing for a specific toxicity endpoint, acute toxicity, by *in vitro* methods (13). Ekwall also emphasised that cell culture methods can be used to assess either basal toxicity or cell type-specific toxicity (14). Another significant promoter for *in vitro* tests was recognition of the role of metabolism to create metabolites more toxic than the parent compound. The biotransformation of compounds and their conjugation had already been known in the 1800s, but Williams' book, *Detoxification Mechanisms: The Metabolism of Drugs and Allied Organic Compounds*, published in 1947 (15), was an important milestone in this area. The use of hepatocytes and hepatocyte extracts, e.g. microsomes and S-9 fractions, significantly advanced the use of *in vitro* systems in identifying the underlying mechanisms and the key components involved in metabolism, including glutathione-S-transferases, identified in 1961, and cytochrome P450s, in 1962.

The development of pharmaceuticals and investigations of disease mechanisms, aimed at the improved cure and treatment of humans, is the biggest single promoter of cell culture methods and technologies. The first medicines were extracts, of which the toxicologically most well-known is sulphanilamide elixir, which, in a product formation with diethylene glycol, caused the death of more than 100 people. This led to the enactment of the US *Federal Food, Drug and Cosmetic Act 1938*, which gave responsibilities to the Food and Drug Administration (FDA) concerning pre-market notification for new drugs, which involved a massive increase in the safety information required. In addition, mechanisms of action had to be considered with new pharmaceuticals, and discoveries concerning mechanisms of carcinogenesis and mutagenesis led to the need for new tests. For instance, the discovery of chemical carcinogenesis and mutagenesis mechanisms raised the need for new tests. Many different bacterial and cellular mutagenicity tests were developed during the 1960s and 1970s, including the Chinese hamster ovary cell test (16).

2.2 Primary and Secondary Cells and Permanent Cell Lines

Cell cultures can be divided into three main types: primary cultures, secondary cultures and continuous cell lines. The primary and secondary cells are usually diploid cells. Primary cultures are derived directly from intact tissue, such as liver or kidney, whereas secondary cultures are derived from primary cultures. These types usually involve diploid cells, but continuous cell lines, often derived from malignant tissues, tend to be aneuploid.

The early cultures were tissue explants, but, after trypsinisation was introduced in 1916, the subculturing of dissociated cells greatly promoted the development and use of monolayer cultures in glass flasks and dishes. Another prerequisite for successful cell cultures was the development of defined media. The following are some of the main cell lines used for a variety of purposes.

The isolations of human HeLa cells (8) and WI-38 fibroblasts (17) were milestones in the development and use of *in vitro* monolayer tests. In 1961, an important finding with human fibroblasts was that diploid cells have a finite lifespan in culture, unless they transform into an immortal aneuploid state (17).

WI-38 cells, isolated in 1962 from human fetal lungs by Leonard Hayflick's research group (17), became one of the most important cell lines in history, because they were used to develop vaccines, which have saved millions of human lives. The Jurkat cell line was one of several leukaemic cell lines developed for screening purposes at the Fred

Hutchinson Cancer Research Center, Seattle, WA, USA. Gillis and Watson found that Jurkat cells were particularly robust producers of IL-2 after stimulation with phytohaemagglutinin (PHA; 18). Cancer cell lines, such as the breast cancer cell line, MCF-7, which was isolated in 1970 and is hormone responsive, have been invaluable in the development of anti-cancer drugs.

CHO cells from the Chinese hamster ovary have been widely used in genotoxicity testing, and mouse embryonic 3T3 fibroblasts have been used in cytotoxicity test procedures accepted by the OECD.

2.3 Stem Cells and iPS Cells

Although the unlimited growth potential of continuous cell lines is an advantage, their immortalisation is not, as they are karyotypically abnormal and accumulate mutations that may affect the value of the data they provide. For these reasons, novel model systems are being developed, based on cells that are expandable, but remain representative of their tissues of origin. The establishment of permanent cell lines through induction of the overexpression of telomerase could be helpful, but it has not been very successful so far. Another option is to establish models based on cells that naturally have high telomerase activity, i.e. stem cells, which can be induced to differentiate into a variety of phenotypically and genetically 'normal' cells, representative of *in vivo* conditions (19).

2.3.1 The Discovery of Stem Cell Populations

The first indications of the activity of stem cells were derived from the research in the 1950s, when an enormous regenerative capacity of the blood system was linked to activity in the bone-marrow, and this was useful for the treatment of anaemia, leukaemia and radiation. Thomas *et al.* were the first to show the benefits of bone-marrow transplantation for the restoration of the blood system after radiotherapy, thus paving the way for an anti-cancer therapy which is still used today (20). The regenerative capacities of the bone-marrow were finally attributed to haematopoietic stem cells (HSCs) in the 1960s, mainly through the work of McCulloch and Till, who described a very rare cell population, which was able to undergo differentiation to the different blood cell types. HSCs could be maintained in the bone-marrow in a quiescent state, then, after injury, could proliferate extensively and form progenitor colonies in the spleen (21, 22). The subsequent isolation of HSCs from different sources has enabled HSC transplantation to remain a standard therapy today (23).

Stem cells have now been identified in many other adult tissues, including the gastrointestinal tract, the epidermis, the liver and even the brain (24). Like HSCs, these adult stem cells possess an enormous expansion and differentiation capacity, but only to cells appropriate for their tissues of origin, and they still undergo senescence when forced to proliferate extensively. The use of adult stem cells in toxicology studies *in vitro* has been very limited up to now, mainly because of difficulties in stem cell isolation, and because of expansion-based exhaustion. The isolation of an even more potent stem cell population is therefore needed.

2.3.2 The Isolation and Generation of Induced Pluripotent Stem Cells

All the body's cells are ultimately derived from the fertilised oocyte during development. The cells of the developing blastocyst therefore represent a stem cell population that is not limited to a specific tissue. In fact, they are the ultimate stem cell population. Given their capacity to differentiate into the capacities to all types of cells, they are called pluripotent stem cells, whereas adult stem cell populations are multipotent. In 1981, George Martin was the first to succeed in isolating these pluripotent stem cells from the developing mouse blastocyst and culturing them *in vitro* (25). Pluripotent embryonic stem cells (ESCs) were first isolated and cultured from a primate blastocyst in 1995 (26), and from a human blastocyst in 1998 (27). Since these early years, ESCs have been shown to represent the ideal cell source for use in generating reproducible batches of cells for studying human development and disease. Pluripotent stem cells do not undergo culture-based senescence, thus permitting their unlimited expansion. With the development of modern high-throughput genetic and epigenetic screening tools, it has been shown that ESCs can be expanded with long-term, full genetic stability, although some culture-induced and stress-induced effects have been reported (28).

Although ESCs can provide 'off-the-shelf' human cells at any given time, their use does have important drawbacks. They will always remain autologous, derived from embryonic material from one individual, but different from that of any other. This greatly hinders their use for regenerative therapy, but also creates problems for *in vitro* toxicology, as no clear toxicological phenotypic profile is known for the donor. Furthermore, the destruction of the developing embryo during ESC isolation poses important ethical questions.

It had long been a central dogma that development is a one-way street, and that stem cells can only lose potency during differentiation (29), but the possibility of generating cells with pluripotent characteristics from adult material, and therefore from human patients, was very attractive. Already in 1962, even before the characterisation of HSCs, John Gurdon disproved the one-way street view of cellular differentiation, by showing that the nuclei of an adult and terminally-differentiated frog epithelial cells could be 'reprogrammed' to a stem cell state when transferred into enucleated eggs (30). Indeed, by this he created the first cloned animals (31), an accomplishment which was followed by the generation of 'Dolly', the first cloned mammal, nearly 40 years later (32).

These essential breakthroughs meant that the generation of a patient-derived pluripotent cells was possible. This was achieved in 2006 by Shinya Yamanaka, who showed that many types of adult differentiated cells could be dedifferentiated and 'induced' to become pluripotent. With his co-workers, he showed that the overexpression of only four pluripotency-associated transcription factors, i.e. Oct4, Sox2, CMYC and KLF4, was sufficient for the complete reprogramming of mouse (33) and human (34) cells into what they called induced pluripotent stem cells (iPSCs).

Gurdon and Yamanaka shared the 2012 Nobel Prize for Physiology or Medicine. As a result of their work, it is now possible to indefinitely expand donor-specific stem cells without any genomic abnormalities and to induce their differentiate into all the cell types of the human body, thus permitting the generation of donor-specific organ models and even large population-driven biobanks.

2.4 The Historical Evolution of *In Vitro* Toxicity Testing

2.4.1 Mounting Criticism of Animal Testing

In the 1920s, J.W. Trevan and other scientists described methods for generating dose-dependent toxicity curves for the effects of novel chemicals on animal models. Acute toxicity was expressed as the LD50, the median lethal dose which caused the death of 50% of the test animals (35). Along with the Draize eye test for ocular irritancy, the LD50 test increasingly became the focus of criticism, not only from animal rights activists, but also from experienced toxicologists (e.g. 36). Given the progress being made in cellular and molecular biology, and later in computer science, interest began to be focused on replacing these and other animal tests with human-focused *in vitro* and *in silico* systems. The development of high-throughput systems and more-effective ways of taking account of the wide variation in human responsiveness were other potential advantages of a move away from reliance on traditional animal tests. A prime example of this historical evolution is the modelling of liver toxicity and biotransformation. Given the important role of the liver as the major site for xenobiotic drug metabolism, the establishment of hepatocyte-based cell models for studying toxicity has been a primary target from the outset.

2.4.2 From Cell Lines to Primary Isolates

Over the years, several hepatic cell lines, often derived from human liver tumours, have been isolated and cultured to form stable line. Of these, the HepG2 cell line came to be widely used, as it provided an excellent *in vitro* model for studying plasma protein secretion (37), hepatotropic viral infection (38, 39), metabolism (40) and liver disease (41). In the 1990s, the first reports of studies on drug metabolism using HepG2 cells were published (42, 43). However, it later became clear that HepG2 cells could not recapitulate drug metabolism and sensitivity *in vitro*, as the expression levels of the drug-metabolising cytochrome P450 enzymes this, and in other hepatic cell lines, were insignificant when compared with hepatocytes *in vivo* (44). In 2002, a new human hepatoma cell line, termed HepaRG, was isolated, which was an expandable cell type with metabolism capacities which much more closely resembled those of primary hepatocytes (45).

Nevertheless, recent studies have underlined the need for better systems (46), and novel immortalisation techniques, including the overexpression of oncogenes and telomerase, are being investigated to establish expandable cell lines derived from primary hepatocytes instead of from cancerous tissue (47). Such cell lines display different phenotypes, depending on the donor and oncogene involved, which could be useful in some circumstances, but the general applicability of the information they can provide is limited. Also, they still lack some essential capacities for drug metabolism.

Primary hepatocytes continue to represent the gold standard for modelling hepatic cellular response to drugs and toxins, as they possess a sufficiently high expression of phase I and II drug metabolism enzymes (48). They can recapitulate donor variability in drug metabolism and clearance, and models are being established to translate *in vitro* screening data to the *in vivo* situation (49, 50). However, primary hepatocytes have two major limitations: they are very unstable *in vitro*, and they lose important characteristics within 12–72 hours in culture, as was recognised in early studies (51). As a result, primary hepatocytes are of limited value for repeat-dose studies. The hope for solving this problem lies mainly in the use of human ESCs and iPSCs to provide differentiated hepatocytes with the capacity for longer-term functioning *in vitro*.

2.4.3 PSC Differentiation for the Modelling of Liver Toxicity

Since the first description of ESC lines, several groups have published protocols for differentiating ESCs, and later also for iPSCs, into cells with hepatocyte features. During the early evaluation of the potential of mouse ESCs, researchers showed the induction of most, if not all, cell types of the body during spontaneous differentiation in embryoid bodies (EBs; 52). These experiments were performed by removing the factors necessary to maintain pluripotency and allowing the ESCs to 'develop' normally in culture. Because this method yields a very heterogeneous population, comprising cells of all three germ layers, researchers soon began to optimise protocols for directed differentiation to specific lineages, e.g. of endoderm cells. In 2001, Hamazaki *et al.* developed a protocol to differentiate mouse ESCs into cells with hepatocyte features in a 3-D EBs, by adding hepatocyte-inducing cytokines (53). The first protocols to differentiate human ESCs into the hepatocyte lineage were reported in 2003 (54). Since then, the protocols used have changed considerably, The homogeneity of the differentiated cell populations was greatly increased by switching from EB culture to monolayer culture (55), and the cytokine cocktails used were improved (56, 57). However, even today, human hepatocytes differentiated from iPSCs only partially resemble the primary hepatocytes, so they are called hepatocyte-like cells. Nevertheless, iPSC-derived hepatocytes have been shown to recapitulate some liver diseases *in vitro*, including steatosis and fatty liver disease (58). They can also model the toxicity of some drug-induced liver injury compounds (59). Finally, a comparison between isolated primary hepatocytes and iPSC-generated hepatocytes from the same donors demonstrated that the individual drug-metabolising profiles were maintained (60). As for primary hepatocytes, the *in vitro* culture conditions used to differentiate PSCs into functional hepatocytes did not support a fully-mature cellular phenotype. The PSC-derived progeny often display fetal features, and therefore do not fully represent donor adult phenotype. Further rapid developments in this field can be expected, which will offer great benefits in the prediction of human *in vivo* toxicity (61).

2.5 Recapitulation of the *In Vivo* Niche

In 2009, Hans Clevers *et al.* described a novel system for the isolation and long-term culture of gut stem cells in self-assembling organoids, which were found to greatly recapitulate the epithelial compartment of the *in vivo* tissue (62). Organoid cultures have also been established for other cell types, including hepatocytes (63). These models are interesting, because they are derived from adult tissues and can therefore represent a specific donor phenotype, and also because they represent a much higher level of differentiation when compared with monolayer cultures. It is now considered that only a full recapitulation of the *in vivo* microenvironment will permit the full recapitulation of the hepatocyte profile *in vitro*. Studies have also shown the importance of the non-parenchymal compartment of the liver in influencing hepatocyte behaviour, and have underlined the necessity for co-cultures with endothelial cells and stellate cells (64–66). Furthermore, increasingly-complicated bio-reactors, in which the *in vivo* blood flow and tissue architecture are recapitulated, have been shown to provide for the more-complete differentiation of hepatocytes.

2.6 The Extracellular Matrix

The extracellular matrix (ECM) is a non-cellular macromolecular 3-D network structure, composed of elastin, fibronectin, laminins, proteoglycans/glycosaminoglycans and other glycoproteins, as well as numerous soluble factors (67). The matrix components bind to each other and to cell receptors, forming a complex network which is the 'home environment' for the cells of tissues and organs. The ECM plays a critical role in cellular signalling and regulates diverse functions, such as cell survival, growth, migration and differentiation, and is therefore vital for maintaining normal homeostasis (68, 69). Its composition differs from one tissue to another, where it represents a highly dynamic network, which continuously undergoes remodelling during normal and pathological conditions. Therefore, consideration of the ECM is critical to understanding functional aspects or diseases of particular tissues. Hence, the creation of the complex 3-D *in vivo* tissue architecture is crucial in the development of relevant and efficient drug screen models *in vitro* (70, 71).

2.6.1 Historical Perspective of the Use of the ECM in 3-D Culture Systems

Since the early 19th century, researchers have wanted to recapitulate organogenesis, and the first 3-D culture system was the hanging-drop method developed by Ross Harrison in 1906 (72). He studied nerve fibres in a drop of lymph on a coverslip inverted and sealed over a hollow depression in a glass slide. This technique was adopted by many scientist, and by the 1950s, tissues from many organs were cultured by using similar techniques. Knowing that collagen is a universal component of connective tissues, Huzella *et al.* grew cells on a layer of collagen (73), and Ehrmann and Gey developed a method for producing a gel from rat tail collagen (74). Cells were shown to grow and survive better on a layer of dried collagen than on a glass surface or on plasma clots. In 1969, Berry and Friend perfused livers with collagenase and produced millions of hepatocytes (75). These hepatocytes grew better in collagen, but still lost the hepatocyte phenotype (76). In 1975, Michalopoulos and Pitot demonstrated that it was possible to trigger the differentiation of hepatocytes, by modifying the substratum by creating thick gels of collagen (77). Similar studies were performed by Emerman and Pitelka for normal mammary epithelial cells (74), which maintained the expression of some milk proteins for a month. In 1977, Richard Swarm and his group isolated a gel with the characteristics of the basement membrane, from a sarcoma cell line. Initially called the EHS matrix, based on the names of its developers (78, 79), it is now known as Matrigel (80).

In 1982, Bissel *et al.* showed that the ECM regulates gene expression (81), and they later produced evidence that a 3-D microenvironment could be produced *in vitro* that sufficiently recapitulated the *in vivo* setting and could support the growth of primary human breast cells and carcinoma cells (82). As the 1990s progressed, other researchers established that tissue-specific phenotypes required multiple factors, including metalloproteinases (MMPs), growth factors and ECM components. Since then, methods have been developed for culture in multi-well plates and for a wide range of cells and tissues, including intestinal stem cells, intestinal crypts and villi, stomach and colon epithelia, pancreas, liver and brain.

2.6.2 The Rationale for Using 3-D Matrices for Drug Screening and Toxicity Testing

Cell-based assays have been an important pillar of the drug discovery process, to provide a relatively simple, fast and cost-effective tool to avoid large-scale and cost-intensive animal testing. Until recently, most of the research for drug discovery or *in vitro* toxicology was based on 2-D culture systems or animal testing. However, only about 8% of the compounds proceed to the clinical development stage, and many drugs fail in clinical trials, largely due to limited clinical efficacy or unpredicted and unacceptable toxicity. As 2-D cultures cannot preserve most differentiated cellular functions, it is believed that *in vitro* 3-D culture systems will permit better preservation of differentiated cell phenotypes and will contribute to improving the prediction of drug metabolism and toxicity (83).

The two most-common forms of 3-D cell culture system involve the use of prefabricated scaffolds and hydrogels (84, 85). Scaffolds can be made from natural or synthetic materials, and can be engineered to have a great variation in pore size, structure and fibres, to allow cells to migrate and grow within the scaffold network (86). A hydrogel is a biocompatible polymer network with a high water content and physical properties that closely mimic the ECM. Like the prefabricated scaffolds, hydrogels can be made from either natural or synthetic materials, and can be produced with various pore sizes. Both these types of 3-D culture systems can be tailored as required, and can be used to grow and differentiate many cell types (87).

Cells cultured in 3-D systems can maintain their differentiated behaviour and expression profiles much better than can cells cultured in 2-D systems, and better reflect the *in vivo* situation (88,89), not least by the availabilty of ECM cues and the mechanical environment of the *in vivo* microenvironment (89—91).

3-D matrices fall into three broad categories: biologically-derived matrices, synthetically-derived matrices and biologically inspired synthetic matrices or hybrids.

2.6.3 Biologically-Derived Matrices

The most commonly used 3-D matrices are derived from the ECM of biological sources. They have the advantage that the 3-D matrix itself initiates cell signalling in various situations (92). In addition, ECM molecular components can themselves function as bioactive molecules, and can act as ligands for a number of cell surface (adhesion) receptors. This can result in the activation of the downstream signalling pathways of these receptors (93).

Matrigel, a mouse tumour-derived membrane that is liquid at low temperatures and solidifies at 37°C, contains all of the most-common ECM molecules found in the basement membrane *in vivo*, and has the advantage of being relatively easy to use and being commercially available (80, 94). It is used to culture cancer cells, stem cells and their progeny, and in many organoid culture systems.

Collagen I and gelatin are also common ECM molecules that can be isolated from various biological sources, including bovine skin, rat tail and human placenta (95—98). Hyaluronic acid is another ubiquitous ECM component, which is used in tissue engineering (99, 100).

The biggest advantage of biologically derived matrices is that they are more biologically relevant than their synthetic counterparts, so the cells cultured on them better reflect the *in vivo* situation. Their disadvantage is that their sources vary in composition, so they are not readily reproducible.

2.6.4 Synthetic Matrices

Synthetic matrices have gained popularity, because they are chemically defined and can be tailored for specific biological systems. Poly(D,L-lactic-*co*-glycolic acid) (PLGA or PLG), polylactide (PLA) and poly(ε-caprolactone) (PCL) are biodegradable polymers, which have been approved by the FDA for biomedical applications (101–103). Polyvinyl alcohol (PVA) is another biocompatible synthetic polymer that is frequently used for the production of synthetic scaffolds (104). Various combinations of co-polymers/composites of these biomaterials have been used in tissue engineering and in drug discovery.

Polyethylene glycol (PEG) hydrogels are also used in tissue engineering. PEG is commercially available with different molecular weights and with various modifications (105, 106). It is highly biocompatible, easy modifiable and relatively inexpensive. Unlike pre-formed scaffolds that require a separate step to load cells into the matrix, many PEG-based hydrogels are engineered to allow for cell encapsulation, thus simplifying the experimental procedures. Various cell types, including kidney cells, osteoblasts, hepatocytes and stem cells, have been successfully grown in PEG hydrogels.

The advantages of synthetically-produced matrices are that they are chemically defined, contain no uncharacterised growth factors or other contaminants and can be tailor-made for particular purposes. Their main disadvantage is that they are not as biologically relevant as biologically-derived matrices and they do not provide the signalling effects, which the ECM naturally provides.

2.6.5 Biologically-Inspired Synthetic (Hybrid) Matrices

Biologically-inspired matrices combine biologically-derived and synthetic matrix technologies to provide a scaffold that is chemically defined and easily engineered, and also contains the relevant biological cues for the cells. Although synthetic 3-D matrices can provide the mechanical cues for cellular proliferation and differentiation, the matrix itself does not permit the activation of the cell receptors which initiate cellular signalling. For these reasons, biologically-inspired peptides, classically the arginylglycylaspartic acid (RGD) peptides, which are responsible for cell adhesion to the ECM, are often added to the synthetic matrices to promote cell adhesion, migration and proliferation. Novel biologically-inspired synthetic peptides have been in tissue engineering (107). Peptide scaffolds are synthetically prepared peptides produced in biologically-inspired sequences that are physiologically relevant and permit cell encapsulation within the scaffold (108, 109). Some examples include the self-assembling peptide, hydrogel (110), PuraMatrix (111), peptide amphiphiles (112) and β-hairpin peptides (113).

Hybrid hydrogel materials, consisting of synthetic polymers and bioactive peptide segments, have recently gained popularity as tissue-engineering matrices. PEG-based hydrogel matrices have been engineered to contain adhesion receptor-binding peptide and enzyme-sensitive cross-linkers, the functional groups on PEG that allow for cross-linking. These types of hydrogels are also known as bioactive hydrogels or cell responsive hydrogels. They permit cell attachment, migration, proliferation and/or differentiations (114, 115). Hybrid matrices have the advantage of being chemically defined and easy to engineer, while still providing biological signals to the encapsulated cells. They allow for some integration of biological signalling peptides, but matrices still are lacking when compared with biologically-derived scaffolds. In addition, peptide-based scaffolds cannot be produced in large quantities, and they can be mechanically weak and prone to falling apart.

2.6.6 Current Challenges and Future Directions

Although 3-D matrix-based cell cultures represent the actual microenvironment of tissues more accurately than 2-D cultures can, they require further development to better mimic the *in vivo* architecture. 3-D cultures are more complex, leading to uncontrollable reproducibility, and sometimes to the introduction of chemical impurities. Another challenge is to scale up the 3-D cell culture approach for automated high-throughput applications.

In the near future, the complexity of the tissue scaffold constructs will increase. This will permit more cell types to be introduced in a single scaffold. This development, along with the addition of perfusion systems, should then permit more of the characteristics of organs to be made available. Another revolution in 3-D technology will be bioprinting and the miniaturisation of tissue constructs for high-throughput applications in drug discovery.

The quality and variety of research now being carried out with 3-D scaffold-based *in vitro* cell culture models is astounding. Although there is still much work to be done, the translation of laboratory-scale model systems into robust and reproducible high-throughput systems, their routine use with a variety of assays will improve the quality and predictive accuracy of preclinical drug development and drug-related toxicology in the near future.

2.7 Omics

The traditional dogma is that DNA is transcribed to messenger RNA, which is translated into the proteins involved in cell structures and functions. However, while they have the same gene complements, the cells of multicellular organisms have diverse phenotypes and functions, as well as showing diverse responses to internal and external stimuli, as a result of the differential regulation of gene expression and downstream molecular activities.

'Omics' is a relatively new collective term, which refers to the components of certain interrelated fields of study in biology, such as genomics, epigenomics, transcriptomics, proteomics and metabolomics. Omics technologies have developed from the need to understand the molecular and cellular mechanisms involved in normal cellular structures and functions, understand the adverse effects of chemicals and the mechanisms underlying diseases, and to develop new drugs with known and targeted mechanisms of action. They can also provide the basis for the shift from reliance on animal studies to more-relevant risk assessment based on human-derived *in vitro* test systems.

Genomics is aimed at the structure, function and mapping of the genome, the complete set of genes within an organism, in contrast to genetics, which is focused on individual genes, genetic variation and heredity. The use of high-throughput DNA sequencing and bioinformatics has resulted in dramatic progress in systems biology. Of particular interest for this chapter is *pharmacogenomics*, the study of the effects of genetic variation on the efficacy and toxicity of drugs.

DNA sequencing technology was developed in the mid-1970s. The first full genome to be sequenced was that of the phiX174 virus (1977), followed by that of a bacterium, *Haemophilus influenza* (1995; 116), a yeast, *Saccharomyces cerevisiae* (1996; 117), a nematode, *Caenorhabditis elegans* (1998; 118), an insect, *Drosophila melanogaster* (2000; 119), the laboratory mouse, *Mus musculus* (2002; 120), a human being, *Homo sapiens* (2003; 121), and a chimpanzee, *Pan troglodytes* (2005; 122).

Epigenomics is the study of the reversible epigenetic modifications that affect gene expression and regulation without altering the DNA sequence itself. These modifications, which include DNA methylation and histone modification, are involved in many cell functions and are controlled by the action of various factors, including repressor proteins. Epigenetic changes are inherited through cell divisions and are fundamental to the process of cell differentiation.

Transcriptomics involves the study of an organism's transcriptome, the sum of all its RNA transcripts or specific sets of transcripts, which represents the consequences of controlled gene expression. It can be focused on the examination of messenger RNAs, but it can also involve transfer RNAs, ribosomal RNA and other non-coding RNAs. It is expected that transcriptomics will provide key information for risk assessment in relation to adverse outcome pathways (11).

Proteomics is concerned with the proteome, the full set of proteins produced or modified by an organism or system, which changes with time, according to normal functions or the effects of various factors, including xenobiotics.

Metabolomics is the study of chemical processed involving metabolites. Its history goes back as far as ancient China, when the presence of glucose in urine was used to diagnose diabetes. The importance of metabolism in toxicology was recognised in the 1800s. The concept of the metabolic profile of an individual was introduced in the 1940s, and the ability to quantitatively measure metabolic profiles became possible in the 1060s, at the time when the key enzymes involved in metabolism, including the glutathione-DS-transferases (123) and cytochrome P450s (124), were discovered.

The metabolome represents the aggregated metabolites of a cell, a tissue, an organ or an organism. A crucial milestone was the publication in 2007 of the human metabolome database (125), a comprehensive, high-quality, freely accessible, online database of small molecule metabolites found in the human body. It facilitates human metabolomics research, including the identification and characterisation of human metabolites, via the use of techniques such as NMR spectroscopy, GC-MS spectrometry and LC/MS spectrometry. The database contains three kinds of data, namely, chemical data, clinical data and molecular biology/biochemistry data.

The integration in systems biology and functional genomics of epigenomics, transcriptomics, proteomics and metabolomics is a challenge which could greatly enhance our understanding of many aspects of molecular biology and cell biology, including toxicology, which could take human variation into account, resulting in greater protection and more-effective treatments for individual human beings.

3. CONCLUSIONS

Thanks to the great achievements in cell culture research and supporting technologies, in addition to the need for cheaper and higher throughput methods than animal experiments and the presence of permissive legislation, which permit the use of human cells, human-relevant cellular models and tests are now believed to be the ideal tools, instead of animal procedures, in toxicity hazard prediction and risk assessment, modelling of diseases, and other types of biomedical research. At present, further great technological developments can be foreseen to help to achieve the final goal of replacing animal experiments with human-oriented non-animal approaches.

The research to find conditions for maintaining homogenous and genetically stable populations of differentiated cells from iPSCs is actively ongoing. This technology can also be applied to produce disease-specific iPSCs. The ultimate goal is to produce human-like organ-on-a-chip systems. *In vivo* cells are in 3-D microenvironments, where they are exposed to cell interactions and interstitial fluids with tissue-specific properties. Active research is ongoing to obtain a medium suitable for all cell types that could be used in many tissue and organ constructs. 3-D bioprinting is being developed as a technology to facilitate the production of multi-tissue, 3-D-structures with human tissue-like microphysiological environments, which mimic their *in vivo* counterparts. There are already microsensors that could be used to control physicochemical conditions and non-invasive technologies to measure biological read-outs.

REFERENCES

1. Hargrave, J.G. (2016). *Paracelsus. Encyclopædia Britannica.* Available at: https://www.britannica.com/biography/Paracelsus.
2. Dewolf, W.C. (1977). Sydney Ringer (1835—1910). *Investigative Urology* **14**, 500—501.
3. Rous, P. & Jones, F.S. (1916). A method for obtaining suspensions of living cells from the fixed tissues, and for the plating out of individual cells. *Journal of Experimental Medicine* **23**, 549—555.
4. Carrel, A. (1923). A method for the physiological study of tissues in vitro. *Journal of Experimental Medicine* **38**, 407—418.
5. Carrel, A. & Rivers, T.M. (1927). La fabrication du vaccin in vitro. *Comptes Rendus des Seances de la Societé de Biologie* **96**, 848.
6. Alkan, S.S. (2004). Monoclonal antibodies: the story of a discovery that revolutionized science and medicine. *Nature Reviews Immunology* **4**, 153—156.
7. Eagle, H. (1955). Nutrition needs of mammalian cells in tissue culture. *Science, New York* **122**, 501—514.
8. Silberman, S. (2010). The woman behind HeLa. *Nature, London* **463**, 610.
9. Russell, W.M.S. & Burch, R.L. (1929). *The Principles of Humane Experimental Technique*, 238pp. London, UK: Methuen
10. NRC. (2007). *Toxicity Testing in the 21st Century: A Vision and a Strategy*, 216pp. Washington, DC, USA: The National Academies Press
11. OECD. (2017). Revised Guidance Document on Developing and Assessing Adverse Outcome Pathways. In *Series on Testing and Assessment No. 184*. Paris, France: OECD, 32pp.
12. EP. (2017). *European Citizens Initiative*, 1p. Brussels, Belgium: European Parliament. Available at: http://www.europarl.europa.eu/committees/en/envi/events-citizint.html?id=20150424CHE00301
13. Bondesson, I., Ekwall, B., Hellberg, S., *et al.* (1989). MEIC a new international multicenter project to evaluate the relevance to human toxicity of *in vitro* cytotoxicity tests. *Cell Biology and Toxicology* **5**, 331—348.
14. Ekwall, B. (1983). Correlation between cytotoxicity data and LD50-values. *Acta Physiologica et Toxicologica* **52**(Suppl. II), 80—99.
15. Williams, R.T. (1947). *Detoxification Mechanisms: The Metabolism of Drugs and Allied Organic Compounds*, 288pp. New York, NY, USA: J. Wiley
16. Chu, E.H. & Malling, H.V. (1968). Mammalian cell genetics. II. Chemical induction of specific locus mutations in Chinese hamster cells in vitro. *Proceedings of the National Academy of Sciences of the USA* **61**, 1306—1312.
17. Hayflick, L. & Moorhead, P.S. (1961). The serial cultivation of human diploid cell strains. *Experimental Cell Research* **25**, 585—621.
18. Gillis, S. & Watson, J. (1980). Biochemical and biological characterization of lymphocyte regulatory molecules. V. Identification of an interleukin 2-producing human leukemia T cell line. *Journal of Experimental Medicine* **152**, 1709—1719.
19. Jennings, P. (2015). The future of *in vitro* toxicology. *Toxicology in Vitro* **29**, 1217—1221.
20. Thomas, E.D., Lochte, H.L.J., Lu, W.C., *et al.* (1957). Intravenous infusion of bone marrow in patients receiving radiation and chemotherapy. *New England Journal of Medicine* **257**, 491—496.
21. McCulloch, E.A. & Till, J.E. (1960). The radiation sensitivity of normal mouse bone marrow cells, determined by quantitative marrow transplantation into irradiated mice. *Radiation Research* **13**, 115—125.
22. Becker, A.J., Mcculloch, E.A. & Till, J.E. (1963). Cytological demonstration of the clonal nature of spleen colonies derived from transplanted mouse marrow cells. *Nature, London* **197**, 452—454.
23. Thomas, E.D., Buckner, C.D., Banaji, M., *et al.* (1977). One hundred patients with acute leukemia treated by chemotherapy, total body irradiation, and allogeneic marrow transplantation. *Blood* **49**, 511—533.
24. Barker, N., Bartfeld, S. & Clevers, H. (2010). Tissue-resident adult stem cell populations of rapidly self-renewing organs. *Cell Stem Cell* **7**, 656—670.
25. Martin, G.R. (1981). Isolation of a pluripotent cell line from early mouse embryos cultured in medium conditioned by teratocarcinoma stem cells. *Proceedings of the National Academy of Sciences of the USA* **78**, 7634—7638.
26. Thomson, J.A., Kalishman, J., Golos, T.G., *et al.* (1995). Isolation of a primate embryonic stem cell line. *Proceedings of the National Academy of Sciences of the USA* **92**, 7844—7848.
27. Thomson, J.A., Itskovitz-Eldor, J., Shapiro, S.S., *et al.* (1998). Embryonic Stem Cell Lines Derived from Human Blastocysts. *Science, New York* **282**(5391), 1145—1147.

28. Lund, R.J., Narva, E. & Lahesmaa, R. (2012). Genetic and epigenetic stability of human pluripotent stem cells. *Nature Reviews Genetics* **13**, 732−744.

29. Waddington, C.H. (1957). *The Strategy of the Genes; A Discussion of Some Aspects of Theoretical Biology*, 262pp. London, UK: Allen & Unwin

30. Gurdon, J.B. (1962). The developmental capacity of nuclei taken from intestinal epithelium cells of feeding tadpoles. *Journal of Embryology and Experimental Morphology* **10**, 622−640.

31. Gurdon, J.B. & Uehlinger, V. (1966). 'Fertile' intestine nuclei. *Nature, London* **210**, 1240−1241.

32. Wilmut, I., Schnieke, A.E., McWhir, J., et al. (2007). Viable offspring derived from fetal and adult mammalian cells. *Cloning and Stem Cells* **9**, 3−7.

33. Takahashi, K. & Yamanaka, S. (2006). Induction of pluripotent stem cells from mouse embryonic and adult fibroblast cultures by defined factors. *Cell* **126**, 663−676.

34. Takahashi, K., Tanabe, K., Ohnuki, M., et al. (2007). Induction of pluripotent stem cells from adult human fibroblasts by defined factors. *Cell* **131**, 861−872.

35. Trevan, J.W. (1927). The error of determination of toxicity. *Proceedings of the Royal Society of London Series B* **101**, 483−514.

36. Zbinden, G. & Flury-Roversi, M. (1981). Significance of the LD50 test for the toxicological evaluation of chemical substances. *Archives of Toxicology* **47**, 77−99.

37. Knowles, B.B., Howe, C.C. & Aden, D.P. (1980). Human hepatocellular carcinoma cell lines secrete the major plasma proteins and hepatitis B surface antigen. *Science, New York* **209**, 497−499.

38. Sureau, C., Romet-Lemonne, J.L., Mullins, J.I., et al. (1986). Production of hepatitis B virus by a differentiated human hepatoma cell line after transfection with cloned circular HBV DNA. *Cell* **47**, 37−47.

39. Mabit, H., Dubanchet, S., Capel, F., et al. (1994). In vitro infection of human hepatoma cells (HepG2) with hepatitis B virus (HBV): spontaneous selection of a stable HBV surface antigen-producing HepG2 cell line containing integrated HBV DNA sequences. *Journal of General Virology* **75**, 2681−2689.

40. Davit-Spraul, A., Pourci, M.L., Soni, T., et al. (1994). Metabolic effects of galactose on human HepG2 hepatoblastoma cells. *Metabolism* **43**, 945−952.

41. Elbein, S.C., Hoffman, M.D., Matsutani, A., et al. (1992). Linkage analysis of GLUT1 (HepG2) and GLUT2 (liver/islet) genes in familial NIDDM. *Diabetes* **41**, 1660−1667.

42. Le Bot, M.A., Glaise, D., Kernaleguen, D., et al. (1991). Metabolism of doxorubicin, daunorubicin and epirubicin in human and rat hepatoma cells. *Pharmacological Research* **24**, 243−252.

43. Roe, A.L., Snawder, J.E., Benson, R.W., et al. (1993). HepG2 cells: an in vitro model for P450-dependent metabolism of acetaminophen. *Biochemical and Biophysical Research Communications* **190**, 15−19.

44. Dai, Y. & Cederbaum, A.I. (1995). Cytotoxicity of acetaminophen in human cytochrome P4502E1-transfected HepG2 cells. *Journal of Pharmacology and Experimental Therapeutics* **273**, 1497−1505.

45. Gripon, P., Rumin, S., Urban, S., et al. (2002). Infection of a human hepatoma cell line by hepatitis B virus. *Proceedings of the National Academy of Sciences of the USA* **99**, 15655−15660.

46. Bell, C.C., Lauschke, V.M., Vorrink, S.U., et al. (2017). Transcriptional, functional, and mechanistic comparisons of stem cell-derived hepatocytes, HepaRG cells, and three-dimensional human hepatocyte spheroids as predictive in vitro systems for drug-induced liver injury. *Drug Metabolism Disposition* **45**, 419−429.

47. Ramboer, E., De Craene, B., De Kock, J., et al. (2014). Strategies for immortalization of primary hepatocytes. *Journal of Hepatology* **61**, 925−943.

48. Bell, C.C., Hendriks, D.F., Moro, S.M., et al. (2016). Characterization of primary human hepatocyte spheroids as a model system for drug-induced liver injury, liver function and disease. *Science Reports* **6**, 25187.

49. Tsamandouras, N., Kostrzewski, T., Stokes, C.L., et al. (2017). Quantitative assessment of population variability in hepatic drug metabolism using a perfused three-dimensional human liver microphysiological system. *Journal of Pharmacology and Experimental Therapeutics* **360**, 95−105.

50. Wilk-Zasadna, I., Bernasconi, C., Pelkonen, O., et al. (2015). Biotransformation in vitro: An essential consideration in the quantitative in vitro-to-in vivo extrapolation (QIVIVE) of toxicity data. *Toxicology* **332**, 8−19.

51. Tompa, A. & Langenbach, R. (1980). Promoting effect of feeder cells in maintenance of adult rat hepatocytes. *Acta Morphologia Academiae Scientiarum Hungaricae* **28**, 393−405.

52. Doetschman, T.C., Eistetter, H., Katz, M., et al. (1985). The in vitro development of blastocyst-derived embryonic stem cell lines: formation of visceral yolk sac, blood islands and myocardium. *Journal of Embryology and Experimental Morphology* **87**, 27−45.

53. Hamazaki, T., Iiboshi, Y., Oka, M., et al. (2001). Hepatic maturation in differentiating embryonic stem cells in vitro. *FEBS Letters* **497**, 15−19.

54. Rambhatla, L., Chiu, C.-P., Kundu, P., et al. (2003). Generation of hepatocyte-like cells from human embryonic stem cells. *Cell Transplantation* **12**, 1−11.

55. Ishii, T., Fukumitsu, K., Yasuchika, K., et al. (2008). Effects of extracellular matrixes and growth factors on the hepatic differentiation of human embryonic stem cells. *American Journal of Physiology − Gastrointestinal and. Liver Physiology* **295**, G313−G321.

56. Rossi, J.M., Dunn, N.R., Hogan, B.L., et al. (2001). Distinct mesodermal signals, including BMPs from the septum transversum mesenchyme, are required in combination for hepatogenesis from the endoderm. *Genes & Development* **15**, 1998−2009.

57. Hay, D.C., Fletcher, J., Payne, C., et al. (2008). Highly efficient differentiation of hESCs to functional hepatic endoderm requires ActivinA and Wnt3a signaling. *Proceedings of the National Academy of Sciences of the USA* **105**, 12301−12306.

58. Ignatius Irudayam, J., Contreras, D., French, S., *et al.* (2015). Modeling steatosis and lipid-mediated cell injury using induced pluripotent stem cell-derived-hepatocytes. Abstract 611.2. *Federation of American Societies for Experimental Biology Journal* **29**, 611.2.

59. Choudhury, Y., Toh, Y.C., Xing, J., *et al.* (2017). Patient-specific hepatocyte-like cells derived from induced pluripotent stem cells model pazopanib-mediated hepatotoxicity. *Science Reports* **7**, 46391.

60. Takayama, K., Morisaki, Y., Kuno, S., *et al.* (2014). Prediction of interindividual differences in hepatic functions and drug sensitivity by using human iPS-derived hepatocytes. *Proceedings of the National Academy of Sciences of the USA* **111**, 16772–16777.

61. Bell, C.C., Lauschke, V.M., Vorrink, S.U., *et al.* (2017). Transcriptional, functional and mechanistic comparisons of stem cell-derived hepatocytes, HepaRG cells and 3D human hepatocyte spheroids as predictive in vitro systems for drug-induced liver injury. *Drug Metabolism Disposition* **45**, 419–429.

62. Sato, T., Vries, R.G., Snippert, H.J., *et al.* (2009). Single Lgr5 stem cells build crypt–villus structures *in vitro* without a mesenchymal niche. *Nature, London* **459**, 262–265.

63. Huch, M., Gehart, H., van Boxtel, R., *et al.* (2015). Long-term culture of genome-stable bipotent stem cells from adult human liver. *Cell* **160**, 299–312.

64. Chan, K.-M., Fu, Y.-H., Wu, T.-J., *et al.* (2013). Hepatic stellate cells promote the differentiation of embryonic stem cell-derived definitive endodermal cells into hepatic progenitor cells. *Hepatology Research* **43**, 648–657.

65. Du, C., Narayanan, K., Leong, M.F., *et al.* (2014). Induced pluripotent stem cell-derived hepatocytes and endothelial cells in multi-component hydrogel fibers for liver tissue engineering. *Biomaterials* **35**, 6006–6014.

66. Soto-Gutiérrez, A., Navarro-Alvarez, N., Zhao, D., *et al.* (2007). Differentiation of mouse embryonic stem cells to hepatocyte-like cells by co-culture with human liver nonparenchymal cell lines. *Nature Protocols* **2**, 347–356.

67. Frantz, C., Stewart, K.M. & Weaver, V.M. (2010). The extracellular matrix at a glance. *Journal of Cell Science* **123**, 4195–4200.

68. Lu, P., Takai, K., Weaver, V.M., *et al.* (2011). Extracellular matrix degradation and remodeling in development and disease. *Cold Spring Harbor Perspectives in Biology* **3**, a005058.

69. Yue, B. (2014). Biology of the extracellular matrix: An overview. *Journal of Glaucoma* **23**, S20–S23.

70. Wang, F., Weaver, V.M., Petersen, O.W., *et al.* (1998). Reciprocal interactions between β1-integrin and epidermal growth factor receptor in three-dimensional basement membrane breast cultures: A different perspective in epithelial biology. *Proceedings of the National Academy of Sciences of the USA* **95**, 14821–14826.

71. Weaver, V.M. & Bissell, M.J. (1999). Functional culture models to study mechanisms governing apoptosis in normal and malignant mammary epithelial cells. *Journal of Mammary Gland Biology and Neoplasia* **4**, 193–201.

72. Harrison, R.G. (1906). Observations on the living developing nerve fiber. *Proceedings of the Society for Experimental Biology and Medicine* **4**, 140–143.

73. Huzella, T. (1932). Orientation de la croissance des cultures de tissus sur la trame fibrillaire artificielle coagulée de la solution de collagène. *Comptes Rendus des Seances de la Societé de Biologie* **109**, 515–518.

74. Emerman, J.T. & Pitelka, D.R. (1977). Maintenance and induction of morphological differentiation in dissociated mammary epithelium on floating collagen membranes. *In Vitro* **13**, 316–328.

75. Berry, M.N. & Friend, D.S. (1969). High-yield preparation of isolated rat liver parenchymal cells: A biochemical and fine structural study. *Journal of Cell Biology* **43**, 506–520.

76. Bissell, D.M. & Tilles, J.G. (1971). Morphology and function of cells of human embryonic liver in monolayer culture. *Journal of Cell Biology* **50**, 222–231.

77. Michalopoulos, G. & Pitot, H.C. (1975). Primary culture of parenchymal liver cells on collagen membranes. Morphological and biochemical observations. *Experimental Cell Research* **94**, 70–78.

78. Swarm, R.L. (1963). Transplantation of a murine chondrosarcoma in mice of different inbred strains. *Journal of the National Cancer Institute* **31**, 953–975.

79. Orkin, R.W., Gehron, P., McGoodwin, E.B., *et al.* (1977). A murine tumor producing a matrix of basement membrane. *Journal of Experimental Medicine* **145**, 204–220.

80. Kleinman, H.K. & Martin, G.R. (2005). Matrigel: Basement membrane matrix with biological activity. *Seminars in Cancer Biology* **15**, 378–386.

81. Bissell, M.J., Hall, H.G. & Parry, G. (1982). How does the extracellular matrix direct gene expression? *Journal of Theoretical Biology* **99**, 31–68.

82. Petersen, O.W., Rønnov-Jessen, L., Howlett, A.R., *et al.* (1992). Interaction with basement membrane serves to rapidly distinguish growth and differentiation pattern of normal and malignant human breast epithelial cells. *Proceedings of the National Academy of Sciences of the USA* **89**, 9064–9068.

83. Antoni, D., Burckel, H., Josset, E., *et al.* (2015). Three-dimensional cell culture: A breakthrough *in vivo*. *International Journal of Molecular Sciences* **16**, 5517–5527.

84. Loh, Q.L. & Choong, C. (2013). Three-dimensional scaffolds for tissue engineering applications: Role of porosity and pore size. *Tissue Engineering Part B Reviews* **19**, 485–502.

85. Hoffman, A.S. (2012). Hydrogels for biomedical applications. *Advanced Drug Delivery Reviews* **64**, 18–23.

86. Wade, R.J. & Burdick, J.A. (2012). Engineering ECM signals into biomaterials. *Materials Today* **15**, 454–459.

87. Kharkar, P.M., Kiick, K.L. & Kloxin, A.M. (2013). Designing degradable hydrogels for orthogonal control of cell microenvironments. *Chemical Society Reviews* **42**, 7335–7372.

88. Edmondson, R., Broglie, J.J., Adcock, A.F., *et al.* (2014). Three-dimensional cell culture systems and their applications in drug discovery and cell-based biosensors. *Assay and Drug Development Technologies* **12**, 207–218.

89. Humphrey, J.D., Dufresne, E.R. & Schwartz, M.A. (2014). Mechanotransduction and extracellular matrix homeostasis. *Nature Reviews Molecular Cell Biology* **15**, 802–812.

90. Lesman, A., Rosenfeld, D., Landau, S., *et al.* (2016). Mechanical regulation of vascular network formation in engineered matrices. *Advanced Drug Delivery Reviews* **96**, 176–182.

91. De Leon Rodriguez, L.M., Hemar, Y., Cornish, J., *et al.* (2016). Structure-mechanical property correlations of hydrogel forming [small beta]-sheet peptides. *Chemical Society Reviews* **45**, 4797–4824.

92. Carletti, E., Motta, A. & Migliaresi, C. (2011). Scaffolds for tissue engineering and 3D cell culture. In J.W. Haycock (Ed.), *3D Cell Culture: Methods and Protocols* (pp. 17–39). Totowa, NJ, USA: Humana Press.

93. Taylor, P.M. (2007). Biological matrices and bionanotechnology. *Philosophical Transactions of the Royal Society B: Biological Sciences* **362**, 1313–1320.

94. Benton, G., Arnaoutova, I., George, J., *et al.* (2014). Matrigel: From discovery and ECM mimicry to assays and models for cancer research. *Comptes Rendus des Seances de la Societé de Biologie* **80**, 3–18.

95. Chevallay, B. & Herbage, D. (2000). Collagen-based biomaterials as 3D scaffold for cell cultures: Applications for tissue engineering and gene therapy. *Medical and Biological Engineering and Computing* **38**, 211–218.

96. Glowacki, J. & Mizuno, S. (2008). Collagen scaffolds for tissue engineering. *Biopolymers* **89**, 338–344.

97. Echave, M.C., Saenz Del Burgo, L., Pedraz, J.L., *et al.* (2017). Gelatin as Biomaterial for Tissue Engineering. *Current Pharmaceutical Design* **23**, 3567–3584.

98. Kang, H.W., Tabata, Y. & Ikada, Y. (1999). Fabrication of porous gelatin scaffolds for tissue engineering. *Biomaterials* **20**, 1339–1344.

99. Collins, M.N. & Birkinshaw, C. (2013). Hyaluronic acid based scaffolds for tissue engineering—A review. *Carbohydrate Polymers* **92**, 1262–1279.

100. Hemshekhar, M., Thushara, R.M., Chandranayaka, S., *et al.* (2016). Emerging roles of hyaluronic acid bioscaffolds in tissue engineering and regenerative medicine. *International Journal of Biological Macromolecules* **86**, 917–928.

101. Silva, E.A. & Mooney, D.J. (2004). Synthetic extracellular matrices for tissue engineering and regeneration. *Current Topics in Developmental Biology* **64**, 181–205.

102. BaoLin, G.U.O. & Ma, P.X. (2014). Synthetic biodegradable functional polymers for tissue engineering: A brief review. *Science China Chemistry* **57**, 490–500.

103. Asti, A. & Gioglio, L. (2016). Natural and synthetic biodegradable polymers: Different scaffolds for cell expansion and tissue formation. *The International Journal of Artificial Organs* **37**, 187–205.

104. Kumar, A. & Han, S.S. (2017). PVA-based hydrogels for tissue engineering: A review. *International Journal of Polymeric Materials and Polymeric Biomaterials* **66**, 159–182.

105. Hoffman, A.S. (2002). Hydrogels for biomedical applications. *Advanced Drug Delivery Reviews* **54**, 3–12.

106. Drury, J.L. & Mooney, D.J. (2003). Hydrogels for tissue engineering: scaffold design variables and applications. *Biomaterials* **24**, 4337–4351.

107. Zhu, J. & Marchant, R.E. (2011). Design properties of hydrogel tissue-engineering scaffolds. *Expert Review of Medical Devices* **8**, 607–626.

108. Chrzanowski, W. & Khademhosseini, A. (2013). Biologically inspired 'smart' materials. *Advanced Drug Delivery Reviews* **65**, 403–404.

109. Chen, F.-M. & Liu, X. (2016). Advancing biomaterials of human origin for tissue engineering. *Progress in Polymer Sciences* **53**, 86–168.

110. Koutsopoulos, S. (2016). Self-assembling peptide nanofiber hydrogels in tissue engineering and regenerative medicine: Progress, design guidelines, and applications. *Journal of Biomedical Materials Research Part A* **104**, 1002–1016.

111. Kyle, S., Aggel, I.A., Ingham, E., *et al.* (2009). Production of self-assembling biomaterials for tissue engineering. *Trends in Biotechnology* **27**, 423–433.

112. Harrington, D.A., Cheng, E.Y., Guler, M.O., *et al.* (2006). Branched peptide-amphiphiles as self-assembling coatings for tissue engineering scaffolds. *Journal of Biomedical Materials Research Part A* **78**, 157–167.

113. Seow, W.Y. & Hauser, C.A.E. (2014). Short to ultrashort peptide hydrogels for biomedical uses. *Materials Today* **17**, 381–388.

114. Lutolf, M.P., Raeber, G.P., Zisch, A.H., *et al.* (2003). Cell-responsive synthetic hydrogels. *Advanced Materials* **15**, 888–892.

115. Raeber, G.P., Lutolf, M.P. & Hubbell, J.A. (2005). Molecularly engineered PEG hydrogels: A novel model system for proteolytically mediated cell migration. *Biophysical Journal* **89**, 1374–1388.

116. Fleischmann, R.D., Adams, M.D., White, O., *et al.* (1995). Whole-genome random sequencing and assembly of *Haemophilus influenzae* Rd. *Science, New York* **269**, 496–512.

117. Goffeau, A., Barrell, B.G., Bussey, H., *et al.* (1996). Life with 6000 genes. *Science, New York* **274**(546), 563–567.

118. C. elegans Sequencing Consortium. (1998). Genome sequence of the nematode *C. elegans*: A platform for investigating biology. *Science, New York* **282**, 2012–2018.

119. Adams, M.D., Celniker, S.E., Holt, R.A., *et al.* (2000). The genome sequence of *Drosophila melanogaster*. *Science, New York* **287**, 2185–2195.

120. Mouse Genome Sequencing Consortium. (2002). Initial sequencing and comparative analysis of the mouse genome. *Nature, London* **420**, 520–562.

121. Collins, F.S., Green, E.D., Guttmacher, A.E., *et al.* (2003). A vision for the future of genomics research. *Nature, London* **422**, 835–847.

122. Chimpanzee Sequencing and Analysis Consortium. (2005). Initial sequence of the chimpanzee genome and comparison with the human genome. *Nature, London* **437**, 69–87.

123. Booth, J., Boyland, E. & Sims, P. (1961). An enzyme from rat liver catalysing conjugations with glutathione. *Biochemical Journal* **79**, 516−524.

124. Estabrook, R.W. (2003). A passion for P450s (rememberances of the early history of research on cytochrome P450). *Drug Metabolism and Disposition: The Biological Fate of Chemicals* **31**, 1461−1473.

125. Wishart, D.S., Tzur, D., Knox, C., *et al.* (2007). HMDB: The Human Metabolome Database. *Nucleic Acids Research* **35**, D521−D526.

Chapter 5.2

Biologically-Inspired Microphysiological Systems

Eva-Maria Dehne[1], James Hickman[2] and Michael Shuler[3]

[1]TissUse GmbH, Berlin, Germany; [2]NanoScience Technology Center, University of Central Florida, Orlando, FL, USA; [3]Meinig School of Biomedical Engineering, Cornell University, Ithaca, NY, USA

SUMMARY

Microphysiological multi-organ devices are designed to mimic the physiological interaction of various interconnected organ models, by successfully imitating organismal functionality and response to substances. The first concepts of *in vitro* multi-organ systems were put forward in the late 1980s, demonstrating that such systems could provide mechanistic insight into toxicology questions. In 2010, governmental grants and initiatives in Europe and the United States strongly accelerated the development of microphysiological systems. The rapid increase in the number of laboratories and spin-off companies working on these devices, and the commitment of big pharma and cosmetics companies, has led to the generation of a diversity of systems for various applications. In conjunction with regulatory science-driven efforts, high-quality data derived from these devices laid the foundation for later qualification studies. Further advancements to include more organs and functionalities lead the way toward systemic micro-organisms on a chip — so-called body-on-a-chip devices. These systems will eventually establish a completely new substance testing paradigm.

1. INTRODUCTION

Advances in *in vitro* methods have led to the development of static human cell culture models of increasing physiological relevance. However, limitations in predicting true human response to drugs and chemicals, in terms of both efficacy and toxicity, have led to the development of more-complex microfluidic culture models, often called microphysiological systems (MPSs). These systems are designed to support an *in vivo*-like environment for *in vitro* cell cultures and to mimic human biology on the smallest acceptable scale, to include flow, functional readouts and multi-organ systems.

Microfabrication and nanofabrication techniques have enabled the development of these systems. With a comprehensive field of application, ranging from the study of physiology to pharmacology and/or toxicology, the biological background of MPSs is comparably broad. Similarly, technological features, such as the mode of pumping (external pumps (1), on board pumps (2, 3) or passive gravity driven flow (4, 5)) or the format of the devices, are often designed for a particular purpose. Plate-based systems with a standardised footprint are mostly designed to be compatible with robotic pipetting and high-throughput screening (6, 7). Organ-on-a-chip systems focus on the generation of organ-specific microenvironments or the integration of additional features, such as the mechanical and electrophysiological stimulation of tissues. The stretching of lung epithelial cells (8) or the stimulation of cardiac models (9) are prominent examples. Mechanical and electrophysiological constructs can also be used for functional readouts of tissue activity, as demonstrated with cardiac cells in a serum-free medium (10). Comprehensive studies on current achievements in the field of MPSs have been published by Marx *et al.* (11) and Wang *et al.* (12).

The integration of multiple tissues into one device allows for the study of inter-organ communication via soluble factors. These multi-organ MPSs not only permit the interaction of distant cells, but also enable the study of complex, time-dependent concentration profiles of the compounds administered and their metabolites. The absorption, distribution, metabolism and excretion (ADME) profiles of substances can be quantitatively described by a mathematical modelling technique called physiologically based pharmacokinetics (PBPK). Using these models in conjunction with pharmacodynamic (PD) models allows them to be effective guides in constructing multi-organ systems for the prediction of potential drug efficacy and toxicity, as well as dose adjustment. The use of serum-free medium removes an unknown variable from the system, especially for the evaluation of compounds for efficacy and toxicity. The proper design principles and scaling rules for multi-organ MPSs are critical for the direct interpretation of results. Generally, when the scaling of the organs integrated into one device becomes more physiological, and liquid-to-cell ratios are closer to those found *in vivo*, metabolite concentration profiles are more likely to be accurate and to replicate the effects found *in vivo* with higher probability. Various scaling approaches for MPSs have been published (13, 14). Finally, the most complex systems — human body-on-a-chip devices — are envisioned to mimic entire organismal functionality through the interactions of a variety of organs. Here, we discuss the important milestones and main achievements in the development of multi-organ MPSs and a vision of the achievement of a human body-on-a-chip.

2. HISTORICAL DEVELOPMENT

The concept of an *in vitro* multi-organ system based on a PBPK-PD model to predict the response of mammals to drugs or environmental chemicals was conceived by Shuler in 1989, leading to US Patent 5,612,188. The first paper describing such a system (15) was followed by a series of papers from Cornell University on macroscale systems. Advances in microfluidics and microfabrication allowed the miniaturisation of the concept and the development of MPSs (see US Patent 7,288,405).

2.1 Pioneering MPSs

Several reviews of the development of MPSs are available. Many of the early developments have been described by Baker (16) and recently by Zhang and Radisic (17) on progress toward the commercialisation of such systems.

The first MPS was directed toward proof of principle by demonstrating that the new technology could predict responses seen in rodent studies. A preliminary description of an MPS was given in 2001 (18), followed by a series of three papers in 2004 (19–21) that clearly established that such systems could provide mechanistic insight into a toxicology problem, namely, why mice are 10 times more sensitive to naphthalene than rats. These papers demonstrated that the reactive metabolite of naphthalene, naphthoquinone, was generated in the liver and circulated to the lung, causing lung cell death. The presence of a fat compartment provided some protection due to adsorption of the reactive metabolite. It was later shown, by using a PBPK model based on the MPS, that rats were less sensitive to naphthalene than mice, because of differences in the kinetics of glutathione synthesis, as glutathione combines with the reactive metabolite resulting in an excretable non-reactive complex. This early work demonstrated not only that creating MPSs was feasible, but also that such systems can provide insight into a toxicological issue.

Other examples of early MPSs include a GI tract–liver model (1), which probed the response to the ingestion of acetaminophen, demonstrating the dose-dependent production of toxic metabolites. Tatosian *et al.* (22) probed the response to treatment of uterine cancer (both sensitive and multidrug resistant (MDR)) by using a multi-organ system that included liver, bone-marrow and other tissue compartments. In this study, responses to the anticancer agent, doxorubicin, and the MDR suppressors, cyclosporin and nicardipine, were shown to act synergistically in the treatment of MDR cancer. Sung *et al.* (5) established the first 'pumpless' multi-organ MPS that facilitated ease of set-up, robust operation and low cost. Since 2010, the pumpless system has been used exclusively by the Cornell group, and the spin-off company, Hesperos, and others have adopted it.

2.2 Examples of Systems Providing Functional Assessments and Serum-Free Medium

Hickman has developed a defined-base serum-free medium system that permits the culture of a wide range of cell types up to several months and removes a major variable (serum) in the system. He published the first serum-free, defined culture system for neuronal systems in 1995 (23), and in most cases, the cells have been shown to maintain functionality for at least 2–3 months. This system can satisfactorily support cardiac cells, hippocampal neurons, motoneurons, sensory neurons, muscle cells, NMJ formation, hepatocytes, and endothelial and epithelial cells. The incorporation of electrical and mechanical readouts for functional hybrid systems substantially decreases the number and frequency of biomarker measurements, also enabling non-invasive chronic functional analysis, which is critical for repeat-dose studies in these systems. The four-organ system has been published (24), with specific functional systems for cardiac cells, for muscle cells, for neurons and for hepatocytes.

2.3 The GO-Bio Multi-Organ-Chip Initiative

A GO-Bio grant from the German Ministry of Education and Research was awarded in 2010 to Uwe Marx's laboratory at the Technische Universität Berlin, its spin-off, TissUse GmbH, the Fraunhofer IWS in Dresden and the Fraunhofer IGB in Stuttgart. The two-phase project aimed at the development of a chip platform mimicking human biology at an entire organismal level.

The ultimate goal of establishing a human-like mini-organism *in vitro*, the human-on-a-chip, was approached by first designing a versatile multi-organ-chip (MOC) platform for various two-organ and four-organ co-cultures, and, in a second step, proceeding to combine more organs. A consistent scaling approach, reflecting the organoid structure of a human, was applied throughout the entire programme. A 28-day human 3D liver–skin culture, including repeated-dose substance exposure in the MOC, represented a first proof of long-term viability and gave first insights into possible organ–organ interactions (3). Further studies showing the integration of biological vasculature (25) or microcapillaries (26), co-cultures of liver-intestine (27), and liver–neurosphere (28) models, were presented. Further platform improvements resulted in a four organ ADMET chip connecting a human primary intestinal model and a skin biopsy in a common media circulation with liver spheroids and a kidney model (29). The viability of all four organ models over 28 days in co-culture and the generation of a reproducible homoeostasis among the cultures were achieved. The creation of a bone-marrow-on-a-chip system permitted the long-term cultures of human haematopoietic stem and progenitor cells to stay in their primitive state and retain their capability of GEMM colony formation (30).

The second phase dedicated to the generation of the human-on-a-chip was initiated in 2015 and will continue until 2018. The final vision is illustrated in Fig. 1 and is currently under evaluation.

2.4 US Programmes

In 2010, the US Food and Drug Administration (FDA) and the National Institutes of Health (NIH) instituted the FDA's Advancing Regulatory Science Initiative, building on the achievements of existing programmes, primarily the Critical Path Initiative, established in 2004, that was designed to transform the way medical products are developed, evaluated and manufactured. This initiative funded three programmes, including the initial work from Harvard for a lung–heart construct (8) that built on previous examples of federal funding of individual projects by the NIH and the National Science

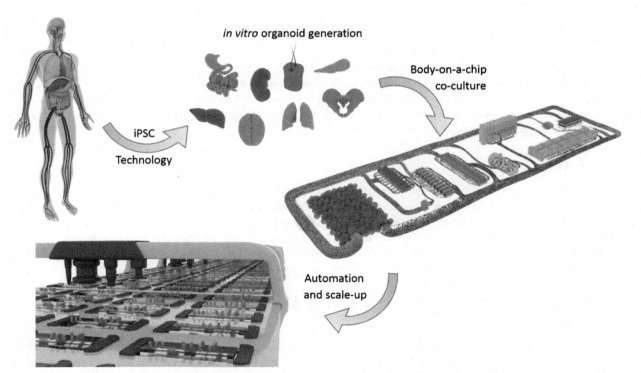

FIGURE 1 Vision of the human body-on-a-chip leading to a new paradigm in substance testing. This platform would permit systemic safety testing and the on-chip modelling of aspects of clinical trials. *iPSC*, induced pluripotent stem cell.

Foundation (NSF). This was further expanded in 2012 by the National Center for Advancing Translational Sciences (NCATS) at the NIH, in collaboration with the Defence Advanced Research Projects Agency (DARPA), and funded a cluster of projects (19 at the NIH), and two large grants (by DARPA) at Harvard and MIT, for the development of platforms able to integrate 10 organ systems. In addition, the Defense Threat Reduction Agency (DTRA) funded a large project led by Wake Forest to construct a seven-organ system. This large input of resources has led to a rapid increase in the number of US laboratories with an interest in developing this technology. This effort has led to the spin-off of many small companies (see 17); Hesperos was the first spin-off from the NIH efforts, whereas Emulate came from the Harvard DARPA effort and CN Bio Innovations from the MIT DARPA studies. The underlying technology has advanced, such that the programmes of many federal research agencies (e.g. NIH, NSF, the National Aeronautics and Space Administration (NASA) and the Department of Defense (DOD)) include calls for such research. This broad base of funding demonstrates the rapid recognition by these agencies of the opportunities that this technology provides and the need to support its expanded development.

2.5 The European 'Body-on-a-Chip' Consortium

Two years later, the European Commission awarded a 3-year grant under the seventh Framework programme (STREP #296257) to a 'Body-on-a-chip' consortium consisting of InSphero AG and the ETH Zurich, Switzerland, Technische Universität Dortmund, Germany, KU Leuven, Belgium, and Astra Zeneca Pharmaceutical, UK. The consortium came up with a 96-well format aggregate-based multi-tissue chip, with the aim of developing an *in vitro* model facilitating the identification of multi-organ toxicity and decreased efficacy due to metabolic activity. In this system, 10 parallel micro-fluidic channels interconnect six culturing compartments, in which microtissues of different types can be loaded. In a coherent study, it could be shown that the co-cultivation of rat liver and colorectal tumour microtissues in the presence of the prodrug, cyclophosphamide, showed a significant reduction in tumour growth after bioactivation by the liver. This effect could only be observed in the microfluidic device (7).

2.6 The Netherlands Institute for Human Organ and Disease Model Technologies

The Netherlands Institute for Human Organ and Disease Model Technologies (hDMT) was formed in 2015 as a pre-competitive, non-profit technological research institute. Today, scientists from 14 Dutch organisations, including academic research centres, research institutes, university medical centres and biotech companies, work together to develop organs-on-chips by using human stem cells. The two main scientific programmes include the development of: (a) human tissue and disease models of vessels-, heart-, cancer- and brain-on-chip; and (b) organ-on-chip technology platforms. Six hDMT researchers recently received a Gravitation grant of almost 19 million Euros from the Netherlands Organisation of Scientific Research (NOW). In their project, called NOCI (Netherlands Organ-on-Chip Initiative), they aim to generate miniature organs from patients and use them to study the development and treatment of diseases. Therefore, models of human brain, heart, intestine and blood vessels will be generated on microfluidic chips. Subsequently, up to three organ-on-chip systems will be linked to study how they influence each other.

2.7 EU-ToxRisk

The European H2020-supported project, EU-ToxRisk, which started in 2016, gathered an international consortium of 39 partners from academia, industry, contract research organisations and regulatory bodies. This 300 million Euro project aimed to integrate new concepts for regulatory chemical safety assessment, such as *in silico* and human-relevant *in vitro* methods. The end-goal is to deliver the reliable, animal-free hazard and risk assessment of chemicals. A multi-organ intestine-liver-neuronal-kidney-toxicity-chip will also be qualified and used to analyse repeated dose toxicity. This evaluation of MOCs under European programmes will encourage regulatory acceptance.

3. CURRENT ACHIEVEMENTS IN INDUSTRIAL ADOPTION AND REMAINING CHALLENGES

Governmental projects and regulatory decisions, such as the European Cosmetics Directive, the European REACH regulation and the new amendment to the US Toxic Substances Control Act, have stimulated the industrial adoption of alternative methods within the last decade. Even though the field of MPS research is still very young and therefore lacks models accepted by regulatory bodies, major pharmaceutical and cosmetics companies are investing heavily in these systems. The diversity of systems being developed in research institutes and newly-formed companies allows for the testing of these devices within the various stages of the drug development process. Plate-based systems, for example, are applicable in early screening studies, due to their compatibility with higher throughput testing. Single-organ MPSs are similarly useful for studying the effects on the target tissue or ruling out specific toxicities at an early stage. Emulate Inc., for example, announced research collaborations with Johnson & Johnson Innovation to enhance their drug candidate design and selection. In a collaboration with Seres Therapeutics Inc., their Intestine-Chip is aimed at identifying novel bacterial compositions with therapeutic potential. Similarly, CN Bio Innovations announced research collaborations with 25 undisclosed pharmaceutical companies, to perform studies within drug discovery and safety programmes. These and other systems show great potential in drug development and early toxicity studies. However, they will only answer specific questions with regard to predefined organs. Multi-organ systems or organismal body-on-a-chip devices are mandatory for the prediction of more-complex effects and human pharmacokinetics.

Hesperos has licensed technology from the University of Central Florida and Cornell for a base 4-organ pumpless system developed with L'Oréal (24), involving liver, skeletal muscle, neuronal and cardiac tissue, which is the first example of a continuously recirculating system in a serum-free medium. This system can be modified by the addition of other tissue compartments, such as barrier tissues (e.g. skin, gastrointestinal tract, kidney blood—brain barrier). Each organ module can be developed separately and combined with other tissues, making the system modular. A key feature is the use of functional measurement of the electrical and mechanical responses of 'target' tissues (e.g. cardiac, neuromuscular junction). The ability to measure functions as well as biomarkers and viability permits sensitive and rapid assessment that is non-destructive. These systems can operate for up to 28 days. The pumpless format allows for a relatively rapid set-up, a robust operation (e.g. absence of gas bubbles) at a low cost, as an inexpensive rocker platform can handle multiple units (up to 12 per platform and 4 platforms per rocker are possible). The system has been used to test more than 30 compounds for customers.

The industrial adoption of multi-organ MOC-based MPSs from TissUse takes place in a stepwise manner, starting with feasibility studies and finally resulting in technology transfers and in-house validation of the MOC platform. Recent feasibility examples were the co-culture of lung airway and liver to study nicotine metabolites, in collaboration with Philip Morris International R&D, and the co-culture of healthy full-thickness skin and lung tumour to develop a combined safety and efficacy ('safficacy') assay for testing oncology drug candidates of Bayer AG. Furthermore, after successful feasibility studies, a technology transfer and in-house validation of the MOC platform has been successfully completed with Astra Zeneca, for a single-organ bone marrow model and a co-culture of pancreatic islets and liver and with Beiersdorf for a co-culture model of skin and liver.

These industrial co-operation and feasibility studies are highly valuable for understanding the benefits and limitations of the respective technologies. Major challenges to be solved for the creation of a body-on-a-chip have so far included the installation of a fully closed biological vasculature, penetrating and interconnecting the various organ models. That having been achieved, the integration of a common recirculating medium transporting nutrients and soluble factors at a physiologically-relevant level, establishing crucial gradients and even carrying parts of the immune system might be less of an issue. Furthermore, the compartmentalisation of complex organs, such as the liver, segregating bile acids into a separated canalicular network away from the blood stream, will be crucial for long-term homoeostasis and tissue survival. Groundwork answering some of these questions has already been carried out, but combining the solutions into one functional device requires the efforts of many different experts and disciplines.

4. A ROAD MAP TOWARD THE REGULATORY ACCEPTANCE OF BODY-ON-A-CHIP SYSTEMS

Insights recently gained in single-organ and multi-organ MPSs have affirmed the potential of these systems to lead to a new paradigm in substance testing, reducing and finally replacing animal trials. More than a dozen companies are evaluating MPS models today and, in some cases, are using them for in-house decision-making during the drug development process. These studies provide high-quality data, which lay the foundation for later qualification studies (Fig. 2). Together with insights gained from MPS-based regulatory science, they might lead to the first validated regulatory safety assays within the next 5—15 years. On this point, the American Institute for Medical and Biological Engineering (AIMBE) has collaborated with the NIH to run six Workshops on Validation and Qualification of MPSs. These workshops have established that the hurdles to be overcome for toxicity evaluations will be different than those for efficacy and that applications to rare diseases is a natural starting point. However, various innovative solutions to the challenges described

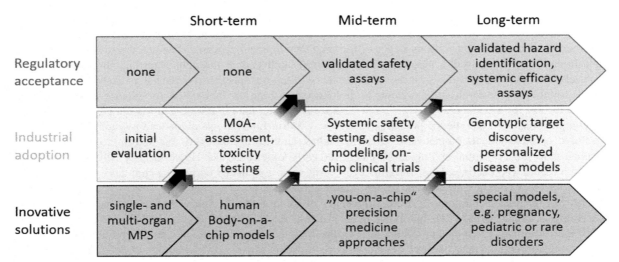

FIGURE 2 Anticipated further developments of microphysiological systems and their progression through stages of industrial adoption and regulatory acceptance.

earlier are essential to achieving the final paradigm shift. Furthermore, comprehensive studies to compare the predictive validity of results with those from other approaches (especially human data) need to be shown. Here, the possibility of using MPSs to answer questions that cannot be addressed in animal models will be beneficial.

Corresponding to current developments, future scientific achievements generated by research institutes or MPS companies are expected to be tested by the industries. Multi-organ MPSs already currently allow for ADME profiling and the study of physiological and pathological multi-organ interactions. Furthermore, the accomplishment of a human body-on-a-chip will permit systemic safety testing and the on-chip modelling of aspects of clinical trials. In the long-term, this might nearly eliminate the need for animal trials in preclinical development and the involvement of healthy volunteers in phase I testing. The restructuring of the preclinical discovery phase might lead to systems that are truly predictive of human responses at an early stage, thus reducing clinical attrition rates, shortening the whole process and greatly reducing costs.

REFERENCES

1. Mahler, G.J., Esch, M.B., Glahn, R.P., et al. (2009). Characterization of a gastrointestinal tract microscale cell culture analog used to predict drug toxicity. *Biotechnology and Bioengineering* **104**, 193–205.
2. Coppeta, J.R., Mescher, M.J., Isenberg, B.C., et al. (2016). A portable and reconfigurable multi-organ platform for drug development with onboard microfluidic flow control. *Lab on a Chip* **17**, 134–144.
3. Wagner, I., Materne, E.M., Brincker, S., et al. (2013). A dynamic multi-organ-chip for long-term cultivation and substance testing proven by 3D human liver and skin tissue co-culture. *Lab on a Chip* **13**, 3538–3547.
4. Kim, J., Fluri, D.A., Kelm, J.M., et al. (2015). 96-well format-based microfluidic platform for parallel interconnection of multiple multicellular spheroids. *Journal of Laboratory Automation* **20**, 274–282.
5. Sung, J.H., Kam, C. & Shuler, M.L. (2010). A microfluidic device for pharmacokinetic-pharmacodynamic (PK-PD) model on a chip. *Lab on a Chip* **10**, 446–455.
6. Trietsch, J.S., Israëls, G., Joore, J., et al. (2013). Microfluidic titer plate for stratified 3D cell culture. *Lab on a Chip* **13**, 3548–3554.
7. Kim, J., Fluri, D.A., Marchan, R., et al. (2015). 3D spherical microtissues and microfluidic technology for multi-tissue experiments and analysis. *Journal of Biotechnology* **205**, 24–35.
8. Huh, D., Matthews, B.D., Mammoto, A., et al. (2010). Reconstituting organ-level lung functions on a chip. *Science, New York* **328**, 1662–1668.
9. Maidhof, R., Tandon, N., Lee, E.J., et al. (2012). Biomimetic perfusion and electrical stimulation applied in concert improved the assembly of engineered cardiac tissue. *Journal of Tissue Engineering and Regenerative Medicine* **6**, 1–21.
10. Stancescu, M., Molnar, P., McAleer, C., et al. (2015). In vitro model of whole heart function. *Biomaterials* **60**, 20–30.
11. Marx, U., Andersson, T.B., Bahinski, A., et al. (2016). Biology-inspired microphysiological system approaches to solve the prediction dilemma of substance testing. *ATLA* **33**, 272–321.
12. Wang, Y., Oleaga, C., Long, C., et al. (2017). Self-contained, low-cost body-on-a-chip systems for drug development. *Experimental Biology and Medicine Online* **0**, 1–13.
13. Marx, U., Walles, H., Hoffmann, S., et al. (2012). Human-on-a-chip developments: A translational cutting-edge alternative to systemic safety assessment and efficiency evaluation of substances in laboratory animals and man. *ATLA* **40**, 235–257.

14. Abaci, H.E. & Shuler, M.L. (2015). Human-on-a-chip design strategies and principles for physiologically based pharmacokinetics/pharmacodynamics modeling. *Integrative Biology* **7**, 383–391.
15. Sweeney, L.M., Shuler, M.L., Quick, D.J., *et al.* (1996). A preliminary physiologically-based pharmacokinetic model for naphthalene and naphthalene oxide in mice and rats. *Annals of Biomedical Engineering* **24**, 305–320.
16. Baker, M. (2011). Tissue models: A living system on a chip. *Nature, London* **471**, 661–665.
17. Zhang, B. & Radisic, M. (2017). Organ-on-a-chip devices advance to market. *Lab on a Chip* **17**, 2395–2420.
18. Sin, A., Baxter, G.T. & Shuler, M. (2001). Animal on a chip: A microscale cell culture analog device for evaluating toxicological and pharmacological profiles. *Proceedings of SPIE 4560, Microfluidics and BioMEMS*, 98–101.
19. Sin, A., Chin, K.C., Jamil, M.F., *et al.* (2004). The design and fabrication of three-chamber microscale cell culture analog devices with integrated dissolved oxygen sensors. *Biotechnology Progress* **20**, 338–345.
20. Viravaidya, K., Sin, A. & Shuler, M.L. (2004). Development of a microscale cell culture analog to probe naphthalene toxicity. *Biotechnology Progress* **20**, 316–323.
21. Viravaidya, K. & Shuler, M.L. (2004). Incorporation of 3T3-L1 cells to mimic bioaccumulation in a microscale cell culture analog device for toxicity studies. *Biotechnology Progress* **20**, 590–597.
22. Tatosian, D.A. & Shuler, M.L. (2009). A novel system for evaluation of drug mixtures for potential efficacy in treating multidrug resistant cancers. *Biotechnology and Bioengineering* **103**, 187–198.
23. Schaffner, A.E., Barker, J.L., Stenger, D.A., Hickman, J.J., *et al.* (1995). Investigation of the factors necessary for growth of hippocampal neurons in a defined system. *Journal of Neuroscience Methods* **62**, 111–119.
24. Oleaga, C., Bernabini, C., Smith, A.S., *et al.* (2016). Multi-organ toxicity demonstration in a functional human in vitro system composed of four organs. *Scientific Reports* **6**, 1–17.
25. Schimek, K., Busek, M., Brincker, S., *et al.* (2013). Integrating biological vasculature into a multi-organ-chip microsystem. *Lab on a Chip* **13**, 3588–3598.
26. Hasenberg, T., Mühleder, S., Dotzler, A., *et al.* (2015). Emulating human microcapillaries in a multi-organ-chip platform. *Journal of Biotechnology* **216**, 1–10.
27. Maschmeyer, I., Hasenberg, T., Jaenicke, A., *et al.* (2015). Chip-based human liver-intestine and liver-skin co-cultures – A first step toward systemic repeated dose substance testing in vitro. *European Journal of Pharmaceutics and Biopharmaceutics* **95**, 77–87.
28. Materne, E.M., Ramme, A.P., Terrasso, A.P., *et al.* (2015). A multi-organ chip co-culture of neurospheres and liver equivalents for long-term substance testing. *Journal of Biotechnology* **205**, 36–46.
29. Maschmeyer, I., Lorenz, A.K., Schimek, K., *et al.* (2015). A four-organ-chip for interconnected long-term co-culture of human intestine, liver, skin and kidney equivalents. *Lab on a Chip* **15**, 2688–2699.
30. Sieber, S., Wirth, L., Cavak, N., *et al.* (2018). Bone marrow-on-a-chip: Long-term culture of human hematopoietic stem cells in a 3D microfluidic environment. *Journal of Tissue Engineering and Regenerative Medicine* **12**, 479–489.

Chapter 5.3

Computational Methods to Predict Toxicity

Mark T.D. Cronin[1] and Miyoung Yoon[2]

[1]School of Pharmacy and Biomolecular Sciences, Liverpool John Moores University, Liverpool, United Kingdom; [2]ToxStrategies Inc., Cary NC, United States of America

SUMMARY

Going back to the 19th century, there is a long history of developing an understanding of how the physicochemical properties and chemical structure of a molecule affect its biological activity. Such approaches, commonly now referred to as being *in silico*, are formalised into (quantitative) structure—activity relationships ((Q)SARs) and read-across to predict toxicity and Physiologically-Based Pharmacokinetic models, to predict the distribution of chemicals *in vivo* and to allow for the extrapolation from *in vitro* effects. There have been many drivers for the development of *in silico* approaches to predict toxicity, fate and distribution. Notable among these have been the needs of various industrial sectors to assess the hazard of chemicals rapidly and efficiently, in terms of cost and animal use. These needs have been amplified globally by legislation aiming to improve animal welfare, and to respond to ethical concerns, as well as to regulate new and existing chemicals. In addition, key advances in chemoinformatics, computational power, and the connectivity of the internet have all played a role in the advancement of *in silico* approaches.

1. INTRODUCTION

Many computational techniques have been applied to replace animal tests for the evaluation of toxicity. The focus of this chapter is on the role that chemistry plays in making a molecule potentially toxic, and influencing where it may be distributed in the body. The terms *in silico* and 'computational' have been used interchangeably to describe these varied, and increasingly diverse, techniques. This chapter is not a full, or even partial, review or overview of these techniques, and should not be considered as such. The reader is referred elsewhere (1—3) as a starting point for an overview of computational toxicology and allied techniques. The chapter draws on the authors' personal experience, and no inference should be drawn from inclusion or exclusion of a particular method.

For this chapter, the following, trivial, definitions of the various techniques may be useful, but these are not official definitions:

- Structure—Activity Relationship (SAR): the relationship between chemical structure (or the relevant part of a molecule) and toxicity. It is often defined in terms of structural alerts, i.e. the (sub-)molecular fragment that causes toxicity.
- Quantitative Structure—Activity Relationship (QSAR): a quantitative relationship between descriptors of chemical structure or properties and toxic potency.
- (Quantitative) Structure—Activity Relationship ((Q)SAR): a generic term to capture either SARs or QSARs or both of them.
- Read-Across: the process of inferring the toxicity or effect of one molecule from knowledge of another, similar, molecule. It usually involves grouping of similar molecules into a category (or analogue, if it is a single similar molecule).

The History of Alternative Test Methods in Toxicology. https://doi.org/10.1016/B978-0-12-813697-3.00031-7

● Chemoinformatics: at the basic level, the application of informatics to capture and manipulate knowledge of chemical structure. For computational toxicology in this chapter, this definition includes the development of databases, models and usable software to make predictions.

● Physiologically-Based Pharmacokinetic (PBPK) Models: a mechanistically-based mathematical representation of biological processes that determine chemical absorption, distribution, metabolism and excretion in the body in humans and in animal species. It integrates independent knowledge on the physiology, biology and chemical properties, permitting prediction of chemical kinetics *in vivo* on the basis of *in vitro* and *in silico* information.

2. DRIVING FORCES FOR THE CURRENT STATE-OF-THE-ART OF *IN SILICO* TOXICOLOGY

No single driving force exists for the development of *in silico* or computational approaches to predict toxicity and the distribution of a chemical *in vivo*, and it is instinctive to rationalise a (biological) response to obtain knowledge about it. Thus, when 19th century chemistry evolved into a more formal understanding of chemical structure and properties, it was intuitive to consider how they affect activity *in vivo*. There are many other reasons for the development of computational approaches, ranging from commercial priorities to the desire to record the knowledge of experts to be used by others, along with advances in technology.

2.1 Driving Forces From Legislation and Regulation

There is much global legislation and many regulations, relating to the use of chemicals in various industrial sectors, that has prompted the use of alternatives and computational methods, in particular. It is not the intention of this chapter to review all of the relevant regulations in detail — some of which have been captured historically (e.g. see Refs. 4—8). The regulations are split into those that promote animal welfare (and thus implicitly encourage the development and use of alternatives) and those which regulate chemicals directly. The EU has stood at the forefront of initiatives to promote animal welfare, almost certainly as a direct response to public pressure. While the significance of the outcome of such legislation is debatable, it has, at least, stimulated the release of significant funds at the European level for research through several decades of the EU Framework Programmes, as well as the Marie Curie Mobility funding, and several other sources.

With regard to computational methods, the biggest driver has undoubtedly been legislation that requires the registration and/or safety assessment of new and existing compounds, in areas such as industrial chemicals and cosmetics ingredients, and, to a lesser extent for *in silico* approaches, pharmaceuticals and pesticides. For instance, in the USA, the *Toxic Substances Control Act* (1986) specified a 'Pre-Manufactory Notification' procedure requiring a rapid decision regarding risk to be made on environmental chemicals, even when no data were supplied (9). In Europe, the 2001 White Paper setting out a 'strategy for a future chemicals policy' was implemented through the Registration, Evaluation, Authorisation and Restriction of Chemicals (REACH) legislation, stimulating an enormous uptake in techniques such as read-across (10).

The European Cosmetics Legislation, that led to a full ban on the marketing and sale of cosmetics ingredients tested after 2013 (even for the most-complex endpoints), has also stimulated the use of computational methods (11). Elsewhere, significant legislation in Canada (e.g. the screening and prioritisation of the Domestic Substance List (DSL; 12)), Japan and Australia has also created much interest in the use of (Q)SAR, and read-across methods to predict toxicity (13).

2.2 Driving Forces From Industry and Commercial Pressures

The requirements of various industries to assess their chemicals, to maximise safety for numerous uses, have also been a driver in the development of alternatives. The requirements of producers and manufacturers are often themselves driven by legislation (the European cosmetics industry being an excellent example) and commercial pressures. The rational design of molecules is a process that has been undertaken since the advent of the modern pharmaceutical industry in the 20th century. Traditionally, this was to identify novel active chemistries, and optimise activity in chemicals, or chemical series. By the 1990s, it became apparent that the traditional methods of drug development were at best inefficient, if not ineffective (14), with many molecules being highly active, when designed and tested *in vitro*, but having no activity *in vivo*, due to problems such as solubility (15).

The desire to avoid toxicity, and the 'fail early, fail fast, fail cheap' mantra meant that new *in silico* methods to screen out candidate molecules with toxicity, while retaining those with high bioavailability, were required. while pharmaceutical companies could obtain some *in silico* resources commercially, they have also had to spend considerable efforts and resources to develop in-house capabilities, the majority of which are not available publicly. There are many successes in these combined capabilities, particularly in areas such as identifying direct-acting mutagens, and screening out cardiotoxicity and other significant organ level effects (16—18). In addition, there has been substantial growth in the use of (Q)SAR methods, to screen for genotoxic impurities according to the ICH M7 regulation (19).

Other non-pharmaceutical industries have utilised *in silico* methods routinely to predict environmental toxicities since the 1980s (20). This was possible, in part, due not only to some of the excellent science and QSAR approaches for, for example, non-polar narcotics (21), but also to other legislative drivers, such as TSCA. It should be remembered that TSCA was the driver for other productive initiatives, resulting in important advances, such as the development of the fathead minnow acute toxicity database in the 1980s (cf. 22), and a better understanding of mechanisms of action (e.g. through the Fish Acute Toxicity Syndromes; 23). Since the 1980s, QSARs have been used for the prediction of acute, and to some extent chronic, toxicity as a result of the free distribution of the US EPA's ECOSAR software, as part of EPISuite (24).

The use of *in silico* methods in the pesticide industry is broadly analogous to that in the pharmaceutical industry, in that for several decades they were most-commonly used to identify new compounds and optimise activity. There are, however, important differences between the types of information that may be considered for pesticides and pharmaceuticals. Naturally there is not only a greater consideration of target and non-target species in the environment (cf. 25) but, possibly, also a greater reluctance to replace animal tests with alternatives. As these alternatives became cheaper, their use became more-predictive and greater confidence could be assigned to the outputs, there has been greater uptake, especially for human health effects such as skin sensitisation, and/or endocrine disruption (26).

Naturally, the cosmetics and personal products industries have supported the use of *in silico* methods for some time, particularly as these are often viewed as 'vanity' or non-essential items, thus not justifying animal experimentation. Even before the EU ban on the testing of cosmetics ingredients, there was widespread use of *in silico* approaches to predict endpoints, such as skin irritation and corrosion, skin sensitisation and mutagenicity. This support for the approaches assisted in the development of a number of the commercial models, and freely available software. The cosmetic industry, in struggling with the challenges of replacing animal tests, has also placed reliance on the development of *in vitro* assays (especially for the local dermal toxicities) and the use of strategies to combine the information obtained from them. As with many players in this area of science, the cosmetics industry also recognised the difficulty in using alternatives to replace the more-complex endpoints such as chronic, reproductive and developmental toxicities (27). In part, to address these challenges, the cosmetics industry responded to public pressure by supporting alternatives, giving significant financial support, e.g. through COLIPA/ Cosmetics Europe, and co-funding initiatives such as SEURAT-1 (28). Many cosmetics companies have shown a willingness to work with others in industry and academia, and with regulators, through these recent funding initiatives.

2.3 Drivers From Academic Research

Many early (Q)SAR studies — especially those that reached the peer-reviewed literature — were from academic researchers. This was perhaps because (Q)SAR analysis provides a greater opportunity to rationalise, model and comprehend the data, than simply reporting results alone. If data for a series of compounds are available, it makes good sense to model those to confirm or deny an underlying hypothesis, or mechanism of action. As data availability increased, along with descriptor calculation becoming freely available (e.g. in the early 1990s), academics were drawn to the area of models — especially those with a chemometrics background.

Many academics exploited increasingly multivariate statistical approaches, such as neural networks and support vector machines, to model larger data sets. However, some of these studies were inappropriate, and resulted in models that fitted the data very well (often beyond the statistical relevance of the original biological data) but had limited predictive capability (29). The ease of modelling enabled a solid supply of (Q)SARs to be developed, but this was hampered by a lack of appreciation for how the models would be used, and the requirements of industry and regulators. This came to a head after the publication of the OECD Principles for the Validation of (Q)SARs in the mid-2000s (30), when modelling became polarised between statistical and mechanistic approaches (31).

It is now acknowledged that there is a need for a broad spectrum of models. Interestingly, the past 5—10 years has seen the focus of *in silico* model development take a more mechanistic approach, as read-across and the use of Adverse Outcome Pathways (AOPs) became driving forces (10,32—34).

2.4 Socio-Economic Drivers

There are at least two main socio-economic drivers, possibly, competing, role. On the one hand, the 1960s crystallised movements against animal testing, but without any clear vision of how this could be achieved. There was also a realisation that environmental changes were occurring in many countries, resulting in polluted rivers, and the extinction of species.

The public demanded to know what the effects of chemicals were, and in addition to a cleaner environment, they wanted safer drugs, in the wake of the thalidomide disaster.

Thus, a desire for better and more-relevant information eventually resulted in legislation in the 1970s and 1980s (such as US TSCA and EU REACH). Because, initially, the information was likely to be available only from animal testing, this was rather at odds with the welfare movement. However, eventually, animal welfare NGOs facilitated progress, and have supported the deployment of *in silico* models. In addition, they have provided funding for more work in this area and, at times, have proved effective at raising the awareness of *in silico* resources, and potential to regulators, and the broader scientific community (35). Increasing globalisation has helped NGOs to promote the use of *in silico* alternatives and data resources, by using webinars and other training, and dissemination means (36).

2.5 The Visionaries Who Drove the Science

A technology can have the best concepts, but without the visionaries to tell us how it can be implemented and the leaders to take us there, little will be achieved.

Rightly, Corwin Hansch is recognised for his pioneering work in the development of QSARs (37), and, along with Al Leo (who made several thousand fundamental measurements of the logarithm of the octanol−water partition coefficient [log P] − a fundamental physicochemical property controlling the uptake, distribution, metabolism and elimination of a chemical; 38), laid the foundations of the science. When work on QSARs was somewhat unfashionable and a speciality, several researchers took it forward and championed it by establishing it on good science. Especially for environmental science, Gil Veith at the US EPA (39), Joop Hermens at Utrecht University (40), and Terry Schultz at University of Tennessee (41), demonstrated the crucial importance of high-quality data, mechanistic understanding and good science to succeed. For human health effects, John Ashby (with Ray Tennant) demonstrated how aspects of chemistry could be identified that are mechanistically related to mutagenicity (42).

A further note should also be made of scientists elsewhere. There is evidence of very significant progress in understanding the chemical basis of toxicology in the USSR in the 1970s − however, much of this work has been lost, or is not currently obtainable. For instance, a significant publication of structure activity relationships for toxicity appeared in 1975 (43), and several QSAR models were developed for predicting significant toxicity endpoints, and much useful data were accumulated refs. 44 and 45 being just two examples of what undoubtedly must be much more research conducted during this period. Some attempt was made to harvest data published in Russian (46). A mention should also be made of the agencies and institutions that enabled progress and development of *in silico* modelling. The US EPA provided enormous resources to support fundamental science in this area, and the development of software that has become the 'standard', e.g. EPISuite (24) and OncoLogic (47, 48).

In the EU, Walter Karcher, head of the (then) European Chemicals Bureau (7, 49), and Michael Balls, the first head of the European Centre for the Validation of Alternative Methods (ECVAM), both supported *in silico* models, and the creation of databases. Mention must be made of the previous work, guidance and tools that have come out of the European Commission's (EC's) Joint Research Centre (JRC), which have proved influential in Europe (and beyond), and have provided a real centre of excellence for science and training (cf. 50−52). This, in turn, must have influenced the EC to plough hundreds of millions of euros into funding, which created not only models but also networks and communities of workers with the overall objective of building capacity.

3. PREDICTION OF TOXICITY

3.1 Structure−Activity Relationships

Knowledge of the relationship between chemical structure and toxicity has evolved for well over a century, with no formal process other than the need to create new chemicals or optimise the activity of existing ones, or to understand and rationalise why a chemical causes toxicity. Nerve gases were used in World War I, undoubtedly, because the structure−activity relationships of some acutely toxic compounds were known, even if the exact mechanism of action was unknown. The implicit structure−activity of these chemicals is still relevant to this day (53). Better definitions of chemicals and their relationship to toxicity began to emerge in the 1950s, with the understanding of, for instance, the K region and bay region toward determining the carcinogenic potencies of polycyclic aromatic hydrocarbons (54), as well as requirements for the metabolic activation of compounds. The latter example, in particular, gave rise to what would become the concept of a toxicophore, i.e. a 3-D molecular configuration that is responsible for toxicity (55). Knowledge of such SARs became well known, but this knowledge was seldom − publicly, at least − compiled.

The Cramer classification system for 'toxicity' is an early example of how numerous SARs could be combined (56). The problem was that the SARs were often poorly described and defined (much of the knowledge was held by held by their developers), and without a mechanistic basis. The late 1980s brought publications describing groups of alerts for mutagenicity (42) and skin sensitisation (57–59). The change here was that the alerts were better defined and placed in the context of mechanistic toxicology and, for these particular endpoints, electrophilic chemistry. The 1980s also saw usable software — often called expert systems in those days, as they intended to capture the knowledge of experts — that could utilise these compilations of alerts (60).

Since the early 1990s, the concept of applying compilations of structural alerts to evaluate and predict toxicity has progressed rapidly, with the expansion to other endpoints and effects. Independently of the work on human health effects, a body of evidence, in the form of SARs, and particularly focusing on electrophilic reactivity, and specific mechanisms of acute toxicity, was built up to assign compounds to modes/mechanisms of action or groupings, for (acute) environmental effects. The scheme, published by Verhaar *et al.* (61), is still commonly applied today, albeit with a small number of updates (62). With regard to human health effects, and/or mammalian toxicity, many endpoints are covered, with the focus now moving from 'toxicity', as proposed by Cramer (56), to apical endpoints, e.g. carcinogenicity (63), and more recently, to organ level toxicity, for instance, focusing on alerts that attempt to define and unravel the mechanistic complexity of liver toxicity (32). Different types of information are being sought, to extract the data for alerts ranging from the traditional use of animal tests (e.g. ref. 42) to human data (e.g. respiratory sensitisation 64, 65), through to approaches, where large volumes of *in vitro* and high-throughput and/or content data can help the development of SARs (66, 67).

The development of compilations of structural alerts has also been stimulated by the availability of software that can capture them, and allow users to apply that knowledge. Bearing in mind that, until the late 1980s, the alerts were available only on paper, e.g. in journal articles or book chapters, they were difficult to use and open to misinterpretation, and may have been applied differently by different users. As noted above, in the late 1980s, systems such as DEREK (now called Derek Nexus from Lhasa Ltd) were becoming better known (60). Derek Nexus, and several other systems like it, have built up knowledge bases of well-documented toxicological SARs for a number of key endpoints. They are used across many industrial sectors and in academia.

Elsewhere, the 1990s saw free software being developed that gave the user access to SARs, such as the OncoLogic system (47, 48), which is still in use today. The last decade has given us many more resources, such as oChem, an on-line system that has attempted to compile as many SARs as possible (68), but does lack, at times, curation and mechanistic understanding. The JRC's Toxtree software has also incorporated a number of freely available sets of rules into a freely available and easy-to-use programme (69). The OECD QSAR Toolbox has many different sets of rules, organised by endpoint and mechanism — this is a remarkable compilation (70).

Overall, we have seen the development of SARs from a 'one chemical — one effect' scenario to compilations of alerts by endpoint, effect and, latterly, mechanism of action. The use of SARs is changing — they were originally intended to be predictions of hazard, and, indeed, systems such as Derek Nexus still fulfil this role. More-recently (see Section 4), read-across has become more-prominent, and software, such as the OECD QSAR Toolbox, has been designed to facilitate the categorisation of chemicals and, search for analogues. There is a need to better understand the role of SARs, and also to provide resources for curation, definition and mechanistic description.

3.2 Quantitative Structure–Activity Relationships

The technique of developing QSARs has been used, in part at least, to predict potency. QSARs are more reliant on large data sets of reliable toxicity values than are SARs, owing to the respective nature of the models; therefore, their development has often been limited, or even hampered, because of the requirement for data. This has, in part at least, led to differences of opinion as to whether they should be used for large 'global' data sets potentially covering many mechanisms and/or chemical classes or should be restricted to 'local' data sets, with more definable domains, chemical classes and mechanisms (31). There is no single or simple answer to this question — it depends on the endpoint being modelled, the type of data, the chemistry and mechanism(s) involved. As more data, and more approaches for modelling, have become available, there has been a growth in the development and publication of QSARs. However, much of this increase in modelling is a result of data availability, rather than being motivated by animal concerns, or the requirements of toxicologists and/or risk assessors.

From the mid-19th century until Hansch's publications in the 1960s (cf. 37, 38), a small number of key breakthroughs occurred in understanding the quantitative relationship between toxicological potency and chemical structure (71). Richet (72) showed that the more (water) soluble a molecule is, the less toxic it is, and Overton (73) and Meyer (74) placed anaesthetic potency (what we may now term non-polar narcosis, or basal cytotoxicity) in the context of hydrophobicity, quantified by partitioning between olive oil and water. Hansch's breakthrough (37) was to coin the term QSAR, and use regression analysis, to quantify biological activity in terms of descriptors for the hydrophobic, electronic and steric properties of molecules.

In terms of usable QSARs to predict toxicity, while a small amount of work was undertaken in the 1970s, the 1980s saw a growth in QSARs for endpoints such as acute environmental toxicity — for instance, Könemann's classic 1980 paper on a QSAR for non-polar narcosis (21) This approach could be described as being local, in that it covered a small number of compounds (about 50) and a single mechanism of action, although the chemical domain was broad, covering a number of classes. This 'local' QSAR approach was extended to human health endpoints in the 1990s, for instance, in Benigni's modelling of the mutagenicity of aromatic amines (75).

The early 1990s saw an increase in computational power that made the use of multivariate statistical analysis and, in particular, neural networks, practically possible. There were many attempts, and too many false dawns, to use neural networks to model toxicity — particularly for the larger, global data sets. They are attractive in terms of providing very high levels of statistical fit but are very prone to overfitting. Since the initial use of neural networks, increasing numbers of types of statistical analysis have been attempted, many simply with the ambition of creating the most-predictive model at the expense of transparency and mechanistic credibility. Techniques such as 'deep learning' are now being applied, but they must be used very cautiously, so as to avoid generating "irrelevant" models with little or no practical utility.

QSARs have, naturally, been amenable to being incorporated into computational software. The US EPA developed its own software, e.g. ECOSAR, in the late 1980s, which was eventually made freely available; the first author of this chapter remembers ECOSAR being distributed on 3-inch floppy disks at a conference in 1994, before the advent of the Internet. Also, companies such as Health Designs Inc (in the late 1980s) and MultiCase Inc (in the early 1990s), with their products TOPKAT and MultiCASE, respectively, led the way in terms of computational toxicology. By the late 1980s, Health Designs Inc had developed a PC-based product that contained models for a variety of mammalian and environmental toxicity endpoints. A prediction could be made from a SMILES string with some form of explanatory text, and 'similar' structures could be identified. Both these companies developed large data sets, and their own proprietary models. This was at a time of considerable scepticism toward these approaches, but they undoubtedly laid the groundwork for what is now a substantial commercial market. The modern approaches to predict toxicity, e.g. ChemTunes from Molecular Networks-Altamira (MN-AM), use the best parts of all approaches, combining SARs with QSARs, supported by large databases (76).

In some ways, the use of (Q)SARs for regulatory purposes has exposed some of their shortcomings. This is despite efforts to better describe the models, by using the QSAR Model Reporting Format and formalising their use through the application of the OECD Principles for the Validation of QSARs (30, 77). (Q)SARs have now become integral components of strategies for toxicity prediction, and making read-across more quantitative.

3.3 Read-Across

Read-across is the simplest of *in silico* techniques to predict toxicity and is, in many ways, inseparable from SARs and QSARs. The premise is straightforward — if two or more chemicals are similar, and toxicity data for one or more are available, then it could be assumed that the toxicity profiles of the molecules concerned closely overlap (78). The use of categories (or groups of similar chemicals) for regulatory assessment became established in the 1990s, if not before (78). Read-across was applied to various categories, especially within the High Production Volume Chemicals at OECD and other agencies. Early use was not well-documented or, by today's standards, well-justified. Early publications on read-across, e.g. Hathaway and Evans (79), report simply that it is possible within well-defined groups of chemicals.

Interest in read-across grew as a result of the REACH regulation and the EU ban on the animal testing of cosmetics. REACH encouraged the use of non-test methods, and by the late 2000s, considerable resources were placed into developing guidance (from the JRC, the ECHA and the OECD, among others), and the OECD QSAR Toolbox — which has been in continual development since version 1.0 was released in 2008 — became available. The Toolbox changed perceptions of read-across, and also provided a freely available tool for grouping and finding data. There was a much greater take-up of read-across for REACH submission than originally had been anticipated (10). At the same time, the need for better methods to predict, from structure if necessary, chronic and developmental and reproductive toxicity (DART) endpoints was recognised (27). Read-across rapidly came to be recognised as one of the solutions to this challenge, and stimulated a considerable research effort (80). In addition, the OECD Toolbox provided a more-mechanistic platform for read-across — where chemical similarity is only one of several means to group compounds; others means, in line with the guidance, include mechanisms, mode of action and metabolic similarity (78, 81).

The main issue with the regulatory use of read-across involved the interpretation of the legislation, which stated that an alternative must provide the same information as the original test. In evaluating read-across predictions for REACH, the ECHA was unable to satisfy itself of this criterion and inevitably rejected some submissions. This prompted an understandable outcry from some quarters (cf. 81–83), and a better understanding of why read-across predictions were being rejected (84). This inevitably has raised expectations from read-across, and has improved it in terms of scientific credibility. To assist with the assessment of read-across, various strategies have been proposed. Schultz *et al.* (85) and the Read-Across Assessment Framework (RAAF), published in 2017 by the ECHA (86), are good examples. There has been much discussion concerning read-across, characterised in four case studies (87–90), and a "lessons learned" paper (80) that have arisen from the SEURAT-1 research cluster.

The intense interest in read-across has also been a time when the development of other software has occurred, such as the freely available Toxmatch (91) and ToxRead (92) programmes. Read-across has now become the basis of constructing hypotheses on mechanisms of toxicity, having advanced from simply considering whether two chemicals are similar in structure. The ECHA (93) introduced the term 'New Approach Methodology' (NAM) data as a line of evidence – these include any relevant *in silico*, *in vitro*, -omics or HTC information. Related to this, the concept of 'chemical read-across' is now supported by the concept of 'biological read-across', where chemicals may be considered to be similar, if they have similar mechanistic or other profiles (94). In addition, the AOP framework provides a mechanistic basis to justify read-across hypotheses (32, 33).

4. CHEMOINFORMATICS

The development and availability of *in silico* models for toxicology is intrinsically linked to computational capabilities and tools. The obvious increase in computational power, and in access to computers, has had several effects. It has allowed computational calculations (e.g. for quantum chemistry), which hitherto would have been impossible, to be commonplace, and has provided all scientists with access to software and models. Graphical User Interfaces for chemistry are now standard, again allowing for the development of software, where a scientist can draw in a chemical structure. The Internet provides ready access to models and to data.

Because adequate computational power, access to computers and the Internet have been available for about 20 years, it is also worth considering the chemoinformatics changes and advances that have allowed for the development of this field. It was possible, albeit at great difficulty, and high cost, to show chemical structures on a computer screen by the 1960s. However, it was not until the late 1980s that colour graphics became more common, and a whole suite of computational chemistry software (e.g. through the Quantum Chemistry Program Exchange (QCPE)) became available. In those days, of course, software was distributed on tapes that had to be sent through the post! The real problem was the easy representation of chemical structure, such that it could be entered into a computer – this was solved, in part at least for 2-D structures, by the development of the Simplified Molecular-Input Line-Entry System strings – known ubiquitously as SMILES strings – thanks to funding from the US EPA, as part of Dr Gil Veith's vision, and the brilliance of the Weininger brothers (two California-based computer scientists; 95). SMILES permits the writing of a string of alphanumeric characters for chemical structure by using a standard keyboard alone – hence the double bond is represented by '=' and the triple bond by '#'. It was developed to allow for the calculation of log P, but is now (one of) the standard means of recording 2-D chemical structure, and allowing it to be entered into computational software.

Over the past decade, there has been increasing access to toxicological data. This is both in terms of the volume of data available and access to it. Even as recently as the 1980s, larger databases such as the Registry of Toxic Effects of Chemical Substances (RTECS) were distributed on microfiche, or as hard copy (e.g. the volumes that comprised the US EPA fathead minnow acute toxicity database). Modellers had to either spend months trawling through these compilations, or rely on the open literature. It was often months of hard work, or pure chance, which enabled sufficient publicly available data sets, which were suitable for modelling, to be found. The advent of the Internet, as a means of distributing information, was not enough. Free access to data also required investment in the data-basing technologies, and the cooperation of industry, regulators and other scientists to release information.

One of the first publicly available databases (even predating the Internet), which is still being updated, is the US EPA's ECOTOX compilation, which attempts to bring together all the literature and regulatory submissions for environmental toxicity (96). Current (publically available) data resources range from COSMOS DB for cosmetics ingredients (97, 98) and eChemPortal (99), which gives access to the ECHA and regulatory data to Internet compilations such as ChEMBL (100) and PubChem (101). The numbers of data range from the 10,000s to the 10,000,000s. In addition, more-sophisticated databases are becoming available, that capture greater depth of the study information and effects at different doses. For example, the eTox database has very detailed granularity in the relative effects of drugs at all dose levels (102). Recent advances in recording data have benefitted from progress in ontologies, and the better structuring of relational databases. The overall effect, particularly in the past 5 years, is that many more data, and much more mechanistic information, are now available.

The recent decades have seen a growth in free-to-use software for descriptor calculation and statistical modelling. Allied to the growth in databases, the modellers have much of what they need to proceed to create models. What was lacking, until about 5 years ago, was a means of successfully transferring models. Recently technologies, such as the KNIME data analytics pipeline, have greatly facilitated access to chemoinformatics tools and GUIs, with the result that models can be easily built and made publically available, without the need of proprietary software (66, 67).

5. PHYSIOLOGICALLY-BASED PHARMACOKINETIC MODELS

5.1 Introduction

Pharmacokinetics is the quantitative study of factors that determine the time-course of chemicals within the body, with regard to their absorption, distribution, metabolism and excretion (ADME). The goal of pharmacokinetic modelling in toxicology is to relate the internal concentrations of active entities at their sites of biological actions to the doses of the compound actually given to an animal or a human. The purpose of using internal exposure is due to the fundamental tenet in toxicology or pharmacology that both the efficacy and the toxicity of chemicals are related to the free concentrations of active compounds reaching target sites, e.g. tissues, cells and macromolecules, rather than the amount of compound at the site of absorption.

PBPK modelling offers a quantitative framework for integrating mechanistic data for physiological and biochemical processes, and serves as a tool to predict internal exposure at the target tissue/site for a wide range of exposure conditions in animals or humans. The mechanistic basis of PBPK models enhances their predictive power, permitting various applications in toxicity testing or the risk assessment context.

5.2 PBPK Modelling — Interspecies Extrapolation

The concept of PBPK modelling, also referred to as whole-body pharmacokinetic modelling, was first described in the context of drug disposition, and the literature on PBPK models dates back to the research of Haggard (103, 104), Teorell (105, 106), Kety (107), Mapleson (108), Riggs (109), Bischoff *et al.* (110) and Fiserova-Bergerova (111). These early PBPK modelling applications with volatile anaesthetics and chemotherapeutics provided clear examples of PBPK modelling concepts and strategies, and paved the way for applying PBPK modelling to toxicology questions in later years, when supported by increasing computational power and capabilities. Even though the primary developments in PBPK approaches by the chemical engineering community were with pharmaceuticals, the real expansion of the application of digital computation to creating PBPK models of increasing complexity since the 1980s occurred when these tools were applied to environmental chemicals and to risk assessment.

The pioneering work by Ramsey and Andersen (112) was based on the inter-institutional collaboration between the Dow Chemical Company and Wright-Patterson Air Force Base. This highlighted the ability of PBPK models to support the extrapolations of tissue dosimetry across dose, dose route and species. The ability of PBPK modelling to support extrapolation to untested or untestable conditions is an essential part of risk assessment. This has made PBPK modelling an attractive tool in human health risk assessments, leading to widespread acceptance of the models of various compounds by regulators (113–116).

PBPK models have played important roles in unravelling dose-response behaviours based on the estimates of tissue dose, and have revolutionised low dose and interspecies extrapolations in risk assessment (reviewed in several publications, e.g. Refs. 117–121). These PBPK models encompass a wide range of volatile compounds of occupational and environmental significance and can also be applied to many other classes of chemicals, including metals, inorganic chemicals, pesticides, persistent organic pollutants, drugs and the metabolites of these classes of chemicals (see the PBPK model knowledge base compiled by Lu *et al.* (122)).

5.3 PBPK Modelling — *In Vitro* to *In Vivo* Extrapolation

In addition to the above 'traditional' applications, PBPK modelling has now emerged as a critical translational tool for linking *in vitro* and *in silico* toxicity estimates to *in vivo* conditions. These applications are essential to support modern toxicological testing and new approaches to 21st century safety assessments. This area of work has been referred as quantitative *in vitro* to *in vivo* extrapolation (QIVIVE; reviewed by Yoon *et al.* (123) and in a special issue on QIVIVE in Toxicology, edited by Yoon, Clewell and Blaauboer (124)). Curiously, the physiological and mechanistic basis of these models are both strengths (the mechanistic basis provides exceptional utility) and limitations. For instance, PBPK models can be expensive and time-consuming to construct, depending on the data sets available, or necessary for their construction/validation.

Obtaining chemical-specific parameters, and those for metabolism, in particular, has been a significant bottleneck in expanding the use of PBPK models to a wider range of chemicals and in gaining acceptance by regulatory agencies even for their 'traditional' applications of PBPK models to chemical-specific toxicity testing and risk assessments (125, 126). Additionally, there is the frequent concern of specificity with individual compounds versus the need to evaluate pharmacokinetics of a large number of chemicals. In adapting the new toxicity testing and safety assessment methods, it is essential to improve the 'throughput' of QIVIVE with 'rapid' PBPK modelling capabilities. The example of the recent rise in PBPK modelling and simulation in drug discovery and development (127−129) shows similar driving forces of increased efficiency in decision-making. For the pharmaceutical industry, there has been increasing pressure to accelerate the drug development process. PBPK modelling has been repeatedly shown as an enabling technology for this transition (130−132).

Recent advances with *in silico/in vitro*-based prediction tools, and in particular those for absorption, distribution and hepatic clearance, and the emergence of 'ready to use' PBPK software tools, such as SimCyp, have illustrated the above developments (133). The work on *in vitro* and *in silico*-based parameterisation strategies with a number of environmental chemicals (reviewed by Yoon *et al.* (123)) shows great progress with the promise of applying those tools to build 'generic' PBPK modelling platforms dedicated to environmental chemicals that are similar in design to SimCyp. In fact, there has been a significant surge in the development of generic PBPK model platforms in the USA and the EU. PLETHEM (134, 135), Httk (136) and RVis (137) are some examples of such platforms, which aim to support the rapid PBPK modelling of environmental chemicals in support of new toxicity testing directions, which emphasise *in vitro* and tiered risk assessment approaches.

6. FUTURE DEVELOPMENTS

There is no doubt that *in silico* methods to predict toxicity are here to stay. There is more than adequate computational capability and even freely available software. The methods behind (Q)SAR are well established and, in reality, need little further development. Read-across as an application of this knowledge is increasing and, is likely to grow further, especially with regard to the chronic and DART endpoints − both for human health and environmental species.

Areas of further meaningful growth are likely to be as follows:

- Further compilation of toxicity data from different sources.
- Better organisation of the data in terms of the level of information that is recorded (i.e. going beyond the paradigm of 'chemical name and toxicity' to something that takes full advantage of relational databases to extract meaningful information).
- Further building of models based around the information contained within an AOP.
- Mining and modelling the enormous data compilations with a mechanistic background, e.g. Tox21, ChEMBL and PubChem.
- Better understanding and quantification of uncertainty within (Q)SARs and read-across, as well as in their predictions.
- Furthering the read-across paradigm to allow for better justifications of similarity hypotheses.
- Development of well-defined groups of chemicals for which read-across is achievable.
- Learning from industrial sectors, such as pharmaceutical sector, which have a rich history and knowledge base in the use of *in silico* methods to predict toxicity.
- Better application of all *in silico* methods as part of strategies or IATA to predict toxicity.
- Development of generic PBPK modelling platforms to rapidly predict *in vivo* kinetics based on *in vitro* and *in silico* data.

Of all these, it is the final issue of how we best use *in silico* methods for a particular decision that will require the most effort. This is being considered, in part, in relation to read-across, but we must also consider the stand-alone evaluation of chemicals for product development and regulatory purposes.

7. CONCLUSIONS

Computational techniques to predict toxicity from structure have been alluring for decades. The possibility of entering a chemical structure into a piece of software, to obtain the same information as from an *in vivo* test, is immensely advantageous. There are a number of well-established (Q)SAR techniques and tools that can be applied to predict toxicity. For some endpoints (e.g. mutagenicity and fish acute toxicity), for some chemicals and/or mechanisms of action, these work relatively well. However, they require better development for complex effects such as chronic and DART endpoints.

Read-across has offered the possibility of real progress to predict toxicity from structure, although it must be noted that its transparency has laid bare many of the deficiencies of this whole area. It is essential that, in the future, we understand the limitations and uncertainties of computational methods to predict toxicity.

Rapid prediction of *in vivo* pharmacokinetics, supported by *in silico* prediction of chemical specific ADME data, including biotransformations, can provide a quantitative bridge between *in silico* predicted toxicity and human safe exposure. In addition, computational methods must be at the heart of 21st century toxicology, rather than being considered to be at the periphery or a mere add-on.

REFERENCES

1. Cronin, M.T.D. & Livingstone, D.J. (Eds.). (2004). *Predicting Chemical Toxicity and Fate*. Boca Raton FL, USA: CRC Press, 445pp.
2. Cronin, M.T.D. & Madden, J.C. (Eds.). (2010). *In Silico Toxicology: Principles and Applications*. Cambridge, UK: The Royal Society of Chemistry, 669pp.
3. Cronin, M.T.D., Madden, J.C., Enoch, S.J., *et al.* (2013). *Chemical Toxicity Prediction: Category Formation and Read-Across*, 191pp. Cambridge, UK: The Royal Society of Chemistry.
4. Cronin, M.T.D., Walker, J.D., Jaworska, J.S., *et al.* (2003). Use of QSARs in international decision-making frameworks to predict ecologic effects and environmental fate of chemical substances. *Environmental Health Perspectives* **111**, 1376−1390.
5. Cronin, M.T.D., Jaworska, J.S., Walker, J.D., *et al.* (2003). Use of QSARs in international decision-making frameworks to predict health effects of chemical substances. *Environmental Health Perspectives* **111**, 1391−1401.
6. Richard, A.M. (1998). Commercial toxicology prediction systems: a regulatory perspective. *Toxicology Letters* **103**, 611−616.
7. Karcher, W. & Karabunarliev, S. (1996). The use of computer based structure-activity relationships in the risk assessment of industrial chemicals. *Journal of Chemical Information and Computer Sciences* **36**, 672−677.
8. Worth, A.P., van Leeuwen, C.J. & Hartung, T. (2004). The prospects for using (Q)SARs in a changing political environment-high expectations and a key role for the European Commission's Joint Research Centre. *SAR and QSAR in Environmental Research* **15**, 331−343.
9. United States Environmental Protection Agency. (2016). *Summary of the Toxic Substances Control Act 1976*, 1p. Washington, DC, USA: Environmental Protection Agency.
10. Spielmann, H., Sauer, U.G. & Mekenyan, O. (2011). A critical evaluation of the 2011 ECHA reports on compliance with the REACH and CLP regulations and on the use of alternatives to testing on animals for compliance with the REACH regulation. *ATLA* **39**, 481−493.
11. European Commission. (2009). Regulation (EC) No 1223/2009 of the European Parliament and of the Council of 30 November 2009 on cosmetic products. *Official Journal of the European Union* **L343**, 59−209.
12. Environment and Climate Change Canada. (1994). *Domestic Substances List (DSL)*, 1pp. Gatineau, QC, Canada: Environment and Climate Change Canada.
13. Tunkel, J., Mayo, K., Austin, C., *et al.* (2005). Practical considerations on the use of predictive models for regulatory purposes. *Environmental Science and Technology* **39**, 2188−2199.
14. Paul, S.M., Mytelka, D.S., Dunwiddie, C.T., *et al.* (2010). How to improve R&D productivity: the pharmaceutical industry's grand challenge. *Nature Reviews Drug Discovery* **9**, 203−214.
15. Lipinski, C.A., Lombardo, F., Dominy, B.W., *et al.* (1997). Experimental and computational approaches to estimate solubility and permeability in drug discovery and development settings. *Advanced Drug Delivery Reviews* **23**, 3−25.
16. Kruhlak, N.L., Benz, R.D., Zhou, H., *et al.* (2012). (Q)SAR modelling and safety assessment in regulatory review. *Clinical Pharmacology & Therapeutics* **91**, 529−534.
17. Yang, C.H., Valerio, L.G. & Arvidson, K.B. (2009). Computational toxicology approaches at the US Food and Drug Administration. *ATLA* **37**, 523−531.
18. Arvidson, K.B., Chanderbhan, R., Muldoon-Jacobs, K., *et al.* (2010). Regulatory use of computational toxicology tools and databases at the United States Food and Drug Administration's Office of Food Additive Safety. *Expert Opinion on Drug Metabolism and Toxicology* **6**, 793−796.
19. Fioravanzo, E., Bassan, A., Pavan, M., *et al.* (2012). Role of *in silico* genotoxicity tools in the regulatory assessment of pharmaceutical impurities. *SAR and QSAR in Environmental Research* **23**, 257−277.
20. Bradbury, S.P., Russom, C.L., Ankley, G.T., *et al.* (2003). Overview of data and conceptual approaches for derivation of quantitative structure-activity relationships for ecotoxicological effects of organic chemicals. *Environmental Toxicology and Chemistry* **22**, 1789−1798.
21. Könemann, H. (1981). Quantitative structure-activity relationships in fish toxicity studies. 1. Relationship for 50 industrial pollutants. *Toxicology* **19**, 209−221.

22. Russom, C.L., Bradbury, S.P., Broderius, S.J., *et al.* (1997). Predicting modes of toxic action from chemical structure: Acute toxicity in the fathead minnow (*Pimephales promelas*). *Environmental Toxicology and Chemistry* **16**, 948–967.

23. McKim, J.M., Bradbury, S.P. & Niemi, G.J. (1987). Fish Acute Toxicity Syndromes and their use in the QSAR approach to hazard assessment. *Environmental Health Perspectives* **71**, 171–186.

24. Card, M.L., Gomez-Alvarez, V., Lee, W.H., *et al.* (2017). History of EPI Suite((TM)) and future perspectives on chemical property estimation in US Toxic Substances Control Act new chemical risk assessments. *Environmental Science - Processes and Impacts* **19**, 203–212.

25. Porcelli, C., Boriani, E., Roncaglioni, A., *et al.* (2008). Regulatory perspectives in the use and validation of QSAR. A case study: DEMETRA model for Daphnia toxicity. *Environmental Science and Technology* **42**, 491–496.

26. Orton, F., Rosivatz, E., Scholze, M., *et al.* (2011). Widely used pesticides with previously unknown endocrine activity revealed as *in vitro* anti-androgens. *Environmental Health Perspectives* **119**, 794–800.

27. Adler, S., Basketter, D., Creton, S., *et al.* (2011). Alternative (non-animal) methods for cosmetics testing: current status and future prospects-2010. *Archives of Toxicology* **85**, 367–485.

28. Gocht, T. & Schwarz, M. (Eds.). (2016). *Towards the Replacement of in vivo Repeated Dose Systemic Toxicity Testing,* Vol. 6, 421pp. Paris, France: COACH Consortium.

29. Dearden, J.C., Cronin, M.T.D. & Kaiser, K.L.E. (2009). How not to develop a quantitative structure-activity or structure-property relationship (QSAR/QSPR). *SAR and QSAR in Environmental Research* **20**, 241–266.

30. Worth, A.P. (2010). The role of QSAR methodology in the regulatory assessment of chemicals. In T. Puzyn, J. Lesczynski & M.T.D. Cronin (Eds.), *Recent Advances in QSAR Studies: Methods and Applications*, pp. 367–382. Dordrecht, The Netherlands: Springer.

31. Enoch, S.J., Cronin, M.T.D., Schultz, T.W., *et al.* (2008). An evaluation of global QSAR models for the prediction of the toxicity of phenols to Tetrahymena pyriformis. *Chemosphere* **71**, 1225–1232.

32. Cronin, M.T.D., Enoch, S.J., Mellor, C.L., *et al.* (2017). *In silico* prediction of organ level toxicity: linking chemistry to adverse effects. *Toxicological Research* **33**, 173–182.

33. Cronin, M.T.D. & Richarz, A.-N. (2017). Relationship between Adverse Outcome Pathways and chemistry-based *in silico* models to predict toxicity. *Applied In Vitro Toxicology* **3**, 286–297.

34. Delrue, N., Sachana, M., Sakuratani, Y., *et al.* (2016). The Adverse Outcome Pathway concept: a basis for developing regulatory decision-making tools. *ATLA* **44**, 417–429.

35. Sullivan, K.M., Manuppello, J.R. & Willett, C.E. (2014). Building on a solid foundation: SAR and QSAR as a fundamental strategy to reduce animal testing. *SAR and QSAR in Environmental Research* **25**, 357–365.

36. ChemicalWatch. (2014). Six alternative testing webinars. Available at. https://chemicalwatch.com/peta-webinars/.

37. Hansch, C., Maloney, P.P., Fujita, T., *et al.* (1962). Correlation of biological activity of phenoxyacetic acids with Hammett substituent constants and partition coefficients. *Nature, London* **194**, 178–180.

38. Leo, A., Hansch, C. & Elkins, D. (1971). Partition coefficients and their uses. *Chemical Reviews* **71**, 525–616.

39. Schultz, T.W. (2014). Gilman D. Veith (1944-2013) - A dedication. *SAR and QSAR in Environmental Research* **25**, 249–251.

40. Hermens, J.L.M. (1990). Electrophiles and acute toxicity to fish. *Environmental Health Perspectives* **87**, 219–225.

41. Cronin, M.T.D. (2013). International QSAR Award Winner 2012: Prof Terry Wayne Schultz. *SAR and QSAR in Environmental Research* **24**, 521–523.

42. Ashby, J. & Tennant, R.W. (1988). Chemical-structure, *Salmonella* mutagenicity and extent of carcinogenicity as indicators of genotoxic carcinogenesis among 222 chemicals tested in rodents by the United States NCI/NTP. *Mutation Research* **204**, 17–115.

43. Ljublina, E.I. & Filov, V.A. (1975). Chemical structure physical and chemical properties and biological activity. In *Methods used in the USSR for Establishing Biologically Safe Levels of Toxic Substances — Meeting. Moscow, USSR, 12–19 December 1972*, pp. 19–44. Geneva, Switzerland: WHO.

44. Belik, A.V. & Lebedeva, M.N. (1988). Prediction of acute toxicity of benzimidazole series compounds by electron structure of their molecules. *Farmakologiya i Toksikologiya* **51**, 100–104.

45. Izmerov, N.F., Sanotsky, I.V. & Sidorov, K.K. (1982). *Toxicometric Parameters of Industrial Toxic Chemicals Under Single Chemical Exposure*, 160pp. Moscow, USSR: United Nations Environment Programme (UNEP). International Register of Potentially Toxic Chemicals (IPRTC).

46. Sihtmaee, M., Blinova, I., Aruoja, V., *et al.* (2010). E-SovTox: An online database of the main publicly-available sources of toxicity data concerning REACH-relevant chemicals published in the Russian language. *ATLA* **38**, 297–301.

47. Woo, Y.T. & Lai, D.Y. (2005). OncoLogic: A mechanism-based expert system for predicting the carcinogenic potential of chemicals. In C. Helma (Ed.), *Predictive Toxicology*, pp. 385–413. New York, NY, USA: Dekker.

48. Woo, Y.T., Lai, D.Y., Argus, M.F., *et al.* (1995). Development of structure-activity relationship rules for predicting carcinogenic potential of chemicals. *Toxicology Letters* **79**, 219–228.

49. Karcher, W. & Devillers, J. (1990). SAR and QSAR in environmental chemistry and toxicology - scientific tool or wishful thinking? In W. Karcher & J. Devillers (Eds.), *Practical Applications of Quantitative Structure-Activity Relationships (QSAR) in Environmental Chemistry and Toxicology*, pp. 1–12. Brussels, Belgium: Eurocourses - Chemical and Environmental Science.

50. Worth, A.P., Hartung, T. & van Leeuwen, C.J. (2004). The role of the European Centre for the Validation of Alternative Methods (ECVAM) in the validation of (Q)SARs. *SAR and QSAR in Environmental Research* **15**, 345–358.

51. Worth, A.P. & Mostrag-Szlichtyng, A. (2012). Towards a common regulatory framework for computational toxicology: current status and future perspectives. In A.G.E. Wilson (Ed.), *New Horizons in Predictive Toxicology: Current Status and Application*, pp. 38–69. Cambridge, UK: The Royal Society of Chemistry.

52. Pavan, M. & Worth, A.P. (2008). Publicly-accessible QSAR software tools developed by the Joint Research Centre. *SAR and QSAR in Environmental Research* **19**, 785–799.

53. Kovacic, P. (2003). Mechanism of organophosphates (nerve gases and pesticides) and antidotes: Electron transfer and oxidative stress. *Current Medicinal Chemistry* **10**, 2705–2709.

54. Loew, G.H., Sudhindra, B.S. & Ferrell, J.E. (1979). Quantum chemical studies of polycyclic aromatics hydrocarbons and their metabolites - correlations to carcinogenicity. *Chemico-biological Interactions* **26**, 75–89.

55. Madden, J.C. & Cronin, M.T.D. (2010). Three-dimensional molecular modelling of receptor-based mechanisms in toxicology. In M.T.D. Cronin & J.C. Madden (Eds.), *In silico toxicology: Principles and applications*, pp. 210–227. Cambridge, UK: The Royal Society of Chemistry.

56. Cramer, G.M., Ford, R.A. & Hall, R.L. (1978). Estimation of toxic hazard - decision tree approach. *Food and Cosmetics Toxicology* **16**, 255–276.

57. Payne, M.P. & Walsh, P.T. (1994). Structure-activity relationships for skin sensitization potential - development of structural alerts for use in knowledge-based toxicity prediction systems. *Journal of Chemical Information and Computer Sciences* **34**, 154–161.

58. Barratt, M.D., Basketter, D.A., Chamberlain, M., *et al.* (1994). An expert-system rulebase for identifying contact allergens. *Toxicology in Vitro* **8**, 1053–1060.

59. Cronin, M.T.D. & Basketter, D.A. (1993). A QSAR evaluation of an existing contact allergy database. In C.G. Wermuth (Ed.), *Trends in QSAR and Molecular Modelling*, Vol. 92, 297–298pp. Leiden, The Netherlands: Escom.

60. Sanderson, D.M. & Earnshaw, C.G. (1991). Computer prediction of possible toxic action from chemical structure; the DEREK system. *Human & Experimental Toxicology* **10**, 261–273.

61. Verhaar, H.J.M., van Leeuwen, C.J. & Hermens, J.L.M. (1992). Classifying environmental pollutants. 1. Structure-Activity Relationships for prediction of aquatic toxicity. *Chemosphere* **25**, 471–491.

62. Ellison, C.M., Madden, J.C., Cronin, M.T.D., *et al.* (2015). Investigation of the Verhaar scheme for predicting acute aquatic toxicity: Improving predictions obtained from Toxtree ver. 2.6. *Chemosphere* **139**, 146–154.

63. Benigni, R., Andreoli, C. & Giuliani, A. (1989). Quantitative structure-activity relationships - principles, and applications to mutagenicity and carcinogenicity. *Mutation Research* **221**, 197–216.

64. Enoch, S.J., Seed, M.J., Roberts, D.W., *et al.* (2012). Development of mechanism-based structural alerts for respiratory sensitization hazard identification. *Chemical Research in Toxicology* **25**, 2490–2498.

65. Enoch, S.J., Roberts, D.W. & Cronin, M.T.D. (2009). Electrophilic reaction chemistry of low molecular weight respiratory sensitizers. *Chemical Research in Toxicology* **22**, 1447–1453.

66. Steinmetz, F.P., Mellor, C.L., Meinl, T., *et al.* (2015). Screening chemicals for receptor-mediated toxicological and pharmacological endpoints: using public data to build screening tools within a KNIME workflow. *Molecular Informatics* **34**, 171–178.

67. Mellor, C.L., Steinmetz, F.P. & Cronin, M.T.D. (2016). Using molecular initiating events to develop a structural alert based screening workflow for nuclear receptor ligands associated with hepatic steatosis. *Chemical Research in Toxicology* **29**, 203–212.

68. Sushko, I., Novotarskyi, S., Koerner, R., *et al.* (2011). Online chemical modelling environment (OCHEM): web platform for data storage, model development and publishing of chemical information. *Journal of Computer-aided Molecular Design* **25**, 533–554.

69. Patlewicz, G., Jeliazkova, N., Safford, R.J., *et al.* (2008). An evaluation of the implementation of the Cramer classification scheme in the Toxtree software. *SAR and QSAR in Environmental Research* **19**, 495–524.

70. Diderich, R. (2010). Tools for category formation and read-across: Overview of the OECD (Q)SAR Application Toolbox. In M.T.D. Cronin & J.C. Madden (Eds.), *In Silico Toxicology: Principles and Applications*, pp. 385–407. Cambridge, UK: The Royal Society of Chemistry.

71. Schultz, T.W., Cronin, M.T.D., Walker, J.D., *et al.* (2003). Quantitative structure-activity relationships (QSARs) in toxicology: a historical perspective. *Journal of Molecular Structure - Theochem* **622**, 1–22.

72. Richet, C. (1893). Sur le rapport entre la toxicité et les propriétés physiques des corps. *Comptes Rendus des Séances de la Société de Biologie (Paris)* **45**, 775–776.

73. Overton, C.E. (1901). *Studien über die Narkose zugleich ein Beitrag zur allgemeinen Pharmakologie*, 195pp. Jena, Switzerland: Gustav Fischer.

74. Meyer, H. (1901). Zur Theorie der Alkoholnarkose. Der Einfluss wechselnder Temperatur auf Wirkungsstärke und Theilungscoefficient der Narcotica. *Archiv für Experimentelle Pathologie und Pharmakologie* **46**, 338–346.

75. Benigni, R., Andreoli, C. & Giuliani, A. (1994). QSAR models for both mutagenic potency and activity - application to nitroarenes and aromatics amines. *Environmental and Molecular Mutagenesis* **24**, 208–219.

76. Anon. (2017). *ChemTunes - Platform and Toxicity Database*. Columbus, OH, USA: Altamira LLC.

77. Hewitt, M., Ellison, C.M., Cronin, M.T.D., *et al.* (2015). Ensuring confidence in predictions: A scheme to assess the scientific validity of *in silico* models. *Advanced Drug Delivery Reviews* **86**, 101–111.

78. Cronin, M.T.D. (2013). Evaluation of categories and read-across for toxicity prediction allowing for regulatory acceptance. In M.T.D. Cronin, J.C. Madden, S.J. Enoch & D.W. Roberts (Eds.), *Chemical Toxicity Prediction: Category Formation and Read-Across*, pp. 155–167. Cambridge, UK: The Royal Society of Chemistry.

79. Hanway, R.H. & Evans, P.F. (2000). Read-across of toxicological data in the notification of new chemicals. *Toxicology Letters* **116**(Suppl. 1), 61.

80. Schultz, T.W. & Cronin, M.T.D. (2017). Lessons learned from read-across case studies for repeated-dose toxicity. *Regulatory Toxicology and Pharmacology* **88**, 185–191.

81. Patlewicz, G., Ball, N., Booth, E.D., *et al.* (2013). Use of category approaches, read-across and (Q)SAR: General considerations. *Regulatory Toxicology and Pharmacology* **67**, 1–12.

82. Ball, N., Bartels, M., Budinsky, R., *et al.* (2014). The challenge of using read-across within the EU REACH regulatory framework; how much uncertainty is too much? Dipropylene glycol methyl ether acetate, an exemplary case study. *Regulatory Toxicology and Pharmacology* **68**, 212–221.

83. Patlewicz, G., Ball, N., Boogaard, P.J., *et al.* (2015). Building scientific confidence in the development and evaluation of read-across. *Regulatory Toxicology and Pharmacology* **72**, 117–133.

84. Ball, N., Cronin, M.T.D., Shen, J., *et al.* (2016). Toward Good Read-Across Practice (GRAP) guidance. *ALTEX* **33**, 149–166.

85. Schultz, T.W., Amcoff, P., Berggren, E., *et al.* (2015). A strategy for structuring and reporting a read-across prediction of toxicity. *Regulatory Toxicology and Pharmacology* **72**, 586–601.

86. European Chemicals Agency (ECHA). (2017). *Read-across Assessment Framework (RAAF)*, 60pp. Helsinki, Finland: ECHA.

87. Przybylak, K.R., Schultz, T.W., Richarz, A.-N., *et al.* (2017). Read-across of 90-day rat oral repeated-dose toxicity: A case study for selected β-olefinic alcohols. *Computational Toxicology* **1**, 22–32.

88. Mellor, C.L., Schultz, T.W., Przybylak, K.R., *et al.* (2017). Read-across for rat oral gavage repeated-dose toxicity for short-chain mono-alkyl-phenols: A case study. *Computational Toxicology* **2**, 1–11.

89. Schultz, T.W., Przybylak, K.R., Richarz, A.-N., *et al.* (2017). Read-across of 90-day rat oral repeated-dose toxicity: A case study for selected n-alkanols. *Computational Toxicology* **2**, 12–19.

90. Schultz, T.W., Przybylak, K.R., Richarz, A.-N., *et al.* (2017). Read-across of 90-day rat oral repeated-dose toxicity: A case study for selected 2-alkyl-1-alkanols. *Computational Toxicology* **2**, 28.

91. Patlewicz, G., Jeliazkova, N., Saliner, A.G., *et al.* (2008). Toxmatch - a new software tool to aid in the development and evaluation of chemically similar groups. *SAR and QSAR in Environmental Research* **19**, 397–412.

92. Gini, G., Franchi, A.M., Manganaro, A., *et al.* (2014). ToxRead: A tool to assist in read across and its use to assess mutagenicity of chemicals. *SAR and QSAR in Environmental Research* **25**, 999–1011.

93. European Chemicals Agency (ECHA). (2016). New approach methodologies in regulatory science. In *Proceedings of a Scientific Workshop, 19–20 April 2016, Helsinki*. Helsinki, Finland: ECHA, 65pp.

94. Zhu, H., Bouhifd, M., Donley, E., *et al.* (2016). Supporting read-across using biological data. *ALTEX* **33**, 167–182.

95. Weininger, D. (1988). SMILES, a chemical language and information system. 1. Introduction to methodology and encoding rules. *Journal of Chemical Information and Modelling* **28**, 31–36.

96. United States Environmental Protection Agency (US EPA). (2017). *ECOTOX Database*. Duluth, MN, USA: US EPA. https://cfpub.epa.gov/ecotox/.

97. Yang, C., Hristozov, D., Tarkhov, A., *et al.* (2015). COSMOS DB as an international share point for exchanging regulatory and toxicity data of cosmetics ingredients and related substances. *Toxicology Letters* **238**, S382.

98. Mostrag-Szlichtyng, A. (2017). *Development of Knowledge Within a Chemical-Toxicological Database to Formulate Novel Computational Approaches for Predicting Repeated Dose Toxicity of Cosmetics-Related Compounds*. PhD Thesis, Liverpool John Moores University (UK), 162pp. available at: http://researchonline.ljmu.ac.uk/6798/1/2017mostrag-szlichtyngphd.pdf.

99. Organisation for Economic Cooperation and Development (OECD). (2017). *eChemPortal Database*. Paris, France: OECD.

100. Gaulton, A., Bellis, L.J., Bento, A.P., *et al.* (2012). ChEMBL: a large-scale bioactivity database for drug discovery. *Nucleic Acids Research* **40**, D1100–D1107.

101. Wang, Y., Xiao, J., Suzek, T.O., *et al.* (2009). PubChem: a public information system for analysing bioactivities of small molecules. *Nucleic Acids Research* **37**, W623–W633.

102. Briggs, K., Cases, M., Heard, D.J., *et al.* (2012). Inroads to predict *in vivo* toxicology - an introduction to the eTOX Project. *International Journal of Molecular Sciences* **13**, 3820–3846.

103. Haggard, H.W. (1924). The absorption, distribution, and elimination of ethyl ether II. Analysis of the mechanism of absorption and elimination of such a gas or vapor as ethyl ether. *Journal of Biological Chemistry* **59**, 753–770.

104. Haggard, H.W. (1924). The absorption, distribution, and elimination of ethyl ether iii. The relation of the concentration of ether, or any similar volatile substance, in the central nervous system to the concentration in the arterial blood, and the buffer action of the body. *Journal of Biological Chemistry* **59**, 771–781.

105. Teorell, T. (1937). Kinetics of distribution of substances administered to the body, I: The extravascular modes of administration. *Archives Internationales de Pharmacodynamie et de Therapie* **57**, 205–225.

106. Teorell, T. (1937). Kinetics of distribution of substances administered to the body, II: the intravascular modes of administration. *Archives Internationales de Pharmacodynamie et de Therapie* **57**, 226–240.

107. Kety, S.S. (1951). The theory and applications of the exchange of inert gas at the lungs and tissues. *Pharmacological Reviews* **3**, 1–41.

108. Mapleson, W.W. (1963). An electric analogue for uptake and exchange of inert gases and other agents. *Journal of Applied Physiology* **18**, 197–204.

109. Riggs, D.S. (1963). *The Mathematical Approach to Physiological Problems: A Critical Primer*, 445pp. Cambridge, MA, USA: MIT Press.

110. Bischoff, K.B., Dedrick, R.L., Zaharko, D.S., *et al.* (1971). Methotrexate pharmacokinetics. *Journal of Pharmaceutical Sciences* **60**, 1128–1133.

111. Fiserova-Bergerova, V. (1976). Mathematical modelling of inhalation exposure. *Journal of Combustion Toxicology* **3**, 201–210.

112. Ramsey, J.C. & Andersen, M.E. (1984). A physiologically based description of the inhalation pharmacokinetics of styrene in rats and humans. *Toxicology and Applied Pharmacology* **73**, 159–175.

113. Clewell, H.J. & Andersen, M.E. (1985). Risk assessment extrapolations and physiological modelling. *Toxicology and Industrial Health* **1**, 111–131.

114. Clewell, R.A. & Clewell, H.J. (2008). Development and specification of physiologically based pharmacokinetic models for use in risk assessment. *Regulatory Toxicology and Pharmacology* **50**, 129–143.

115. Anon. (1987). Pharmacokinetics in Risk Assessment. In *Drinking Water and Health,* Vol. 8, 512pp. Washington, DC, USA: The National Academy Press.

116. Loizou, G., Spendiff, M., Barton, H.A., *et al.* (2008). Development of good modelling practice for physiologically based pharmacokinetic models for use in risk assessment: the first steps. *Regulatory Toxicology and Pharmacology* **50**, 400–411.

117. Clewell, H.J., Andersen, M.E. & Barton, H.A. (2002). A consistent approach for the application of pharmacokinetic modelling in cancer and noncancer risk assessment. *Environmental Health Perspectives* **110**, 85–93.

118. Krishnan, K. & Andersen, M.E. (2007). Physiologically based pharmacokinetic modelling in toxicology. In A.W. Hayes (Ed.), *Principles and Methods of Toxicology*, pp. 193–241. New York NY, USA: Taylor and Francis.

119. Lipscomb, J.C. & Ohanian, E.V. (Eds.). (2006). *Toxicokinetics and Risk Assessment.* New York, NY, USA: Informa Healthcare.

120. Reddy, M., Yang, R.S., Clewell, H.J., *et al.* (2005). *Physiologically Based Pharmacokinetic Modelling: Science and Applications*, 420pp. Hoboken, NJ, USA: John Wiley & Sons, Inc.

121. EPA. (2006). *Approaches for the Application of Physiologically Based Pharmacokinetic (PBPK) Models and Supporting data in Risk Assessment, EPA 600/R-05/043A,* 123pp. Washington, DC, USA: US EPA.

122. Lu, J., Goldsmith, M.R., Grulke, C.M., *et al.* (2016). Developing a physiologically-based pharmacokinetic model knowledgebase in support of provisional model construction. *PLoS Computational Biology* **12**, e1004495.

123. Yoon, M., Campbell, J.L., Andersen, M.E., *et al.* (2012). Quantitative *in vitro* to *in vivo* extrapolation of cell-based toxicity assay results. *Critical Reviews in Toxicology* **42**, 633–652.

124. Quantitative *in vitro* to *in vivo* extrapolation (QIVIVE): An essential element for *in vitro*-based risk assessment. Yoon, M., Clewell, H.J. & Blaauboer, B.J. (Eds.). *Toxicology* **332**, (2015), 1–124.

125. Coecke, S., Pelkonen, O., Leite, S.B., *et al.* (2013). Toxicokinetics as a key to the integrated toxicity risk assessment based primarily on non-animal approaches. *Toxicology in Vitro* **27**, 1570–1577.

126. Bessems, J.G., Loizou, G., Krishnan, K., *et al.* (2014). PBTK modelling platforms and parameter estimation tools to enable animal-free risk assessment: recommendations from a joint EPAA–EURL ECVAM ADME workshop. *Regulatory Toxicology and Pharmacology* **68**, 119–139.

127. Bouzom, F., Ball, K., Perdaems, N., *et al.* (2012). Physiologically based pharmacokinetic (PBPK) modelling tools: how to fit with our needs? *Biopharmaceutics & Drug Disposition* **33**, 55–71.

128. Chen, Y., Jin, J.Y., Mukadam, S., *et al.* (2012). Application of IVIVE and PBPK modelling in prospective prediction of clinical pharmacokinetics: strategy and approach during the drug discovery phase with four case studies. *Biopharmaceutics & Drug Disposition* **33**, 85–98.

129. Jones, H.M., Chen, Y., Gibson, C., *et al.* (2015). Physiologically based pharmacokinetic modelling in drug discovery and development: a pharmaceutical industry perspective. *Clinical Pharmacology & Therapeutics* **97**, 247–262.

130. Peck, C.C., Barr, W.H., Benet, L.Z., *et al.* (1992). Opportunities for integration of pharmacokinetics, pharmacodynamics, and toxicokinetics in rational drug development. *Journal of Pharmaceutical Sciences* **81**, 605–610.

131. Charnick, S.B., Kawai, R., Nedelman, J.R., *et al.* (1995). Physiologically based pharmacokinetic modelling as a tool for drug development. *Journal of Pharmacokinetics and Biopharmaceutics* **23**, 217–229.

132. Rowland, M., Balant, L. & Peck, C. (2004). Physiologically based Pharmacokinetics in Drug Development and Regulatory Science: a Workshop Report. In *AAPS PharmSci* **6**, pp. 56–67. Washington, DC: Georgetown University. May 29–30, 2002.

133. Rostami-Hodjegan, A. (2012). Physiologically based pharmacokinetics joined with *in vitro–in vivo* extrapolation of ADME: a marriage under the arch of systems pharmacology. *Clinical Pharmacology & Therapeutics* **92**, 50–61.

134. Moreau, M., Leonard, J., Phillips, K.A., *et al.* (2017). Using exposure prediction tools to link exposure and dosimetry for risk-based decisions: A case study with phthalates. *Chemosphere* **184**, 1194–1201.

135. Pendse, S.N., Efremenko, A., McMullen, P.D., *et al.* (2017). PLETHEM: An interactive open-source platform for bridging the source-to-outcome continuum. *The Toxicologist, Supplement to Toxicological Sciences* **150**. Abstract 3184.

136. Pearce, R.G., Setzer, R.W., Strope, C.L., *et al.* (2017). Httk: R package for high-throughput toxicokinetics. *Journal of Statistical Software* **79**, 1–26.

137. Loizou, G. (4 February 2016). *A Free to Use PBPK Modelling Platform, SOT-BMSS Webinar*, 8pp. London, UK: Health & Safety Laboratory, Health & Safety Executive.

Chapter 5.4

Integrated Approaches to Testing and Assessment

Andrew P. Worth[1] and Bas J. Blaauboer[2]

[1]Joint Research Centre, European Commission, Ispra, Italy; [2]Utrecht University, Utrecht, The Netherlands

SUMMARY

Integrated Approaches to Testing and Assessment (IATA) are a flexible tool for chemical safety assessment, based on the integration and translation of data derived from multiple methods and sources. In addition to traditional *in vitro* and *in vivo* tests, IATA are increasingly incorporating new approach methods, such as high-throughput screening and high-content imaging methods, along with computational approaches that are used as a means of data generation, interpretation and integration. In this chapter, we describe the historical development of IATA, from both conceptual and practical perspectives, and we assess the current status of IATA in toxicological decision-making.

1. THE NEED FOR INTEGRATED TESTING

For the regulatory assessment of chemicals, very few alternative methods have been accepted as full replacements of the traditional animal toxicity tests, and to date these have been limited to methods for the classification of topical effects (e.g. skin corrosion and irritation). Because of the limitations of individual methods, it is generally considered that the assessment of the 'more-complex' biological endpoints, including sensitisation and systemic toxicities, will require the use of multiple methods and information sources, to adequately cover the full range of toxicological responses and the intended chemical space. For this reason, there have been considerable efforts to develop Integrated Approaches to Testing and Assessment (IATA), to apply them in the development of chemicals and products, and to implement them within regulatory frameworks.

The possible applications of IATA include priority setting, hazard identification, hazard classification and labelling and risk assessment. The increasing use of IATA in the assessment of chemicals is expected to have numerous benefits, including the reduction, refinement and replacement of animal testing, increased efficiencies in testing and assessment, the safer design of innovative chemical products, and improvements in the protection of human health and the environment.

2. EVOLUTION OF THE IATA CONCEPT

As illustrated in Table 1, integrated approaches have been referred to different ways, including Intelligent or Integrated Testing Strategies (ITS) and, more recently, Integrated Approaches to Testing and Assessment (IATA). While definitions also vary, most emphasise the Three Rs and/or efficiencies in testing as the overall purpose, and some make reference to the underlying design (e.g. tiered approaches). In general, historical definitions have not distinguished between integrated approaches that are entirely prescriptive (rule-based) and those that are entirely or partially based on expert judgement. However, the most recent definition of IATA by the OECD (1) makes a clear distinction between rule-based approaches that generate predictions, termed 'defined approaches' (DAs) to testing and assessment, and flexible, judgement-based

The History of Alternative Test Methods in Toxicology. https://doi.org/10.1016/B978-0-12-813697-3.00032-9

TABLE 1 Selected Definitions of Integrated Testing Strategy (ITS) and Integrated Approaches to Testing and Assessment (IATA)

Definition/Explanation of ITS or IATA
'An integrated testing strategy is any approach to the evaluation of toxicity which serves to reduce, refine or replace an existing animal procedure, and which is based on the use of two or more of the following: physicochemical data, *in vitro* data, human data (for example, epidemiological, clinical case reports), animal data (where unavoidable), computational methods (such as quantitative structure-activity relationships [QSAR]) and biokinetic models.' (14)
'In the context of safety assessment, an Integrated Testing Strategy is a methodology which integrates information for toxicological evaluation from more than one source, thus facilitating decision-making. This should be achieved whilst taking into consideration the principles of the Three Rs (reduction, refinement and replacement).' (32)
'A tiered approach to data gathering, testing, and assessment that integrates different types of data (including physicochemical and other chemical properties as well as *in vitro* and *in vivo* toxicity data). When combined with estimates of exposure in an appropriate manner, the IATA provides predictions of risk. In an IATA, unsuitable substances are screened out early in the process. This reduces the number of substances that are subjected to the complete suite of regulatory tests. Plausible and testable hypotheses are formulated based on existing information and/or information derived from lower tier testing and only targeted testing is performed in the higher tiers. Failure to satisfy the toxicity requirements at a lower tier typically precludes further testing at a higher tier.' (45)
'An integrated test strategy is an algorithm to combine (different) test result(s) and, possibly, non-test information (existing data, *in silico* extrapolations from existing data or modeling) to give a combined test result. They often will have interim decision points at which further building blocks may be considered.' (10)
'An approach based on multiple information sources used for the hazard identification, hazard characterisation and/or safety assessment of chemicals. An IATA integrates and weights all relevant existing evidence and guides the targeted generation of new data, where required, to inform regulatory decision-making regarding potential hazard and/or risk. Within an IATA, data from various information sources (i.e. physicochemical properties, *in silico* models, grouping and read-across approaches, *in vitro* methods, *in vivo* tests and human data) are evaluated and integrated to draw conclusions on the hazard and/or risk of chemicals.' (1)

approaches that lead to safety conclusions, termed IATA. Within such IATA, there can be one or more DAs, and a greater or lesser degree of expert judgement. The distinction between DAs and IATA was motivated by the need to distinguish between those elements that can in principle be validated and standardised (DAs) and those elements that can only be partially harmonised (expert judgement).

A related concept that has been widely used is 'weight-of-evidence'. According to Linkov *et al.* (2), this term can be found in the scientific literature with a variety of meanings, ranging from the purely colloquial use of the word to structured approaches to data integration and interpretation. Focusing on the structured approaches, Linkov *et al.* identified a variety of weight-of-evidence methods, ranging from qualitative approaches to increasingly more quantitative ones. The need to apply weight-of-evidence considerations within IATA is commonly expressed in regulatory guidance documents, often in a qualitative or semi-quantitative manner. Guidance on how to conduct weight-of-evidence within regulatory assessments has been provided by ECHA (3) and by EFSA (4, 5). In addition, the OECD initiated a guidance development project in 2017.

Various reviews and commentaries on IATA have been published (6–10).

3. THE EARLY DAYS OF IATA AND THE IMPACT OF REACH

Efforts to develop and evaluate IATA have been published in the scientific literature since the early 1990s. A pioneering example was the ECITTS project, which illustrated the integration of biokinetic modelling with *in vitro* testing for the prediction of systemic toxicity (11–13). Subsequently, the European Centre for the Validation of Alternative Methods (ECVAM) proposed some generic and endpoint-specific strategies for assessing systemic toxicity (14). Subsequent efforts by ECVAM focused on the development of tiered strategies for local toxicity (skin and eye irritation/corrosion), as well as on the development of a generic approach for evaluating these strategies (15–18). Around the same time, the Dutch Health Council published a generic tiered exposure-driven approach to toxicity assessment, emphasising the need to use mechanistic information (19). Most of the proposals at this time focused on IATA hazard identification and classification, although a few were also considering the use of *in vitro* methods for risk assessment purposes (20).

During this period, there were two major policy drivers for the development of IATA for regulatory assessments. The first was the EU initiative to prohibit animal testing on cosmetics, which took legal effect through the 7th Amendment to

TABLE 2 EU-Funded Research Projects That Have Contributed to Integrated Approaches to Testing and Assessment (IATA) Development

Project	Endpoint(s)
AcuteTox (January 2005—June 2010), ref. 74080	Acute systemic toxicity
ChemScreen (January 2010—December 2013), ref. 93580	Reproductive and developmental toxicity
CADASTER (January 2009—December 2012), ref. 89337	Aquatic toxicity, bioaccumulation, biodegradation
EUToxRisk (January 2016—present)	Repeat-dose toxicity, developmental toxicity
OSIRIS (April 2007—September 2011), ref. 81288	Skin sensitisation, repeat-dose toxicity, mutagenicity, carcinogenicity
PREDICT-IV (May 2008—October 2013), ref. 86700	Liver, kidney and central nervous system toxicity
ReProTect (July 2004—June 2009), ref. 75291	Reproductive and developmental toxicity
SensiTiv (October 2005—March 2011), ref. 84805	Skin and respiratory sensitisation
SEURAT-1 (January 2011—December 2016)	Repeat-dose toxicity

Information about these projects can be obtained from the cordis.europa.eu project website by using the project reference numbers, except for the SEURAT-1 project, where enquiries should be made to http://www.seurat-1.eu/.

the Cosmetics Directive (21). The second was the European Commission's proposal (White Paper) for a new chemicals legislation in 2001 (22), which led to the adoption in 2006 of the REACH regulation, which includes a number of provisions for avoiding animal testing (23).

Stimulated by these policy developments, several EU-funded research projects focused on the development of building blocks and testing strategies for the main regulatory endpoints as summarised in Table 2. Within the UK, a DEFRA-funded project resulted in proposed decision trees for all the major human health and environmental effects required under REACH (24). During the same period, the European Commission's Joint Research Centre coordinated the formulation of testing strategies for human health and environmental effects that ultimately became part of ECHA's guidance on fulfilling information requirements under REACH (25).

4. IATA DEVELOPMENT IN THE POST-REACH ERA AND THE IMPACT OF TOX21

In 2007, the US National Academy of Sciences (NAS) published its vision of Toxicology in the 21st Century (26), recognising that the regulatory assessment of chemical safety needs to move away from the use of 'one-size-fits-all' and largely pre-defined batteries of standard toxicity tests and exposure studies, toward the use of hypothesis-driven approaches that are tailored to the characteristics and intended use of the chemical. The NAS vision foresaw a 'paradigm shift' away from toxicity testing in animals toward the use of pathway-based approaches that capture an understanding of chemical fate (in the environment and in biological organisms) and the underlying mechanisms of toxicity in exposed organisms. To fulfil this vision, it would be necessary to make better use of mechanistic data derived from high-throughput and high-content screening (HTS/HCS) assays in cell lines, cell cultures and/or tissue surrogates, combined with the application of a range of computational methods for data analysis and predictive modelling. The US developments are also described in Chapter 2.13.

Within the OECD, the so-called paradigm shift has led to efforts to develop Adverse Outcome Pathways (AOPs) and provide guidance on how to use AOPs in the development of IATA (27). In 2015, the OECD initiated an IATA Case Studies project as a means of developing and exchanging experience in IATA. The studies are put forward by one or more lead countries and reviewed by others. They are published following endorsement by the Working Party on Hazard Assessment, but without the binding commitment associated with OECD Test Guidelines (TGs). To date, case studies have focused on grouping and read-across for human health and environmental endpoints, as well as on a workflow for risk assessment based entirely on alternative approaches.

Within the EU, the Tox21 philosophy has been embraced by major EU-funded research programmes such as SEURAT-1 and EUToxRisk (Table 2). A common feature of the IATA proposed in the Tox21 era is an increased emphasis on risk assessment (in addition to hazard identification) based on the use of *in vitro* tests providing mechanistic information and *in vitro* points of departure combined with the use of biokinetic modelling to carry out *in vitro* to *in vivo* extrapolation (28—30).

5. THE VALIDATION OF IATA

An important aspect of IATA is that the assessment is based on a weight-of-evidence approach, which implies some degree of expert judgement. At one extreme, IATA can be explicitly described and prescriptive, leaving little room for expert choices. At the other extreme, IATA can be loosely described and flexible, allowing multiple options for the assessor. The optimal choice of IATA, for a given regulatory application, is highly context dependent, making a one-size-fits-all solution difficult or impossible. The context is defined by the type of chemical, its exposure route, the endpoint being assessed and the regulatory context in which safety decisions are made. In view of these differences, IATA for regulatory decision-making can rarely be fully standardised and harmonised. However, certain IATA components can be standardised, and these have been recently termed 'Defined Approaches to Testing and Assessment' by the OECD (1). DAs are based on a fixed set of information sources and a fixed Data Interpretation Procedure (DIP), based on inputs from different information sources. The concept of DIP was 'resurrected' from the 2005 guidance on validation (31), to capture algorithms that make extrapolations (prediction models), as well as those that directly interpret measurements of an endpoint (e.g. classification of sensitisation potential based on animal data).

The need to validate IATA, and the choice of validation approach, has been discussed extensively (10, 32, 33). There are three main issues concerning the practical validation of IATA: (a) the extent to which they can in principle be validated, depending on their degree of standardisation; (b) the scientific feasibility of the exercise, given that most available data have generally been used already in developing the approach and its component parts; and (c) the nature and formality of the validation process. This debate has been confused, primarily by the fact that IATA represent very different types of regulatory solution, which are more or less standardised. However, the recent distinction between DAs and IATA has led to the broad recognition that only standardised components of IATA (i.e. DAs) can be meaningfully validated, even though possible outcomes of applying of an entire IATA (resulting from different combinations of expert choices) can be simulated.

6. THE ACCEPTANCE AND USE OF IATA

IATA for the hazard identification and classification of skin irritation and corrosion were among the first IATA to be recognised by the OECD (in 2002 as a non-binding appendix to TG 404 (34), updated in 2015 as a separate guidance document (35)). These are relatively well-defined in terms of how the component parts are combined (within tiered approaches), when many of these components are officially accepted physicochemical and *in vitro* tests.

IATA for the hazard identification and classification of eye irritation have taken longer to gain international regulatory acceptance, with OECD guidance being adopted in 2017 (36). This can be attributed to the longer time-frames needed for the development and validation of component *in vitro* tests, which need to cover different mechanisms of eye toxicity and different potency ranges.

The next milestone is expected to be regulatory acceptance of IATA for the hazard identification and classification of skin sensitisation. This is because the mechanistic basis of this endpoint is well established, and there have been many efforts to develop computational models and tests for the individual key events within the skin sensitisation AOP. For the early key events (haptenation, keratinocyte and dendritic cell activation), relevant *in chemico* or *in vitro* tests have been formally validated and gained regulatory acceptance as OECD TG 442C (37), TG 442D (38) and TG 442E (39). For later key events (T-cell activation and proliferation), *in vitro* tests are either lacking or not yet validated.

Numerous IATA for skin sensitisation have been proposed, representing different applications (hazard identification, classification, potency assessment) and different integration approaches. These have been reviewed elsewhere (40). Some are already being used in-house within individual companies (e.g. Unilever; (41)), and a generic IATA is recommended for the purposes of REACH (25). However, there is no guidance on the use of skin sensitisation IATA at the international level. To partially bridge this gap, an OECD project was initiated in 2017 to develop a performance-based TG for skin sensitisation DAs. For the most part, these DAs seek to replace animal testing by optimising the ability to predict skin sensitisation (potential or potency), irrespective of financial cost. Recently, research has also taken cost-effectiveness into account, recognising the constraints faced by industry in the product development (42). The international acceptance of IATA for skin sensitisation appears achievable in the coming years.

For systemic toxicities, including acute and repeat-dose toxicity, reproductive toxicity and carcinogenicity (see Chapter 3.6), generic IATA are proposed in REACH guidance, but there is no guidance at the OECD level. In some sectors (e.g. food), the Threshold of Toxicological Concern (TTC) approach, which can be regarded as an IATA for carcinogenicity and repeat-dose toxicity, has been accepted for the risk screening or assessment of chemicals present at low exposure levels in the diet and in consumer products (see also Chapter 3.4).

7. CONCLUSIONS

Since the early 1990s, considerable research investments have been made into the development of IATA for a range of (eco)toxicological effects, with emphasis on endpoints required by chemicals legislation. Within the EU, major policy drivers have been legislative developments related to assessment of cosmetic products and industrial chemicals (REACH), which prohibit and restrict animal testing, respectively. At the time of writing (June 2017), there is a huge and growing body of so-called 'new approach methodologies (NAMs)' (43).

While these methods are increasingly being used by companies for in-house product development purposes, very few have translated into regulatory solutions. The international harmonisation of IATA for human health effects is currently limited to a handful of endpoints that are inherently more 'predictable', such as local toxicities (skin and eye effects), with skin sensitisation being a near-term prospect.

The rise of high-throughput and high-content *in vitro* testing methods, combined with increasingly transparent and accessible computational methods to support integration of diverse data streams (44, 45), means that IATA are increasingly being conceived as flexible, scientifically justified combinations of primarily non-standard studies. This poses a growing challenge to a regulatory assessment paradigm that so far has been based on a prescribed set of animal TGs and/or standardised non-animal tests. At the same time, there is an opportunity to apply new assessment methods to help address societal challenges for which there are no standard chemical testing requirements (e.g. metabolic disorders, cognitive impairments and rare diseases). Ultimately, the mismatch between regulatory needs and the availability of scientific solutions will need to be resolved in a creative way. In other words, a paradigm shift is needed not only in the way that chemical safety assessments are conducted but also in the way that regulatory decisions are taken. A new generation of assessment methods will only be able to meet a new generation of regulatory needs if they are credible in the eyes of decision-makers and if this credibility can be established without the need to demonstrate the ability of new methods to directly predict the results of traditional animal tests, which are themselves poorly reproducible and in many cases of questionable human relevance. This implies a need to establish confidence in new methods in terms of their scientific robustness and mechanistic relevance to the biological effect (toxicity) of interest, whereas confidence in IATA should be established by means of a systematic and comprehensive characterisation of the underlying uncertainties in the assessment process (46). Accordingly, international harmonisation efforts will need to focus more on developing consistent frameworks for treating uncertainties in regulatory assessments and less on developing prescriptive solutions for specific endpoints.

REFERENCES

1. OECD. (2016). *Guidance Document on the Reporting of Defined Approaches to be used within Integrated Approaches to Testing and Assessment.* Series on Testing and Assessment No. 255, 23pp. Paris, France: OECD.
2. Linkov, I., Loney, D., Cormier, S., *et al.* (2009). Weight-of-evidence evaluation in environmental assessment: Review of qualitative and quantitative approaches. *The Science of the Total Environment* **407**, 5199—5205.
3. ECHA. (2016). *Practical Guide: How to Use Alternatives to Animal Testing to Fulfil the Information Requirements for REACH Registration*, 42pp. Helsinki, Finland: ECHA.
4. EFSA. (2017). Guidance on the assessment of the biological relevance of data in scientific assessments. *EFSA Journal* **15**(4970), 73.
5. EFSA. (2017). Guidance on the use of the weight of evidence approach in scientific assessments. *EFSA Journal* **15**(4971), 69.
6. Van Leeuwen, C., Patlewicz, G. & Worth, A. (2007). Intelligent testing strategies. In C. van Leeuwen, & T. Vermeire (Eds.), *Risk Assessment of Chemicals. An Introduction*, pp. 467—509. Berlin/Heidelberg, Germany: Springer.
7. Ahlers, J., Stock, F. & Werschkun, B. (2008). Integrated testing and intelligent assessment-new challenges under REACH. *Environmental Science and Pollution Research International* **15**, 565—572.
8. Schaafsma, G., Kroese, E.D., Tielemans, E.L.J.P., *et al.* (2009). REACH, non-testing approaches and the urgent need for a change in mind set. *Regulatory Toxicology and Pharmacology* **53**, 70—80.
9. Jaworska, J. & Hoffmann, S. (2010). Integrated testing strategy (ITS) — opportunities to better use existing data and guide future testing in toxicology. *ALTEX* **27**, 231—242.
10. Hartung, T., Luechtefeld, T., Maertens, A., *et al.* (2013). Integrated testing strategies for safety assessments. *ALTEX* **30**, 3—18.
11. Walum, E., Balls, M., Bianchi, V., *et al.* (1992). ECITTS: an integrated approach to the application of in vitro test systems to the hazard assessment of chemicals. *ATLA* **20**, 406—428.
12. Blaauboer, B.J., Balls, M., Bianchi, V., *et al.* (1994). The ECITTS integrated toxicity testing scheme: The application of in vitro test systems to the hazard assessment of chemicals. *Toxicology in Vitro* **8**, 845—846.
13. DeJongh, J., Forsby, A., Houston, J., *et al.* (1999). An integrated approach to the prediction of systemic toxicity using computer-based biokinetic models and biological in vitro test methods: Overview of a prevalidation study based on the ECITTS project. *Toxicology in Vitro* **13**, 549—554.
14. Blaauboer, B.J., Barratt, M.D. & Houston, J.B. (1999). The integrated use of alternative methods in toxicological risk evaluation. ECVAM Integrated Testing Strategies Task Force Report 1. *ATLA* **27**, 229—237.

15. Worth, A.P., Fentem, J.H., Balls, M., *et al.* (1998). An evaluation of the proposed OECD testing strategy for skin corrosion. *ATLA* **26**, 709–720.

16. Worth, A.P. & Fentem, J.H. (1999). A general approach for evaluating stepwise testing strategies. *ATLA* **27**, 161–177.

17. Worth, A.P. (2000). *The Integrated Use of Physicochemical and In Vitro Data for Predicting Chemical Toxicity* (Ph.D. thesis), 375pp. Liverpool, UK: Liverpool John Moores University.

18. Worth, A.P. (2004). The tiered approach to toxicity assessment based on the integrated use of alternative (non-animal) tests. In M.T.D. Cronin, & D. Livingstone (Eds.), *Predicting Chemical Toxicity and Fate*, pp. 389–410. Boca Raton, FL, USA: CRC Press.

19. Dutch Health Council. (2001). *Toxicity Testing: A More Efficient Approach. Publication no. 2001/24E*, 70pp. The Hague, The Netherlands: Health Council of the Netherlands.

20. Eisenbrand, G., Pool-Zobel, B., Baker, V., *et al.* (2002). Methods of in vitro toxicology. *Food and Chemical Toxicology* **40**, 193–236.

21. EC. (2003). Directive 2003/15/EC of the European Parliament and of the Council of 27 February 2003 amending Council Directive 76/768/EEC on the approximation of the laws of the Member States relating to cosmetic products. *Official Journal of the European Union* **L66**, 26–35.

22. EC. (2001). *White Paper: Strategy for a Future Chemicals Policy*, 32pp. Brussels, Belgium: European Commission.

23. EC. (2006). Regulation (EC) No 1907/2006 of the European Parliament and of the Council of 18 December 2006 concerning the Registration, Evaluation, Authorisation and Restriction of Chemicals (REACH), establishing a European Chemicals Agency, amending Directive 1999/45/EC and repealing Council Regulation (EEC) No 793/93 and Commission Regulation (EC) No 1488/94 as well as Council Directive 76/769/EEC and Commission Directives 91/155/EEC, 93/67/EEC, 93/105/EC and 2000/21/EC. *Official Journal of the European Union* **L396**, 1–849.

24. Grindon, C., Combes, R., Cronin, M.T.D., *et al.* (2008). Integrated testing strategies for use with respect to the requirements of the EU REACH legislation. *ATLA* **36**(Supplément, Le 1), 7–27.

25. ECHA. (2017). *Guidance on Information Requirements and Chemical Safety Assessment. Chapter R.7a: Endpoint Specific Guidance*. Version 6.0, 610pp. Helsinki, Finland: ECHA.

26. NRC. (2007). *Toxicity Testing in the 21st Century: A Vision and a Strategy*, 216pp. Washington, DC, USA: The National Academies Press.

27. OECD. (2016). *Guidance Document for the Use of Adverse Outcome Pathways in Developing Integrated Approaches to Testing and Assessment (IATA)*. Series on Testing and Assessment No. 260, 25pp. Paris, France: OECD.

28. Blaauboer, B.J., Boekelheide, K., Clewell, H.J., *et al.* (2012). The use of biomarkers of toxicity for integrating in vitro hazard estimates into risk assessment for humans. *ALTEX* **29**, 411–425.

29. Blaauboer, B.J., Boobis, A.R., Bradford, B., *et al.* (2016). Considering new methodologies in strategies for safety assessment of foods and food ingredients. *Food and Chemical Toxicology* **91**, 19–35.

30. Thomas, R.S., Philbert, M.A., Auerbach, S.S., *et al.* (2013). Incorporating new technologies into toxicity testing and risk assessment: moving from 21st century vision to a data-driven framework. *Toxicological Sciences* **136**, 4–18.

31. OECD. (2005). *Guidance Document on the Validation and International Acceptance of New or Updated Test Methods for Hazard Assessment*. Series on Testing and Assessment no. 34, 96pp. Paris, France: OECD.

32. Kinsner-Ovaskainen, A., Akkan, Z., Casati, S., *et al.* (2009). Overcoming barriers to validation of non-animal partial replacement methods/integrated testing strategies: the report of an EPAA-ECVAM workshop. *ATLA* **37**, 437–444.

33. Kinsner-Ovaskainen, A., Maxwell, G., Kreysa, J., *et al.* (2012). Report of the EPAA-ECVAM workshop on the validation of integrated testing strategies (ITS). *ATLA* **40**, 175–181.

34. OECD. (2002). *OECD TG No. 404: Acute Dermal Irritation/Corrosion*, 13pp. Paris, France: OECD.

35. OECD. (2014). *Guidance Document on an Integrated Approach on Testing and Assessment (IATA) for Skin Corrosion and Irritation*. Series on Testing and Assessment No. 203, 64pp. Paris, France: OECD.

36. OECD. (2017). *Guidance Document on an Integrated Approach on Testing and Assessment (IATA) for Serious Eye Damage and Eye Irritation*. Series on Testing & Assessment No. 263, 90pp. Paris, France: OECD.

37. OECD. (2015). *OECD TG No. 445C: In Chemico Skin Sensitisation: Direct Peptide Reactivity Assay (DPRA)*, 19pp. Paris, France: OECD.

38. OECD. (2015). *OECD TG No. 445D: In Vitro Skin Sensitisation: Human Cell Line Activation Test (h-CLAT)*, 20pp. Paris, France: OECD.

39. OECD. (2016). *OECD TG No. 442E: In Vitro Skin Sensitisation: ARE-Nrf2 Luciferase Test Method*, 20pp. Paris, France: OECD.

40. Ezendam, J., Braakhuis, H.M. & Vandebriel, R.J. (2016). State of the art in non-animal approaches for skin sensitization testing: from individual test methods towards testing strategies. *Archives of Toxicology* **90**, 2861–2883.

41. Maxwell, G., MacKay, C., Cubberley, R., *et al.* (2014). Applying the skin sensitisation adverse outcome pathway (AOP) to quantitative risk assessment. *Toxicology in Vitro* **28**, 8–12.

42. Leontaridou, M. (2017). *An Economic Approach to Non-animal Toxicity Testing for Skin Sensitisation* (Ph.D. thesis), 151pp. Wageningen, The Netherlands: Wageningen University

43. ECHA. (2016). *New Approach Methodologies in Regulatory Science. Proceedings of a Scientific Workshop*, 65pp. Helsinki, Finland: ECHA.

44. NAS. (2016). *Using 21st Century Science to Improve Risk-Related Evaluations*, 200pp. Washington, DC, USA: The National Academies Press.

45. Council of Canadian Academies. (2012). *Integrating Emerging Technologies into Chemical Safety Assessment*, 324pp. Ottawa, ON, Canada: Council of Canadian Academies.

46. EFSA. (2018). Guidance on Uncertainty Analysis in Scientific Assessments. *EFSA Journal* **16**(5123), 39.

Chapter 5.5

The Validation of Alternative Test Methods

Michael Balls[1], Andrew P. Worth[2] and Robert D. Combes[3]

[1]University of Nottingham, Nottingham, United Kingdom; [2]Joint Research Centre, European Commission, Ispra, Italy; [3]Independent Consultant, Norwich, United Kingdom

SUMMARY

As non-animal toxicity tests began to be developed in the late 1980s, the need for their validation, i.e. the independent assessment of their relevance and reliability for particular purposes, was recognised, and international discussions on the principles of validation and their practical application took place, notably, in Europe and the USA. This came to involve recognition of a prevalidation stage to ensure that a method was ready for formal validation and of a prediction model, an unambiguous algorithm for converting test data into a prediction of a relevant *in vivo* pharmacotoxicological endpoint. By the mid-1990s, validated non-animal methods could be proposed for the development of test guidelines and for regulatory acceptance. Meanwhile, the validation process itself evolved as a result of practical experience, and processes such as catch-up validation, weight-of-evidence validation, QSAR model validation and integrated testing strategies came to be seen as important. Major roles in these developments were played by ECVAM in Europe, ICCVAM in the USA, JaCVAM in Japan, and the OECD, but validation centres now operate in a number of other countries.

1. ESTABLISHING THE PRINCIPLES

The validation of a test method is the process by which its relevance and reliability for a particular purpose are independently assessed. It is an essential stage in the evolution of the method from its development to its acceptance and application for regulatory purposes. The principles according to which alternative tests should be validated have been agreed at an international level, although there is some variation among different validation authorities on how the actual validation process is conducted.

There is already a vast literature on the subject of validation, which ranges across a spectrum from reports on successful studies leading eventually to regulatory acceptance, to misunderstandings about the process itself or attempts to manipulate it in the service of vested interests. This review will mainly be focused on events in Europe, as those in other parts of the world will be discussed in other chapters.

The first tests to be validated and accepted for regulatory purposes were those for the determination of genotoxicity caused by damage to the DNA of bacterial cells, such as those of *Salmonella typhimurium* in the Ames test, and *in vitro* cytogenetics tests for chromosomal damage and aberrations in mammalian cells. These tests were evaluated in the 1970s, in inter-laboratory 'round robin' trials coordinated by various national and international authorities and societies, which involved the blind testing of coded chemicals according to strictly-defined protocols and standardised methods for data recording and interpretation.

In the early 1980s, the primary focus was on the development of *in vitro* tests that might eventually replace the LD50 test and the Draize rabbit skin and eye irritation tests, which had become the aim of animal rights campaigners on both sides of the Atlantic.

The History of Alternative Test Methods in Toxicology. https://doi.org/10.1016/B978-0-12-813697-3.00033-0

Having organised an inter-laboratory collaboration which led to the kenacid blue cytotoxicity test, FRAME organised a multi-centre validation study involving independently classified, coded and distributed test chemicals. Realising that the lessons learned might be helpful to others, FRAME set up an international test validation scheme, with the support of the UK Government Home Office (1).

Shortly afterwards, in 1986, an excellent conference on *Approaches to Validation* took place in Baltimore, Maryland, the proceedings of which were published in 1987 as the fifth volume in the CAAT series on *Alternative Methods in Toxicology* (2).

The year 1999 was to be particularly significant, as John Frazier, from CAAT, having completed a report on validation for the OECD (3), had met some ERGATT members at a conference in Berlin, where it was agreed that an international workshop on the principles of validation should be organised. The workshop, later to become known as Amden I, was held in Amden, Switzerland, in January 1990, with the support of Procter & Gamble and FRAME (4). Later that year, ERGATT organised a workshop on the regulatory acceptance of alternative methods, which was held in Vouliagmeni, Greece, and funded by DGXI of the European Commission (5).

In 1991, DGXI and the UK Home Office contracted FRAME to manage a validation study on alternatives to the Draize eye test, but the management of the study was transferred to Ispra, when Michael Balls became head of the newly-created ECVAM. The EC/HO study involved 9 tests, 60 test items and 37 laboratories in nine countries (6). It is often said that the study was a failure, but that is not true — it was the alternative methods that failed to predict the Draize test scores, but, on reflection, it was realised that that was not surprising, given the poor reproducibility of the *in vivo* test results. Many important lessons were learned from the study, which were applied in subsequent validation studies.

A study organised by COLIPA on alternatives to the Draize eye test for cosmetic ingredients led to the conclusion that the tests had performed no better than in the EC/HO study, but its value was that it illustrated the importance of applying a prediction model, an unambiguous algorithm for converting test data into a prediction of a relevant *in vivo* pharmaco-toxicological endpoint (7). The concept of the prediction model had been discussed previously by Bruner *et al.* (8), and in a discussion on the validation of prediction models, Archer *et al.* (9) described an alternative test as the combination of a test system and a prediction model, both of which needed to be validated.

2. LEARNING FROM PRACTICAL EXPERIENCE

In the light of these and other developments, a second workshop was held at Amden in 1994 (Amden II), organised by ERGATT for ECVAM, to discuss practical aspects of the application of the validation process. The workshop report emphasised the need for clearly defined stages, namely, test development, prevalidation, validation, independent assessment, and progress toward regulatory assessment (10). It contained 25 conclusions and recommendations, and of particular importance was guidance on the design, management and organisation of validation studies, with emphasis on the roles of various partners, including the sponsors, contractors, management team, steering committee, participating laboratories, lead laboratories, and those responsible for test item selection, for their coding and distribution, and for data collection and analysis. This guidance was closely followed in a number of successful international validation studies, including the EC/COLIPA study on the 3T3 NRU *in vitro* test for phototoxicity (11) and the ECVAM study on *in vitro* tests for skin corrosivity.

The importance of the prevalidation step was emphasised by Curren *et al.* (12) as a means of ensuring that candidate tests were likely to be relevant to their stated purpose and were ready for formal validation. The step involved three stages, namely, protocol refinement, protocol transfer and protocol performance, and it was even envisaged that the satisfactory outcome of the third stage might in some circumstances be sufficient for the method to be recommended for regulatory acceptance and application.

A number of other concepts and systems evolved along the way, including the application of structural and performance criteria and catch-up validation, as a means of increasing the efficiency of the validation process and of avoiding complications arising from the patenting of methods or the withdrawal of methods.

Skin^2, a reconstituted human skin product, had been withdrawn from the market, after it had been accepted by the US Department of Transport for classifying chemicals in terms of their skin corrosivity. The withdrawal of Skin^2 and also of EPISKIN, a similar product, took place during a formal validation study, which, as in the case of the withdrawal of another human skin product, Organogenesis, a few years earlier, caused considerable frustration and annoyance. It was proposed that this kind of problem could be avoided, if, rather than validating a particular protocol or specific commercial product, clearly-defined structural and performance criteria would be defined, and any methods which met these criteria could be subject to fast-track prevalidation and formal validation (13). Thereafter, any new method which met the criteria could be considered scientifically valid and acceptable, albeit with the need for a small and independent catch-up validation study in some circumstances.

An early example of a successful catch-up study, conducted at the request of the Scientific Committee on Cosmetology of the EC, involved an evaluation of whether the validated 3T3 NRU phototoxicity test (PT) could be applied to UV filter chemicals used in cosmetics (14).

3. THE EVOLUTION OF THE ECVAM VALIDATION PROCESS

The ECVAM validation process, as it had developed up to that time, was summarised at the ECVAM Status Seminar, which took place in June 2002, held at the time of the retirement of Michael Balls, the first Head of ECVAM (15). It included ECVAM's criteria for test development, prevalidation, and formal validation, and the process of independent assessment leading to ESAC statements in the case of successful outcomes, as had previously been discussed in detail (16). At that point, ESAC statements had been published on 10 alternative methods.

A number of important developments took place over the next few years, and a number of significant reports were published, including the following:

1. Increased recognition of the importance of biostatistical aspects of the validation process, particularly as a result of the validation of the 3T3 NRU phototoxicity test, as discussed by the ECVAM Biostatistics Task Force (17) and Hothorn (18), and in a special ATLA supplement (19).
2. Balls and Combes (20) suggested that a formal *invalidation* process was necessary, because many currently accepted animal tests and candidate animal and non-animal tests did not, and could never, meet the agreed criteria for necessity, test development, prevalidation, validation and acceptance. We therefore needed an invalidation process to parallel and protect the validation process, so that such methods could be independently reviewed and declared irrelevant and/or unreliable for their claimed purposes. An additional advantage of such a process would be that valuable resources would no longer be wasted in attempts to secure the acceptance of inherently inadequate tests. They listed a number of OECD test guidelines which ought to be reviewed. An ECVAM workshop on invalidation took place at Ispra in 2006, but no workshop report was published.
3. Where it was not necessary, or even possible, to conduct a practical laboratory study to establish the validity of tests or testing strategies, a weight-of-evidence (WoE) approach could be employed to use already-available information in a structured, systematic, independent and transparent retrospective evaluation. Crucial aspects would include study management and design; selection of experts without vested interests; collection of data and data quality control; differential weighting of various types of evidence, alone and in combination; evaluation of test performance in terms of reliability and relevance in relation to purpose; and publication of outcome and peer reviews. These principles were discussed in 2004 at ECVAM Workshop 58 (21). This report is especially important, because it contains detailed proposals about how the WoE approach could be conducted, together with outlines of the modular ECVAM validation scheme in operation at that time (22), the ESAC peer-review process and the ICCVAM process for test method validation assessments, as well as a list of the practical and WoE assessments that had been conducted by ECVAM, ICCVAM and the OECD.
4. A number of comments were made over the years on problems with the validation process (e.g. (23, 24)), including a report by a working group of the European Partnership for Alternative Approaches to Animal Testing (EPAA) on barriers to validation and ways of overcoming them (25).
5. Points of reference in the validation process were considered in 2006, at ECVAM workshop 66 (26), at which reference methods, reference chemicals and reference results were considered. One of the ongoing and unsolved problems is identifying test items for use in validation studies, for which toxicological data of sufficient relevance and of sufficiently high quality are available. Ideally, such data should have come from human experience, as data from animal tests are not relevant or reliable because of species differences, strain differences within the animal species used and human variation — problems further compounded by the use of unreasonable dose levels and dosing schemes (as in the rodent bioassay for chemical carcinogenicity). It should be noted that the importance of the independent selection of appropriate test items and, where appropriate, their coding and distribution, was realised early in the development of the validation process. Paul Brantom and his colleagues at BIBRA International played an important role in this respect (27). Also, one of the reasons that the validation of the 3T3 NRU PT was successful was that the selection of the test items used was not based on animal data, but on the advice of independent human toxicologists.
6. In 2006, the optimisation of the post-validation process was considered at ECVAM Workshop 67. A number of recommendations were made in the workshop report (28), including the establishment of a partnership with the newly established European Partnership for Alternative Approaches to Animal Testing (EPAA) and the setting up of an

ECVAM Regulatory Advisory Panel, a role which has been given to, the Preliminary Assessment of Regulatory Relevance Network (PARERE), in line with Article 47(5) of *Directive 2010/63/EU* on the protection of animals used for scientific purposes (see Chapter 2.13).

The EURL ECVAM validation process has been streamlined and standardised over recent years, to adapt to new requirements and priorities (29). Today it can be summarised as follows.

The validation process starts with the receipt of test method submissions via the standard test submission procedure (i.e. through the EURL ECVAM website) or in reply to a specific call. The test methods are assessed by EURL ECVAM with regard to scientific and technical aspects, their regulatory relevance and their impact on the Three Rs. For most health effects or 'endpoints', the relevance of a single test method is typically evaluated with respect to its potential usefulness when combined with complementary methods; for example, within an integrated testing strategy. Ideally, the test method is assessed within the framework of an EURL ECVAM strategy that has been defined for each toxicological area, or, if that is not available, to a conceptual framework that has broadly been accepted. These EURL ECVAM strategies typically address different regulatory domains and related needs, review the progress made to date, identify gaps and opportunities in relation to method development and validation, and outline what actions should be taken to deliver solutions that carry Three Rs impact. Whilst formulating these strategies, EURL ECVAM usually consults with its regulatory and scientific advisory bodies (PARERE and the ESAC) and its stakeholder forum (ESTAF), as well as with international cooperation partners also involved in method validation (ICATM). In some cases, EURL ECVAM also consults its advisory and stakeholder bodies with regard to the merits of individual methods if deemed appropriate.

If the submitted test methods are found to be sufficiently developed and relevant for entering validation, a study is launched if suitable resources are available. A validation study may be executed by third parties, or in some cases, the method is transferred to the EURL ECVAM laboratories, where the test method protocols are reviewed and refined, if necessary, in close collaboration with the test method submitters. If the validation study foresees the need for a ring trial to demonstrate the reliability and relevance of the method, then EURL ECVAM launches a call with ECVAM's Network of Validation Laboratories (EU-NETVAL).

If the validation trial has been completed successfully, a validation study report is drafted and submitted to the ESAC for independent peer review. The ESAC issues an opinion on the test method's scientific validity in the context of its intended purpose. On the basis of ECVAM's own evaluation, the ESAC opinion and regulatory/stakeholder input, EURL ECVAM drafts its recommendation on the validity of the test method, which then undergoes a public commentary round before being published on the EURL ECVAM website and communicated to the European Commission services and other stakeholders.

4. INTERNATIONAL COLLABORATION IN APPLYING THE VALIDATION PROCESS

ECVAM was established in 1991, and the US Interagency Coordinating Committee on Validation of Alternative Methods (ICCVAM) was set up in 1995, when it was hoped that the validation criteria for replacement alternative and *animal* tests could be harmonised. An informal collaboration between the two authorities was established, and, for example, the ESAC endorsed ICCVAM's acceptance of the CORROSITEX method for skin corrosivity.

The Japanese Center for the Validation of Alternative Methods (JaCVAM) was set up in 2005, and is located in the office of New Testing Method Assessment, Division of Pharmacology, Biological Safety Research Center of the National Institute of Health Sciences, Tokyo. Its purpose and activities are similar to those of ECVAM and ICCVAM, i.e. to promote the use of alternative methods to animal testing in regulatory studies, thereby expanding application of the Three Rs to animal testing wherever possible, whilst meeting the responsibility to ensure the protection of the public by assessing the safety of chemicals and other materials.

The South Korean Centre for the Validation of Alternative Methods (KoCVAM) was set up in 2010, as part of the National Institute of Food and Drug Safety Evaluation of the South Korean Food and Drug Administration.

The Brazilian Centre for the Validation of Alternative Methods (BraCVAM) was established in 2013, as the Brazilian focal point to identify promising methods for validation. BraCVAM's activities are supported by the Brazilian National Network on Alternative Methods (RENaMA).

The establishment of the Canadian Centre for Alternatives to Animal Methods (CCAAM) was announced on 15 July 2017. CCAAM and its subsidiary, the Canadian Centre for the Validation of Alternative Methods (CaCVAM), aim to promote the use of non-animal methodologies in biomedical research, education and chemical toxicity testing.

Since 2009, collaboration among the different validation authorities has been encouraged on a more formal basis, via the International Cooperation on Alternative Test Methods (ICATM). The ICATM includes governmental organisations from the EU (EURL ECVAM), US (ICCVAM), Japan (JaCVAM), Canada (Health Canada, CCAAM and CaCVAM), South Korea (KoCVAM), Brazil (BraCVAM) and China (CFDA and the Institute of Toxicology, Guangdong Provincial Center for Disease Control and Prevention). The ICATM Members (EU, US, Japan, Canada and South Korea) and Observers (Brazil and China) are working are working together to promote enhanced international cooperation and coordination on the scientific development, validation and regulatory use of alternative approaches.

Collaboration on validation has also taken place under the auspices of the OECD, and this has played an important role in the development of OECD test guidelines, as discussed by Gourmelon and Delrue ((30), see also Chapter 2.15).

5. THE VALIDATION OF QSARS

In 2005, the OECD published its long-awaited "Guidance Document on the Validation and International Acceptance of New or Updated Test Methods for Hazard Assessment" (31). This completed an activity which started in 1998 as a follow-up to the 1996 Solna Workshop on the Harmonisation of Validation and Acceptance Criteria for Alternative Toxicological Test Methods (32) and which also led to the 2002 Stockholm Conference on "Validation and Regulatory Acceptance of New and Updated Methods in Hazard Assessment" (33).

The 2005 guidance reiterated the principles of validation and provided a series of recommendations for the conduct of validation studies. It defined validation as '*the process by which the reliability and relevance of a particular approach, method, process or assessment is established for a defined purpose*'. This wide-ranging definition was intended to cover all kinds of traditional and alternative testing methods, although its application to computational models, such as QSARs, and approaches based on multiple data streams, such as Integrated Testing Strategies, was not elaborated.

The beginnings of an internationally agreed framework for establishing the validity of QSARs for regulatory purposes can be traced to an ICCA-LRI workshop held in 2002 in the Portuguese coastal town of Setubal. This brought together a broad international stakeholder group to formulate guiding principles for the development and application of QSARs for regulatory purposes (34—36). The fact that the Setubal workshop and Stockholm conference were held during the same week is perhaps a reflection of how distinct the QSAR and *in vitro* method communities were at the time. The principles agreed upon during the workshop, which became known as the "Setubal principles", were based on the ECVAM principles for test development (37) and some early ECVAM publications on the validation of computational methods (38, 39).

The Setubal principles, along with evidence (case studies) of their utility, were subsequently considered by the OECD and adopted, with some modifications, as the "OECD principles for (Q)SAR validation for regulatory purposes" (40) at the 37th Joint Meeting of the Chemicals Committee and Working Party on Chemicals, Pesticides and Biotechnology in November 2004. The five OECD principles are very succinct: *To facilitate the consideration of a (Q)SAR model for regulatory purposes, it should be associated with the following information: (a) a defined endpoint; (b) an unambiguous algorithm; (c) a defined domain of applicability; (d) appropriate measures of goodness-of-fit; and (e) a mechanistic interpretation, if possible.*

In reaching consensus on these principles, there was considerable disagreement about the choice of statistical approach to validation (hence the generic wording of principle 4), and on the need to demonstrate mechanistic relevance (hence the weak wording of principle 5). The need for practical guidance on how to apply the principles was subsequently fulfilled by the JRC (European Chemicals Bureau), which developed a preliminary guidance document in consultation with a QSAR Working Group of Member State nominees (41). This laid the foundation for the eventual OECD guidance document (42) and regulatory guidance on the application of QSARs under REACH (43). Importantly, for a number of practical considerations, the process of establishing the acceptability of QSAR models did not depend on formalised validation and adoption procedures, but rather on providing convincing argumentation to regulatory bodies such as the European Chemicals Agency (ECHA), based on structured and transparent documentation (the QSAR Model Reporting Format, QMRF). This recognises that model "validity" is in the "eye of the beholder" (the regulatory body) and that acceptability is highly context dependent (44). Similar guidance was subsequently developed by the JRC for the European Food Safety Authority (EFSA) (45) and has been applied in EFSA guidance on the dietary risk assessment of pesticide residues (46).

6. THE VALIDATION OF INTEGRATED TESTING STRATEGIES

Starting in the late 1990s, the recognition that one-to-one replacements of animal tests would be the exception rather than the rule prompted the development of methodological solutions based on multiple data streams (16, 47). These methodologies have been referred to in various ways, including test batteries, intelligent or integrated testing strategies (ITS), and more recently, Integrated Approaches to Testing and Assessment (IATA; see also, Chapter 5.4).

The need to validate these integrated approaches, and the choice of validation approach, has been discussed extensively (48–50). There are three main practical considerations: (a) the extent to which a given approach can in principle be validated, depending on its degree of standardisation; (b) the scientific feasibility of the exercise, given that most available data have generally been used already in developing the approach; and (c) the nature and formality of the validation process. This debate has been confused primarily by the fact that integrated approaches represent very different types of assessment, which can be more or less standardised. However, the recent distinction between defined approach (DA) and IATA (51) has led to the broad recognition that validation efforts can only be meaningfully applied to standardised components of IATA (i.e. DAs), even though possible outcomes of applying of an entire IATA (resulting from different combinations of expert choices) can be simulated.

Drawing on the successful experience of the QMRF as a reporting standard for QSAR models, the JRC (ECVAM) developed a similar template (and associated principles) for characterising DAs (51, 52). Following on from this work, the EU (ECVAM), US (ICCVAM) and Canada (Health Canada) started a new OECD project in 2017 to develop a Performance-based Test Guideline (PBTG) for Defined Approaches (DA) suitable for the assessment of skin sensitisation. The resulting PBTG is expected to comprise a series of DAs that are considered suitable replacements for the standard animal test (the local lymph node assay).

7. THE ULTIMATE QUESTIONS

It is clear from this brief review of a vast literature that a huge amount of effort has gone into working out the principles of the validation process and applying them in practical studies and evaluation aims at establishing the relevance and reliability of alternative tests and testing strategies for particular purposes. In recent years, with the rapid rise of new technologies and methodologies (e.g. computational models, high-throughput screening, toxicogenomics), the basic principles of validation remain sound and useful, even though this has prompted discussions with regard to the practical aspects of the validation process (53, 54). A recent and comprehensive overview of best practices and new perspectives regarding the validation of alternative methods is given by Eskes and Whelan (55).

Ultimately, however, a validation study is not an end in itself, but a means of independently confirming that new methods are relevant and reliable for their stated purposes. This leads to two inescapable questions. First, for how many alternative methods are there internationally agreed protocols and guidelines which are accepted for regulatory purposes? Second, how many animal test guidelines have been withdrawn, because there is no longer a need for them, as replacement alternatives are now available?

There is a supplementary question — despite national and international laws which stipulate the general principle that an animal experiment may not be performed if a suitable non-animal procedure is available, are regulations in force which nevertheless permit or require a specific animal test to be carried out?

REFERENCES

1. Balls, M. & Clothier, R. (2009). FRAME and the validation process. *ATLA* **37**, 631–640.
2. Goldberg, A.M. (Ed.). (1987). *In Vitro Toxicology: Approaches to Validation,* 521pp. New York, NY, USA: Mary Ann Liebert, Inc.
3. Frazier, J. (1990). *Scientific Criteria for Validation of In Vitro Toxicity Tests.* Environment Monograph No. 36, 62pp. Paris, France: OECD.
4. Balls, M., Blaauboer, B., Brusick, D., *et al.* (1990). Report and recommendations of the CAAT/ERGATT workshop on the validation of toxicity test procedures. *ATLA* **18**, 313–337.
5. Balls, M., Botham, P., Cordier, A., *et al.* (1990). Report and recommendations of an international workshop on promotion of the regulatory acceptance of validated non-animal toxicity test procedures. *ATLA* **18**, 339–344.
6. Balls, M., Botham, P.A., Bruner, L.H., *et al.* (1995). The EC/HO international validation study on alternatives to the Draize eye irritation test. *Toxicology in Vitro* **9**, 871–929.
7. Brantom, P.G., Bruner, L.H., Chamberlain, M., *et al.* (1997). A summary report of the COLIPA international validation study on alternatives to the Draize rabbit eye irritation test. *Toxicology in Vitro* **11**, 141–179.
8. Bruner, L.H., Carr, G.J., Chamberlain, M., *et al.* (1996). No prediction model — no validation study. *Toxicology in Vitro* **10**, 479–501.
9. Archer, G., Balls, M., Bruner, L.H., *et al.* (1997). The validation of toxicological prediction models. *ATLA* **25**, 505–516.
10. Balls, M., Blaauboer, B.J., Fentem, J.H., *et al.* (1995). Practical aspects of the validation of toxicity test procedures. The report and recommendations of ECVAM Workshop 5. *ATLA* **23**, 129–147.
11. Spielmann, H., Balls, M., Dupuis, J., *et al.* (1998). The international EU/COLIPA *In vitro* phototoxicity validation study: results of phase II (blind trial), part 1: the 3T3 NRU phototoxicity test. *Toxicology in Vitro* **12**, 305–327.

12. Curren, R.D., Southee, J.A., Spielmann, H., *et al.* (1995). The role of prevalidation in the development, validation and acceptance of alternative methods. *ATLA* **23**, 211–217.
13. Balls, M. (1997). Defined structural and performance criteria would facilitate the validation and acceptance of alternative test methods. *ATLA* **25**, 483–484.
14. Spielmann, H., Balls, M., Dupuis, J., *et al.* (1998). A study on UV filter chemicals from Annex VII of the European Union *Directive 76/768/EEC*, in the *in vitro* 3T3 NRU phototoxicity test. *ATLA* **26**, 679–708.
15. Worth, A.P. & Balls, M. (2002). The principles of validation and the ECVAM validation process. *ATLA* **30**(Suppl. 2), 15–22.
16. Worth, A.P. & Balls, M. (2002). The role of ECAM in promoting the regulatory acceptance of alternative methods in the European Union. *ATLA* **29**, 525–535.
17. Holzhütter, H.-G., Archer, G., Dami, N., *et al.* (1996). Recommendations for the application of biostatistical methods during the development and validation of alternative toxicological methods. *ATLA* **24**, 511–530.
18. Hothorn, L.A. (2002). Selected biostatistical aspects of the validation of *in vitro* toxicological assays. *ATLA* **30**(Suppl. 2), 93–98.
19. Balls, M. (Ed.). (2003). Biostatistical Methods and the Development, Validation and Application of *In Vitro* Toxicity Tests. *ATLA* **31**(Suppl. 1), 1–103.
20. Balls, M. & Combes, R. (2005). The need for a formal invalidation process for animal and non-animal tests. *ATLA* **33**, 299–308.
21. Balls, M., Amcoff, P., Bremer, S., *et al.* (2006). The principles of weight of evidence validation of test methods and testing strategies. The report and recommendations of ECVAM Workshop 58. *ATLA* **34**, 603–620.
22. Hartung, T., Bremer, S., Casati, S., *et al.* (2004). A modular approach to the ECVAM principles on test validity. *ATLA* **32**, 467–472.
23. Balls, M. (1998). Why is it proving to be so difficult to replace animal tests? *Lab Animal* **5**, 44–47.
24. Hartung, T. (2007). Food for thought ... on validation. *ALTEX* **24**, 67–73.
25. Ahr, H.-J., Alepée, N., Breier, S., *et al.* (2008). Barriers to validation. A report by EPAA Working Group 5. *ATLA* **36**, 459–464.
26. Hartung, T., Edler, L., Gardner, I., *et al.* (2008). Points of reference in the validation process. The report and recommendations of ECVAM Workshop 66. *ATLA* **36**, 343–352.
27. Brantom, P.G., Aspin, P. & Thompson, C. (1995). Supply, coding and distribution of samples for validation studies. *ATLA* **23**, 348–351.
28. Bottini, A.A., Alepée, N., Phillips, B., *et al.* (2008). Optimisation of the post-validation process. *ATLA* **36**, 353–366.
29. Zuang, V., Schäffer, M., Tuomainen, A.M., *et al.* (2013). *EURL ECVAM Progress Report on the Development, Validation and Regulatory Acceptance of Alternative Methods (2010–2013)*. JRC Report EUR 25981, 63pp.
30. Gourmelon, A. & Delrue, N. (2016). Validation in support of internationally harmonised OECD test guidelines for assessing the safety of chemicals. In C. Eskes, & M. Whelan (Eds.), *Advances in Experimental Medicine and Biology* **856**. *Validation of Alternative Methods for Toxicity Testing*, pp. 9–32. Basel, Switzerland: Springer Verlag.
31. OECD. (2005). *Guidance Document on the Validation and International Acceptance of New or Updated Test Methods for Hazard Assessment*. OECD Series on Testing and Assessment No. 34, 67pp. Paris, France: OECD.
32. OECD. (2009). *Final Report of the OECD Workshop on "Harmonization of Validation and Acceptance Criteria for Alternative Toxicological Test Methods" (Solna Report)*. ENV/MC/CHEM/TG(96)9, 53pp. Paris, France: OECD.
33. OECD. (2002). In *Report of the OECD Conference on "Validation and Regulatory Acceptance of New and Updated Methods in Hazard Assessment" That Was Held in Stockholm, Sweden, 6–8 March 2002, ENV/JM/TG/M(2002)2*, 133pp. Paris, France: OECD.
34. Cronin, M.T.D., Jaworska, J.S., Walker, J.D., *et al.* (2003). Use of QSARs in international decision-making frameworks to predict health effects of chemical substances. *Environmental Health Perspectives* **111**, 1391–1401.
35. Eriksson, L., Jaworska, J.S., Worth, A.P., *et al.* (2003). Methods for reliability and uncertainty assessment and for applicability evaluations of classification- and regression-based QSARs. *Environmental Health Perspectives* **111**, 1361–1375.
36. Jaworska, J.S., Comber, M., Auer, C., *et al.* (2003). Summary of a workshop on regulatory acceptance of (Q)SARs for human health and environmental endpoints. *Environmental Health Perspectives* **111**, 1358–1360.
37. Balls, M. & Karcher, W. (1995). The validation of alternative test methods. *ATLA* **23**, 884–886.
38. Dearden, J.C., Barratt, M.D., Benigni, R., *et al.* (1997). The development and validation of expert systems for predicting toxicity. The report and recommendations of an ECVAM/ECB workshop (ECVAM workshop 24). *ATLA* **25**, 223–252.
39. Worth, A.P., Barratt, M.D. & Houston, J.B. (1998). The validation of computational prediction techniques. *ATLA* **26**, 241–247.
40. OECD. (2005). *Report From the Expert Group on (Q)SARs on the Validation of (Q)SARs*. Series on Testing and Assessment No. 49, 154pp. Paris, France: OECD.
41. Worth, A.P., Bassan, A., Gallegos, A., *et al.* (2005). *The Characterisation of (Quantitative) Structure-Activity Relationships: Preliminary Guidance*. JRC Report EUR 21866, 93pp.
42. OECD. (2007). *Guidance Document on the Validation of (Quantitative) Structure-activity Relationships [(Q)SAR] Models*. Series on Testing and Assessment No. 69, 154pp. Paris, France: OECD.
43. ECHA. (2011). *Guidance on Information Requirements and Chemical Safety Assessment, Chapter R.5 : Adaptation of Information Requirements*, 28pp. Helsinki, Finland: ECHA
44. Worth, A.P. & Mostrag-Szlichtyng. (2011). Towards a common regulatory framework for computational toxicology: Current status and future perspectives. In A.G.E. Wilson (Ed.), *New Horizons in Predictive Toxicology: Methods and Applications*, pp. 38–69. Cambridge, UK: The Royal Society of Chemistry.

45. Worth, A., Lapenna, S., Lo Piparo, E., *et al.* (2011). *A Framework for Assessing In Silico Toxicity Predictions: Case Studies With Selected Pesticides.* JRC Report EUR 24705, 52pp.

46. EFSA. (2016). Guidance on the establishment of the residue definition for dietary risk assessment. *EFSA Journal* **14**(4549), 129.

47. Worth, A.P. (2000). *The Integrated Use of Physicochemical and In Vitro Data for Predicting Chemical Toxicity* (Ph.D. thesis). Liverpool, UK: Liverpool John Moores University.

48. Kinsner-Ovaskainen, A., Akkan, Z., Casati, S., *et al.* (2009). Overcoming barriers to validation of non-animal partial replacement methods/integrated testing strategies: The report of an EPAA-ECVAM workshop. *ATLA* **37**, 437−444.

49. Kinsner-Ovaskainen, A., Maxwell, G. & Kreysa, J. (2012). Report of the EPAA-ECVAM workshop on the validation of integrated testing strategies (ITS). *ATLA* **40**, 175−181.

50. Hartung, T., Luechtefeld, T., Maertens, A., *et al.* (2013). Integrated testing strategies for safety assessments. *ALTEX* **30**, 3−18.

51. OECD. (2016). *Guidance Document on the Reporting of Defined Approaches to be Used Within Integrated Approaches to Testing and Assessment.* Series on Testing and Assessment No. 255, 23pp. Paris, France: OECD.

52. OECD. (2016). *Guidance Document on the Reporting of Defined Approaches and Individual Information Sources to be Used Within Integrated Approaches to Testing and Assessment (IATA) for Skin Sensitisation.* Series on Testing and Assessment No. 256, 24pp. Paris, France: OECD.

53. Judson, R., Kavlock, R., *et al.* (2013). Perspectives on validation of high-throughput assays supporting 21st century toxicity testing. *ALTEX* **30**, 1/13.

54. Piersma, A.H., Burgdorf, T., Louekari, K., *et al.* (2018). Workshop on acceleration of the validation and regulatory acceptance of alternative methods and implementation of testing strategies. *Toxicology in Vitro* **50**, 62−74.

55. Eskes, C. & Whelan, M., Eds. (2016). Validation of alternative methods for toxicity testing. In *Advances in Experimental Medicine and Biology* **856**, 407pp. Basel, Switzerland: Springer Verlag.

Current Status of Alternatives and Future Prospects

Chapter 6.1

Alternative Toxicity Test Methods: Lessons Learned and Yet to Be Learned

Michael Balls[1], Robert D. Combes[2] and Andrew P. Worth[3]

[1]University of Nottingham, Nottingham, United Kingdom; [2]Independent Consultant, Norwich, United Kingdom; [3]Joint Research Centre, European Commission, Ispra, Italy

SUMMARY

The development of alternative methods to living animals, originally in the area of toxicity testing for chemical safety assessment, and more recently in biomedical research, has a rich history going back to the 1950s. In the early days, the drivers for change were mostly based on animal welfare concerns, but the evidence has increasingly pointed to the scientific and practical limitations of reliance on traditional animal methods. As toxicology transitioned into the 21st century, the need to assess an ever increasing range of chemicals, products and exposure scenarios has been accompanied by a plethora of new tools and assessment approaches. This rapid pace of change, both in terms of societal expectations for safety assessment science and the need to evaluate and intelligently apply the emerging technologies, continues to present challenges, as well as opportunities. This chapter highlights a number of lessons learned from a historical review of the field, and reflects on how far we have come since the seminal work of Russell and Burch in 1959.

1. INTRODUCTION

While editing this book, we have found ourselves overwhelmed by the variety and volume of efforts being invested, all over the world, in the development of relevant and reliable alternative methods for use in predictive toxicity testing. It has been impossible to do justice to it all, even in a book which is much longer than was originally foreseen. For example, we regret that there is insufficient coverage of what is going on in certain countries, such as Canada, India, the Baltic States and Eastern European countries.

We can be hopeful that the future will see dramatically-new technological developments, which will lead to the better protection of humans and the environment from risks associated with exposure to chemicals and chemical products, and to more-effective and safer medicines. However, this can only happen, if all concerned are willing to recognise the mistakes that have been made in the past, as well as the successes, and to learn the important lessons to be gained from the shared experience. We must also be open to learning lessons which have yet to be acquired, some of which have either not yet been recognised or are being ignored.

The aim of toxicity testing is to identify and quantify potential hazards (hazard assessment), taking into account the probability that they will have serious adverse effects in a variety of circumstances (risk assessment). This means dealing, not with mere possibilities, but with probabilities in real situations, leading to effective and reliable risk assessment, then to effective risk avoidance or risk management.

One lesson is that we must beware of making generalisations from specific cases, recognising the importance of taking into account variation in relation to both exposure and the population being exposed.

It must also be recognised that much greater understanding is needed at all levels, not only about the properties of the chemicals and products themselves, but also about their interactions with cells, tissues and organs, and their effects on individual organisms and populations. That is where the limitations of traditional animal *in vivo* testing cannot be overcome. Responses in laboratory animal species are often profoundly different from each other, as well as from humans, and there is also much variation between and within different sub-populations of the same species. Also, the animals cannot be exposed to all the circumstances which humans will meet.

The single human target, who is the focus of the attention of the toxicologist and the regulator, does not, in fact, exist. Factors such as genetic make-up, age, sex, ethnicity, occupation, residential location, lifestyle, current or historical diseases, and use of medicines, can have profound effects on the outcome of exposure to chemicals or chemical products. This greatly complicates the risk assessment process. Identifying human sub-populations with differences in terms of relevance to susceptibility to toxic effects, such as differences in the enzymes involved in the metabolism of drugs and other chemicals, must be a high priority for the future. Risk assessment for human health is not only about identifying hazard and estimating exposure. It also involves having sufficient knowledge of the individual who may be at risk.

Extrapolation from animal *in vivo* to human *in vivo* involves looking into one black box in the hope of understanding what could happen in another black box. This is a classic example of failure to understand the nature and design of models. A model cannot be useful, if there is insufficient knowledge about the model itself and what is being modelled. Despite this, Russell and Burch's 1959 stern warning of the danger of the high fidelity fallacy has largely been ignored (1).

Scientifically-advanced *in silico* and *in vitro* methods, described in earlier chapters of this book, can be of vital importance in overcoming this problem, by providing essential knowledge of modes of action (MoAs) and adverse outcome pathways (AOPs) in a variety of circumstances. Of course, these methods need to be used selectively and appropriately, in an ethically acceptable and scientifically rational way, possibly along with human volunteer studies. In general, it is unlikely that these methods will be used in isolation, but in the context of intelligent and manageable integrated testing strategies for particular and clearly-defined purposes. For example, the human cells used *in vitro* could be selected to be relevant to the specific sub-population of patients in need of the new drug in the course of development.

2. PRESSURE FOR CHANGE

Originally, the demands for reducing or eliminating the reliance of biomedical research and testing on the use of animals, came primarily from individuals and organisations concerned about the welfare of the animals used in potentially painful procedures, rather than about the better protection of humans and the environment. In general, the scientists involved appear to have been content with the *status quo*, and animal experimentation has long been assumed to be the normal, acceptable and conventional approach in biomedical research, testing and education. There have been exceptions to this, of course. Weil and Scala's frank exposé of the limitations of the Draize eye irritation test in 1971 (2), and Zbinden and Fluri-Roversi's 1981 criticism of the LD50 acute toxicity test (3), had some impact on toxicologists, as well as greatly encouraging the animal welfare campaigners. However, much of what was to be achieved in the next 30 years was because some scientists came to be employed by the campaigning organisations or to work in collaboration with them, and politicians began to take notice of what they had to say.

Nevertheless, in contrast to what has happened in some scientific fields, such as physics and chemistry, where transformational changes in thinking have led to genuine insights and new theories, the conceptual understanding in toxicology has hardly changed at all. Dose and effect are still being measured within the same traditional paradigm (i.e. external rather than internal doses, and apical effects rather than upstream mechanistic ones). A fundamental principle is that all chemicals are toxic at some level, and that the degree of effect is proportional to the exposure level (monotonic relationship). However, for chemicals with certain (e.g. endocrine-related) effects, it has been reported that more-complex (i.e. non-monotonic) dose responses may occur (4). There is, however, no scientific consensus on the reproducibility and toxicological relevance of this phenomenon.

Some ideas are being imported from other fields, however, such as approaches to complex systems and unpredictable (chaotic) behaviour (5), as in systems biology, but a great deal of fundamental research in toxicology is taking place without any obvious influence of Russell and Burch's Three Rs concept or its implications.

3. TESTING NEEDS AND THE PROBLEM OF DOSAGE

As discussed in Chapter 5.3, with further discussion in Chapters 3.1–3.4 and 3.7, the nature of chemicals and their uses determines what kind of testing is required. Industrial chemicals are used for many purposes, which do not require that they interact with the human body, and depending on the hazards they may represent, exposure to them can be avoided, limited or controlled in various ways. By contrast, biologically-active chemicals, such as medicines and biologicals, including vaccines, are designed for use by humans, as are cosmetic ingredients and products and food additives. Pesticides and biocides are designed to be toxic to certain types of organisms, and this is an area where species differences between humans and animals are a great advantage.

In the case of drugs, biologicals, cosmetics and food additives, rational calculations of human exposure are possible, which can result in the application of reasonable doses in tests. By contrast, very high doses have tended to be used in testing industrial chemicals on a 'worst-case scenario' basis, which can mean that the results have questionable relevance for humans. That was part of Zbinden and Fluri-Roversi's criticism of the LD50 test, where more-sensible, dose-limited testing eventually came to be used. However, daily, life-time dosage at the maximum tolerated dose has survived as the regimen used in the rodent bioassay for chemical carcinogens. It is doubtful whether the results have any meaning in relation to chemical carcinogenesis in rodents, let alone in humans.

One advantage of the emerging *in silico* and *in vitro* methods and strategies is that they can involve the high-throughput testing of very large numbers of samples within a reasonable time-frame. This also makes possible the study of the effects of combinations of chemicals (6), in a wide variety of circumstances, with a wide range of doses and with cells from different human sub-populations or patient groups. Another very promising development, as discussed in Chapter 3.8, is the undertaking of first-in-human volunteer studies through the administration of microdoses of drug candidates (<100 µg/each administration) in Phase 0 trials, coupled with ethical, sufficiently safe and ultra-sensitive analytical detection methods.

4. THE THREE RS AND REPLACEMENT

The Three Rs concept introduced by Russell and Burch has had a profound effect on the progress made in the development, acceptance and use of alternative test methods in toxicology. They considered toxicity testing in animals to be 'an urgent humanitarian problem, both numerically and in terms of severity, for it regularly involves a finite and large incidence of distress which is often considerable and sometimes acute' (1). They were particularly concerned about the application of high doses, at which 'a very large number of substances [would be] toxic'. As pointed out in 2014 (7), their comment that 'in theory, we should be able to classify all the ways in which toxic and lethal symptoms are produced' must be seen as embarrassing, 55 years after *The Principles* was published. It is possible that much of this knowledge already exists, but, if so, it is dispersed throughout the scientific literature and described in different ways by different scientific communities. Making this knowledge more accessible, and to do so in a consistent and quality-controlled manner, is the motivation behind the OECD's AOP Knowledge Base project, which aims to provide a collaborative platform for knowledge sharing on mechanisms of toxicity.

Although a number of national and international laws are based on the Three Rs, and although national Three Rs centres are still being established in the 2010s, it can be argued that the Three Rs concept has served its purpose and that the focus in future should be on relevant research for human and environmental benefit, with animal welfare as a secondary beneficial consequence (8). *Reduction* is really about good experimental design, and *Refinement* is about treating animals properly. It is *Replacement* that should be the main and ultimate goal.

In the case of pharmaceuticals, humans are suffering greatly because of the inability of the traditional animal-based approach to testing to provide the understanding needed about what is likely to happen in humans. More than 95% of new drugs have to be withdrawn after their acceptance for clinical use, as a result of lack of efficacy or unacceptable side-effects not detected in pre-clinical testing (9). If that is true of pharmaceuticals, where details of *human* toxicity become available, and their comparison with the animal data is possible, why should we believe that data from animal toxicity tests are more relevant to humans for industrial chemicals, pesticides, cosmetic ingredients or food additives?

One important lesson is that we should not expect, or advocate, the *direct replacement* of animal procedures by non-animal equivalents (10). Seeking *indirect replacement* is much more intelligent. It involves defining what information is needed, then using advanced, non-animal techniques and strategies to obtain it, bypassing animal testing altogether. This implies that attempts to predict specific endpoints in specific animal species are flawed, especially when a given animal test is only partially predictive of itself, as a result of species differences and/or inherent reproducibility limitations (e.g.11). A good example of interspecies differences is biotransformation — whether or not it happens with a particular compound, and if so, what enzymes are involved and what metabolites are produced. The evidence is that the enzymes involved in biotransformation are different in humans and laboratory animals, and that they are also the subject of much human variation (12). In this situation, the only way to provide the necessary information on this situation is to use well-characterised human *in vitro* procedures. The other kinetic processes of absorption, distribution and elimination also vary within and between species. Mathematical (physiologically-based kinetic) models can be used in attempts to describe such variations in toxicokinetics, provided that the underlying absorption, distribution, metabolism and elimination (ADME) properties are known or can be approximated (see also Chapter 5.3).

It would be difficult to replace the use of the word 'alternative' in referring to a *Replacement* method (see also Chapter 1.1), but it is preferable to regard the new, scientifically advanced methods as *different* ways of tackling problems according to new approaches with *different* foundations at the molecular, cell, tissue and organ levels. They offer new ways of tackling complex problems in complex dynamic systems, via, for example, omics approaches (Chapter 5.1), and the use of organ-on-a-chip, or even body-on-a-chip, devices (Chapter 5.2), coupled with increasing understanding of specific MoAs and AOPs, with integration of data increasingly facilitated by mathematical modelling (see also Chapter 5.3). In recent years, there has been a growing tendency to refer to replacement methods and approaches as 'New Approach Methodologies' (NAMs; 13). On the one hand, this appears to be coining a new word for an old idea, but on the other hand, it reflects a new attitude to the use of non-animal methods, which are credible in their own right, rather than being seen as second-best and used only for animal welfare reasons.

Of no less importance are integrated approaches to testing and assessment (IATA, Chapter 5.4), which involve the intelligent, selective and manageable application of computational and test methods, for example, by using decision-tree approaches applicable to particular situations. It should not be necessary to perform every possible test in a strategy. For example, if a drug in development is found to be sufficiently toxic to the liver to halt its progress, its effects on the kidney or on the cardiac or nervous systems would not need to be investigated.

5. VALIDATION

The principles of validation developed in the early 1990s are still applicable today, despite attempts to elaborate them and to use new terminology to describe the same concepts (see Chapter 5.5).

Validation was first considered in relation to genotoxicity testing, because of its purported link with carcinogenicity, but the process was then elaborated for application to the testing of cosmetic ingredients and products, because of pressure from the general public and politicians, who wanted to see an end of animal tests for eye and skin irritancy and for sensitisation. With the introduction of the EU REACH regulation, the focus changed to chemicals, partly because of fears that very large numbers of animals would be used.

The ways in which validation is practised have evolved (e.g. for the validation of *in silico* methods), and will continue to evolve, as the new technologies discussed in Chapters 5.1–5.3 are developed and applied. This will be a particular challenge, for example, in the rapidly developing field of microphysiological systems.

One unresolved problem has been the use of animal test data as gold standards to be matched by alternative test methods. Their use at the beginning of the 1990s was simply because the regulators and regulatory toxicologists at the time would accept no other way, as they were satisfied with the *in vivo* procedures employed at that time and were not convinced by the reasons for change. A major lesson was learned in the EC/HO validation study on alternatives to the Draize eye irritancy test (14). The test samples and the *in vivo* data were selected by a panel linked to the European Centre for the Ecotoxicology and Toxicology of Chemicals (ECETOC), and it was not discovered until after the study had been completed that the *in vivo* data were so variable that almost any result in one of the *in vitro* tests would have matched the score in at least one rabbit! Subsequent experience has shown that it is very difficult to obtain sets of reference chemicals for use in validation studies, for which sufficient data of high-quality and relevance are available.

Nevertheless, the most pressing need is to replace the reliance of the pre-clinical testing of drugs in animals with human-relevant tests and strategies. The need is obvious, as most drugs have to be withdrawn after their acceptance for clinical use, because of unacceptable side-effects not detected in pre-clinical testing or because of lack of therapeutic efficacy. This offers a unique advantage for the further development and critical evaluation of the validation process — there are, or will be, human data against which the performance of a test or testing strategy can be judged.

Björn Ekwall was well aware of this, and combed the poisons centres of the world for acute human toxicity data for comparison with the results of *in vitro* cytotoxicity tests for the test items used in the Multicenter Evaluation of *In Vitro* Cytotoxicity (MEIC) project (see Chapter 2.5). A different approach was used in relation to the successful validation of the 3T3 NRU *in vitro* phototoxicity test, for which a group of experts, meeting at an ECVAM workshop, agreed to use their experience with humans, as well as animals, to select and classify a set of reference test items. The use of expert elicitation in selecting reference chemicals should be explored further, and experience with humans should be taken into account, wherever possible.

There is a danger that validation studies can become too complicated by trying to evaluate too many tests and reference test items and for too many purposes. This is despite what was learned in the EC/HO study, and in subsequent studies, particularly in ECVAM validation studies, where the need to satisfy criteria for necessity and test development, and a pre-validation study, came to be seen as essential steps before a formal multi-centre validation study was undertaken. The validation process should characterise the strengths and weaknesses of tests and defined approaches based on multiple tests, so that optimal and efficient decision-making solutions can be found. Nevertheless, the process should not be regarded as a kind of pass—fail examination, leading to an unchangeable qualification. The design, conduct and outcomes of validation studies themselves need to be independently evaluated, and the relevance and reliability of tests and testing strategies need to be kept under constant review, after they have been accepted and applied to many more test items and by many more laboratories than were involved in the original validation study.

Independence from bias is an essential component of the validation process, but it has not always been achieved. It is here that national and international validation centres, such as ECVAM, ICCVAM and JacVAM, plus the newer centres (see Chapter 5.5) have an important role to play, not least through their involvement in the International Cooperation on Alternative Test Methods (ICATM), which was established in 2009.

It has been suggested (15) that a formal *invalidation* process is necessary because many currently accepted animal tests and candidate animal and non-animal tests do not, and could never, meet the agreed criteria for necessity, test development, scientific validity and acceptance. However desirable this might seem from a scientific perspective, it would be difficult to accomplish in practice, as it would need to be conducted at the highest policy level, such as by the OECD, where enormous effort is put into the drafting and acceptance of test guidelines, but comparatively little effort is invested in their subsequent re-evaluation. Invalidation would require international acceptance, which would not be easy to obtain. One of the lessons from the past was that some OECD Member Countries were reluctant to accept *in vivo* acute toxicity tests not involving lethality as alternatives to the LD50 test. Nevertheless, a way needs to be found of ceasing to accept and use a test guideline, when the test concerned has been shown to be inadequate, or a better test that should replace it has been validated.

6. ACCEPTANCE

It is clear that the acceptance of non-animal tests and testing strategies requires more than good science. It also involves regulatory, commercial, legal, political and sociological considerations. The interplay between these factors is complicated, but a growing body of research is now focused on analysing how they collectively contribute to barriers to the acceptance and use of new methods (e.g. 16). This type of research is valuable, as it looks at the dynamics in an impartial manner, with a view to informing strategies on how to increase the uptake of new approaches.

Regulatory bodies have a key role to play in this process. Their primary responsibility is to enforce regulations as they stand at the current time. The laws on which regulations are based and enacted by parliaments are the result of the democratic political process, and once a law is in place, it must be enforced. This applies to general aspects of toxicity testing, as well as to the performance of particular tests.

In the 1980s, when there was increasing interest in the potential value of toxicity test methods not involving living animals, the regulatory authorities, industrial companies, industry associations and representatives of OECD Member Countries tended to be suspicious of demands for totally new approaches to hazard and risk assessment. This was not only because they saw them as implying criticism of current practice, but also because they were unfamiliar with the 'alternative science' with which they were presented.

The advocates of change recognised that current practice had to continue until the relevance and reliability of what they proposed had been properly developed, published, independently validated and accepted. By the mid-1980s, cosmetics companies and trade associations in Europe and the USA responded by making positive scientific and financial contributions to the development of alternative methods for cosmetics testing.

In the early 1990s, the European Commission was prompted to use the requirements of *Directive 86/609/EEC* as the justification for setting up ECVAM as part of its Joint Research Centre (JRC) at Ispra (Chapter 2.10).

As time passed, some regulatory authorities became more supportive of the search for better ways of protecting humans and the environment from risks of various kinds, even though some scientists continued to vigorously resist any change from the day-to-day routines to which they were accustomed. This was sometimes linked to commercial interests, as it must also be admitted that animal testing was financially rewarding, and there were companies ready and willing to continue to do it for as long as it was permissible.

As the 21st century got under way, several initiatives by regulatory bodies began to challenge the traditional testing paradigms with new, non-animal approaches, often in the context of collaborative confidence building exercises. Good examples are the work of the US agencies in the Tox21 consortium (Chapter 2.13), the Environmental Protection Agency (EPA) in inhalation testing (Chapter 3.5), and the international project called *Accelerating the Pace of Chemical Risk Assessments* (APCRA; 17; Chapter 2.13). The APCRA project involves the EPA, Health Canada, the European Chemicals Agency (ECHA), the European Food Safety Authority (EFSA) and the JRC, along with other governmental institutions. In addition, predictive toxicology case studies are being developed and peer-reviewed by OECD Member Countries in the Working Party on Hazard Assessment (Chapter 2.15), again with a view to confidence building. At the same time, associations, such as Cosmetics Europe, ECETOC, CEFIC and ILSI, are undertaking similar work. Increasingly, implementing the Three Rs is seen as good scientific practice and a means of increasing innovation, as well as animal welfare (18), just as Russell and Burch foresaw.

The acceptance of new methods and strategies should be a formal requirement in the regulatory process, and a detailed explanation should be made public when a decision is taken not to accept a method or strategy shown scientifically to be valid and useful for its stated purpose.

Where a non-animal test or testing strategy has been accepted for use in hazard or risk assessment and an animal test can no longer be considered necessary or justifiable, the legal position is clear — it should be used. In the EU, according to *Directive 2010/63/EU*, the EU Member States must *ensure that a procedure* [on an animal] *is not carried out, if another method or strategy for obtaining the result sought, not entailing the use of a live animal, is recognised under the legislation of the Union.*

One point is clear — laws and regulations are of no value, unless they are enforced rigorously and fairly. Otherwise, questions will continue to be raised as to why animal tests continue to be performed in the EU, when validated or even recognised alternative methods are available (19).

What is important is not what is said, but what is done. The Three Rs have far more supporters on paper than individuals or institutions genuinely committed to what they offer, for the benefit of both animals and humans, and science.

7. INFORMATION EXCHANGE

We live in a world where we are all in danger of being overwhelmed by the immense amount of information which is available to us. In science, this involves an increasing number of publications and official documents, plus all that is available via the Internet (see also Chapter 4.1). An associated problem is that of quality control, with much of the information not being adequately peer-reviewed, despite initiatives such as ECVAM's DataBase service on ALternative Methods to Animal Experimentation (DB-ALM; Chapter 4.2).

There seems to be a move away from conventional databases toward multi-user platforms for sharing knowledge via social media tools. This has the advantage of being rapid, dynamic and personal, but can suffer from the liability of lack of informed criticism.

There is a risk that we will be overwhelmed by jargon and acronyms for schemes and organisations. It seems that the wheel is regularly being re-invented, irrespective and regardless of what has gone before. This is contrary to the generally accepted scientific method. The series of ECVAM workshop reports contained many key recommendations, only some of which were ever followed up. These should be revisited, and earlier reports and other sources referenced within them should be consulted, before scientists claim that their latest ideas are original.

8. EDUCATION AND TRAINING

The new methodology is inevitably becoming increasingly sophisticated and technically demanding, and in addition to the question of whether a test method is itself relevant and reliable, there is also the question of how often a technician would need to carry out a particular test, to maintain a satisfactory level of performance. A test may 'not work' because of the way it was carried out, not because there is anything wrong with the procedure itself.

This has various consequences. The standard operating procedures for tests must be of a very high standard, and they must include appropriate controls on the quality of the performance of the test each time it is carried out. The technicians involved must have sufficient training, with a route to advice and support in case of need. Training in Good *In Vitro* Method Practices (GIVIMP; 20) is essential.

IATA are likely to involve many different procedures serving a single main purpose. It is likely that only the biggest companies would be able to afford laboratories and staff sufficient for all the tests. One consequence of this is that contract testing laboratories might specialise in offering some, but not all, the available tests, so client companies would have to send test items to a variety of places, to accumulate all the information they needed.

The free movement of research scientists, training sessions associated with scientific conferences and offered by various organisations, including animal welfare charities, plus initiatives by governments and the EU, offer a variety of opportunities for training and financial support. In this respect, the EU initiatives such as the JRC Enlargement Programme (see Chapter 2.10) and the Research Framework Programmes have provided tremendous opportunities for training and scientific exchanges. Nevertheless, there is an ongoing need to provide educational and training opportunities on alternative methodologies and to target different audiences such as schoolchildren, undergraduates, early career scientists, technicians, as well as regulators and decision makers (21).

9. CONCLUSIONS

Replacement alternative (i.e. scientifically advanced, non-animal) methods need to be enthusiastically developed and evaluated and, if shown to be fit-for-purpose, accepted and applied, for the benefit of the biomedical sciences, human health, the environment and animals.

Some of the barriers to the uptake of alternative methods are gradually being overcome. For example, the supply of human cells and tissues has been problematic, because of the ethical and safety issues involved. However, tissues derived from human induced pluripotent stem cells (hiPSCs) provide a promising means of circumventing such problems for the study of chemical toxicity and disease mechanisms (22). Another problem has been that many *in vitro* culture media require animal sera, which is associated with a number of scientific and safety issues and animal welfare concerns due to suffering when the serum is collected (23). However, there are now increasing possibilities of using serum-free media (24).

Of course, challenges still remain. The pace of technological change — the complexity of what is on offer and still being developed — is so great that manageability, the availability of scientific and technical skills, and costs are major issues. And perhaps the biggest challenge of all is psychological — the transformation of toxicology and biomedical research will require conviction, ingenuity and determination.

REFERENCES

1. Russell, W.M.S. & Burch, R.L. (1959). *The Principles of Humane Experimental Technique*, 238pp. London, UK: Methuen
2. Weil, C.S. & Scala, R.A. (1971). Study of intra- and interlaboratory variation in the results of rabbit eye and skin irritation tests. *Toxicology and Applied Pharmacology* **19**, 276—360.
3. Zbinden, G. & Flury-Roversi, M. (1981). Significance of the LD50 test for the toxicological evaluation of chemical substances. *Archives of Toxicology* **47**, 77—99.
4. Beausoleil, C., Beronius, A., Bodin, L., *et al.* (2016). Review of non-monotonic dose-responses of substances for human risk assessment. *EFSA Supporting Publication* **1027**, 290.
5. Sharma, V. (2009). Deterministic chaos and fractal complexity in the dynamics of cardiovascular behavior: Perspectives on a new frontier. *The Open Cardiovascular Medicine Journal* **3**, 110—123.
6. Bopp, S., Berggren, E., Kienzler, A., *et al.* (2015). *Scientific Methodologies for the Assessment of Combined Effects of Chemicals - A Survey and Literature Review*. JRC Report EUR 27471, 64pp.
7. Balls, M. (2014). The Wisdom of Russell and Burch. 9. The toxicity testing problem. *ATLA* **42**, P13—P14.
8. Balls, M. (2014). Animal experimentation and alternatives: Time to say goodbye to the Three Rs and hello to humanity. *ATLA* **42**, 327—333.
9. Asher, M. (2016). Parsing clinical success rates. *Nature Reviews Drug Discovery* **15**, 447.
10. Balls, M. (2013). The Wisdom of Russell and Burch. 6. Replacement. *ATLA* **41**, P52—P53.
11. Dumont, C., Barroso, J., Matys, I., *et al.* (2016). Analysis of the Local Lymph Node Assay (LLNA) variability for assessing the prediction of skin sensitization potential and potency of chemicals with non-animal approaches. *Toxicology in Vitro* **34**, 220—228.
12. Martignoni, M., Groothuis, G.M. & de Kanter, R. (2006). Species differences between mouse, rat, dog, monkey and human CYP-mediated drug metabolism, inhibition and induction. *Expert Opinion on Drug Metabolism and Toxicology* **2**, 875—894.
13. ECHA. (2016). New approach methodologies in regulatory science. In *Proceedings of a Scientific Workshop, 19—20 April 2016, Helsinki*, 65pp. Helsinki, Finland: ECHA.
14. Balls, M., Botham, P.A., Bruner, L.H., *et al.* (1995). The EC/HO international validation study on alternatives to the Draize eye irritation test for classification and labeling of chemicals. *Toxicology in Vitro* **9**, 871—929.
15. Balls, M. & Combes, R. (2005). The need for a formal invalidation process for animal and non-animal tests. *ATLA* **33**, 299—308.
16. Schiffelers, M.J., Blaauboer, B.J., Bakker, W.E., *et al.* (2014). Regulatory acceptance and use of 3R models for pharmaceuticals and chemicals: expert opinions on the state of affairs and the way forward. *Regulatory Toxicology and Pharmacology* **69**, 41—48.
17. Kavlock, R. (2016). *Practitioner Insights: Bringing New Methods for Chemical Safety Into the Regulatory Toolbox; It is Time to get Serious*. BNA Daily Environment Report 223 DEN B-1, 1—3.
18. Holmes, A.M., Creton, S. & Chapman, K. (2010). Working in partnership to advance the 3Rs in toxicity testing. *Toxicology* **267**, 14—19.
19. Bowles, E. (2018). The myth of Replacement and the legal reality. *ATLA* **46**, 39—41.
20. Coecke, S., Bernasconi, C., Bowe, G., *et al.* (2016). Practical aspects of designing and conducting validation studies involving multi-study trials. In A. Bal-Price, & P. Jennings (Eds.), *Advances in Experimental Medicine and Biology* **856**. *In Vitro Toxicology Systems, Methods in Pharmacology and Toxicology*, pp. 133—163. New York, NY, USA: Springer.
21. EURL ECVAM. (2018). *Mapping Education and Training on the 3Rs. JRC Science Update, 27-02-18*. Available at: https://ec.europa.eu/jrc/en/science-update/education-and-training-3rs.
22. Pamies, D., Barreras, P., Block, K., *et al.* (2017). A human brain microphysiological system derived from induced pluripotent stem cells to study neurological diseases and toxicity. *ALTEX* **34**, 362—376.
23. van der Valk, J. & Gstraunthaler, G. (2018). Fetal Bovine Serum (FBS) - A pain in the dish? *ATLA* **45**, 329—332.
24. van der Valk, J., Bieback, K., Buta, C., *et al.* (2017). Fetal bovine serum (FBS): Past - Present - Future. *ALTEX* **35**, 99—118.

Chapter 6.2

The Current Situation and Prospects for Tomorrow: Toward the Achievement of Historical Ambitions

Andrew Rowan[1] and Horst Spielmann[2]

[1]The Humane Society of the United States, Washington, DC, USA; [2]Freie Universität Berlin, Berlin, Germany

SUMMARY

Regulatory toxicology has begun to embrace new hazard characterisation approaches, which can be integrated into regulatory safety assessments. The vision is to fundamentally change the way the safety of chemicals is assessed, by replacing or reducing the use of traditional animal experiments with a predictive toxicology that is based on a comprehensive understanding of how chemicals can cause adverse effects in humans (MoA and AOP), or adversely impact on the environment, and a 'renewed' awareness of the importance of the fate of the chemical in the body (kinetics) for the induction of adverse effects. Integrated Approaches to Testing and Assessment (IATA) will help evaluators to assess data from such novel methods consistently, and to understand their relevance for specific endpoints, to obtain reproducible, understandable and statistically-sound results. To position toxicity data generated by alternative methods in a regulatory context, the need for reliable methods has to be combined with a strategy for how to best integrate the resulting data with computational modelling and existing knowledge and information, in order to provide a prediction with sufficient confidence for acceptance in a safety assessment. The new concept proposed by the US Food and Drug Administration to replace *formal validation* with *qualification for a specific context of use*, seems to be the most promising way forward. Once a new model or assay is considered to be qualified for a specific context of use, industry and other stakeholders can use it for its qualified purpose during product development, and regulators should then be confident in applying it without needing to re-review the underlying data supporting validation and acceptance for specific purposes.

1. CHALLENGES FOR REGULATORY TESTING IN THE 21ST CENTURY

Regulators and the general public are facing increasingly complex challenges that require harnessing the best available science and technology on behalf of patients and consumers. Therefore, we need to develop new tools, standards and approaches that efficiently and consistently assess the efficacy, quality, performance and safety of products. New scientific discoveries and technologies are not being sufficiently applied to ensure the safety of new chemicals, drugs and other products to which consumers are likely to be exposed. In addition, members of the public are demanding that greater attention is paid to many more chemicals and products already in commercial use, but the existing testing systems do not have the capacity to deliver the *in vivo* data required. Thus, we must bring 21st century approaches to 21st century products and problems.

Most of the toxicological methods used for regulatory assessment still rely on high-dose animal studies, and default extrapolation procedures that have remained relatively unchanged for decades, despite the technological revolutions in the biosciences over the past 50 years. The new technologies now have the ability to test tens of thousands of chemicals a year in high-throughput systems, and thousands of chemicals a year in organotypic medium-throughput and low-throughput systems. However, we now need to develop better predictive models, to identify concerns earlier in the product development process, to reduce the time and costs involved in testing, and to reduce the loss of promising biological molecules due to false-positive results. We need to modernise the tools used to identify potential risks to consumers, who are exposed to drugs, new food additives and other chemical products.

The challenge today is that the toxicological evaluation of chemicals must take advantage of the on-going revolution in biology and biotechnology. This revolution now permits the study of the effects of chemicals, by using cellular components, cells and tissues — preferably of human origin — rather than whole animals.

This more-modern regulatory science would take advantage of new tools, including functional genomics, proteomics, metabolomics, high-throughput screening, human organs-on-a-chip, and systems biology, and could then replace current toxicology assays with tests that incorporate a mechanistic understanding of disease and of underlying toxic side-effects. This should allow the development, validation and qualification acceptance of pre-clinical and clinical models that accelerate the evaluation of toxicity during the development of drugs and other chemicals to which humans are exposed. The goals include the development of biomarkers to predict toxicity and screen at-risk human subjects during clinical trials and after new products are made available on the market. The new methods should also enable the rapid screening of chemicals, which could be applied to the large number of industrial chemicals that have not yet been evaluated under the current testing system, e.g. according to the EU chemicals regulations.

Currently, the global capacity to test chemicals thoroughly in traditional animal studies would probably not be more than 50—100 chemicals a year. By contrast, the new high-throughput methods developed in the US Environmental Protection Agency (EPA) *CompTox* programme (1; see also Chapter 2.13), involving the robotic systems at the National Center for Advancing Translational Sciences (NCATS) at the National Institutes of Health (NIH), could test 30,000 or more chemicals in several hundred functional tests within a year, while using human cells and systems. This flood of new biological data would drive the development of more-satisfactory, more-predictive computer algorithms that could assist regulatory decision-making. With the addition of data from new "organs-on-a-chip" technologies (see also Chapter 5.2), the regulatory relevance of the data from the high-throughput systems could be further refined.

2. ADAPTING TOXICITY TESTING TO THE CHALLENGES OF THE 21ST CENTURY IN EUROPE

To adapt toxicity testing to progress in the life sciences and to end toxicity testing in animals, in the 1980s, various government institutions of the European Commission (EC) and EU Member States promoted and funded the development and validation of *in vitro* toxicity tests, which were accepted at the international level by the OECD (see also Chapter 2.15) in the early 2000s. Initially, the research activities in Europe were stimulated by the requirements of the EU Cosmetics Directive ((2); see also Chapter 3.1), and were aimed at ending the suffering of experimental animals in safety tests for cosmetics and especially in local toxicity tests on the skin and eye. The funding of research in the *Alternative Testing Strategies Programme* of the 6th (FP6) and 7th (FP7) EU Framework Programmes of the Research and Innovation Directorate General of the EC was quite successful. For this specific field of toxicology, *in vitro* tests were developed, validated and accepted by regulators, and the full ban on animal testing for cosmetic products manufactured or marketed within the EU finally came into forced on 11 March 2013 (3). Although this was a unique success story and represented a breakthrough from the scientific, regulatory and ethical points of view, which was acknowledged around the world, those *in vitro* toxicity tests were based on the progress with 2-D *in vitro* culture techniques achieved in the 20th century.

To speed up the change to challenges of the 21st century, in collaboration with the cosmetics industry, the EU FP7 multi-centre SEURAT-1 project was established to replace repeat-dose systemic toxicity testing *in vivo* in animals. In addition, the EU launched another FP7 project, Accelerate (XLR8), to implement the transition to a toxicity pathway-based paradigm for chemical safety assessment, a concept proposed in 2007 by the US National Research Council (NRC) report, *Toxicity Testing in the 21st Century: A Vision and a Strategy* (4).

3. THE US VISION TOXICITY TESTING IN THE 21ST CENTURY (TOX21)

The new concept for a regulatory toxicity testing paradigm (see also Chapter 2.13) relies mainly on understanding "toxicity pathways" — the cellular response pathways that can result in adverse health effects when sufficiently perturbed (4). Such a system would evaluate biologically-significant alterations, without relying on studies on whole animals. In addition, "targeted testing" has to be conducted, to clarify and refine information from toxicity pathway tests for use in chemical risk assessments. Increasingly, targeted testing in animals will become less necessary, as better systems are developed to understand how chemicals are metabolised in the human body, when applying only tests on cells and tissues.

Such targeted animal tests could be phased out in the next 10 to 15 years, provided that more resources are devoted to developing this new regulatory toxicology.

A toxicity pathway refers to a chemically-induced chain of events at the cellular level that may ultimately lead to an adverse effect such as tumour formation. Such pathways ordinarily coordinate normal processes, such as hormone signalling or gene expression. For example, a protein that, on chemical binding, blocks or amplifies the signalling of a specific receptor could alter the pathway's normal function and induce a "pathway perturbation." Dose-response and extrapolation modelling will permit the translation of cellular tests to whole human systems. Specifically, the modelling will estimate exposures that would lead to significant perturbations of expected toxicity pathways, observed in cellular tests.

4. THE ADVERSE OUTCOME PATHWAY CONCEPT

An Adverse Outcome Pathway (AOP) is a sequence of key events linking a molecular initiating event (MIE) to an adverse outcome (AO) through different levels of biological organisation. AOPs span multiple levels of biological organisation, and the AO can be at the level of the individual organism, population or ecosystem. Each AOP is a set of chemical, biochemical, cellular or physiological responses, which characterise the biological effects cascade resulting from a particular exposure. The key events in an AOP should be definable and should make sense from a physiological or biochemical perspective. AOPs are the central element of a toxicological knowledge framework being built to support chemical risk assessment based on mechanistic reasoning.

Meanwhile, the new concept has generated much interest, and the OECD launched a new programme on the development of AOPs in 2013 (5, 6). As a consequence, the OECD requires that the AOP concept should be taken into account when new toxicity tests are introduced or existing ones are updated. The AOP knowledge-base (AOP KB), set up by the OECD in 2014, is a formal Internet-based repository (http://aopkb.org) for information on AOPs. The content of the AOP KB, which contained 233 AOPs in March 2018, continues to evolve, as more information is gained on AOPs, their Key Events (KEs) and Key Event Relationships (KERs).

Approaches such as the development of AOPs and the identification of modes of action (MoA), together with the use of Integrated Approaches to Testing and Assessment (IATA) as the means of combining multiple lines of evidence, are seen as the fundamental pathway to the hazard identification and characterisation of a chemical. MoAs and AOPs are conceptually similar: MoAs include the chemical specific kinetic processes of Absorption, Distribution, Metabolism and Elimination (ADME), and describe the mechanism of action of the chemical in the human body, whereas AOPs focus on non-chemical-specific biological pathways, starting with an MIE (e.g. binding to an enzyme), resulting in perturbations (KEs) leading to an AO at the organism level.

5. INTEGRATED APPROACHES TO TESTING AND ASSESSMENT

Complex endpoints cannot be predicted by a single stand-alone non-animal test, as it will never be possible to reproduce a whole organism, mainly due to the lack of kinetic relationships and cross-talk amongst cells, tissues and organs. It is, instead, necessary to use IATA based on a weight-of-evidence (WoE) approach, where information and evidence from a battery of tests can be incorporated. A shift is foreseen towards the use of more human data in terms of biologically significant perturbations in key toxicity pathways.

IATA are scientific approaches to hazard and risk characterisation, based on an integrated analysis of existing information coupled with new information by using testing strategies (see also Chapter 5.4). IATA can include a combination of methods and integrating results from one or many methodological approaches, including ranging from flexible to rule-based ones, so-called defined approaches. IATA should ideally be based on knowledge of the MoA by which chemicals induce their toxicity. Such information is, of course, often missing for complex endpoints, e.g. carcinogenicity or developmental toxicity (see also Chapter 3.7). This approach has been used successfully to partially replace skin sensitisation testing in animals: the first three *in vitro* AOP-based OECD Test Guidelines (TGs) have been adopted, covering the MIE of the skin sensitisation AOP (protein binding, TG 442C; (7)) and the intermediate KEs of keratinocyte activation (TG 442D; (8)) and dendritic cell activation (TG 442E; (9)).

6. THE USE OF ALTERNATIVE TEST FOR THE EU CHEMICALS REGULATION (REACH)

Since 2008, the European Chemicals Agency (ECHA) has been responsible for the regulation of new and existing chemicals in the EU, in compliance with the EU Registration, Evaluation, Authorisation and Restriction of Chemicals (REACH) Regulation (10). ECHA has published several reports on "The use of alternatives to testing on animals for the

REACH Regulation", the most recent one being in 2017 (11). Before starting any higher tier-testing on animals (for endpoints specified in Annexes IX and X of the regulation), registrants must first submit a proposal to ECHA. Therefore, ECHA has been asking registrants what alternative methods they have considered before submitting their testing proposals. Registrants can then consider the feedback received to fulfil their REACH information requirements. For phase-in (formerly-existing) chemicals, registrants have used existing information, and alternatives to animal testing. Of 6290 substances covered in the 2017 report, 89% had at least one data endpoint where an alternative was used instead of a study on animals. Results from *in vitro* toxicity tests are accepted for local toxicity to eye and skin, as well as for skin sensitisation. The most common alternative method for human health data endpoints was using information on similar substances (read-across), for 63% of the analysed substances, followed by combining information from different sources (WoE, 43%) and computer modelling (QSAR prediction, 34%). Read-across was most often used as a key study for higher-tier endpoints, e.g. reproductive toxicity, developmental toxicity and long-term toxicity to fish.

The extensive use of read-across, in comparison with other alternative approaches, was not expected (outside of ECHA), as it did not have high visibility in the academic research community, which was focusing on the development of *in vitro* methods in toxicology. To promote a consistent, and correct scientific use of read-across, in 2015, ECHA published a Read-Across Assessment Framework (RAAF) targeting human health endpoints. The RAAF explains how ECHA evaluates read-across in registration dossiers. In 2017, the RAAF was extended to additionally cover environmental endpoints (12).

7. NEW TECHNOLOGIES

7.1 Human-on-a-Chip (Multi-Organ-Chip) Technology Applied to Toxicity Testing

Pressures to change from the use of traditional animal models to novel technologies arise from their limited value for predicting human health effects and from animal welfare considerations (13). This change depends on the availability of human organ models combined with the use of new technologies in the field of omics and systems biology, as well as respective evaluation strategies. Ideally, this requires an appropriate *in vitro* model for each organ system (see also Chapter 5.2).

In this context, it is important to consider combining individual organ models into systems. The miniaturisation of such systems on the smallest possible chip-based scale is now being achieved, to miniaturise the demand for human tissue and to meet the high-throughput needs of industry (14, 15). A multi-organ-chip technology has been established, based on a self-contained smartphone size chip format, within a German BMBF project (16). An integrated micro-pump supports microcirculation for 28 days under dynamic perfusion conditions. The inclusion of human organ equivalents for liver, intestine, kidney and skin allowed ADME and toxicity (ADMET) testing in a four-organ-chip. The system also holds promise for developing disease models for the pre-clinical efficacy testing of new drugs. An encouraging example is a human microfluidic two-organ-chip model of pancreatic islet micro-tissues and liver spheroids, which maintained a functional feedback loop between the liver and the insulin-secreting islet micro-tissues for up to 15 days, in an insulin-free medium (17), which represents a promising simulation of human type 2 diabetes mellitus.

Since 2012, the NIH and the US Food and Drug Administration (FDA) have been funding a major multi-centre program for development of a technology platform that will mimic human physiological systems in the laboratory by using an array of integrated, interchangeable engineered human tissue constructs — "a human body-on-a-chip" (18). The programme, which is coordinated by the National Center for Advancing Translational Sciences (NCATS), intends to combine the technologies to create a microfluidic platform that can incorporate up to 10 individual engineered human micro-physiological organ system modules in an interacting circuit. The modules will be designed to mimic the functions of specific organ systems representing a broad spectrum of human tissues, including the circulatory, endocrine, gastrointestinal, immune, integumentary, musculoskeletal, nervous, reproductive, respiratory and urinary systems.

The goal of the programme is to create a versatile platform capable of accurately predicting drug and vaccine efficacy, toxicity and pharmacokinetics in pre-clinical testing. The research team anticipates that the platform will be suitable for use in regulatory reviews, amenable to rapid translation to the biopharmaceutical research community, and adaptable for the integration of future technologies, such as advances in stem cell technologies, and in relation to personalised medicine.

In the EU, the Organ-on-Chip development (ORCHID) project started in 2017, as an EU-funded initiative (https://h2020-orchid.eu), coordinated by Leiden University Medical Center and the Dutch Organ-on-Chip consortium (hDMT). The main goal of ORCHID is to create a roadmap for organ-on-chip technology, and to build a network of all relevant stakeholders.

7.2 Virtual Organ Models in Predictive Toxicology

Cell agent-based models are useful for modelling developmental toxicity by virtue of their ability to accept data on many linked components, and implement a morphogenetic series of events. These data can be simulated (e.g. what is the effect of localised cell death on the system?) or the data can be derived from *in vitro* studies. In the latter case, perturbed parameters are introduced as simple lesions or combinations of lesions identified from the data, where the assay features have been annotated, and mapped to a pathway or cellular process implemented in the virtual model. Whereas in the EPA ToxCast programme, predictive models are built with computer-assisted mapping of chemical-assay data to chemical endpoint effects (19), the virtual tissue models incorporate biological structure and thus extend the *in vitro* data to a higher level of biological organisation. A developing system can be modelled and perturbed 'virtually' with toxicological data, then the predictions on growth and development can be compared with real experimental findings.

7.3 Virtual Liver Projects

The goal of the US Virtual Liver project is to develop models for predicting liver injury due to chronic chemical exposure. by simulating the dynamics of perturbed molecular pathways, their linkage with adaptive or adverse processes leading to alterations of cell state, and integration of the responses into a physiological tissue model. When completed, the Virtual Liver Web portal, and accompanying query tools, will provide a framework for the incorporation of mechanistic information on hepatic toxicity pathways, and for characterising interactions spatially and across the various cell types that comprise liver tissue.

The German BMBF-funded Virtual Liver project focuses on the establishment of a 3-D model of the liver that correctly recapitulates alterations of the complex micro-architecture, both in response to, and during, regeneration from chemically-induced liver damage. Currently, there is only limited knowledge on how cells behave in a coordinated fashion to establish functional tissue architecture, and to respond to chemically-induced tissue damage during regeneration. A vision of this project is that the spatial-temporal events during tissue damage and regeneration can be simulated *in silico*. Because the exact position and metabolic capacity of the individual cells of the model are known, it should also be possible to simulate the degree to which a certain pattern of chemically-induced liver damage compromises the metabolic capacity at the organ level. Finally, a long-term goal will be to integrate intracellular mechanisms into each cell of the model, as many of the critical intracellular key mechanisms still need to be elucidated.

7.4 The Virtual Embryo

The EPA programme, the Virtual Embryo Project (v-Embryo) is a computational framework for developmental toxicity, focused on the predictive toxicology of children's health and developmental defects, following prenatal exposure to environmental chemicals. The research is motivated by scientific principles in systems biology, as a framework for the generation, assessment and evaluation of data, tools and approaches in computational toxicology. The long-term objectives are to determine the specificity and sensitivity of biological pathways relevant to human developmental health and disease, to predict and understand key events during embryogenesis leading to adverse foetal outcomes, and to assess the impacts of prenatal exposure to chemicals at various stages of development and scales of biological organisation.

8. THE FUTURE OF TOXICOLOGY IS *IN VITRO*

The process of validation of new approaches needs to be reconsidered in terms of efficiency and time to completion. In particular, the scientific community needs to understand that it is possible for alternative methods to meet some or all regulatory needs, and should not be used only for prioritisation purposes. Furthermore, the fate of the animal testing in this transitional phase towards IATA is unclear.

The progress in replacing regulatory animal tests was based on the intention to replace an animal test for a specific endpoint of toxicity by a single *in vitro* assay, or by applying a testing strategy, involving a few *in vitro* tests. This approach, which had been developed in Europe, proved successful for more than a decade in relation to local toxicity testing, but could not be applied to more-complex and systemic toxicity endpoints. Meanwhile, the AOP concept that was developed by the US National Academy of Sciences (NAS) 10 years ago had significantly changed regulatory safety testing, as it permitted several *in vitro* assays to be combined in IATA for complex endpoints, e.g. for skin sensitisation. In essence, IATA will be developed, which incorporate the results from assays at various levels of biological organisation, such as *in silico* high-throughput screening (HTS), chemical-specific aspects (ADME), and an AOP describing the biological (toxicodynamic) basis of toxicity. Ultimately, a limited amount of information on both the AOP for critical effects and the ADME for a chemical, associated with the AO, should permit the development of IATA and guide more-detailed AOP and ADME research, in cases where higher precision is needed in a specific decision-making context (20). It is encouraging that American and European regulators are reporting that the AOP framework, in the form of a structured AOP knowledge database (21), is increasingly being used to integrate data, based on traditional and emerging toxicity testing paradigms. The promise of AOPs will, however, only be fully realised through the active engagement of multiple stakeholders, requiring substantive and long-term planning (22).

Therefore, it is not surprising, but encouraging, that by the end of 2017, the FDA and the NIH had published new roadmaps for toxicity testing, which were based on the new principles of safety testing without animals by using the novel molecular and computational techniques, e.g. the *FDA Predictive Toxicology Roadmap* ((23), see also Chapter 2.12) and the ICCVAM *Strategic Roadmap for Establishing New Approaches to Evaluate the Safety of Chemicals and Medical Products in the United States"* (24). In this context, the FDA makes the most pragmatic proposal, and suggests that *Rather than validation, an approach we frequently take for biological (and toxicological) models and assays is qualification. Within the stated context of use, qualification is a conclusion that the results of an assessment, using the model or assay, can be relied on to have a specific interpretation and application in product development and regulatory decision-making* (23).

It is also very encouraging that, early in the 21st century, the US regulatory agencies are giving the *long-sought goal of refining, reducing, and replacing testing on animals* the high priority that it deserves, both for scientific and for animal welfare reasons, in accordance with the hopes expressed 60 years ago by the pioneers of the Three Rs concept, William Russell and Rex Burch (25).

The final aim is to combine different 'organoids' to generate a human-on-a-chip, an approach that would allow studies of complex physiological organ interactions. The recent advances in the area of induced pluripotent stem cells (iPSCs; see also Chapter 5.1) provide a range of possibilities that include cellular studies of individuals with different genetic backgrounds (e.g. human disease models; (17)). However, throughput remains a significant limitation, and there will continue to be a need for emphasis on "fit-for-purpose" assays.

In conclusion, 21st century technologies are providing multi-dimensional human data at the molecular and cellular level that will advance predictive toxicology.

REFERENCES

1. Williams, A. (2017). *CompTox chemistry dashboard*, 38pp. Washington, DC, USA: Office of Research and Development, US EPA.
2. EU. (2009). Regulation (EC) No 1223/2009 of the European Parliament and of the Council of 30 November 2009 on cosmetic products. *Official Journal of the European Union* **L342**, 59–210.
3. EC. (2013). *Communication from the Commission to the European Parliament and the Council on the animal testing and marketing ban and on the state of play in relation to alternative methods in the field of cosmetics COM(2013)*, 135 final, 6pp. Brussels, Belgium: European Commission.
4. NRC. (2007). *Toxicity testing in the 21st century: A vision and a strategy*, 216pp. Washington, DC, USA: The National Academies Press.
5. OECD. (2016). Guidance Document for the Use of Adverse Outcome Pathways in Developing Integrated Approaches to Testing and Assessment (IATA), 25pp. *Series on Testing and Assessment no. 260*. Paris, France: OECD.
6. OECD. (2017). Revised Guidance Document on Developing and Assessing Adverse Outcome Pathways, 32pp. *Series on Testing and Assessment no. 184*. Paris, France: OECD.
7. OECD. (2015). *OECD TG No. 445C: In chemico skin sensitisation: Direct peptide reactivity assay (DPRA)*, 19pp. Paris, France: OECD.
8. OECD. (2015). *OECD TG No. 445D: In vitro skin sensitisation: Human cell line activation test (h-CLAT)*, 20pp. Paris, France: OECD.
9. OECD. (2016). *OECD Test No. 442E: In vitro skin sensitisation: ARE-Nrf2 luciferase test method*, 20pp. Paris, France: OECD.
10. EC. (2006). Regulation (EC) No 1907/2006 of the European Parliament and of the Council of 18 December 2006 concerning the Registration, Evaluation, Authorisation and Restriction of Chemicals (REACH), establishing a European Chemicals Agency, amending Directive 1999/45/EC and repealing Council Regulation (EEC) No 793/93 and Commission Regulation (EC) No 1488/94 as well as Council Directive 76/769/EEC and Commission Directives 91/155/EEC, 93/67/EEC, 93/105/EC and 2000/21/EC. *Official Journal of the European Union* **L396**, 1–849.
11. ECHA. (2017). *The use of alternatives to testing on animals for the REACH regulation*. Third report under Article 117(3) of the REACH Regulation, 103pp. Helsinki, Finland: ECHA.
12. ECHA. (2017). *Read-across Assessment Framework (RAAF)*, 60pp. Helsinki, Finland: ECHA.
13. Andersen, M.E. & Krewski, D. (2009). Toxicity testing in the 21st century: bringing the vision to life. *Toxicological Sciences* **107**, 324–330.
14. Esch, M.B., King, T.L. & Shuler, M.L. (2011). The role of body-on-a-chip devices in drug and toxicity studies. *Annual Review of Biomedical Engineering* **13**, 55–72.
15. Huh, D., Hamilton, G.A. & Ingber, D.E. (2011). From 3D cell culture to organs-on-chips. *Trends in Cell Biology* **21**, 745–754.
16. Marx, U., Walles, H., Hoffmann, S., et al. (2012). 'Human-on-a-chip' developments: a translational cutting edge alternative to systemic safety assessment and efficiency evaluation of substances in laboratory animals and man? *ATLA* **40**, 235–257.

17. Bauer, S., Wennberg Huldt, C., Kanebratt, K.P., *et al.* (2018). Functional coupling of human pancreatic islets and liver spheroids on-a-chip: Towards a novel human ex vivo type 2 diabetes model. *Nature Scientific Reports* **8**, 1672.

18. NIH. (2012). *Press Release, 24 July 2012: NIH funds development of tissue chips to help predict drug safety DARPA and FDA to collaborate on groundbreaking therapeutic development initiative*, 2pp. Bethesda, MD, USA: National Institutes of Health.

19. Judson, R.S., Houck, K.A., Kavlock, R.J., *et al.* (2010). In vitro screening of environmental chemicals for targeted testing prioritization: the ToxCast project. *Environmental Health Perspectives* **118**, 485–492.

20. Edwards, S.W., Tan, Y.M., Villeneuve, D.L., *et al.* (2016). Adverse Outcome Pathways: organizing toxicological information to improve decision making. *Journal of Pharmacology and Experimental Therapeutics* **356**, 170–181.

21. Ives, C., Campia, I., Wang, R.L., *et al.* (2017). Creating a structured adverse outcome pathway knowledgebase via ontology-based annotations. *Applied In Vitro Toxicology* **4**, 298–311.

22. Carusi, A., Davies, M.R., De Grandis, G., *et al.* (2018). Harvesting the promise of AOPs: An assessment and recommendations. *The Science of the Total Environment* **628**, 1542–1556.

23. FDA. (2017). *FDA's predictive toxicology roadmap*, 16pp. Silver Spring, MD, USA: US FDA.

24. ICCVAM. (2018). *A strategic roadmap for establishing new approaches to evaluate the safety of chemicals and medical products in the United States*, 13pp. Research Triangle Park, NC, USA: NIEHS.

25. Russell, W.M.S. & Burch, R.L. (1950). *The Principles of Humane Experimental Technique*, 238pp. London, UK: Methuen.

Index

'*Note:* Page numbers followed by "f" indicate figures, "t" indicate tables.'

Printed in the United States
By Bookmasters